THIRD EDITION

Surgical Decision Making

Lawrence W. Norton, M.D.

Professor and Vice-Chairman
Department of Surgery
University of Colorado School of Medicine
Denver, Colorado

Glenn Steele, Jr., M.D.

The William V. McDermott Professor of Surgery
Harvard Medical School
Chairman, Department of Surgery
New England Deaconess Hospital
Boston, Massachusetts

Ben Eiseman, M.D.

Emeritus Professor
Department of Surgery
University of Colorado School of Medicine
Denver, Colorado

W. B. SAUNDERS COMPANY

Harcourt Brace Jovanovich, Inc.   Philadelphia   London   Toronto   Montreal   Sydney   Tokyo

W. B. SAUNDERS COMPANY
Harcourt Brace Jovanovich, Inc.

The Curtis Center
Independence Square West
Philadelphia, Pennsylvania 19106

Library of Congress Cataloging-in-Publication Data

Surgical decision making / [edited by] Lawrence Norton,
Glenn Steele, Jr., Ben Eiseman.—3rd ed.

p. cm.

Includes bibliographical references and index.

ISBN 0–7216–6598–5

1. Surgery—Decision making.   I. Norton, Lawrence W.
  II. Steele, Glenn.   III. Eiseman, Ben.   [DNLM: 1. Decision
  Making.   2. Surgery.   WO 100 S9623]

RD31.5.S87 1993   617—dc20

DNLM/DLC   92–8005

SURGICAL DECISION MAKING, Third Edition

ISBN 0–7216–6598–5
International Edition ISBN 0–7216–4900–9

Printed in the United States of America.

Last digit is the print number: 9   8   7   6   5   4   3   2   1

Contributors

Alan D. Aaron, M.D.
Clinical Instructor, Orthopaedic Oncology Service, Department of Orthopaedics, Georgetown University Hospital, Washington, DC

Jean T. Abbott, M.D.
Assistant Professor of Surgery (Emergency Medicine), University of Colorado School of Medicine; Attending, Emergency Department, University of Colorado Health Sciences Center, Denver, Colorado

Charles Abernathy, M.D.
Professor of Surgery, University of Colorado School of Medicine; Associate Director of Surgery, Denver General Hospital, Denver, Colorado

James T. Anderson, M.D.
Associate Clinical Professor of Surgery (Cardiothoracic), University of Colorado School of Medicine, Denver; Attending, Penrose–St. Francis Affiliated Hospitals, Colorado Springs, Colorado

Henry T. Bahnson, M.D.
Professor of Surgery, University of Pittsburgh School of Medicine; Distinguished Physician, Veterans Affairs; Attending, University of Pittsburgh Medical Center, Pittsburgh, Pennsylvania

Edward J. Bartle, M.D.
Associate Professor of Surgery, University of Colorado School of Medicine, Denver, Colorado

Theodore C. Barton, M.D.
Assistant Clinical Professor of Surgery, Harvard Medical School; Chief of Gynecology, New England Deaconess Hospital and New England Baptist Hospital, Boston, Massachusetts

B. Timothy Baxter, M.D.
Assistant Professor of Surgery, University of Nebraska Medical Center; Chief, Vascular Surgery, Omaha VA Hospital, Omaha, Nebraska

Robert W. Beart, Jr., M.D.
Professor of Surgery, Mayo Medical School; Chief of Surgery, Mayo Clinic Scottsdale, Scottsdale, Arizona

Peter N. Benotti, M.D.
Associate Professor of Surgery, Tufts University; Chief of Gastrointestinal Surgery, New England Medical Center, Boston, Massachusetts

Ross S. Berkowitz, M.D.
Professor of Obstetrics and Gynecology and Reproductive Biology, Harvard Medical School; Director of Gynecology and Gynecologic Oncology, Brigham and Women's Hospital, Boston, Massachusetts

F. William Blaisdell, M.D.
Professor and Chairman, Department of Surgery, University of California School of Medicine, Davis, Sacramento, California

Leslie H. Blumgart, M.D.
Enid A. Haupt Professor of Surgery, Memorial Sloan-Kettering Cancer Center, New York, New York

Bradley C. Borlase, M.D., M.S.
Instructor in Surgery, Harvard Medical School; Attending, New England Deaconess Hospital, Boston, Massachusetts

Edward L. Bradley III, M.D.
Whitaker Professor of Surgery, Emory University School of Medicine; Attending, Emory University Hospital, Piedmont Hospital, and Grady Memorial Hospital, Atlanta, Georgia

Robert E. Breeze, M.D.
Assistant Professor of Surgery (Neurosurgery), University of Colorado School of Medicine; Attending, University Hospital, VA Medical Center, Denver General Hospital, St. Anthony's Hospital Central, and Children's Hospital, Denver, Colorado

Murray F. Brennan, M.D.
Professor of Surgery, Cornell University; Alfred P. Sloan Professor of Surgery and Chairman, Department of Surgery, Memorial Sloan-Kettering Cancer Center, New York, New York

James M. Brown, M.D.
Clinical Instructor, University of Colorado School of Medicine; Resident in Cardiothoracic Surgery, University of Colorado Health Sciences Center, Denver, Colorado

Blake Cady, M.D.
Professor of Surgery, Harvard Medical School; Chief of Surgical Oncology, New England Deaconess Hospital, Boston, Massachusetts

David N. Campbell, M.D.
Associate Professor of Surgery (Cardiothoracic), University of Colorado School of Medicine; Attending, Children's Hospital and Colorado Health Sciences Center, Denver, Colorado

Larry C. Carey, M.D.
Professor and Chairman, Department of Surgery, University of South Florida; Attending, Tampa General Hospital, Moffitt Cancer and Research Center, James A. Haley Veterans Hospital, and Bay Pines Veterans Hospital, Tampa, Florida

Roy E. Carlson, M.D.
Assistant Clinical Professor of Surgery, University of Colorado School of Medicine; Attending, Swedish Medical Center, Englewood, and Porter Memorial Hospital, Denver, Colorado

Peter A. Cataldo, M.D.
Assistant Clinical Professor of Surgery (Colon and Rectal), Wright State School of Medicine and Uniformed Services School for the Health Sciences; Attending, Wright-Patterson USAF Medical Center, Dayton, Ohio

W. Randolph Chitwood, Jr., M.D.
Professor and Chief of Cardiothoracic Surgery, East Carolina University School of Medicine; Director of Heart Center of Eastern North Carolina and Chief of Cardiothoracic Surgery, Pitt County Memorial Hospital, Greenville, North Carolina

David R. Clarke, M.D.
Associate Professor of Surgery, University of Colorado School of Medicine; Chief of Pediatric Cardiothoracic Surgery, The Children's Hospital, Denver, Colorado

Mack L. Clayton, M.D.
Clinical Professor of Orthopedic Surgery, University of Colorado School of Medicine; Attending, VA Medical Center, Denver, Colorado

William Cody, M.D.
Surgical Group of South Jersey, Cherry Hill; Attending, West Jersey Health Systems, Marlton Division, Marlton; Our Lady of Lourdes Medical

Center and the Cooper Hospital University Medical Center, Camden, New Jersey

Max M. Cohen, M.D.
Professor of Surgery, University of Colorado School of Medicine; Chairman, Department of Surgery, Rose Medical Center, Denver, Colorado

John J. Coleman III, M.D.
Professor of Surgery, Indiana University School of Medicine; Director, Division of Plastic Surgery, Indiana University Medical Center, Indianapolis, Indiana

Jack G. Copeland, M.D.
Professor of Surgery, University of Arizona College of Medicine; Attending, University Medical Center, Tucson VA Hospital, Kino Hospital, and Tucson General Hospital, Tucson, and St. Luke's Hospital, Phoenix, Arizona

Stanley Coulthard, M.D.
Clinical Professor of Surgery and Acting Chairman, Section of Otolaryngology, University of Arizona College of Medicine, Tucson, Arizona

James J. Corrigan, Jr., M.D.
Professor of Pediatrics and Clinical Professor of Medicine, Tulane University School of Medicine; Attending, Tulane University Medical Center Hospital; Visiting Physician, Medical Center of Louisiana, New Orleans, Louisiana

E. David Crawford, M.D.
Professor and Chief, Division of Urology, and Associate Director of Cancer Center, University of Colorado School of Medicine; Attending, University of Colorado Health Sciences Center, Denver, Colorado

Jeffrey S. Cross, M.D.
Resident in Surgery, University of Colorado Health Sciences Center, Denver, Colorado

Haile T. Debas, M.D.
Professor and Chairman, Department of Surgery, University of California, San Francisco; Attending, The Medical Center at the University of California, San Francisco, San Francisco, California

Robert E. Donohue, M.D.
Professor of Surgery (Urology), University of Colorado School of Medicine; Chief, Urology Section, Denver VA Medical Center; Attending, Rose Medical Center, Children's Hospital, and Denver General Hospital, Denver, Colorado

Hugh Dougall, M.D.
Attending, Calgary General Hospital, Calgary, Alberta, Canada

George W. Drach, M.D.
Professor of Surgery (Urology), University of Arizona College of Medicine; Attending, University Medical Center; Consulting, VA Medical Center; Courtesy Staff, Tucson Medical Center and El Dorado Hospital; Visiting Consultant, Tucson General Hospital, Tucson, Arizona

William Droegemueller, M.D.
Professor and Chairman, Department of Obstetrics and Gynecology, University of North Carolina School of Medicine, Chapel Hill, North Carolina

Walter H. Dzik, M.D.
Assistant Professor of Medicine, Harvard Medical School; Director, Blood Bank and Tissue Typing Laboratory, New England Deaconess Hospital, Boston, Massachusetts

Robert B. Dzioba, M.D.
Clinical Associate Professor of Surgery, Section of Orthopaedics, University of Arizona College of Medicine; Chief of Staff, University Medical Center, Tucson, Arizona

Michael J. Edwards, M.D.
Assistant Professor of Surgery, University of Louisville, Louisville, Kentucky

Ben Eiseman, M.D.
Emeritus Professor of Surgery, University of Colorado School of Medicine; Attending, Denver VA Hospital, Denver, Colorado

E. Christopher Ellison, M.D.
Director, Ohio Digestive Disease Institute, Grant Medical Center, Columbus, Ohio

Tommy N. Evans, M.D.
Emeritus Professor, Obstetrics and Gynecology, University of Colorado School of Medicine; Attending, Good Samaritan Regional Medical Center, Phoenix, Arizona

Thomas Eyen, M.D.
Resident in Otolaryngology–Head and Neck Surgery, University of Colorado Health Sciences Center, Denver, Colorado

Victor W. Fazio, M.D., FRACS
Professor of Surgery, Ohio State University at Cleveland Clinic; Chairman, Department of Colon and Rectal Surgery, The Cleveland Clinic Foundation, Cleveland, Ohio

Frederick Feit, M.D.
Associate Professor of Medicine, New York University School of Medicine; Director, Cardiac Catheterization, Bellevue Hospital; Attending, New York University and Bellevue Hospitals, New York, New York

David V. Feliciano, M.D.
Professor of Surgery, Emory University School of Medicine, Atlanta; Clinical Professor of Surgery, Uniformed Services University of the Health Sciences, Bethesda, Maryland; Chief of Surgery, Grady Memorial Hospital, Atlanta, Georgia

Carlos Fernández-del Castillo, M.D.
Instructor in Surgery, Harvard Medical School; Assistant in Surgery, Massachusetts General Hospital, Boston, Massachusetts

Richard G. Fiddian-Green, B.M., B.Ch., FRCS
Professor of Surgery, University of Massachusetts Medical School, Worcester, Massachusetts

Josef Fischer, M.D.
Christian R. Holms Professor and Chairman, Department of Surgery, University of Cincinnati College of Medicine, Cincinnati, Ohio

Manson Fok, M.B.B.S.(HK), FRCS(Ed)
Lecturer, Department of Surgery, University of Hong Kong, Queen Mary Hospital, Hong Kong

R. Armour Forse, M.D., Ph.D.
Associate Professor of Surgery, Harvard Medical School; Chief, Division of General Surgery, New England Deaconess Hospital, Boston, Massachusetts

Richard J. Fowl, M.D.
Associate Professor of Surgery, University of Cincinnati School of Medicine; Attending, University of Cincinnati Medical Center, Cincinnati, Ohio

Charles F. Frey, M.D.
Professor and Vice Chairman, Department of Surgery, University of California, Davis; Attending, University of California, Davis Medical Center, Sacramento, California

David A. Fullerton, M.D.
Assistant Professor of Surgery (Cardiothoracic), Unversity of Colorado School of Medicine; Chief, Cardiothoracic Surgery, Denver VA Hospital, Denver, Colorado

Aubrey C. Galloway, M.D.
Associate Professor of Surgery and Director, Cardiac Surgical Research, New York University

School of Medicine; Attending, New York University Hospital and Bellevue Hospital, New York, New York

Donald S. Gann, M.D.
Professor of Surgery and Associate Chairman, Department of Surgery, University of Maryland School of Medicine; Chief, Section of Endocrine Surgery and Section of Trauma and Critical Care, University of Maryland Medical System, Baltimore, Maryland

Glenn W. Geelhoed, M.D., M.P.H.
Professor of Surgery and Professor of International Medical Education, George Washington University, Washington, DC

Philippe Gertsch, M.D.
Reader, Department of Surgery, University of Hong Kong, Queen Mary Hospital, Hong Kong

Howard M. Goodman, M.D.
Assistant Professor of Obstetrics and Gynecology and Reproductive Biology, Harvard Medical School; Attending, Brigham and Women's Hospital, Boston, Massachusetts

Clive S. Grant, M.D.
Associate Professor of Surgery, Mayo Graduate School of Medicine; Consultant in General Surgery, Mayo Clinic, Mayo Foundation, Rochester, Minnesota

Ronald E. Greenberg, M.D.
Assistant Professor of Medicine, Albert Einstein College of Medicine, Bronx; Attending, Division of Gastroenterology, Long Island Jewish Medical Center, New Hyde Park, New York

Roberta J. Hall, M.D.
Assistant Professor of Surgery, University of Colorado School of Medicine; Attending, Transplant Surgery, University Hospital and Children's Hospital, Denver, Colorado

John F. Hansbrough, M.D.
Professor of Surgery, University of California, San Diego, Medical Center; Professor of Surgery and Director, Regional Burn Center, University of California, San Diego, Medical Center, San Diego, California

R. Phillip Heine, M.D.
Fellow, Maternal–Fetal Medicine, Department of Obstetrics and Gynecology, University of Colorado School of Medicine, Denver, Colorado

Richard Heppe, M.D.
Attending, Swedish Medical Center, Englewood, and Porter Memorial Hospital, Denver Presbyterian Hospital, and Children's Hospital, Denver, Colorado

Gilbert Hermann, M.D.
Clinical Professor of Surgery, University of Colorado School of Medicine; Attending, Rose Medical Center, Denver, Colorado

J. Laurance Hill, M.D.
Professor, University of Maryland School of Medicine; Professor, The Johns Hopkins University School of Medicine; Surgeon-in-Chief, University of Maryland Hospital; Attending, Mercy Hospital, Union Memorial Hospital, St. Agnes Hospital, and St. Joseph Hospital, Baltimore, Maryland

Walter D. Holder, Jr., M.D.
Clinical Associate Professor of Surgery, University of North Carolina School of Medicine, Chapel Hill; Chief, Surgical Oncology Division, and Director of Research, Department of General Surgery, Carolinas Medical Center, Charlotte, North Carolina

Alan Hopeman, M.D.
Emeritus Professor of Surgery, University of Colorado School of Medicine; Consulting Cardiothoracic Surgeon, Denver Veterans Administration Hospital and Fitzsimons Army Hospital, Denver, Colorado

Todd K. Howard, M.D.
Director, Surgical Intensive Care Unit, and Assistant Director, Transplant Services, Cedars–Sinai Medical Center, Los Angeles, California

Bradley S. Hurst, M.D.
Assistant Professor, Obstetrics and Gynecology and Reproductive Endocrinology, University of Colorado School of Medicine; Attending, University of Colorado Health Sciences Center, Denver, Colorado

Bruce W. Jafek, M.D.
Professor and Chairman, Department of Otolaryngology–Head and Neck Surgery, University of Colorado School of Medicine; Chief of Otolaryngology–Head and Neck Surgery, University Hospital; Attending, Rose Medical Center, Denver General Hospital, and Denver VA Hospital; Consultant, Children's Hospital and Fitzsimons Army Medical Center, Denver, Colorado

J. Milburn Jessup, M.D.
Associate Professor of Surgery, Harvard Medical School; Attending, New England Deaconess Hospital, New England Baptist Hospital, Southwood Community Hospital, and Goddard Memorial Hospital, Boston, Massachusetts

Michael R. Johnston, M.D.
Head, Division of Thoracic Surgery, Mt. Sinai Hospital, Toronto, Ontario, Canada

Susan L. Jolly, M.D.
Attending, Swedish Medical Center, Porter Memorial Hospital, Littleton Hospital, and Denver VA Hospital, Denver, Colorado

Todd N. Jones, R.N., M.S.
Clinical Instructor of Surgery, University of Colorado School of Medicine, Denver, Colorado; Product Manager—Nutrition, McGaw, Inc., Irvine, California

M. J. Jurkiewicz, M.D.
Professor of Surgery, Emory University School of Medicine; Attending, Division of Plastic Surgery, Emory University Hospital, Atlanta, Georgia

Igal Kam, M.D.
Associate Professor of Surgery, University of Colorado School of Medicine; Chief, Division of Transplantation, University of Colorado Health Sciences Center, Denver, Colorado

Frederick M. Karrer, M.D.
Assistant Professor of Surgery, University of Colorado School of Medicine; Director of Pediatric Transplantation, Children's Hospital; Attending, University of Colorado Health Sciences Center, Denver, Colorado

Glenn Kelly, M.D.
Associate Clinical Professor of Surgery, University of Colorado School of Medicine; Attending, Porter Memorial Hospital, Swedish Medical Center, and Littleton Hospital, Denver, Colorado

Richard F. Kempczinski, M.D.
Professor of Surgery and Chief, Vascular Surgery, University of Cincinnati School of Medicine; Attending, University of Cincinnati Medical Center, Cincinnati, Ohio

Lawrence L. Ketch, M.D.
Assistant Professor, University of Colorado School of Medicine; Chief, Division of Plastic and Reconstructive Surgery, University Hospital; Chief, Pediatric Plastic Surgery, Children's Hospital; Attending, Denver General Hospital; Courtesy Staff, Rose Medical Center and Denver VA Hospital, Denver, Colorado

Robert L. Kormos, M.D.
Assistant Professor of Surgery, University of Pittsburgh; Attending and Director, Artificial Heart Program, University of Pittsburgh Medical Center, Pittsburgh, Pennsylvania

Ann M. Kosloske, M.D., M.P.H.
Professor of Surgery, McGill University Faculty of Medicine; Director, Pediatric Surgical Training Program, Montreal Children's Hospital, Montreal, Quebec, Canada

Stephen J. Lahey, M.D.
Assistant Professor of Surgery, Harvard Medical School; Attending, New England Deaconess Hospital, Boston, Massachusetts

Sidney Levitsky, M.D.
David W. and David Cheever Professor of Surgery, Harvard Medical School; Chief, Division of Cardiothoracic Surgery, New England Deaconess Hospital, Boston, Massachusetts

R. Dale Liechty, M.D.
Professor of Surgery, University of Colorado School of Medicine; Attending, University of Colorado Health Sciences Center, VA Medical Center, and Rose Medical Center, Denver, Colorado

Kevin O. Lillehei, M.D.
Assistant Professor of Surgery (Neurosurgery), University of Colorado School of Medicine; Attending, University of Colorado Health Sciences Center, Denver, Colorado

John R. Lilly, M.D.
Professor of Surgery, University of Colorado School of Medicine; Chief of Pediatric Surgery, Children's Hospital, Denver, Colorado

Robert C. Lim, M.D.
Professor of Surgery, University of California, San Francisco; Attending, University of California, San Francisco, Hospitals, San Francisco, California

Alex G. Little, M.D.
Professor and Chairman, Department of Surgery, University of Nevada School of Medicine; Attending, University Medical Center, Reno, Nevada

Joseph LoCicero III, M.D.
Attending Surgeon, New England Deaconess Hospital and Dana-Farber Cancer Institute, Boston, Massachusetts

Frank W. LoGerfo, M.D.
Professor of Surgery, Harvard Medical School; Chief, Division of Vascular Surgery, New England Deaconess Hospital, Boston, Massachusetts

Jeffrey A. Lowell, M.D.
Clinical Instructor of Surgery, Harvard Medical School, Boston; Attending, Department of General Surgery, Lahey Clinic Medical Center, Burlington, Massachusetts

Steven R. Lowenstein, M.D., M.P.H.
Associate Professor of Medicine, Surgery and Preventive Medicine/Biometrics, University of Colorado School of Medicine; Associate Director, Emergency Medicine and Trauma, University of Colorado Health Sciences Center, Denver, Colorado

James W. Lucarini, M.D.
Instructor in Otolaryngology, Harvard Medical School; Attending, New England Deaconess Hospital, Department of Surgery, Dana-Farber Cancer Institute, Division of Otolaryngology, and Massachusetts Eye and Ear Infirmary, Department of Otolaryngology; Courtesy Staff, The Children's Hospital, Department of Otolaryngology, Boston, Massachusetts

Francis J. Major, M.D.
Associate Professor of Obstetrics and Gynecology, University of Colorado School of Medicine; Attending, Presbyterian-St. Luke's Hospital, Denver, Colorado

Leonard Makowka, M.D., Ph.D., FRCS(C)
Professor of Surgery, University of California, Los Angeles, School of Medicine; Chairman, Department of Surgery, and Director of Transplant Ser-

vices, Cedars-Sinai Medical Center, Los Angeles, California

Ash Mansour, M.D.
Instructor of Surgery, University of Colorado School of Medicine, Denver, Colorado; Attending Surgeon, Martin Army Hospital, Ft. Benning, Georgia

John Marek, M.D.
Resident in Surgery, University of Colorado Health Sciences Center, Denver, Colorado

R. Russell Martin, M.D.
Clinical Assistant Professor of Surgery, University of Hawaii School of Medicine, Director of Trauma, Tripler Army Medical Center, Honolulu, Hawaii; Adjunct Clinical Assistant Professor of Surgery, Baylor College of Medicine, Houston, Texas

Kenneth L. Mattox, M.D.
Professor of Surgery, Baylor College of Medicine; Adjunct Clinical Professor of Surgery, Uniformed Services University for the Health Sciences, Bethesda, Maryland; Chief of Staff and Chief of Surgery, Ben Taub General Hospital, Houston, Texas

W. Patrick Mazier, M.D.
Clinical Professor, Michigan State University; President, Ferguson Clinic; Attending, Ferguson Hospital, Blodgett Memorial Medical Center, Butterworth Hospital, and St. Mary's Hospital, Grand Rapids, Michigan

Kenneth H. McCarley, M.D.
Resident in Otolaryngology–Head and Neck Surgery, University of Colorado Health Sciences Center, Denver, Colorado

Ian McColl, M.S.
Chairman, Department of Surgery, London University at Guy's Hospital; Director of Surgery Guy's Hospital, London, United Kingdom

Douglas E. Merkel, M.D.
Assistant Professor of Medicine, Northwestern University Medical School, Chicago; Attending, Department of Medicine and Department of Pathology, Evanston Hospital, Evanston, Illinois

Arlen Meyers, M.B.A., M.D.
Associate Professor of Otolaryngology–Head and Neck Surgery, University of Colorado School of Medicine; Chief, Otolaryngology–Head and Neck Surgery, Denver VA Medical Center, Denver, Colorado

Marilyn Milkman, M.D.
Clinical Faculty, Department of Obstetrics/Gynecology, University of California, San Francisco; Attending, Mt. Zion Hospital of UCSF, San Francisco, California

Ernest E. Moore, M.D.
Professor and Vice Chairman, Department of Surgery, University of Colorado School of Medicine; Chief, Department of Surgery, Denver General Hospital, Denver, Colorado

Frederick A. Moore, M.D.
Assistant Professor of Surgery, University of Colorado School of Medicine; Chief, Critical Care, Denver General Hospital, Denver, Colorado

Sean J. Mulvihill, M.D.
Associate Professor of Surgery, University of California, San Francisco; Attending, The Medical Center at the University of California, San Francisco, San Francisco, California

Philip T. Neff, M.D.
Resident in Surgery, University of Colorado Health Sciences Center, Denver, Colorado

Cynthia L. Norrgran, M.D.
Attending Neurosurgeon, Colorado Neurological Institute, Englewood, Colorado

Lawrence W. Norton, M.D.
Professor and Vice-Chairman, Department of Surgery, University of Colorado School of Medicine; Chief, Division of General Surgery, University of Colorado Health Sciences Center, Denver, Colorado

Robert T. Osteen, M.D.
Associate Professor of Surgery, Harvard Medical School; Vice-Chairman, Surgery, Brigham and Women's Hospital, Boston, Massachusetts

Edward Passaro, Jr., M.D.
Professor of Surgery, University of California, Los Angeles, School of Medicine; Chief, Surgical Service, VA Medical Center, West Los Angeles: Attending, UCLA Medical Center, Los Angeles, California

Bruce C. Paton, M.D., FRCS(Ed), FRCP(Ed)
Clinical Professor of Surgery, University of Colorado School of Medicine; Attending, Porter Memorial Hospital, Swedish Medical Center, and University Hospital, Denver, Colorado

William H. Pearce, M.D.
Associate Professor of Surgery, Northwestern University Medical School; Attending Surgeon, Northwestern Memorial Hospital; Chief, Vascular Surgery Section, VA Lakeside Medical Center, Chicago, Illinois

Nathan W. Pearlman, M.D.
Professor of Surgery, University of Colorado School of Medicine; Attending, University of Colorado Health Sciences Center and Denver VA Medical Center, Denver, Colorado

Norman E. Peterson, M.D.
Professor, Department of Surgery (Urology), University of Colorado School of Medicine; Associate Director, Surgery, and Chief, Urology Division, Denver General Hospital, Denver, Colorado

Luis G. Podesta, M.D.
Associate Director, Transplant Services, Cedars-Sinai Medical Center, Los Angeles, California

Hiram C. Polk, Jr., M.D.
Ben A. Reid, Sr., Professor and Chairman, Department of Surgery, University of Louisville School of Medicine, Louisville, Kentucky

Joseph H. Rapp, M.D.
Associate Professor of Surgery, University of California, San Francisco; Attending, University of California, San Francisco, Medical Center, San Francisco, California

Scott L. Replogle, M.D.
Clinical Assistant Professor, University of Colorado School of Medicine, Denver; Attending, AVISTA Hospital/Medical Center, Louisville; Boulder Community Hospital, Boulder; McKee Medical Center, Loveland; Longmont United Hospital, Longmont; and St. Anthony's Hospital System, Denver, Colorado; and Regional West Medical Center, Scottsbluff, Nebraska

Jerome P. Richie, M.D.
Elliott C. Cutler Professor of Surgery, Harvard Medical School; Chairman, Harvard Program in Urology; Chief of Urology, Brigham and Women's Hospital, Boston, Massachusetts

William A. Robinson, M.D., Ph.D.
Professor of Medicine and American Cancer Society Professor of Clinical Oncology, University of Colorado School of Medicine, Denver, Colorado

David B. Roos, M.D.
Clinical Professor of Surgery, University of Colorado School of Medicine; Attending, Presbyterian/St. Luke's Medical Center, Denver, Colorado

Alexander S. Rosemurgy II, M.D.
Associate Professor of Surgery, University of South Florida, Tampa, Florida

Robert B. Rutherford, M.D.
Professor of Surgery, University of Colorado School of Medicine; Chief, Vascular Surgery Section, University Hospital, Denver, Colorado

David C. Sabiston, Jr., M.D.
James B. Duke Professor of Surgery and Chairman, Department of Surgery, Duke University Medical Center, Durham, North Carolina

William P. Schecter, M.D.
Associate Clinical Professor of Surgery, University of California, San Francisco; Attending Surgeon, San Francisco General Hospital, San Francisco, California

Michael J. Schutz, M.D.
Assistant Professor of Urology, University of Arkansas for Medical Sciences; Attending, University Hospital and J.L. McClellan VA Medical Center, Little Rock, Arkansas

Robert G. Scribner, M.D.
Assistant Clinical Professor of Surgery, Stanford University, Palo Alto; Chief of Vascular Surgery, Seton Medical Center, Daly City, California

Linda S. Sher, M.D.
Assistant Director, Transplant Services, Cedars-Sinai Medical Center, Los Angeles, California

Walton Shim, M.D.
Professor of Surgery, John A. Burns School of Medicine, University of Hawaii; Chief of Surgery and Director of Surgical Education, Kapiolani Medical Center for Women and Children, Honolulu, Hawaii

Everett E. Spees, M.D., Ph.D.
Professor of Surgery, University of Colorado School of Medicine; Attending, University of Colorado Health Sciences Center and St. Luke's Presbyterian Medical Center, Denver, Colorado

Bruce E. Stabile, M.D.
Professor of Surgery, University of California, San Diego, School of Medicine; Chief, Surgical Service, VA Medical Center; Attending, UCSD Medical Center, San Diego, California

Thomas H. Stanisic, M.D.
Professor of Surgery (Urology), University of Arizona College of Medicine; Attending, University Medical Center, VA Medical Center, and Tucson Medical Center, Tucson, Arizona

Glenn Steele, Jr., M.D.
The William V. McDermott Professor of Surgery, Harvard Medical School; Chairman, Department of Surgery, New England Deaconess Hospital, Boston, Massachusetts

Gianna Stellin, M.D.
Assistant Professor of Surgery, University of California, Irvine; Attending, University of California, Irvine, Medical Center, Irvine, California

Michael D. Stone, M.D.
Assistant Professor of Surgery, Harvard Medical School; Attending, Division of Surgical Oncology, New England Deaconess Hospital, Boston, Massachusetts

Ronald J. Stoney, M.D.
Professor of Surgery, University of California, San Francisco; Attending, University of California, San Francisco, Medical Center, San Francisco, California

Gary Alan Tannenbaum, M.D.
Fellow in Vascular Surgery, Division of Vascular Surgery, New England Deaconess Hospital, Harvard Medical School, Boston, Massachusetts

John Terblanche, Ch.M., FCS(SA), FRCS(Eng)
Professor and Chairman, Department of Surgery, University of Cape Town, and Co-Director, Medical

Research Council Liver Research Centre; Professor and Chairman, Department of Surgery, Groote Schuur Hospital Teaching Hospital Group, Cape Town, South Africa

Norman W. Thompson, M.D.
Henry K. Ransom Professor of Surgery, University of Michigan; Chief, Division of Endocrine Surgery, University of Michigan Hospitals, Ann Arbor, Michigan

J. Brantley Thrasher, M.D.
Staff Urologist, Madigan Army Medical Center, Tacoma, Washington

Gary D. VanderArk, M.D.
Clinical Associate Professor of Surgery (Neurosurgery), University of Colorado School of Medicine, Denver; Attending, Colorado Neurological Institute, Englewood, Colorado

Greg Van Stiegmann, M.D.
Associate Professor of Surgery, University of Colorado School of Medicine; Chief, Surgical Endoscopy, University of Colorado Health Sciences Center and Denver VA Hospital, Denver, Colorado

Hugo V. Villar, M.D.
Professor of Surgery and Radiation Oncology, University of Arizona College of Medicine; Attending, University Medical Center, Tucson, Arizona

Richard Ward, M.D.
Clinical Professor of Surgery, University of California School of Medicine, Davis; Attending, Sutter General Hospital, Sutter Memorial Hospital, and Mercy General Hospital, Sacramento, California

Andrew L. Warshaw, M.D.
Harold and Ellen Danser Professor of Surgery, Harvard Medical School; Associate Chief of Surgery, Massachusetts General Hospital, Boston, Massachusetts

Philip C. Watt, M.D.
Resident in Surgery, University of California, Los Angeles, School of Medicine and VA Medical Center, West Los Angeles, Los Angeles, California

Watts R. Webb, M.D.
Professor of Surgery, Tulane University School of Medicine; Attending, Charity Hospitals of Louisiana, Southern Baptist Hospital, Touro Infirmary, and Tulane University Medical Center, New Orleans; Huey P. Long Regional Hospital, Pineville; St. Jude Medical Center, Kenner, Louisiana; and Gulf Coast Community Hospital, Biloxi, and Memorial Hospital, Gulfport, Mississippi

John Wettlaufer, M.D.
Clinical Professor of Urology, University of Colorado School of Medicine, Denver, Colorado; Chief of Urology, Madigan Army Medical Center, Tacoma, Washington

Paul Wexler, M.D.
Clinical Professor in Obstetrics and Gynecology, University of Colorado School of Medicine; Attending, Rose Medical Center and Lutheran Medical Center; Honorary Staff, Children's Hospital, Denver; Courtesy Staff, Humana Aurora, Porter Hospital, and Swedish Hospital, Aurora, Colorado

Glenn J. R. Whitman, M.D.
Associate Professor and Chief, Cardiothoracic Surgery, The Medical College of Pennsylvania, Philadelphia, Pennsylvania

Jerome D. Wiedel, M.D.
Professor and Chairman, Department of Orthopedic Surgery, University of Colorado School of Medicine; Attending, University Hospital, Presbyterian/St. Luke's Hospital, Denver General Hospital, and Rose Medical Center, Denver, Colorado

William C. Willard, M.D.
Staff Surgeon, Madigan Army Medical Center, Tacoma, Washington

David P. Winchester, M.D.
Associate Professor of Clinical Surgery, Northwestern University Medical School, Chicago; Senior Attending Surgeon and Chief, General Surgery and Surgical Oncology, Evanston Hospital, Evanston, Illinois

William G. Winter, M.D.
Professor of Orthopedic Surgery, University of Colorado School of Medicine; Chief, Orthopedics, Denver VA Medical Center; Attending, University Hospital; Courtesy Staff, Denver General Hospital, Denver, Colorado

Leslie Wise, M.D.
Professor of Surgery, Albert Einstein College of Medicine, Bronx; Chairman, Department of Surgery, Long Island Jewish Medical Center, New Hyde Park, New York

Francis G. Wolfort, M.D.
Associate Professor of Surgery, Harvard Medical School; Chief of Plastic and Reconstructive Surgery, New England Deaconess Hospital, Boston, and Cambridge Hospital, Cambridge; Attending, Children's Hospital, Boston, Massachusetts

John Wong, Ph.D.(Syd), FRACS
Professor and Head, Department of Surgery, University of Hong Kong, Queen Mary Hospital, Hong Kong

Roger Wotkyns, M.D.
Professor of Surgery, University of Colorado School of Medicine; Attending, Denver VA Medical Center, University of Colorado Health Sciences Center, Denver, Colorado

Byron Young, M.D.
Johnston-Wright Chair of Surgery, and Chairman, Department of Surgery, College of Medicine, University of Kentucky; Chief, Division of Neurosurgery, University Hospital, Lexington, Kentucky

Preface

The first two editions of *Surgical Decision Making* had as their objective to provide in the graphic form of an algorithm the preferred approach to managing common surgical problems. Comment accompanying each algorithm provided the rationale for choosing a course of action.

Acceptance of the algorithm as an instrument of decision analysis leads us to introduce another edition of the text. Once again, decisions recommended by authors are based on personal and published experience. Unlike its predecessors, however, this third edition attempts to justify choices on the basis of outcome and cost. Finding reliable data concerning outcome is often difficult. Although the sensitivity and specificity of a laboratory or imaging test can be determined with accuracy, numbers for clinical outcomes such as perioperative mortality, relief of pain, and disease-free survival are far from exact.

Our change in emphasis in this edition is in concert with society's demand for standards of clinical performance by which quality and cost-effectiveness can be measured. Clinicians understandably resist the idea of reducing multifactorial decisions, which are subject to variations of the patient and the provider, to simple line drawings. A cookbook approach to problem solving cannot possibly reflect the circumstances under which the surgeon exercises judgment. This book is not intended to prescribe behavior in every instance. It offers the reader an opportunity to follow the logic of an expert in selecting the best among many competing options of diagnosis and treatment.

Critics challenge medicine to minimize expense and yet to maintain quality care. Health economists recognize that many of the expensive tests clinicians perform are, in retrospect, unnecessary. A surgeon can answer such criticism by determining in advance what decisions are both beneficial and economically prudent. This edition of *Surgical Decision Making* provides some of the data a surgeon needs to determine the number and complexity of management options and the risk of complications associated with treatment.

The new edition has been expanded by adding chapters in the areas of transplantation surgery and perioperative management. More than one-third of the authors are new. They represent many geographic areas and medical centers. As in earlier editions, the range of surgical interests is broad to serve as a resource for both the practicing surgeon and the trainee.

LAWRENCE W. NORTON, M.D.
GLENN STEELE, JR., M.D.
BEN EISEMAN, M.D.

Contents

GENERAL

Preoperative Laboratory Evaluation 2
Bradley C. Borlase, M.D., M.S., and Ben Eiseman, M.D.

Preoperative Cardiac Evaluation 4
Ash Mansour, M.D.

Perioperative Arrhythmia 6
Glenn J. R. Whitman, M.D., and David A. Fullerton, M.D.

Postoperative Monitoring of the Unstable Patient 8
Edward J. Bartle, M.D.

Cardiopulmonary Resuscitation 10
Steven R. Lowenstein, M.D., M.P.H., and Jean T. Abbott, M.D.

Shock 14
R. Armour Forse, M.D., Ph.D., Bradley C. Borlase, M.D., M.S., and Peter N. Benotti, M.D.

Bleeding Disorders 16
James J. Corrigan, Jr., M.D.

Transfusion 18
Walter H. Dzik, M.D.

Postoperative Fever 22
Bradley C. Borlase, M.D., M.S., Peter N. Benotti, M.D., and R. Armour Forse, M.D., Ph.D.

Nutritional Support 24
Todd N. Jones, R.N., M.S., and Frederick A. Moore, M.D.

AIDS and Surgery 26
William P. Schecter, M.D., Ash Mansour, M.D., and Robert C. Lim, M.D.

Hypothermia 28
Bruce C. Paton, M.D., FRCS(Ed), FRCP(Ed)

HEAD AND NECK

Closed Head Injury 32
Gary D. VanderArk, M.D., and Cynthia L. Norrgran, M.D.

Unequal Pupils 34
Kevin O. Lillehei, M.D.

Otorrhea 36
James W. Lucarini, M.D.

Epistaxis 40
Kenneth H. McCarley, M.D., and Bruce W. Jafek, M.D.

Maxillary Fractures 42
Scott L. Replogle, M.D.

Mandibular Fractures 44
Scott L. Replogle, M.D.

Carcinoma of the Lip 46
Lawrence L. Ketch, M.D.

Carcinoma of the Oral Cavity 48
Stanley Coulthard, M.D.

Parotid Tumor 50
John J. Coleman III, M.D., and M. J. Jurkiewicz, M.D.

Neck Mass 52
Thomas Eyen, M.D., and Arlen Meyers, M.B.A., M.D.

Carcinoma of the Larynx 54
Nathan W. Pearlman, M.D.

CARDIOPULMONARY

Chest Injury 58
Alan Hopeman, M.D.

Pulmonary Embolism 60
W. Randolph Chitwood, Jr., M.D., and David C. Sabiston, Jr., M.D.

Pleural Effusion and Empyema 62
Watts R. Webb, M.D.

Lung Abscess 64
Jeffrey S. Cross, M.D., and Michael R. Johnston, M.D.

Carcinoma of the Lung 66
Stephen J. Lahey, M.D.

Patent Ductus Arteriosus 68
Sidney Levitsky, M.D.

Coarctation of the Aorta   70
James T. Anderson, M.D.

Neonatal Cyanosis   72
David R. Clarke, M.D.

Cyanotic Congenital Heart Disease   74
David R. Clarke, M.D.

Congenital Obstructive Cardiac Anomalies   76
David N. Campbell, M.D.

Congenital Septal Defects   78
David N. Campbell, M.D.

Acute Myocardial Infarct   80
Aubrey C. Galloway, M.D., Frederick Feit, M.D., and Ben Eiseman, M.D.

Coronary Artery Disease   82
Jack G. Copeland, M.D.

Aortic Valve Stenosis   84
Bruce C. Paton, M.D., FRCS(Ed), FRCP(Ed)

Mitral Stenosis   86
Glenn J. R. Whitman, M.D.

GASTROINTESTINAL

Blunt Abdominal Trauma   90
James M. Brown, M.D., and Ernest E. Moore, M.D.

Penetrating Abdominal Trauma   92
David V. Feliciano, M.D.

Duodenal Injury   94
R. Russell Martin, M.D., and Kenneth L. Mattox, M.D.

Pancreatic Injury   96
R. Russell Martin, M.D., and Kenneth L. Mattox, M.D.

Penetrating Injury of the Colon   98
Philip T. Neff, M.D., and Ernest E. Moore, M.D.

Achalasia   102
Alex G. Little, M.D.

Carcinoma of the Esophagus   104
Manson Fok, M.B. B.S.(HK), FRCS(Ed), and John Wong, Ph.D.(Syd), FRACS

Gastroesophageal Reflux 106
Joseph LoCicero III, M.D.

Gastric Ulcer 108
Sean J. Mulvihill, M.D., and Haile T. Debas, M.D.

Duodenal Ulcer 112
Max M. Cohen, M.D.

Postgastrectomy Syndrome 114
Bruce E. Stabile, M.D., Edward Passaro, Jr., M.D., and Philip C. Watt, M.D.

Upper Gastrointestinal Bleeding 116
Lawrence W. Norton, M.D.

Bleeding Esophageal Varices 118
Greg Van Stiegmann, M.D.

Jaundice: Diagnostic Workup 120
John Marek, M.D., and Greg Van Stiegmann, M.D.

Obstructive Jaundice: Interventional Options 122
John Marek, M.D., and Greg Van Stiegmann, M.D.

Cholelithiasis 124
Lawrence W. Norton, M.D.

Common Bile Duct Stones 126
Philippe Gertsch, M.D., and Leslie Blumgart, M.D.

Liver Tumor 130
John Terblanche, Ch.M., FCS(SA), FRCS(Eng)

Acute Pancreatitis 132
Alexander S. Rosemurgy II, M.D., and Larry C. Carey, M.D.

Chronic Pancreatitis 134
Charles F. Frey, M.D.

Pancreatic Pseudocyst 138
Edward L. Bradley III, M.D.

Carcinoma of the Pancreas 140
Carlos Fernández-del Castillo, M.D., and Andrew L. Warshaw, M.D.

Small Bowel Obstruction 142
Ian McColl, M.S.

Acute Mesenteric Vascular Occlusion 144
B. Timothy Baxter, M.D., and William H. Pearce, M.D.

Short Bowel Syndrome 146
Leslie Wise, M.D., and Ronald E. Greenberg, M.D.

Enterocutaneous Fistula 148
Josef Fischer, M.D.

Gastrointestinal Lymphoma 150
Robert T. Osteen, M.D., William Cody, M.D., and Ben Eiseman, M.D.

Crohn's Disease of the Small Bowel 152
Victor W. Fazio, M.D., FRACS

Acute Right Lower Quadrant Pain 154
Richard G. Fiddian-Green, B.M., B.Ch., FRCS

Volvulus 156
Hugo V. Villar, M.D.

Diverticular Disease 158
Gilbert Hermann, M.D., and Charles Abernathy, M.D.

Lower Gastrointestinal Bleeding 160
Robert W. Beart, Jr., M.D.

Ulcerative Colitis 162
Robert W. Beart, Jr., M.D.

Carcinoma of the Colon 164
Michael J. Edwards, M.D., and Hiram C. Polk, Jr., M.D.

Carcinoma of the Rectum or Anus 166
J. Milburn Jessup, M.D., and Glenn Steele, Jr., M.D.

Anorectal Abscess/Fistula 168
Peter A. Cataldo, M.D., and W. Patrick Mazier, M.D.

Hemorrhoids 170
Peter A. Cataldo, M.D., and W. Patrick Mazier, M.D.

Pilonidal Disease 172
Ash Mansour, M.D.

BREAST AND SOFT TISSUES

Nipple Discharge 176
Roger Wotkyns, M.D., and Lawrence W. Norton, M.D.

Solitary Breast Mass 178
Lawrence W. Norton, M.D.

Early Breast Carcinoma   180
Lawrence W. Norton, M.D.

Advanced Breast Cancer   182
David P. Winchester, M.D., and Douglas E. Merkel, M.D.

Recurrent Breast Carcinoma   186
Michael D. Stone, M.D., and Blake Cady, M.D.

Hodgkin's Disease   190
Walter D. Holder, Jr., M.D.

Retroperitoneal Mass   194
William C. Willard, M.D., and Murray F. Brennan, M.D.

Melanoma   196
William A. Robinson, M.D., Ph.D.

Burns   198
John F. Hansbrough, M.D.

ENDOCRINE

Hyperthyroidism   202
R. Dale Liechty, M.D.

Thyroid Nodule   204
R. Dale Liechty, M.D.

Thyroid Carcinoma   206
Clive S. Grant, M.D.

Hypercalcemia and Hyperparathyroidism   208
Norman W. Thompson, M.D.

Insulinoma   210
R. Dale Liechty, M.D.

Zollinger-Ellison Syndrome (Gastrinoma)   212
E. Christopher Ellison, M.D.

Pheochromocytoma   214
Glenn W. Geelhoed, M.D., M.P.H.

Cushing Syndrome   216
Donald S. Gann, M.D.

VASCULAR

Thoracic Outlet Syndrome   220
David B. Roos, M.D.

Leg Claudication   222
Richard F. Kempczinski, M.D., and Richard J. Fowl, M.D.

Peripheral Arterial Embolism   224
F. William Blaisdell, M.D., and Richard Ward, M.D.

Abdominal Aortic Aneurysm   226
Ronald J. Stoney, M.D., and Joseph H. Rapp, M.D.

Cerebrovascular Insufficiency   228
Robert G. Scribner, M.D.

Renovascular Hypertension   230
Gary Alan Tannenbaum, M.D., and Frank W. LoGerfo, M.D.

Varicose Veins   232
Robert B. Rutherford, M.D., and Glenn Kelly, M.D.

Venous Stasis Ulcers   234
Roy E. Carlson, M.D.

PEDIATRICS

Tracheoesophageal Fistula   238
Roberta J. Hall, M.D., Frederick M. Karrer, M.D., and John R. Lilly, M.D.

Infantile Pyloric Stenosis   240
Jeffrey A. Lowell, M.D.

Neonatal Bowel Obstruction   242
Frederick M. Karrer, M.D., and John R. Lilly, M.D.

Hirschsprung Disease   246
Walton Shim, M.D.

Imperforate Anus   248
J. Laurance Hill, M.D.

Surgical Jaundice in Infancy   250
Gianna Stellin, M.D., and John R. Lilly, M.D.

Retroperitoneal Mass in Infancy   252
Ann M. Kosloske, M.D.

TRANSPLANTATION

Kidney Transplantation   256
Roberta J. Hall, M.D., and Igal Kam, M.D.

Pancreas Transplantation   258
Roberta J. Hall, M.D., and Everett E. Spees, M.D., Ph.D.

Liver Transplantation   260
Luis G. Podesta, M.D., Linda S. Sher, M.D., Todd K. Howard, M.D.,
and Leonard Makowka, M.D., Ph.D.

Heart Transplantation   262
Robert L. Kormos, M.D., and Henry T. Bahnson, M.D.

UROLOGIC

Traumatic Hematuria   266
Norman E. Peterson, M.D.

Adult Urinary Tract Infection   268
Richard Heppe, M.D.

Renal or Ureteral Calculus   270
George W. Drach, M.D.

Renal Mass   272
Robert E. Donohue, M.D.

Bladder Tumor   274
Thomas H. Stanisic, M.D.

Prostatism   278
John Wettlaufer, M.D., and J. Brantley Thrasher, M.D.

Carcinoma of the Prostate   282
Jerome P. Richie, M.D.

Scrotal Mass   284
Norman E. Peterson, M.D.

Testis Tumor   286
Michael J. Schutz, M.D., and E. David Crawford, M.D.

GYNECOLOGIC

Vaginal Bleeding in Reproductive Years   290
Marilyn Milkman, M.D., and Paul Wexler, M.D.

Vaginal Bleeding in Nonreproductive Years   294
Marilyn Milkman, M.D., and Paul Wexler, M.D.

Pelvic Inflammatory Disease   296
R. Phillip Heine, M.D., and William Droegemueler, M.D.

Endometriosis   298
Bradley S. Hurst, M.D.

Carcinoma of the Cervix   300
Theodore C. Barton, M.D.

Endometrial Carcinoma   302
Howard M. Goodman, M.D., and Ross S. Berkowitz, M.D.

Adnexal Mass   304
Tommy N. Evans, M.D.

Ovarian Mass   306
Francis J. Major, M.D.

ORTHOPEDIC

Cervical Spine Fracture   310
Robert E. Breeze, M.D.

Thoracolumbar Spine Fracture   312
Robert B. Dzioba, M.D.

Pelvic Fracture   314
Alan D. Aaron, M.D.

Hip Fracture   316
Susan L. Jolly, M.D., and Mack L. Clayton, M.D.

Femoral Shaft Fracture   318
Jerome D. Wiedel, M.D., and Hugh Dougall, M.D.

Tibial Shaft Fracture   320
Jerome D. Wiedel, M.D., and Hugh Dougall, M.D.

Knee Fracture   322
William G. Winter, M.D.

Ankle Fracture   324
William G. Winter, M.D.

Hand Fractures   326
Francis G. Wolfort, M.D.

Flexor Tendon Injuries of the Hand   330
Lawrence L. Ketch, M.D.

Back Pain   334
Byron Young, M.D.

INDEX   337

General

Preoperative Laboratory Evaluation

Bradley C. Borlase, M.D., M.S., and Ben Eiseman, M.D.

(A) History (50 percent) and physical examination (17 percent) account for two thirds of the diagnoses made in patients.

(B) Laboratory and special studies such as computed tomography scanning when logically indicated by the history and physical examination contribute only one third of the diagnoses.

(C) Risk factors, particularly the anatomic site of operation, contribute significantly to postoperative mortality.

Operative Site	Postoperative Mortality
Intracranial	9.7%
Intrathoracic	8.6%
Upper abdomen	6.6%
Head and neck (nonthyroid)	6.4%

(D) Preoperative chest x-ray for patients below age 50 years is not required routinely. Indications for preoperative chest x-ray are thoracotomy, known cardiopulmonary disease, high risk for unsuspected tuberculosis, and age over 50 years.

(E) Routine electrocardiogram is warranted in patients over age 50 years or in those with significant risk factors to detect arrhythmias or unsuspected coronary artery disease.

(F) Arterial blood gas levels are measured in patients who have a significant history of chronic pulmonary disease.

(G) Complete blood counts are abnormal in only 3 percent of patients with nonsignificant histories and physical examinations. Clotting profiles (prothrombin time, partial thromboplastin time, platelets, bleeding time) are necessary only in patients with easy bruising, frequent epistaxis, excessive menorrhagia, hematuria, prolonged bleeding after tooth extraction, abnormal bleeding during or after surgery, collagen vascular disease, liver or kidney disease, specific medications (aspirin, nonsteroidal antiinflammatory drugs), and a positive family history.

(H) Urinalysis is used to detect unsuspected urinary infection or disease. Glycosuria occurs in 8 percent, proteinuria in 6 percent, and bacteriuria in less than 1 percent of men and 3 percent of women. Serum chemistries are better screens for diabetes or renal disease than urine examinations because they are more specific.

(I) Serum electrolytes have no proven value as routine preoperative tests unless there is significant history, such as diuretics, renal disease, diarrhea, vomiting, or heart disease. Fasting blood sugar screens should be performed for the 1 percent of patients who have unsuspected diabetes.

(J) Gastrointestinal function is assessed by an expensive array of malabsorption testing. These studies are indicated only by a significant history and physical examination.

(K) Malnutrition significantly increases complications, length of stay, and hospital mortality. Preoperative assessment includes history of weight loss (>10%) and albumin and creatinine-height index (see **P**) testing. Patients who are severely malnourished benefit from a brief period of preoperative nutrition.

(L) Impaired immunofunction increases complications and mortality. Delayed-type hypersensitivity skin testing predicts increased probability of poor outcome. Anergic patients and patients remaining anergic are at high risk.

(M) Evaluation of the vascular system primarily involves a search for cardiac, cerebral, and aortoiliac disease.

(N) Stress tests are diagnostic of myocardial ischemia. Dipyridamole-thallium scans predict cardiac risk in patients with vascular disease or a history of myocardial infarction who are about to undergo abdominal surgery.

(O) Lung volumes are predictive of risk. An FEV_1 less than 1.0 predicts extended postoperative mechanical ventilation and possible respirator dependency.

(P) Creatinine clearance decreases with age, thus increasing the risk of renal insufficiency. A 24-hour urine collection analyzed for creatinine clearance and electrolytes accurately determines kidney function. Results also evaluate stress status (nitrogen balance, catabolic index) and nutritional status (creatinine-height index).

REFERENCES

Borlase BC, Eiseman B. Routine laboratory tests. In: Eiseman E, Stahlgren L, eds. Cost effective surgical management. Philadelphia: WB Saunders, 1987:5.

Christou NV, Tellado-Rodriguez J, Chantnand L, et al. Estimating mortality risk in preoperative patients using immunologic, nutritional, and acute-phase response variables. Ann Surg 1989;1:69–70.

Farrow SC, Fowkes FGR, Lunn JN, et al. Epidemiology in anesthesia: II. Factors affecting mortality in hospital. Br J Anesth 1982;54:811–817.

Fowkes FGR, Lunn JN, Farrow SC, et al. Epidemiology in anesthesia: III. Mortality risk in patients with co-existing physical disease. Br J Anesth 1982;54:819–825.

Savino JA, DelGuencio LRM. Preoperative assessment of high-risk surgical patients. Surg Clin North Am 1985;65:763–790.

Schneider AJL. Assessment of risk factors and surgical outcome. Surg Clin North Am 1983;63:1113–1126.

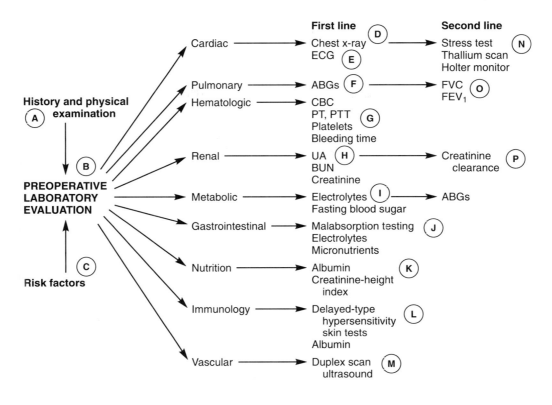

Preoperative Cardiac Evaluation

Ash Mansour, M.D.

(A) A thorough history identifies risk factors predisposing the patient to generalized atherosclerotic disease. The most significant risk factors are a family history of coronary artery disease (CAD), smoking, hypertension, diabetes mellitus, and previous myocardial infarction or history of angina. On physical examination, assessment of the carotid arteries for bruits and the distal circulation for pulses is essential. Special attention is paid to the cardiac examination to rule out an S_3 sound, jugular venous distension, or other signs of congestive heart failure. History and physical examination can give the examiner an idea of the patient's Goldman preoperative risk factor. An electrocardiogram can show evidence of important arrhythmias (heart block, atrial fibrillation), previous myocardial injury, left ventricular hypertrophy, or significant ischemic changes (ST wave changes).

(B) Patients in good physical condition with low risk for heart disease may proceed to surgery without further workup. If the patient has any evidence of atherosclerotic disease and CAD and a major abdominal or thoracic operation is planned, then a preoperative treadmill stress test is advisable.

(C) If the target heart rate and blood pressure are reached on the Bruce protocol, surgery can be done without further workup. A suboptimal test due to the patient's inability to exercise or complete the test for any reason is an indication for obtaining a dipyridamole-thallium scan (DTS).

(D) DTS has been used to identify patients with significant CAD. This test may show one of three findings, including (1) normal scan—no further workup necessary; (2) fixed disease—indicative of significant CAD that probably would not benefit from myocardial revascularization (myocardial function should be assessed by gated blood scan [MUGA]); and (3) evidence of redistribution—indicative of important CAD that may benefit from revascularization (proceed to coronary angiography to determine extent of disease and need for bypass). A normal DTS was once thought to be reliable for identifying low-risk patients for myocardial events. Studies have shown that up to 10 percent of patients with normal scans have nonfatal perioperative myocardial events. Newer tests, such as exercise DTS or dobutamine stress echocardiography, are being investigated to improve the sensitivity of DTS.

(E) Coronary angiography is the standard in evaluating coronary arteries and ventricular function. Approximately one third of patients undergoing aortic aneurysmectomy or peripheral vascular bypass surgery have significant correctable CAD.

(F) MUGA is useful in assessing myocardial function and ejection fraction. If MUGA demonstrates good function, surgery can be performed without further workup. If a patient has poor ejection fraction, further workup with coronary angiography is indicated to determine if revascularization can be done. If CAD is inoperable, careful consideration should be given to canceling elective surgery or choosing a less invasive or palliative procedure.

(G) The detection of correctable CAD is an indication to proceed with coronary artery bypass grafting before another planned operation. There are very few situations where a coronary artery bypass graft may need to be combined with another procedure (eg, resection of a symptomatic abdominal aortic aneurysm).

REFERENCES

Diamond GA, Forrester JS. Analysis of probability as an aid in the clinical diagnosis of coronary artery disease. N Engl J Med 1979; 300:1350–1358.

Ellestad MH, Cooke BM, Greenberg PS. Stress testing: clinical application and predictive capacity. Prog Cardiovasc Dis 1979; 21:431–460.

Gibbons RJ, Lee KL, Cobb FR, et al. Ejection fraction response to exercise in patients with chest pain, coronary artery disease and normal resting ventricular function. Circulation 1982; 66:643–648.

Goldman L. Cardiac risk factors and complications of noncardiac surgery. Ann Intern Med 1983; 98:504–513.

Hertzer NR, Beven EG, Young JR, et al. Coronary artery disease in peripheral vascular patients: a classification of 1,000 coronary angiograms and results of surgical management. Ann Surg 1984; 199:223–233.

McEnroe CS, O'Donnell TF, Yeager A, et al. Comparison of ejection fraction and Goldman risk factor analysis to dipyridamole–thallium 201 studies in the evaluation of cardiac morbidity after aortic aneurysm surgery. J Vasc Surg 1990; 11:497–504.

Reul GJ, Cooley DA, Duncan JM, et al. The effect of coronary bypass on the outcome of peripheral vascular operations in 1,093 patients. J Vasc Surg 1986; 3:788–798.

Rutherford RB. Preoperative cardiac evaluation in vascular surgery patients: a selective approach. Seminars in Vascular Surgery 1991; 4:106–109.

History and physical examination (A)
  Family history of CAD
  Smoker
  Hypertension
  Diabetes
  Previous MI
  Angina
  Bruits
  Venous distension
  CHF

Lab
  ECG

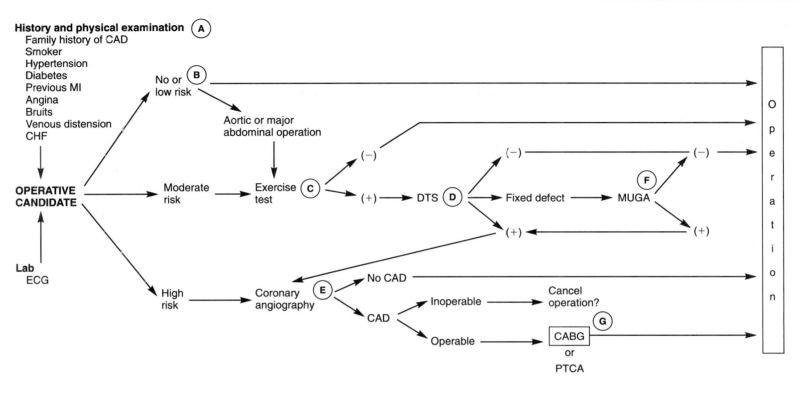

Perioperative Arrhythmia

Glenn J. R. Whitman, M.D., and David A. Fullerton, M.D.

(A) Risk factors for perioperative arrhythmia include hypertension, cigarette smoking, diabetes, hypercholesterolemia, hypertriglyceridemia, and family history of heart disease. Physical examination delineates the emergent nature of the therapy: hypotension requires immediate countershock; a well-tolerated arrhythmia permits deliberate medical therapy.

(B) Causes include (1) ischemia; (2) hypoxia; (3) pulmonary embolus; (4) endogenous or exogenous catecholamines, as occurs with severe pain, intravenous dopamine, respiratory nebulizers using β-agonists such as Alupent, and oral or intravenous theophylline derivatives; (5) electrolyte disturbances (hypokalemia and hypomagnesemia); (6) hypothermia; (7) mechanical problems such as right ventricular stimulation by a Swan-Ganz catheter in the right ventricle or a chest tube making contact with the epicardium; and (8) hyperthyroidism.

(C) Ventricular tachycardia must be differentiated from supraventricular tachycardia (SVT). SVT is probable when the QRS complex is preceded by a premature P wave, is narrow, or, if wide, has a right bundle branch block morphology. Regardless of the cause, countershock is necessary if the patient is in extremis. Medical therapy is appropriate if the patient is hemodynamically stable.

(D) Ventricular asystole is the absence of any ventricular electric activity. It may follow third-degree heart block without a ventricular escape mechanism or result from prolonged ventricular fibrillation and myocardial ischemia. Treatment is cardiopulmonary resuscitation, intravenous epinephrine, sodium bicarbonate, calcium chloride, isoproterenol, and atropine. A ventricular pacemaker may be the only effective form of therapy.

(E) In first-degree atrioventricular (AV) block each atrial impulse is conducted to the ventricle but with a conduction delay, the PR interval being greater than 0.20 second. This benign abnormality requires no therapy.

(F) There are two types of second-degree AV block: Mobitz Type I (Wenckebach) is progressive lengthening of the PR interval until an atrial impulse fails to conduct. The cycle then repeats itself. This generally is benign and requires no therapy. It may occur after an inferior myocardial infarction and is self-limiting. No pacemaker is required. Mobitz Type II involves either repetitive or paroxysmal loss of atrial impulse conduction without progressive lengthening of the PR interval. It can progress to complete heart block. Immediate placement of a temporary pacemaker is warranted.

(G) In third-degree AV block, no atrial impulse is conducted to the ventricle. The ventricular escape mechanism fixes heart rate at approximately 40 beats per minute. Acute onset usually follows anterior myocardial infarction. Treatment is immediate insertion of a pacemaker.

(H) A premature P wave before an expected sinus beat depolarizes the sinoatrial node. This usually produces an interval before the next sinus P wave, which is of normal duration. Premature atrial complexes are generally benign but may herald other atrial tachyarrhythmias. They should be investigated and treated.

(I) Paroxysmal atrial tachycardia (PAT) results from either an ectopic automatic focus stemming from one focus in the atrium (PAT) or from several atrial foci (multifocal atrial tachycardia [MAT]). It usually begins abruptly and lasts minutes to hours. The atrial rate of 160 to 250 beats per minute is often conducted at a ratio of 1:1. There may be variable AV nodal block if the patient is digitalized. Thirty percent of PATs occur in healthy people; other causes are rheumatic heart disease (30 percent) and ischemic heart disease (15 to 20 percent) after acute myocardial infarction. Digitalis intoxication should be ruled out. Management options include digitalis, β-blockers, verapamil, quinidine, and Pronestyl.

(J) MAT has a mortality rate of 50 to 60 percent because of underlying pulmonary disease or cor pulmonale and congestive heart failure. Therapy primarily involves the underlying disease. Antiarrhythmic efficacy is disappointing.

(K) Atrial flutter involves a rapid and regular rate of 250 to 350 beats per minute, usually conducted through the AV node at a ratio of 2:1. Vagal stimulation, digoxin therapy, or β-blockade may change a 2:1 block to a higher-degree block. Treatment is digitalis. If flutter produces hemodynamic instability, synchronized low-energy DC countershock (10 to 40 J) may be effective. Digitalization with or without quinidine or Pronestyl may prevent recurrence. Neither quinidine nor Pronestyl should be given until the patient is fully digitalized because these drugs may increase AV node conduction and lead to a 1:1 ventricular response tachycardia.

(L) In atrial fibrillation discoordinated atrial activity bombards the AV node, producing an irregularly irregular ventricular response. P waves are absent on electrocardiogram, and ventricular response is between 120 and 180 beats per minute. Therapy is aimed at increasing the refractoriness of the AV node, usually by digitalization. As with flutter, after AV node blockade quinidine or Pronestyl may convert the patient to a normal sinus rhythm. Verapamil or β-blockers combined with digoxin slow the ventricular response, permitting increased cardiac output.

(M) Atrioventricular junctional tachycardia may be either paroxysmal or nonparoxysmal. The former has rates of 160 to 250 beats per minute and may occur in healthy people and be tolerated for prolonged periods. Vagal stimulation may stop it. If persistent, β-blockade, verapamil, digitalis, or rarely DC countershock is effective. The nonparoxysmal variety has a slower rate of 70 to 130 beats per minute and is always associated with diseased hearts, for example, in congestive heart failure or after myocardial infarction. In either case the nodal

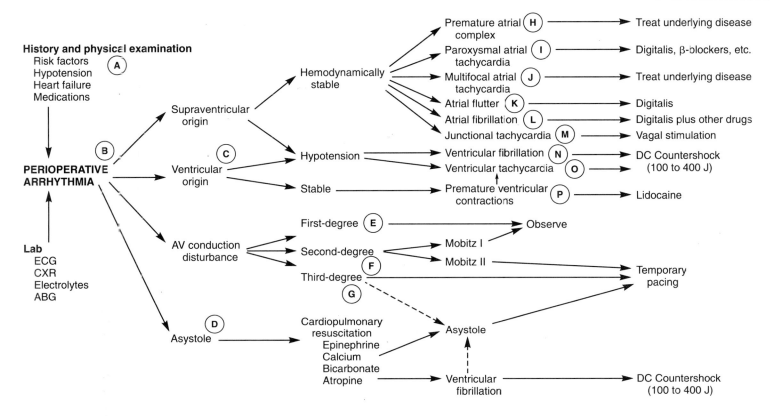

History and physical examination
Risk factors (A)
Hypotension
Heart failure
Medications

Lab
ECG
CXR
Electrolytes
ABG

rhythm may capture both the ventricles and atria, producing a characteristic, narrow QRS complex followed by retrograde P waves. The two most common causes of nonparoxysmal junctional tachycardia are digitalis intoxication (60 percent) and inferior infarction. If over-digitalization is not the cause, digitalis may slow the rate and restore hemodynamic stability.

(N) Ventricular fibrillation is a chaotic ventricular rhythm in which multiple areas of the ventricle depolarize simultaneously, resulting in no cardiac output. It is usually due to ischemia but might also be due to digitalis intoxication. In a witnessed fibrillatory arrest, a precordial thump should precede immediate DC countershock. Cardiopulmonary resuscitation should proceed as long as there is no effective rhythm. Calcium, epinephrine, bicarbonate, DC countershock, and intravenous lidocaine should be administered until a rhythm is established.

(O) Ventricular tachycardia (VT) is defined as more than six successive premature ventricular complexes (PVCs). If it lasts less than 30 seconds it is considered nonsustained. Sustained VT is generally at a regular rate (180 to 250 beats per minute) and is associated with shock. It may be difficult to differentiate VT from SVT with aberrant conduction. Both should be managed with synchronized DC countershock. Electrocardiographic characteristics of VT include a QRS complex greater than 0.14 second, absence of a right bundle branch block, triphasic regular sinus rhythm in lead V_1, and left axis deviation in the frontal plane. Lidocaine is the first intravenous drug of choice, followed by Pronestyl or bretylium.

(P) PVCs originate in the ventricle and depolarize the myocardium without being conducted through the normal conduction pathways. The QRS complex is wide and bizarre, with the ST segment and T wave directed opposite to the QRS

complex. Since the sinus node is frequently unaffected, the interval between the normal beat preceding the PVC and the following beat is usually twice the normal sinus interval. This is a fully compensatory pause. Ventricular fibrillation or tachycardia can result from consecutive PVCs, one that falls on a T wave, or multifocal PVCs. An underlying cause must be sought for PVCs that occur perioperatively. Intravenous lidocaine may prevent a lethal arrhythmia. The principal causes are ischemia, hypokalemia, and catecholamines.

REFERENCES

Chung EK. Quick reference to cardiovascular disease. 2nd edition. Philadelphia: JB Lippincott, 1982.
Chung EK. Principles of cardiac arrhythmias. 4th edition. Baltimore: Williams & Wilkins, 1989.
Wellens JJ, Bar F, Lie KI. The value of the electrocardiogram in the differential diagnosis of a tachycardia with a widened QRS complex. Am J Med 1978;64:27–33.

Postoperative Monitoring of the Unstable Patient

Edward J. Bartle, M.D.

(A) Clinical judgment is necessary to decide when to monitor a patient. It is based on the patient's underlying disease state, the stress event that has occurred, and the risk of adverse consequences.

(B) Certain operations, especially those involving the vascular system (abdominal aortic aneurysmectomy, coronary artery bypass graft), necessitate postoperative ICU monitoring. Some patients require monitoring after extensive operations (pelvic exenteration), when blood loss has been excessive, or when major postoperative fluid shifts are anticipated.

(C) Basic monitoring is also based on severity and prognostic indices. These indices evaluate perfusion and basic physiologic functions. Central venous pressure monitoring and placement of a Foley catheter may not be necessary in all patients.

(D) Remember the five Ps—pain, pulselessness, paresthesias, pallor, and poikilothermia.

(E) Basic nutritional evaluation includes measuring albumin and possibly transferrin and prealbumin. Nitrogen losses are evaluated by the urinary urea nitrogen.

(F) Minimal vascular monitoring can be done by determining the ankle brachial index. Additionally, portable segmental limb pressures and pulse volume recordings can be obtained.

(G) Indications for total parenteral nutrition are numerous. Oxygen consumption, CO_2 production, caloric needs, and respiratory quotient are easily evaluated using the metabolic cart.

(H) Either repeat diagnostic peritoneal lavage or computed tomography scanning may be used in traumatized patients who remain unstable despite previous negative examinations. The computed tomography scan is superior to evaluate retroperitoneal blood and to exclude spleen and liver trauma.

(I) Questions of vessel patency and flow, especially in the carotid artery, can be answered noninvasively by portable duplex scanning.

(J) When gastrointestinal bleeding is considered to be the cause of blood loss, angiography or red blood cell scanning can sometimes localize a site of bleeding. Angiography has the advantage of facilitating the selective infusion of vasopressin to control the bleeding.

(K) A Swan-Ganz catheter is used in patients who have continued volume problems or left-sided heart failure. It helps when the central venous pressure is not reliable for assessing cardiac function.

(L) Calculating pulmonary artery wedge pressure and left ventricular stroke work index and constructing a Starling curve can be useful in managing complex patients.

REFERENCES

Cerra FB, ed. Manual of critical care. St. Louis: CV Mosby, 1987.

Chernow B, ed. The pharmacologic approach to the critically ill patient. Baltimore: Williams & Wilkins, 1983.

Hiatt JR, Harrier HD, Koening BV, et al. Nonoperative management of major blunt liver injury with hemoperitoneum. Arch Surg 1990;125:101–103.

Longo WE, Baker CC, McMillen MA, et al. Nonoperative management of adult blunt splenic trauma. Ann Surg 1989;210:626–629.

Mackersie RC, Tivary AD, Shackford SR, et al. Intra-abdominal injury following blunt trauma. Arch Surg 1989;124:809–813.

Shaw JHF, Wolfe RR. Metabolic intervention in surgical patients. Ann Surg 1988;207:274–282.

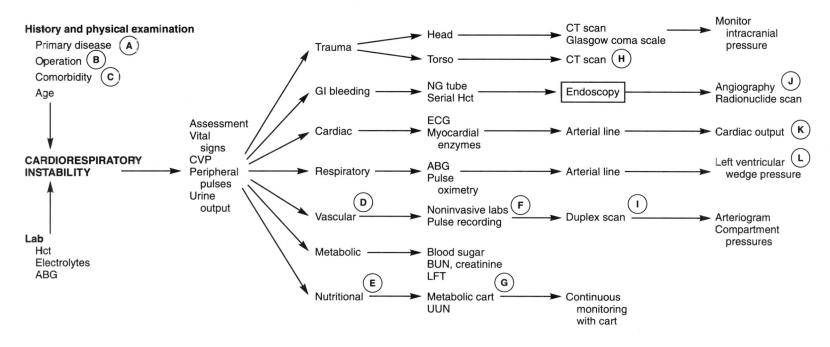

History and physical examination
- Primary disease (A)
- Operation (B)
- Comorbidity (C)
- Age

CARDIORESPIRATORY INSTABILITY

Lab
- Hct
- Electrolytes
- ABG

Assessment
Vital
signs
CVP
Peripheral
pulses
Urine
output

Trauma
- Head → CT scan / Glasgow coma scale → Monitor intracranial pressure
- Torso → CT scan (H)

GI bleeding → NG tube / Serial Hct → Endoscopy → Angiography (J) / Radionuclide scan

Cardiac → ECG / Myocardial enzymes → Arterial line → Cardiac output (K)

Respiratory → ABG / Pulse oximetry → Arterial line → Left ventricular (L) wedge pressure

Vascular (D) → Noninvasive labs (F) / Pulse recording → Duplex scan (I) → Arteriogram / Compartment pressures

Metabolic → Blood sugar / BUN, creatinine / LFT

Nutritional (E) → Metabolic cart (G) / UUN → Continuous monitoring with cart

Cardiopulmonary Resuscitation

Steven R. Lowenstein, M.D., M.P.H., and Jean T. Abbott, M.D.

(A) Verify unresponsiveness by gently shaking or shouting at the patient.

(B) Cardiopulmonary resuscitation (CPR) provides less than 25 percent of prearrest cerebral blood flow and almost no flow to the myocardium. Rapid conversion of a treatable rhythm disturbance therefore is the first priority. Quick-look paddles should be applied at once. Ventricular fibrillation (VF) or pulseless ventricular tachycardia (VT) should be identified and electric defibrillation performed without delay. VF and VT are the most treatable of all the arrest rhythms, but the success of treatment falls 4 percent with every minute of delay. Defibrillation should be attempted *before* airway opening, chest compressions, or intravenous therapy.

(C) To relieve obstruction, displace the mandible (and the attached tongue and epiglottis) anteriorly, using head-tilt and chin-lift. Head-tilt should not be used in trauma patients; jaw-thrust is recommended. Suction the oropharynx, use a finger sweep to remove vomitus and debris, and insert a plastic oral airway.

(D) If breathing is absent or inadequate, administer mouth-to-mouth or mouth-to-pocket mask ventilation. The bag-valve-mask also provides excellent tidal volumes but only if the rescuer is skilled in its use.

(E) Start chest compressions if the patient is pulseless (carotid). Place the heel of one hand on top of the other on the lower half of the sternum. Compress forcefully at a rate of 80 to 100 compressions per minute. Each thrust should depress the sternum 1.5 to 2 inches. Release the sternum completely between compressions.

(F) In patients with rhythms other than VF or VT, and in VF/VT patients in whom initial defibrillation fails, perform tracheal intubation rapidly. Intubation protects the airway from aspiration and provides the most effective ventilation and oxygen delivery. Use orotracheal intubation in apneic patients and nasotracheal intubation in dyspneic, breathing patients. Emergent cricothyrotomy may be necessary for severe craniofacial trauma, foreign body aspiration, anaphylaxis, or epiglottitis. Venous access is critical. Central venous cannulation (internal jugular or subclavian) optimizes drug delivery. In the absence of venous access, the endotracheal tube provides a route to administer epinephrine, atropine, or lidocaine. Fluids and drugs can be administered via the intraosseous route in children.

(G) Electromechanical dissociation (EMD) is characterized by electrocardiographic evidence of electrical activity (QRS complexes) in the absence of effective myocardial contractions. Intraarterial monitoring and echocardiograms often demonstrate cardiac activity, especially when the QRS complex is relatively narrow (a favorable prognostic sign).

(H) In a hospital setting, asystole can result from a hypervagal response to drugs, anesthetics, or invasive procedures.

(I) VF and pulseless VT are treated using electric defibrillation.

(J) Reversible causes and treatments of EMD are hypovolemia (crystalloid infusion), severe acidemia (ventilation and bicarbonate administration), pneumothorax (tube thoracostomy), hyperkalemia (calcium chloride and sodium bicarbonate), cardiac tamponade (pericardiocentesis or thoracotomy), and anaphylaxis (volume infusion and epinephrine).

(K) Asystole artifact must be ruled out by checking cable connections and monitor leads. The monitor leads are rotated to exclude fine VF or "null-plane" VF, which, rarely, may resemble the flat line of asystole in a single lead.

(L) The initial defibrillation dose of 200 watt-seconds maximizes successful defibrillation and minimizes myocardial damage and the development of postcountershock pulseless bradyarrhythmias. The five Ps guide defibrillation technique: use firm paddle *pressure* (approximately 25 lb of force per paddle); use a conducting *paste* or gel; employ the proper paddle *position* (one paddle just beneath the left nipple and the other beneath the right clavicle to the right of the sternum); deliver the shock in the expiratory *phase* of the ventilatory cycle (to minimize resistance caused by air in the lungs); and deliver three consecutive countershock *pulses* (successive electric currents lower skin resistance). Between countershocks pause only long enough to check for return of a spontaneous rhythm.

(M) If defibrillation is successful, administer an antiarrhythmic drug (lidocaine, 1 mg/kg bolus, then 2 to 4 mg/min) to prevent refibrillation. Refibrillation is especially likely in the presence of ischemia, infarction, electrolyte abnormalities (hypokalemia or hypomagnesemia), and other factors that cause ventricular ectopy and temporal dispersion (heterogeneity) of conduction velocities and refractory periods.

(N) Epinephrine (1 to 5 mg intravenously [1:10,000] q 5 min during arrest) should be used in all cases of asystole. Then administer atropine (1 mg intravenously and repeat once 5 minutes later). Patients who have hypervagotonia due to acidemia, oropharyngeal manipulation, inferoposterior myocardial infarction, drugs, anesthetics, or procedures may respond to atropine. Transcutaneous or intravenous pacing can be applied in the asystolic patient. Although electric capture is sometimes seen, pulses are generated

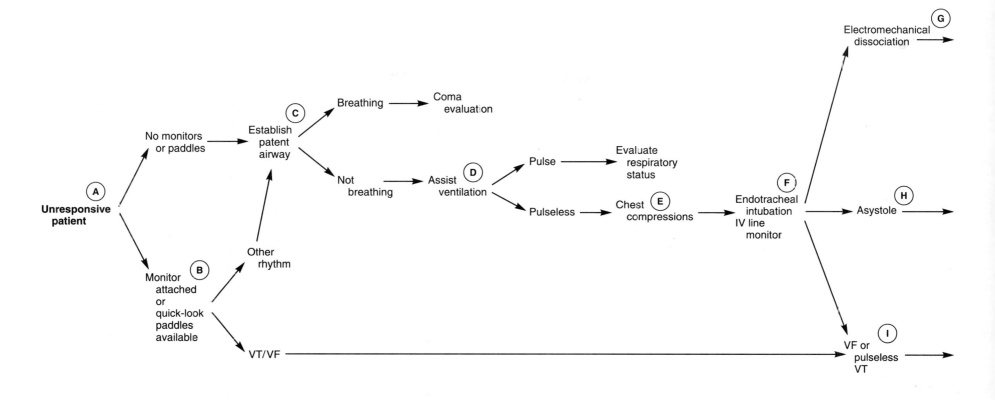

Cardiopulmonary Resuscitation (Continued)

only rarely. Success rates are negligible, except in patients who develop asystole immediately after cardioversion and in selected patients who develop severe heart block or bradyarrhythmias in the setting of acute myocardial infarction or conduction system disease.

(O) Calcium is generally ineffective in patients with EMD, asystole, or VF. Intracellular calcium concentrations may reach toxic levels during arrest and reperfusion. Calcium overload may contribute to reperfusion cellular injury. Calcium may be beneficial, however, to some patients with EMD—those with a wide QRS complex, a prolonged resuscitation effort, hypocalcemia, or hyperkalemia.

(P) If the initial three countershocks fail, begin CPR, administer oxygen, perform endotracheal intubation, and start an intravenous line.

(Q) The α-adrenergic (pressor) properties of epinephrine augment aortic diastolic blood pressure and increase the coronary perfusion pressure. The standard dose of epinephrine is 1 mg repeated every 5 minutes. Higher doses (up to 0.2 mg/kg every 5 minutes) may be needed. After the admin-

istration of epinephrine, countershocks at maximum energy levels should be repeated.

(R) Lidocaine is the first-line antiarrhythmic drug for incessant VF or VT. An initial dose of 1 mg/kg should be administered, followed by repeat boluses of 0.5 mg/kg every 5 minutes to a total dose of 3 mg/kg. For refractory VT use procainamide as the second drug after lidocaine.

(S) Bretylium tosylate may be added (7 to 10 mg/kg) if VF persists.

(T) Magnesium sulfate (4 to 8 g) should be considered for all patients with refractory VF, especially those with acute myocardial ischemia or infarction and those receiving digitalis or diuretics. β-Adrenergic blocking drugs and amiodarone may also be useful for treating patients with refractory VF or VT.

(U) Severe metabolic acidosis impedes treatment of VF. Giving sodium bicarbonate has risks, mainly the generation of new carbon dioxide, which may exacerbate myocardial intracellular acidosis. Sodium bicarbonate is not needed in the first 10 to 15 minutes of cardiac arrest if adequate ventilation is maintained. If severe metabolic acidosis (pH < 7.2) develops, sodium bicarbonate (1

mEq/kg intravenously) may be considered. In general, the acidemia of cardiopulmonary arrest is managed better by aggressive alveolar ventilation than by bicarbonate.

REFERENCES

American Heart Association. Standards and guidelines for cardiopulmonary resuscitation (CPR) and emergency cardiac care (ECC). JAMA 1986;255:2905.
Charlop S, Kahlam S, Lichstein E, et al. Electromechanical dissociation: diagnosis, pathophysiology, and management. Am Heart J 1989;118:355–360.
Lowenstein SR. Cardiopulmonary resuscitation in non-injured patients. In: Wilmore DW, Brennan MF, Harken AH, Holcroft JW, Meakins JL, eds. Care of the surgical patient. Volume 2. New York: Scientific American, 1990;1–24.
Paradis NA, Martin GB, Rivers EP, et al. Coronary perfusion pressure and the return of spontaneous circulation in human cardiopulmonary resuscitation. JAMA 1990;263:1106–1113.
Paradis NA, Martin GB, Rosenberg J, et al. The effect of standard and high-dose epinephrine on coronary perfusion pressure during prolonged cardiopulmonary resuscitation. JAMA 1991;265:1139–1144.
Stempien A, Katz AM, Messineo FC. Calcium and cardiac arrest. Ann Intern Med 1986;105:603–606.
Weil MH, Rackon EC, Trevino R, et al. Difference in acid–base state between venous and arterial blood during cardiopulmonary resuscitation. N Engl J Med 1986;315:153–156.

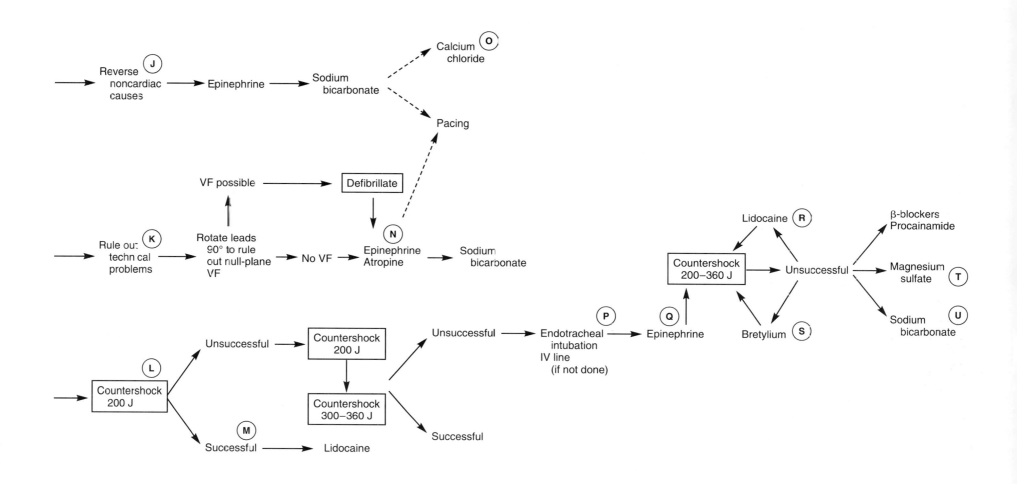

Shock

R. Armour Forse, M.D., Ph.D., Bradley C. Borlase, M.D., M.S., and Peter N. Benotti, M.D.

(A) Pneumothorax must be considered and treated early in the course of resuscitation.

(B) With flat neck veins; low central venous pressure; and a history of fluid loss, blood loss, trauma, or surgery, resuscitation begins with a fluid challenge. The volume given should be based on a quick estimate of the need or 30 mL/kg of an intravascular expander such as Ringer's lactate.

(C) If neck veins are distended, central venous pressure is increased, or an arrhythmia is present, a cardiac cause must be considered.

(D) If shock persists, a pulmonary artery line (Swan-Ganz catheter) should be inserted.

(E) Treatment of arrhythmia is followed by consideration of a pacemaker and long-term pharmacologic support.

(F) If filling pressures are normal or low, the causes include severe hypovolemia, sepsis, severe trauma, or neurogenic shock.

(G) High filling pressures and poor cardiac function suggest several compressive causes. Mechanical causes should be considered and treated early. This may require pericardiocentesis for treatment of cardiac tamponade and pericarditis, ventilation for support of patients with pulmonary embolism, and surgery for some cardiac problems. Therapy for the failing heart is to off-load the intravascular space by diuresis. Subsequent therapy is more specific for the pattern of cardiac failure. During resuscitation, constant monitoring of the level of oxygenation and acid–base balance must be carried out. The use of nitrates for vasodilation is based on the combined cardiac assessment.

(H) If the systemic vascular resistance (SVR) is high and the cardiac output (CO) is low, the patient is hypovolemic and needs volume expansion with attention to acidosis. Be prepared for continued fluid needs with ongoing third-space losses. Treat the cause of blood or fluid loss.

(I) With low SVR, the diagnostic possibilities are either sepsis or neurogenic shock. Primary treatment is to remove the cause of shock, provide fluids (balanced crystalloids), and optimize electrolytes and acid–base balance. Renal dose dopamine often helps to preserve renal function. If CO is very low, use dobutamine, 5 μg/kg/min. Alpha agents should be used to provide vasoconstriction only after failure of previous therapy. Start vasoconstrictive therapy using phenylephrine, 100 μg, to increase resistance, or use norepinephrine starting at 0.01 μg/kg/min. Monitor organ function and peripheral circulation closely.

(J) Diuresis can begin with furosemide, 40 mg, and increase as the patient improves. CO and pulmonary wedge pressure should be monitored. An inotrope can be added.

(K) If shock persists SVR should be reduced. If the heart rate is slow, it should be increased by using isoproterenol, 0.2 μg/kg/min.

(L) If filling pressures (central venous pressure and pulmonary wedge pressure) are normal or low, use an afterload-reducing agent such as sodium nitroprusside, 0.5 μg/kg/min. If filling pressures are high, nitroglycerin, 25 μg/min, can be used.

REFERENCES

Forse RA, Kinney JM. General and metabolic management. In: Meakins, JL, ed. Surgical infections in critical care medicine. New York: Churchill Livingstone, 1985, pp 233–255.

Holcroft JW. Shock. In: Wilmore DW, Brennan MF, Harken AH, et al, eds. Critical care: American College of Surgeons care of the surgical patient. New York: Scientific American, 1989, pp 4-1–4-30.

Parrillo JE. Septic shock in humans: clinical evaluation, pathogenesis, and therapeutic approach. In: Shoemaker WC, Ayres H, Grenvik A, et al, eds. Textbook of critical illness. Philadelphia: WB Saunders, 1989, pp 1006–1024.

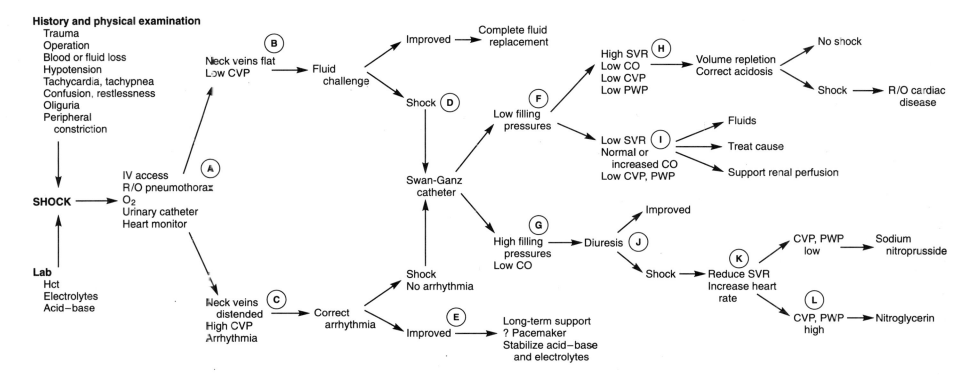

History and physical examination
Trauma
Operation
Blood or fluid loss
Hypotension
Tachycardia, tachypnea
Confusion, restlessness
Oliguria
Peripheral
    constriction

SHOCK

Lab
Hct
Electrolytes
Acid–base

IV access
R/O pneumothorax
O₂
Urinary catheter
Heart monitor

(A)

(B) Neck veins flat
Low CVP → Fluid challenge → Improved → Complete fluid replacement

Shock (D)

(C) Neck veins distended
High CVP
Arrhythmia → Correct arrhythmia → Shock No arrhythmia

Improved (E) → Long-term support
? Pacemaker
Stabilize acid–base
and electrolytes

Swan-Ganz catheter

Low filling pressures (F)

High filling pressures
Low CO (G)

High SVR (H)
Low CO
Low CVP
Low PWP → Volume repletion
Correct acidosis → No shock

Shock → R/O cardiac disease

Low SVR (I)
Normal or increased CO
Low CVP, PWP → Fluids
→ Treat cause
→ Support renal perfusion

Diuresis (J) → Improved

Shock → Reduce SVR
Increase heart rate (K) → CVP, PWP low → Sodium nitroprusside

(L) CVP, PWP high → Nitroglycerin

Bleeding Disorders

James J. Corrigan, Jr., M.D.

(A) Coagulation and platelet screening tests are indicated when there is a history of easy bruising, recurrent mucous membrane bleeding, or bleeding after trauma, biopsies, or previous surgery; a systemic disease known to be associated with a bleeding disorder; or physical signs of bleeding (eg, petechiae, ecchymoses, hematomas). Routine screening tests include the prothrombin time (PT), activated partial thromboplastin time (APTT), platelet count, and bleeding time. The PT evaluates the extrinsic coagulation system (fibrinogen and factors II, V, VII, and X); the APTT tests the intrinsic coagulation system (fibrinogen and factors II, V, VII, IX, XI, and XII). Neither test measures factor XIII activity. Factor XIII is tested by a clot stability technique. The bleeding time measures overall platelet function but is abnormal in thrombocytopenic states.

(B) When the platelet count is below 50,000/μL, abnormal bleeding occurs. Qualitative platelet disorders can be detected by prolonged bleeding time, usually in conjunction with a normal platelet count, and can be further categorized by studies of platelet function (adhesion, aggregation, release, and clot retraction). Abnormal function is most commonly acquired as a result of drugs, immune complexes, and uremia. Drugs involved are those that inhibit the platelet prostaglandin mechanism, such as salicylates and nonsteroidal antiinflammatory agents (eg, indomethacin, phenylbutazone, sulfinpyrazone, and ibuprofen). The duration of the effect is variable and, with aspirin, can last 7 to 10 days. Studies suggest that patients with thrombotic thrombocytopenic purpura respond better to ex-change transfusion, plasma transfusion, or plasma exchange than to steroids and splenectomy. For unknown reasons some patients with qualitative platelet defects (eg, uremia, congenital defects) respond to cryoprecipitate infusions and may not need platelet transfusions.

(C) The presence of a prolonged APTT with normal PT, platelet count, and bleeding time suggests either hemophilia or heparin anticoagulation (or contamination if the sample was obtained from a heparin-containing line). Mixing patient plasma with normal plasma corrects the abnormal APTT in hemophilia, but the APTT of the mixture remains prolonged in the presence of heparin. Specific factor assay is necessary in hemophilia to ascertain the type and severity of the defect. Von Willebrand disease differs from hemophilia A (factor VIII deficiency) in that it is transmitted as an autosomal dominant trait (hemophilia A is X-linked recessive). Prolonged bleeding time is associated with von Willebrand disease.

(D) Vitamin K deficiency is a common cause of acquired coagulopathy in surgical patients. Patients at risk are those receiving antibiotics who have altered intestinal function and are not receiving vitamin K in their diet or in hyperalimentation fluids. Coumarin drugs also produce a vitamin K deficiency state.

(E) In advanced liver disease hepatic synthesis of most of the coagulation factors is reduced. Factor VIII is the exception. These patients do not respond to vitamin K. They may have a mild hyperfibrinolytic state and thrombocytopenia, especially those with splenomegaly secondary to portal hypertension.

(F) Multiple rapid transfusions (over 10 units in 12 hours) cause washout of unstable clotting factors (V, VIII) and platelets. Bank blood, unless freshly drawn, is deficient in these substances. To prevent this coagulopathy, 1 unit of fresh frozen plasma should be administered with every 5 units of bank blood, and units of platelet concentrate given as necessary to maintain counts above 50,000/μL.

(G) A consumption coagulopathy due to disseminated intravascular coagulation can be seen in septic shock, other types of shock, tissue necrosis, massive large-vessel thrombosis, and severe allergic reactions. Consumed in the process are certain clotting factors (especially fibrinogen and factors V and VIII) and platelets. The fibrinolytic mechanism is activated, which removes the fibrin and produces fibrin split products. Fibrin split products can form complexes with fibrinogen and fibrin monomer, giving nonclottable products called soluble fibrin complexes (SFCs). SFCs can be detected by certain paracoagulation tests, such as the protamine precipitation test and the ethanol gelation test.

(H) Primary fibrinolysis is rare. It is most commonly precipitated by prostatic surgery and, occasionally, by thoracotomy and extracorporeal bypass. Epsilon aminocaproic acid (EACA) inhibits fibrinolysis, probably by directly antagonizing plasminogen activators. Used excessively, EACA can produce pathologic clotting.

History and physical examination
 Easy bruising
 Bleeding
 Systemic disease
 Petechiae
 Ecchymoses
 Hematomas

BLEEDING DIATHESIS Ⓐ

Lab
 PT
 APTT
 Platelet count
 Bleeding time
 Clot stability

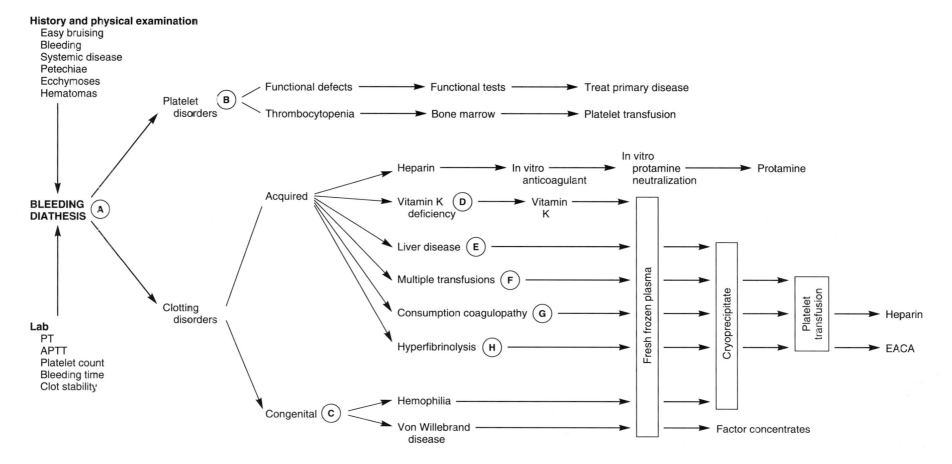

REFERENCES

Ansell JE, Kumar R, Deykin D. The spectrum of vitamin K deficiency. JAMA 1977; 238:40–42.

Feinstein DI. Diagnosis and management of disseminated intravascular coagulation: the role of heparin therapy. Blood 1982; 60:284–287.

Hilgartner MW, Pochedly C. Hemophilia in the child and adult. 3rd Ed. New York: Raven Press, 1989.

Huestis DW, Bove JR, Case J. Practical blood transfusion. 4th Ed. Boston: Little, Brown & Co, 1988.

Janson PA, Jubelirer SJ, Weinstein MJ, et al. Treatment of the bleeding tendency in uremia with cryoprecipitate. N Engl J Med 1980; 303:1318–1322.

Murray DJ, Olson J, Strauss R, et al. Coagulation changes during packed red cell replacement of major blood loss. Anesthesiology 1988; 69:839–845.

Roberts HR, Cederbaum AI. The liver and blood coagulation: physiology and pathology. Gastroenterology 1972; 63:297–320.

Suchman AL, Griner PF. Diagnostic use of the activated partial thromboplastin time and prothrombin time. Ann Intern Med 1986; 104:810–816.

Williams CE, Short PE, George AJ, et al. Critical factors in haemostasis: evaluation and development. Chichester, England, Ellis Horwood Ltd., 1988.

Transfusion

Walter H. Dzik, M.D.

A Blood components include fresh frozen plasma, platelet concentrates, cryoprecipitate, and specialized blood derivatives such as factor VIII:C concentrates. Each "unit" of a blood component carries roughly the same risk for transfusion complications as a unit of packed red cells. Beware of inappropriate use of blood components to prevent bleeding in patients with abnormal laboratory coagulation values or in patients about to undergo bedside procedures. The risk of bleeding in these instances does not correlate well with the results of the prothrombin time, activated partial thromboplastin time, bleeding time, and so on. Decide whether the bleeding is local or generalized. The common error is to transfuse blood components to a patient who has mildly abnormal coagulation results and who is having local bleeding (eg, central line site, duodenal ulcer) in the mistaken belief that the bleeding is due to coagulopathy. Local bleeding is best treated with local measures (stitch on central line site, endoscopic or surgical treatment of ulcer).

B Oxygen supply to tissues depends on perfusion, oxygen content of the blood (hemoglobin mass × % saturation), and oxygen extraction by tissues. Bleeding patients must first receive volume resuscitation with crystalloid or colloid volume expanders to reestablish perfusion. Because of increased oxygen extraction, most tissues that are adequately perfused do not become ischemic even in the presence of severe anemia (Hgb = 7 g/dL).

C The four elements of normal hemostasis are vascular integrity, platelet plugging, coagulation and fibrin formation, and natural fibrinolysis of formed clot. Local vascular disruption remains the most common cause of bleeding. Platelet plugging is essential for the immediate hemostasis seen during surgery. Disorders of coagulation are common in hospitalized patients.

D The degree of oxygen consumption should be considered before transfusions are given to stable patients with a low hematocrit. Patients on bed rest who are not febrile, who do not have congestive heart failure, and who are not hypermetabolic have low oxygen requirements and therefore can tolerate anemia in the range of 7 g/dL. Since the cardiac bed has the highest O_2 extraction, a history of angina should be sought in patients with anemia. Other characteristics of symptomatic anemia are headache, dizziness, and breathlessness. Physical examination reveals pallor (not cyanosis) and tachycardia. Important laboratory data include the arterial and mixed venous oxygen saturation and the cardiac output, in addition to the hematocrit. Bleeding patients who suddenly lower their red cell mass compensate by increasing cardiac output and oxygen extraction, resulting in a lower venous oxygen saturation. Patients with normal or elevated mixed venous oxygen saturations (> 75 percent) are unlikely to profit from additional red cells unless there is isolated critical underperfusion of a selected organ bed (eg, coronary stenosis). Assess a patient, not a hematocrit!

E Platelet hemostasis depends on both function and number. Although the bleeding time may be prolonged in patients with known platelet defects, the test has poor sensitivity and specificity and is a poor preoperative predictor of surgical hemostasis. Decreased platelet function resulting from drugs (especially aspirin-containing compounds and antibiotics), uremia, cardiopulmonary bypass, and liver disease is common in sick, hospitalized patients. Stopping the offending drug and treating the underlying cause is the first step in therapy. Platelet transfusion does not correct the platelet defect in uremia. Desmopressin acetate (DDAVP) has been shown to be an effective adjunct in most syndromes of platelet dysfunction and improves hemostasis by causing release of endogenous stores of von Willebrand factor, thus promoting increased platelet adhesion. Decreased platelet numbers result from decreased production, increased destruction, or both. The best test to evaluate this differential is the bone marrow examination. Known platelet destructive syndromes are often clear from the history and physical examination, and include splenomegaly, immune thrombocytopenic purpura (ITP), disseminated intravascular coagulopathy, and drug effects. Heparin-associated thrombocytopenia is a serious platelet destruction syndrome that often causes arterial thrombosis rather than bleeding. In the absence of platelet destruction, the platelet count in a normal-sized adult should increase by 5000 to 10,000 platelets/μL for each unit transfused.

F Mild prolongations of the prothrombin/activated partial thromboplastin time (over 1.5 times normal) are unlikely to reflect abnormalities that cause bleeding. If prolongation of the prothrombin time is out of proportion to the activated partial thromboplastin time, suspect vitamin K deficiency or liver disease. Vitamin K deficiency, exacerbated by poor nutrition and antibiotics, is the most common coagulation defect among hospitalized patients and should be treated with parenteral vitamin K rather than blood products. Prolongation of the activated partial thromboplastin time out of proportion to the prothrombin time raises the possibility of von Willebrand disease, residual heparin, a lupus-like anticoagulant, or a factor deficiency. This differential can be generally resolved rapidly by repeating the test after mixing in vitro equal parts of the patient's plasma and normal plasma. Desmopressin acetate is useful in mild von Willebrand disease and has a rapid onset of action. Protamine neutralizes residual heparin. Fresh frozen plasma may be most useful in the setting of multifactor deficiency of liver disease, but

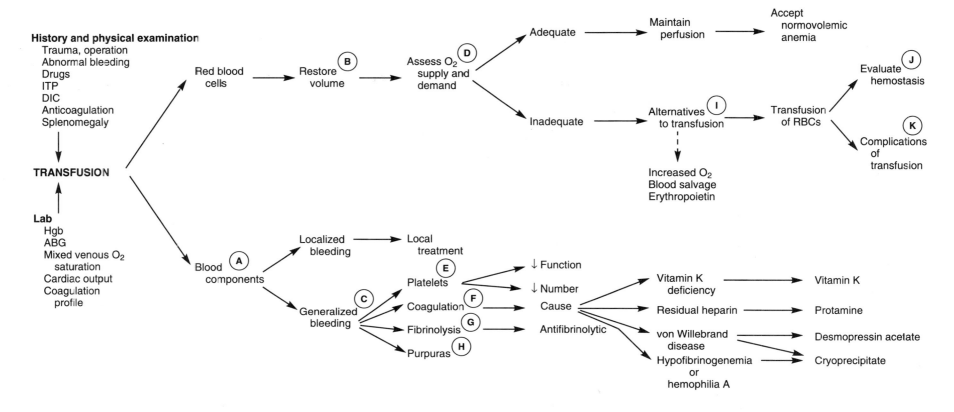

History and physical examination
Trauma, operation
Abnormal bleeding
Drugs
ITP
DIC
Anticoagulation
Splenomegaly

TRANSFUSION

Lab
Hgb
ABG
Mixed venous O₂
    saturation
Cardiac output
Coagulation
    profile

Red blood cells → Restore volume (B) → Assess O₂ supply and demand (D) → Adequate → Maintain perfusion → Accept normovolemic anemia

Assess O₂ supply and demand → Inadequate → Alternatives to transfusion (I) → Transfusion of RBCs → Evaluate hemostasis (J)
Transfusion of RBCs → Complications of transfusion (K)
Alternatives to transfusion ⤍ Increased O₂ / Blood salvage / Erythropoietin

Blood components (A) → Localized bleeding → Local treatment
Blood components → Generalized bleeding (C)
Generalized bleeding → Platelets (E) → ↓ Function / ↓ Number
Generalized bleeding → Coagulation (F) → Cause
Generalized bleeding → Fibrinolysis (G) → Antifibrinolytic
Generalized bleeding → Purpuras (H)

Cause → Vitamin K deficiency → Vitamin K
Cause → Residual heparin → Protamine
Cause → von Willebrand disease → Desmopressin acetate
Cause → Hypofibrinogenemia or hemophilia A → Cryoprecipitate / Desmopressin acetate

---

treatment should be guided chiefly by bleeding, not laboratory valves. Cryoprecipitate is not a concentrate of all plasma coagulation factors. Cryoprecipitate is rich in fibrinogen and factor VIII and should be reserved for patients with bleeding who have severe hypofibrinogenemia (< 100 mg/dL) or for patients with hemophilia A or severe von Willebrand disease.

(G) Pure fibrinolytic syndromes are rare. Patients with hepatic cirrhosis exhibit chronic low-grade fibrinolysis and have decreased defenses against sudden increases in blood fibrinolytic activity. Inhibitors of fibrinolysis, such as ε-amino caproic acid (Amicar), may be more valuable in some patients than transfusion of blood components.

(H) Some conditions result in excessive bleeding in the face of normal blood coagulation. Examples include systemic amyloidosis, angiodys-

plasia, and the hemorrhagic purpuras such as cryoglobulinemia, myeloma, and vasculitis.

(I) Immediate alternatives to transfusion of red cells include increasing O₂ supply (supplemental oxygen) if the arterial O₂ saturation is low and decreasing oxygen demand. Blood salvage techniques are useful adjuncts to blood transfusion in bleeding patients. For stable patients with renal failure, anemia should be treated with recombinant erythropoietin rather than red cell transfusions.

(J) Bleeding patients may have coexisting coagulopathies or may develop coagulopathies during resuscitation. Patients actively bleeding whose resuscitation required more than one blood volume are likely to require blood components for coagulation in addition to red cell transfusions.

(K) Despite the increasing safety of blood products, transfusions still carry the risk of numer-

ous complications, some of which are fatal. Each additional unit transfused carries an independent risk of complication. Well-known complications of transfusion include

Febrile nonhemolytic reaction:	1 in 100
Alloantibody sensitization:	1 in 100
Hepatitis C virus:	1 in 1000
Delayed hemolytic reaction:	1 in 1000
Hepatitis B virus:	1 in 10,000
HIV-1 virus:	1 in 100,000
Fatal ABO hemolysis:	1 in 100,000

Of the numerous complications that may accompany massive transfusion, metabolic abnormalities and coagulopathy are particularly important. Metabolic changes promoting depressed left ventricular function include hypothermia from refrigerated blood products, citrate toxicity, lactic acidosis from underperfusion, and hyperkalemia from tissue is-

Transfusion (Continued)

chemia and acidemia. Hemostasis abnormalities include dilutional coagulopathy, disseminated intravascular coagulopathy, shock liver and platelet dysfunction.

REFERENCES

Channing RP, Rodgers MD, Levin J. A critical reappraisal of the bleeding time. Semin Thromb Hemost 1990; 16:1–20

Dzik WH. Massive transfusion. In: Churchill H, Kurtz S, eds. Clinical blood transfusion. Oxford: Blackwell Scientific Publications, 1988.

Eschbach JW, Egrie JC, Downing MR, et al. Correction of the anemia of end-stage renal disease with recombinant human erythropoietin: results of a combined phase I and phase II trial. N Engl J Med 1987; 316:773–783.

Ewe K. Bleeding after liver biopsy does not correlate with indices of peripheral coagulation. Dig Dis Sci 1981; 36:388–393.

Gould SA, Rice CL, Moss GS. The physiologic basis for the use of blood and blood products. Surg Annu 1984; 16:13–21.

National Blood Resource Education Program. The use of autologous blood. JAMA 1990; 263:414–417.

NIH Consensus Conference. FFP: indications and risks. JAMA 1985; 253:551–553.

NIH Consensus Conference. Perioperative red cell transfusion. JAMA 1988; 260:2700–2703.

NIH Consensus Conference. Platelet transfusion therapy. JAMA 1987; 259:1777–1780.

Stump DC, Taylor FB, Nesheim ME, et al. Pathologic fibrinolysis as a cause of clinical bleeding. Semin Thromb Hemost 1990; 16:260–273.

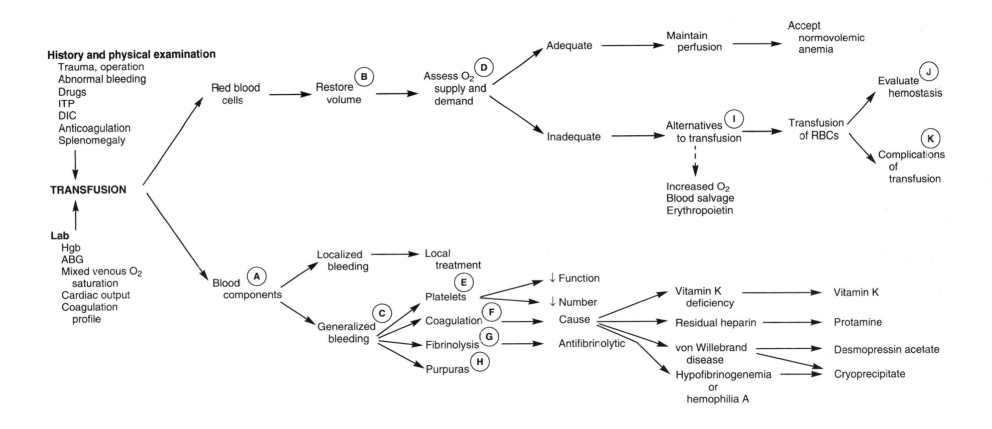

History and physical examination
  Trauma, operation
  Abnormal bleeding
  Drugs
  ITP
  DIC
  Anticoagulation
  Splenomegaly

TRANSFUSION

Lab
  Hgb
  ABG
  Mixed venous O_2
    saturation
  Cardiac output
  Coagulation
    profile

Red blood cells → Restore volume (B) → Assess O_2 supply and demand (D)

Adequate → Maintain perfusion → Accept normovolemic anemia

Inadequate → Alternatives to transfusion (I) → Transfusion of RBCs

Increased O_2
Blood salvage
Erythropoietin

Evaluate hemostasis (J)

Complications of transfusion (K)

Blood components (A)

Localized bleeding → Local treatment

Generalized bleeding (C)

Platelets (E) → ↓ Function / ↓ Number

Coagulation (F) → Cause

Fibrinolysis (G) → Antifibrinolytic

Purpuras (H)

Vitamin K deficiency → Vitamin K

Residual heparin → Protamine

von Willebrand disease → Desmopressin acetate

Hypofibrinogenemia or hemophilia A → Cryoprecipitate

Postoperative Fever

Bradley C. Borlase, M.D., M.S., Peter N. Benotti, M.D., and
R. Armour Forse, M.D., Ph.D.

(A) History and physical examination will lead to diagnosis and management in 66 to 75 percent of patients with postoperative fever. A history significant for preexisting conditions (preoperative fever, heart valve disease, foreign body), transfusion, need for central access, and type and class of operation (clean vs. contaminated) predicts the source of postoperative fever.

(B) The diagnosis of postoperative fever (> 38° C) depends on postoperative day and severity of patient illness (American Society of Anesthesiology [ASA] physical status classification; APACHE II). The most common sources of fever are extraabdominal (60 to 80 percent). Therefore, evaluation should first exclude extraabdominal disease. Intraabdominal sources are common in patients in the ICU (30 to 66 percent).

(C) Urinary tract infection (40%), wounds (25%), and pulmonary complications (15%) are frequently responsible for postoperative fever. White blood cells, blood urea nitrogen, trauma, postoperative day ($\geq$ 3), ASA class ($\geq$ III), and severity of temperature elevation ($\geq$ 38° C) are useful predictors when establishing the cause of postoperative fever.

(D) ICU patients are likely to have an intraabdominal focus for postoperative fever (50 to 60 percent if $\geq$ 39° C). Bacteremia, leukocytosis ($\geq$ 12,000), ileus, pain, mental status changes, and operative contamination suggest an intraabdominal focus.

(E) Computed tomography scanning has a 90 percent sensitivity and specificity for intraabdominal sepsis, common duct dilation, and intra- and extrahepatic masses. Ultrasound is 95 percent diagnostic of gallstones. Radionuclide scan is 90 to 95 percent sensitive in detecting cholecystitis in the postoperative patient.

REFERENCES

Borlase BC, Eiseman B. Routine laboratory tests. In: Eiseman S, ed. Cost-effective surgical management. Philadelphia: WB Saunders, 1987, pp 5–12.

Borlase BC, Simon JS, Hermann G. Abdominal surgery in patients undergoing chronic hemodialysis. Surgery 1987; 102:15–18.

Freischlasg J, Busuttil RW. The value of postoperative fever evaluation. Surgery 1983;94:358–363.

Galicier C, Richet H. A prospective study of postoperative fever in a general surgery department. Infect Control 1985;6:487–490.

Hoogewood HM, Rubli E, Terrier F, et al. The role of computerized tomography in fever, septicemia, and multiple system organ failure after laparotomy. Surg Gynecol Obstet 1986;162:539–543.

Jorgensen FS, Sorense CG, Kjergaard J. Postoperative fever after major abdominal surgery. Ann Chir Gynaecol 1988;77:47–50.

Legall JR, Fagniez PL, Meakins J, et al. Diagnostic features of early high post-laparotomy fever: a prospective study of 100 patients. Br J Surg 1982;69:452–455.

Mellors JW, Kelly JJ, Gusberg RJ, et al. A simple index to estimate the likelihood of bacterial infection in patients developing fever after abdominal surgery. Am Surg 1988;54:558–564.

History and physical examination (A)
- Preoperative fever
- Foreign body
- Heart valve
- Diabetes
- Immunosuppression
- Renal failure
- Venous access
- Transfusion
- Ear, throat, chest, abdominal, leg examination

POSTOPERATIVE FEVER (B)

Lab
- WBC and differential
- Chest x-ray
- Urinalysis
- Blood cultures

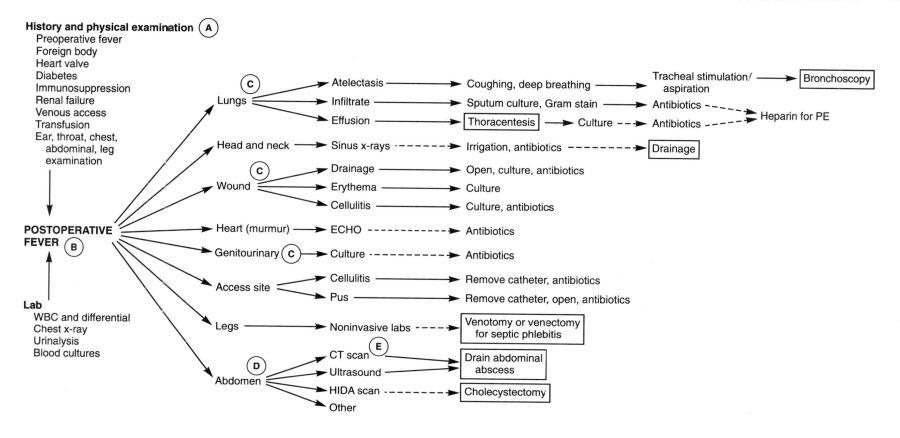

Lungs (C)
- Atelectasis → Coughing, deep breathing → Tracheal stimulation/aspiration → Bronchoscopy
- Infiltrate → Sputum culture, Gram stain → Antibiotics --→ Heparin for PE
- Effusion → Thoracentesis → Culture --→ Antibiotics --→ Heparin for PE

Head and neck → Sinus x-rays -----→ Irrigation, antibiotics -----→ Drainage

Wound (C)
- Drainage → Open, culture, antibiotics
- Erythema → Culture
- Cellulitis → Culture, antibiotics

Heart (murmur) → ECHO -----→ Antibiotics

Genitourinary (C) → Culture -----→ Antibiotics

Access site
- Cellulitis → Remove catheter, antibiotics
- Pus → Remove catheter, open, antibiotics

Legs → Noninvasive labs --→ Venotomy or venectomy for septic phlebitis

Abdomen (D)
- CT scan (E) → Drain abdominal abscess
- Ultrasound → Drain abdominal abscess
- HIDA scan -----→ Cholecystectomy
- Other

Nutritional Support

Todd N. Jones, R.N., M.S., and Frederick A. Moore, M.D.

(A) Patients who are either malnourished or at risk for developing malnutrition because they are unable to ingest or absorb nutrients require nutritional assessment. This includes a medical history (eg, weight loss, anorexia, chronic disease) and a physical examination to assess lean body mass and subcutaneous fat stores.

(B) Laboratory measurements include visceral protein markers, lymphocyte count, and urinary nitrogen output. The degree of malnutrition can be classified by the following measurements:

	Mild	Moderate	Severe
Albumin	2.8–3.2	2.5–2.8	<2.5
Transferrin	180–200	150–180	<150
Total lymphocyte count	1500–1800	1000–1500	<1000
Urinary N_2 output	8–10 g	10–12 g	>12 g

(C) Preoperative nutritional repletion of high-risk surgical patients is an attractive concept, but prospective randomized trials show that only severely malnourished patients benefit from this expensive therapy. Mildly to moderately malnourished patients should begin nutritional support once postoperative resuscitation is complete. Well-nourished patients who undergo major surgery or sustain significant trauma or burns may benefit from early (within 48 hours) postoperative nutrition.

(D) When the oral route is unavailable for nutritional support, the enteral route is preferred because it is cheaper and safer. It also offers physiologic benefits. Substrates are better utilized, gut muscosal integrity is maintained, and immunologic competence is enhanced. Combining enteral and parenteral feeding in patients with excessive metabolic demands (eg, burns) or mild gastrointestinal intolerance is gaining acceptance.

(E) Total parenteral nutrition (TPN) tends to be more convenient in critically ill patients. In terminally ill patients with no therapeutic options, TPN may be considered futile.

(F) The stomach is accessed by blind nasal intubation. Jejunal access may require endoscopic or radiologic guidance. Displacement of a nasoenteric tube into the stomach can cause serious pulmonary aspiration. The optimum tube should be 8 to 12 French, have a weighted tip, be radiopaque, and be large enough to aspirate gastrointestinal contents. After gastric feedings, residuals should be measured initially every 4 hours, then every 8 hours. An acceptable residual volume is less than twice the hourly rate of feeding. Bolus feeding is reserved for patients with an established gag reflex and proven tolerance to continuous, full-dose infusion.

(G) Percutaneous endoscopic gastrostomy, with or without jejunal tube, is a safe, cost-effective, and time-saving alternative to traditional operative gastrostomy.

(H) Despite a gastric ileus (1 to 2 days) and impaired colon peristalsis (3 to 5 days), small bowel motility and absorption remain intact after laparotomy. Enteral feeding through needle-catheter jejunostomy can begin within 12 hours of operation. Full nutritional support is possible in over 85 percent of patients.

(I) Peripheral parenteral nutrition is used when a central venous catheter is contraindicated or as a short-term therapy pending either oral or enteral diet. A combination of oral and enteral nutrition and peripheral parenteral nutrition can provide full nutritional support when central TPN is unavailable.

(J) Patients requiring parenteral nutritional support for more than 7 days should receive central TPN. A subclavian line is reserved exclusively for TPN infusion. The TPN solution is mixed as a 3-in-1 admixture (ie, amino acids, dextrose, and fat) to be infused over 24 hours. Alternatively, the solution, with or without lipids, can be prepared for 8- to 12-hour infusion.

(K) Isotonic diets are polymeric formulas designed for use in patients with complete digestive ability. Typically they are used for gastric feedings.

(L) Diets with added fiber improve diarrhea by decreasing transit time and adding bulk. They are useful in chronically tube-fed patients who have altered bowel habits.

(M) Stress formulas are designed for hypermetabolic, catabolic patients. The protein source is generally simple amino acids. Nonprotein calories are provided as 70 to 75 percent carbohydrates and 25 to 30 percent fat. The nonprotein calorie-to-nitrogen ratios tend to be low (100:1). Stress formulas are enhanced with branched-chain amino acids and medium-chain triglycerides.

(N) This new class of enteral formulas are supplemented with glutamine, arginine, omega 3 (ω3) fatty acids, and nucleic acids. Glutamine maintains gut mucosal integrity. The other nutrients are directed at modulating monocyte and lymphocyte function to reverse postoperative immunosuppression.

(O) Elemental formulas contain simple amino acids or dipeptides (as protein source), glucose or dextrin (as source of nonprotein calories), and small amounts of fat (for essential fatty acid requirements). These are easily absorbed and minimize pancreatobiliary secretion. Low viscosity prevents clogging of small-bore feeding tubes. High osmolarity can cause gastrointestinal intolerance. Elemental diets are generally the most expensive enteral formulas.

(P) Standard peripheral parenteral solutions have an osmolarity of less than 800 mOsm/L to minimize phlebitis. The amino acid concentration should not exceed 4.25 percent, and the dextrose concentration ranges from 5 to 11 percent. Lipids are concurrently administered as an important

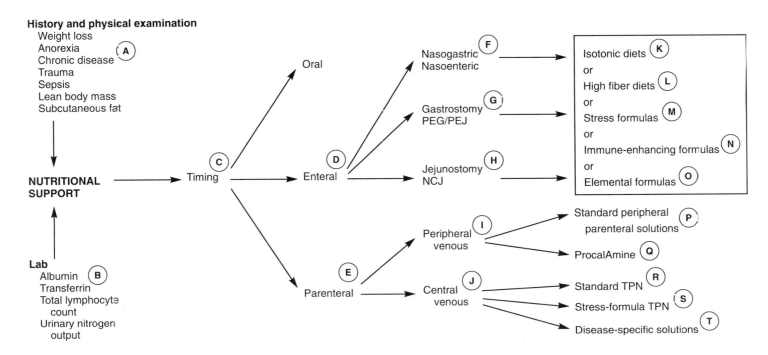

History and physical examination
Weight loss
Anorexia
Chronic disease (A)
Trauma
Sepsis
Lean body mass
Subcutaneous fat

NUTRITIONAL SUPPORT

Lab (B)
Albumin
Transferrin
Total lymphocyte count
Urinary nitrogen output

Timing (C)

Oral

Enteral (D)

Parenteral (E)

Nasogastric Nasoenteric (F)

Gastrostomy PEG/PEJ (G)

Jejunostomy NCJ (H)

Peripheral venous (I)

Central venous (J)

Isotonic diets (K)
or
High fiber diets (L)
or
Stress formulas (M)
or
Immune-enhancing formulas (N)
or
Elemental formulas (O)

Standard peripheral parenteral solutions (P)

ProcalAmine (Q)

Standard TPN (R)

Stress-formula TPN (S)

Disease-specific solutions (T)

source of nonprotein calories and to protect against phlebitis. Electrolytes, vitamins, minerals, and trace elements are added to complete the nutrient profile.

(Q) ProcalAmine is a premade, ready-to-use peripheral parenteral solution that uses glycerol as a caloric source. Glycerol does not require insulin to be transported into the cell and has been shown to be an effective nitrogen-sparing substrate. ProcalAmine provides 30 g protein/L and 250 calories. It is supplemented with maintenance electrolytes. The addition of lipids is recommended to increase nonprotein calories.

(R) Standard TPN formulas traditionally use dextrose for nonprotein calories. Mixed-fuel formulas (30 to 40 percent of calories as lipid) are now popular. The amino acid concentration in standard TPN solution is 40 to 50 g/L (4.0 to 5.0

percent) and the branched-chain amino acid content is 18 to 23 percent. The nonprotein calorie-to-nitrogen ratio is approximately 150:1. Each TPN formula is supplemented with electrolytes, vitamins, minerals, and trace elements.

(S) Stress-formula TPN has a lower nonprotein calorie-to-nitrogen ratio (100 to 125:1) and increased branched-chain amino acids (45 percent). Approximately 25 percent of calories are given as lipid (0.5 to 1.0 g/kg) and the rest as dextrose. Stress-formula TPN is recommended for hypermetabolic, catabolic patients (eg, major trauma or burns) and for septic patients with multiple organ failure.

(T) These solutions are designed to meet age- and disease-specific requirements. Hepatic-failure (high branched-chain amino acids, low aromatic amino acids), renal-failure (high essential

amino acids), and pediatric formulas are available. The efficacy of pediatric formulas is established. The hepatic-failure formula improves encephalopathy but otherwise is no better than standard amino acid therapy. Renal-failure formulas do not improve nutritional status or outcome when compared with standard amino acid solutions.

REFERENCES

Cerra F. Hypermetabolism, organ failure and metabolic support. Surgery 1987; 101:1–14.

Gilder H. Parenteral nourishment of patient undergoing surgical or traumatic stress. JPEN 1986; 10:88–99.

Hassett J, Border J. The metabolic response to trauma and sepsis. World J Surg 1983; 7:125–131.

Lemoyne M, Jeejeebhoy K. Total parenteral nutrition in the critically ill patient. Chest 1986; 89:568–575.

Moore FA, Moore EE, Jones TN, et al. TEN versus TPN following major abdominal trauma: reduced septic mortality. J Trauma 1987; 29:916–923.

AIDS and Surgery

William P. Schecter, M.D., Ash Mansour, M.D., and Robert C. Lim, M.D.

(A) Most HIV-infected people are asymptomatic. Many patients show no evidence of immune deficiency until the onset of clinical AIDS. Other patients develop generalized lymphadenopathy, oral thrush, thrombocytopenia, or weight loss before a diagnosis of AIDS.

(B) Risk factors include homosexuality, prostitution, intravenous drug use, multiple sexual partners, hemophilia, and blood transfusion received between 1978 and 1985.

(C) Infectious agents commonly associated with AIDS include cytomegalovirus, *Pneumocystis carinii* pneumonia, and other opportunistic organisms including Candida, atypical mycobacteria, and toxoplasma.

(D) Non-Hodgkin's lymphoma and Kaposi sarcoma are common neoplasms in HIV-infected patients. The presence of these neoplasms is sufficient for a diagnosis of AIDS.

(E) In the asymptomatic phase, the hemogram is usually normal. The T4 helper lymphocyte count is a useful measure of immune function. A T4 count less than 200 mm^3 indicates significant immunodeficiency.

(F) The enzyme-linked immunosorbent assay (ELISA) is a highly sensitive screening test for HIV infection. A Western blot test is used to confirm a positive enzyme-linked immunosorbent assay. The window of seronegativity after infection may be several years but is usually a matter of weeks.

(G) The lag time between HIV seroconversion and the onset of clinical AIDS can be 10 years or longer. Mean survival from the onset of AIDS has improved in recent years.

(H) If fine-needle aspiration cytology of an enlarged lymph node is negative, the patient can be observed. If it is positive for lymphoma, open biopsy may be required to determine the cell type. This information guides chemotherapy.

(I) Thrombocytopenia associated with immune deficiency rarely responds to steroids. If a patient has not yet developed clinical AIDS, response to splenectomy is usually good. Splenectomy in a patient with AIDS has a high risk of morbidity and mortality.

(J) Open lung biopsy of a pulmonary infiltrate is seldom used. *Pneumocystis carinii* pneumonia is suspected radiologically and identified by obtaining induced sputum specimens or by transbronchial biopsy.

(K) HIV-seropositive patients are a risk to surgical personnel in the operating room. The operating team and nursing staff must exercise strict body fluid precautions such as double gloving and the use of face shields, double sleeves, and water-impermeable gowns and boots. Single-glove puncture occurs in 17 percent of surgical procedures. Careful surgical technique is essential to prevent puncture or laceration.

(L) Anorectal pathology includes proctalgia, fissures, anal ulcer, proctitis, fistula, warts, and hemorrhoids. HIV-infected patients with good muscle mass tolerate anorectal surgery well. Most AIDS patients can be managed without surgery. Carefully selected AIDS patients who do not respond to medical management have benefited from limited anorectal surgery.

(M) Abdominal pain not associated with peritonitis may be due to abscess, lymphadenopathy, thickened small bowel, or lymphoma.

(N) Lesions in the liver may be either infectious (abscess or granuloma) or neoplastic. Diagnosis is made by needle biopsy and computed tomography scan. Formal laparotomy is rarely indicated for diagnosis.

(O) Medical management of *Pneumocystis carinii* pneumonia includes pentamidine and trimethoprim-sulfamethoxazole.

(P) Clinical findings at laparotomy for peritonitis might be small-bowel perforation from cytomegalovirus ulcer, small-bowel obstruction from lymphoma, or more common illnesses such as appendicitis, cholecystitis, and perforated peptic ulcer.

(Q) Medical management of toxoplasmosis is with pyrimethamine and sulfadiazine.

REFERENCES

Barone JE, Gingold BS, Nealon TF, et al. Abdominal pain in patients with acquired immune deficiency syndrome. Ann Surg 1986; 204:619–623.

Cello JP. Acquired immunodeficiency syndrome cholangiopathy: spectrum of disease. Am J Med 1989; 86:539–546.

Ferguson CM. Surgical complications of human immunodeficiency virus infection. Am Surg 1988; 54:4–9.

Potter DA, Danforth DN Jr, Macher AM, et al. Evaluation of abdominal pain in AIDS patient. Ann Surg 1984; 199:332–339.

Wilson SE, Robinson G, Williams RA, et al. Acquired immune deficiency syndrome (AIDS): indications for abdominal surgery, pathology and outcome. Ann Surg 1989; 210:428–434.

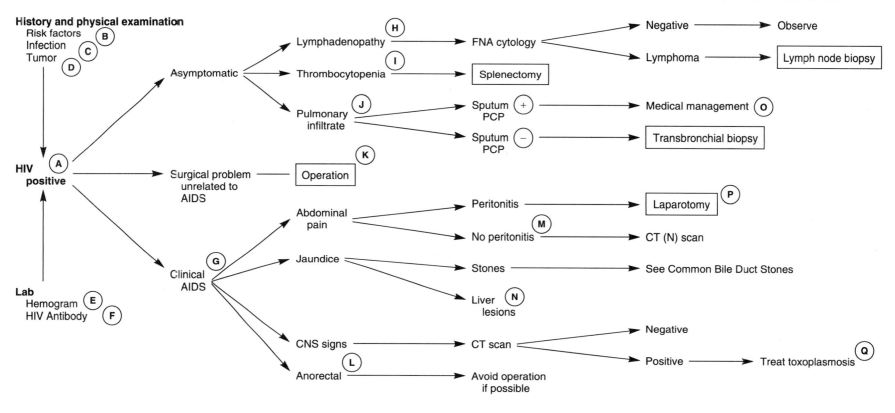

History and physical examination
Risk factors (B)
Infection (C)
Tumor (D)

HIV positive (A)

Lab
Hemogram (E)
HIV Antibody (F)

Asymptomatic
→ Lymphadenopathy (H) → FNA cytology → Negative → Observe
                                      → Lymphoma → Lymph node biopsy
→ Thrombocytopenia (I) → Splenectomy
→ Pulmonary infiltrate (J) → Sputum PCP (+) → Medical management (O)
                          → Sputum PCP (−) → Transbronchial biopsy

Surgical problem unrelated to AIDS → Operation (K)

Clinical AIDS (G)
→ Abdominal pain → Peritonitis → Laparotomy (P)
                → No peritonitis (M) → CT (N) scan
→ Jaundice → Stones → See Common Bile Duct Stones
          → Liver lesions (N)
→ CNS signs → CT scan → Negative
                      → Positive → Treat toxoplasmosis (Q)
→ Anorectal (L) → Avoid operation if possible

Hypothermia

Bruce C. Paton, M.D., F.R.C.S. (Ed.), F.R.C.P. (Ed.)

(A) Any core temperature (esophageal, high rectal, bladder, tympanic membrane) below 35°C constitutes hypothermia. Accepted classifications include mild, 35 to 32°C; moderate, 32 to 28°C; deep, 28 to 25°C; and profound, under 25°C.

(B) History includes circumstances of exposure (eg, obvious accidental exposure, old age, social circumstances). It also notes associated diseases (neurologic, cardiovascular, or endocrine), drug or alcohol intoxication, and psychiatric disorders.

(C) Hypothermia produces unconsciousness, bradycardia, and hypotension. Peripheral pulses are often impalpable. Inability to feel a pulse, obtain a blood pressure, or hear a heart beat does not equate with death in the cold patient. Unconsciousness with a core temperature higher than 32°C may be due to associated drugs or head injury and not to hypothermia. Bradycardia (even to 4 beats per minute) and atrial fibrillation are common arrhythmias when temperature falls below 30°C. Ventricular fibrillation or asystole can occur with a temperature lower than 25°C.

(D) Abnormalities of serum K^+, Na^+, and glucose are found frequently. Blood urea nitrogen and creatinine are elevated if there is renal shutdown. Acidosis is common especially during rewarming. Measurements of pH should not be corrected for temperature. A toxicant screen is essential to exclude drugs or alcohol as the cause of hypothermia.

(E) Barring head injury or drug overdose, unconsciousness in a cold patient is considered to be caused by hypothermia (temperature usually lower than 32°C). Those who arrive in the emergency room conscious should survive.

(F) Unconscious cold patients must be admitted to the ICU or operating room (if extracorporeal circulation is to be used), and treatment of both hypothermia and associated conditions must be started.

(G) Passive rewarming consists of removing wet clothing, covering with warm blankets, monitoring the electrocardiogram and temperature, and allowing endogenous metabolism to rewarm the body. This can be done in the emergency room, the ICU, or a hospital room.

(H) Arrhythmias with ineffective cardiac output may occur during rewarming. Most arrhythmias disappear with normothermia. Active rewarming is frequently necessary before ventricular defibrillation is possible. Rewarming may cause relative hypovolemia, which should be treated with volume replacement as indicated by standard criteria.

(I) Determination of heart beat can be difficult. Shivering conflicts with electrocardiogram monitoring, and pulse and blood pressure may not be palpable. An arterial cutdown is necessary to measure blood pressure.

(J) If the heart is beating, the patient should be treated with full intensive care monitoring. Treatment must be carefully controlled and cautious rather than overenthusiastic. Handle the patient gently. Endotracheal intubation and the insertion of Swan-Ganz catheters must be done gently but should not be withheld for fear of inducing ventricular fibrillation. Correct acidosis and electrolyte abnormalities slowly and on the basis of specific hypotension due to vasodilation during rewarming.

(K) Cardiopulmonary resuscitation is started as soon as absence of heart beat is confirmed. Cardiopulmonary resuscitation started in the field must be continued until cardiac action can be definitively determined and treated.

(L) Active rewarming may be external or internal. External methods are less traumatic than internal ones, and they are more readily available but less efficient. The method chosen should be appropriate to the situation and, if possible, should allow resuscitation during rewarming. External rewarming may include hot water bottles, piped suits or blankets, radiant heat, warmed circulating air, or warm water tub (45°C). Immersion in warm water is the most efficient method. Internal rewarming begins with the administration of warm, humidified oxygen to all patients. This prevents further heat loss and provides additional heat. Body cavity lavage (peritoneum, pleura) is efficient and requires minimal equipment. Femorofemoral or total cardiopulmonary bypass with a heat exchanger is the most efficient method of rewarming but requires special equipment in a cardiac center. It is the optimal treatment for profound hypothermia with cardiac arrest.

(M) Survival depends more on associated diseases and injuries than on the depth of hypothermia. Mild hypothermia should not cause death. Deep hypothermia with cardiac arrest treated by cardiopulmonary bypass has a 50 percent mortality. Elevated blood urea nitrogen or K^+ and the need for resuscitation outside a hospital have a bad prognosis. Serum K^+ over 10 mEq/L signifies inability to resuscitate. Hypothermia incidental to severe trauma adds significantly to mortality.

REFERENCES

Auerbach PS, Geehr EC, eds. Management of wilderness and environmental emergencies. 2nd ed. St. Louis: CV Mosby, 1989.

Danzl DF, Pozos RS, Auerbach PS, et al. Multicenter hypothermia survey. Ann Emerg Med 1987; 16:1042–1055.

Lloyd EL. Hypothermia and cold stress. Rockville, MD: Aspen, 1986.

Paton BC. Accidental hypothermia. Pharmacol Ther 1983; 22:331–377.

Pozos RS, Wittmers LE, eds. The nature and treatment of hypothermia. Minneapolis: University of Minnesota Press, 1983.

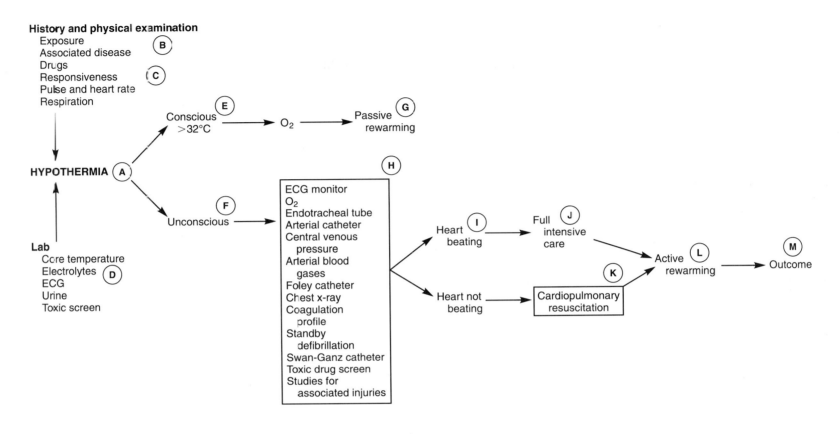

History and physical examination
- Exposure
- Associated disease   (B)
- Drugs
- Responsiveness   (C)
- Pulse and heart rate
- Respiration

HYPOTHERMIA (A)

Lab
- Core temperature
- Electrolytes   (D)
- ECG
- Urine
- Toxic screen

Conscious >32°C (E) → O₂ → Passive rewarming (G)

Unconscious (F) →

(H)
- ECG monitor
- O₂
- Endotracheal tube
- Arterial catheter
- Central venous pressure
- Arterial blood gases
- Foley catheter
- Chest x-ray
- Coagulation profile
- Standby defibrillation
- Swan-Ganz catheter
- Toxic drug screen
- Studies for associated injuries

Heart beating (I) → Full intensive care (J)

Heart not beating → Cardiopulmonary resuscitation (K)

→ Active rewarming (L) → Outcome (M)

Head and Neck

Closed Head Injury

Gary D. VanderArk, M.D., and Cynthia L. Norrgran, M.D.

(A) The cardinal sign of increased intracranial pressure is loss of consciousness. Deterioration to unconsciousness may be due to systemic causes (cardiopulmonary dysfunction or infection) or direct injury to the brain (hematoma or brain edema). Neurologic examination includes evaluation of eye opening, verbal response, and motor response. On the Glascow Coma Scale (GCS) a rating of 8 or less is considered coma.

(B) Increased intracranial pressure can present with an increase in blood pressure and a decrease in heart rate (the Cushing reflex). This response is opposite to that of hypovolemic shock. Head injury often produces electrocardiographic changes and can cause cardiac arrhythmias that further decrease cardiac output and brain perfusion.

(C) Because hypoxia increases brain swelling, anything that blocks the unconscious patient's airway is disastrous. Obstruction can be caused by the tongue, blood, or gastric contents. Providing a patent airway and giving oxygen are important in the early treatment of patients with head injury.

(D) Any patient unconscious from a closed head injury is assumed to have a broken neck until proven otherwise. The patient should be immobilized with a collar and transported with the head taped to a backboard. A lateral cervical spine x-ray should be done on arrival at the emergency department.

(E) The unconscious patient who develops hypoxia or hypercarbia requires intubation and mechanical ventilation. Nasotracheal intubation is preferred if a neck injury is suspected. The stomach is aspirated before intubation.

(F) Scalp lacerations or puncture wounds must be evaluated for underlying injuries (depressed skull fracture or penetrating brain injury).

(G) Amnesia indicates previous unconsciousness.

(H) Hemotympanum, otorrhea, or rhinorrhea is diagnostic of basilar skull fracture. Prophylactic antibiotics are not indicated. Patients usually recover with only elevation of the head of their bed.

(I) Dilation and fixation of one or both pupils is an ominous sign. It represents third nerve dysfunction secondary to tentorial herniation from increased pressure. If this pressure is not reduced quickly, irreversible damage occurs. If pupillary responses to light are absent bilaterally, the mortality rate is 65 percent for patients with mass lesions and 82 percent for those with diffuse brain injury.

(J) Treatment consists of cleansing and sterile probing to rule out penetration or depression. If neither exists, suturing can be done using local anesthesia.

(K) Skull x-rays can diagnose a depressed skull fracture. A compound skull fracture must be debrided to the depth of the wound. The presence of a skull fracture increases a conscious patient's chances of developing intracranial bleeding 400-fold.

(L) Hyperventilation is the most rapid method of decreasing intracranial pressure. A P_{CO_2} of 25 mmHg is ideal. Mannitol, 1 g/kg, and furosemide, 1 mg/kg, are effective hyperosmotic agents. Steroids do not decrease intracranial pressure in the acute situation.

(M) The risk of increased intracranial pressure in patients with normal computed tomography scans is low.

(N) The incidence of seizures after head injury is 5 percent. This rises to 35 percent with an acute intracranial hematoma and is as high as 70 percent with a depressed skull fracture causing dural laceration. For adults with amnesia of less than 24 hours' duration and no intracranial hematoma, the incidence of seizures is virtually zero.

(O) Craniotomy is necessary in 5 to 10 percent of patients with closed head injury. Acute hemorrhage requires a large craniotomy, whereas subacute or chronic hematomas can be treated with twist drill or burr hole evacuation.

(P) One third of patients with diffuse brain injury have elevated intracranial pressure. All patients with a GCS score of 7 or less should have their intracranial pressure monitored.

(Q) Prognosis need not be ominous. Patients with mild head injury (GCS score 13 to 15) have no mortality and few (7 percent) residual aftereffects. After moderate injury (GCS score 8 to 12), 93 percent of patients are discharged and only 10 percent require continuing medical care. After severe injury (GCS score 3 to 7), 42 percent are discharged and have mostly poor outcomes. Age is the most important pretrauma factor affecting outcome.

REFERENCES

Becker DP, Gade GF, Young HF, et al. Diagnosis and treatment of head injuries in adults. In: Youmans JR, ed. Neurological surgery. 3rd ed. Philadelphia: WB Saunders, 1989:2017–2148.

Becker DP, Gudeman SK. Textbook of head injury. Philadelphia: WB Saunders, 1989.

Hoff JT, Anderson TE, Cole TM, eds. Mild to moderate head injury: contemporary issues in neurological surgery. Boston: Blackwell Scientific Publishers, 1989.

Jennet G, Teasdale G. Management of head injuries. Philadelphia: FA Davis, 1981.

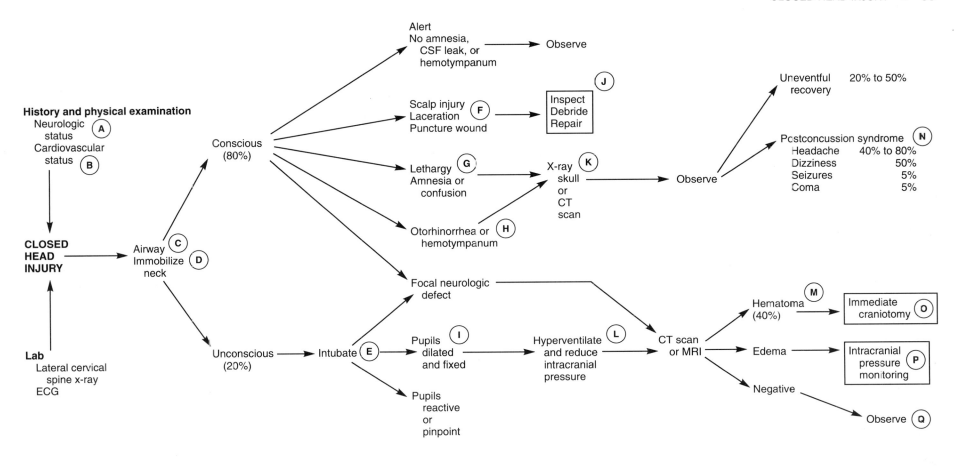

History and physical examination
Neurologic (A)
  status
Cardiovascular
  status (B)

**CLOSED
HEAD
INJURY**

Airway (C)
Immobilize (D)
neck

Lab
Lateral cervical
  spine x-ray
ECG

Conscious
(80%)

Alert
No amnesia,
  CSF leak, or
  hemotympanum → Observe

Scalp injury (F)
Laceration
Puncture wound → Inspect (J)
Debride
Repair

Lethargy (G)
Amnesia or
confusion

Otorhinorrhea or (H)
hemotympanum

X-ray (K)
skull
or
CT
scan

→ Observe

Uneventful   20% to 50%
recovery

Postconcussion syndrome (N)
  Headache   40% to 80%
  Dizziness   50%
  Seizures   5%
  Coma   5%

Unconscious
(20%)

Intubate (E)

Focal neurologic
defect

Pupils (I)
dilated
and fixed

Pupils
reactive
or
pinpoint

Hyperventilate (L)
and reduce
intracranial
pressure

CT scan
or MRI

Hematoma (M)
(40%) → Immediate (O)
craniotomy

Edema → Intracranial
pressure (P)
monitoring

Negative → Observe (Q)

Unequal Pupils

Kevin O. Lillehei, M.D.

(A) Elements important in the history of anisocoria include time of onset (if known); association with events, activities, or environmental exposures; age; illnesses (diabetes, cerebrovascular disease, cancer); and systemic or neurologic complaints.

(B) Examine the eyes for pupillary size, shape, and reactivity to direct and consensual illumination and to near fixation. If anisocoria is present, pupillary size should be recorded under both bright and dim illumination. The best corrected visual acuity should be determined. Extraocular muscle function is assessed by testing eye movement in the cardinal positions of gaze. A funduscopic examination is performed. The integrity of the globe is ascertained from the anterior segment to the posterior pole.

(C) Anisocoria, other than simple anisocoria, rarely occurs as an isolated event. A thorough neurologic examination that pays attention to the cranial nerves should be performed.

(D) Pupil size is governed by the balance of sympathetic innervation to the iris dilator muscle and parasympathetic innervation to the iris sphincter muscle. Sympathetic innervation involves a three-neuron chain. First-order neurons arise in the hypothalamus and run through the brainstem and ipsilateral cervical cord to synapse at the cervicothoracic junction. Second-order neurons exit the spinal cord along the first thoracic nerve root and enter the sympathetic chain, synapsing at the superior cervical ganglion. Third-order (postganglionic) neurons travel along the internal carotid artery, cross into the ophthalmic division of the trigeminal nerve, and finally reach the iris dilator muscle as the long ciliary nerves. Parasympathetic innervation arises in the Edinger-Westphal nucleus of the midbrain and travels along the surface of the oculomotor nerve to synapse at the ciliary ganglion located in the posterior aspect of the orbit. Postganglionic fibers, the short ciliary nerves, run to the iris sphincter muscle. Both the sympathetic and parasympathetic innervation run ipsilateral, with anisocoria being the result of a focal dysfunction of one pathway.

(E) The normal pupillary size is 2 to 6 mm (average 3 mm). In the elderly the pupils tend to be smaller (senile miosis) and reaction to light can be more difficult to see.

(F) A parasympathetic abnormality results in the larger pupil being pathologic.

(G) A sympathetic abnormality results in the smaller pupil being pathologic.

(H) The cocaine test is used to confirm the presence of a Horner's syndrome. It is unnecessary if ptosis or anhidrosis is present. If unsure, cocaine (4 to 10 percent) is instilled in both eyes and the pupillary size under similar illumination is measured in 30 minutes. Cocaine blocks the reuptake of norepinephrine by postganglionic fibers. Failure of the iris to dilate confirms the presence of a sympathetic abnormality somewhere in the three-neuron chain. It provides no help in localizing the abnormality.

(I) The pilocarpine test is used to distinguish pre- and postganglionic parasympathetic denervation from pharmacologic blockade. Postganglionic denervation to the iris sphincter muscle results in the phenomenon of denervation hypersensitivity to cholinergic agents. Administration of a dilute (0.1 percent) concentration of pilocarpine results in miosis. Preganglionic parasympathetic dysfunction does not result in denervation hypersensitivity, and miosis occurs only with a more concentrated (1 percent) solution of pilocarpine. Failure of the pupil to respond to 1 percent pilocarpine is evidence for the presence of pharmacologic blockade (ie, atropine eye drops).

(J) Simple anisocoria is a benign condition affecting 15 to 30 percent of the population. Pupil asymmetry tends to be ≥0.4 mm and persists from bright to dim illumination. The condition may or may not have been noted by the patient previously.

(K) Injury to the orbital floor can affect the inferior ramus of the oculomotor nerve supplying the medial and inferior rectus muscles, the inferior oblique muscle, and the ciliary ganglion. This results in compromise of preganglionic parasympathetic fibers to the iris sphincter muscle.

(L) Injury to the orbital apex can affect the optic nerve running through the optic foramen or structures within the superior orbital fissure (oculomotor, trochlear, and abducens nerves and the ophthalmic division of the trigeminal nerve). Injury to the oculomotor nerve results in anisocoria. Emergent surgical intervention is indicated only when there is a potentially reversible optic nerve injury, usually secondary to a displaced fragment of bone.

(M) Traumatic iridoplegia usually involves both the sphincter and dilator muscles. As a result, the pupil is usually dilated (traumatic mydriasis) but miosis can occur. The deformity may resolve but often is permanent.

(N) Horner's syndrome is characterized by ipsilateral miosis and ptosis, with facial anhidrosis if the lesion is proximal to the superior cervical ganglion.

(O) Adie's tonic pupil is characterized by a large pupil that is poorly reactive to light, both

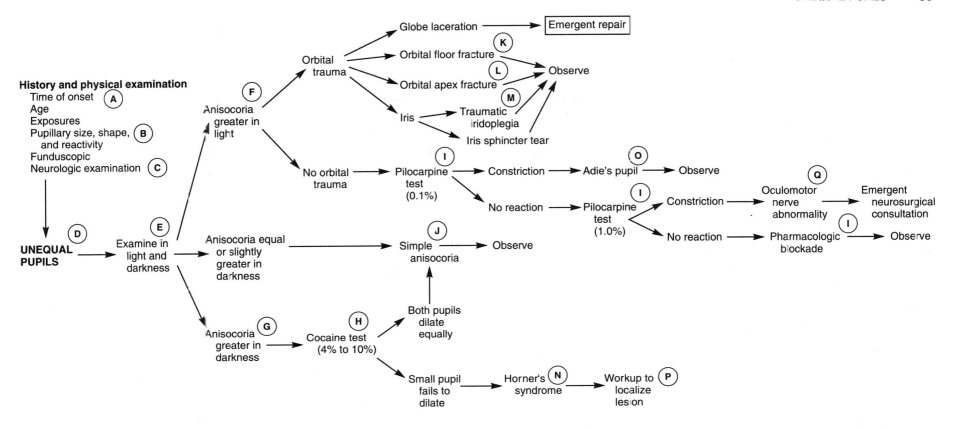

directly and consensually, with preserved miosis to near testing. It is seen most frequently in women ages 20 to 40 years. It may be associated with more diffuse autonomic nervous system dysfunction (diminished deep tendon reflexes, asymmetric sweating, or constipation). This is a benign condition and no treatment is required.

(P) Localizing lesions in the sympathetic pathway involves examining associated structures along the three-neuron chain. Causes affecting first-order neurons include brainstem stroke, brainstem or cervical cord trauma, and spinal cord tumors.

Causes affecting second-order neurons include neck trauma, vertebral metastases, and apical lung lesions. Causes affecting third-order neurons include migraine headache, carotid artery tumor, dissecting carotid aneurysm, or cavernous sinus lesions.

(Q) In most cases the pupil abnormality is associated with ptosis and external deviation of the eye, confirming oculomotor nerve dysfunction. This is a medical emergency that requires ruling out cerebral swelling with unilateral medial temporal lobe herniation and impending brainstem compression or the presence of an ipsilateral posterior communicating artery aneurysm. Less emergent is microvascular ischemia of the oculomotor nerve caused by diabetes, meningovascular syphilis, or atherosclerosis.

REFERENCES

Beck RW, Smith CH, eds. Neuro-ophthalmology: a problem-oriented approach. Boston: Little, Brown & Co, 1988.
Thompson HS, Pilley SFJ. Unequal pupils: a flow chart for sorting out the anisocorias. Surv Ophthalmol 1976; 21:45–48.

Otorrhea

James W. Lucarini, M.D.

A Otorrhea is assessed for color, clarity, viscosity, odor, and temporal pattern. Its relationship to head trauma, hearing loss, pain, fever, or pruritus is determined. Thick, purulent drainage usually indicates bacterial infection. Thin or clear discharge suggests serous fluid or cerebrospinal fluid (CSF). Foul smell is often noted in anaerobic or mixed bacterial infection. Acute, subacute, or chronic courses hint at diagnosis. Head trauma suggests the possibility of CSF leakage. Conductive hearing loss suggests disruption of the canal or middle ear, whereas sensorineural hearing loss and vertigo indicate disruption of the inner ear by infection, tumor, or trauma. Pain and fever accompanying purulent otorrhea indicate acute otitis media, otitis externa, or, less commonly, acute mastoiditis. Chronic or recurrent otorrhea is seen in cholesteatoma or chronic granulation disease and, less commonly, represents cancer or tuberculosis. Pruritus is common and especially noted in eczematous conditions and otomycosis.

B Culture of the drainage should be followed by careful suctioning and examination under the microscope to assess the canal and the integrity of the tympanic membrane.

C If edema prevents visualization of the tympanic membrane, a gauze or mericel wick is placed in the canal and antibiotic or steroidal drops are instilled several times each day. Frequent suctioning and replacement of the wick are performed until the medial canal is patent and the tympanic membrane can be assessed. Oral antibiotics should be started if there is suspicion of acute otitis media.

D Bacterial otitis externa or swimmer's ear is cellulitis of the canal skin caused by *Pseudomonas, Proteus,* or *Staphylococcus.* It is characterized by marked pain that is intensified by manipulation of the auricle or pressure on the tragus. Treatment involves topical antibiotic or steroidal drops, strict avoidance of water in the ear, and repeated suctioning of purulence and debris. Occasionally, narrow canals or obstruction due to exostoses (bony canal protruberances) requires widening of the canal through canalplasty. When the infection becomes localized (furunculosis), it requires incision and drainage along with oral antibiotics to cover *Staphylococcus aureus.*

E Fungal otitis externa or otomycosis is usually caused by *Aspergillus* or other saprophytic fungi in association with a bacterial infection. Itching is the prominent initial symptom, and discharge may be scant and serous. Examination typically reveals gray and black velvety debris covering an erythematous canal. Mycelia and spores are seen under the microscope. Treatment involves thorough cleansing of the canal and application of antifungal agents such as Cresylate or Merthiolate.

F Eczematous external otitis may be associated with similar scalp infections. Local allergens may be introduced by patients who manipulate the canal frequently. Occasionally, there is a local allergy to neomycin in otic drops. Treatment involves removal of local allergens and use of topical steroid drops or creams.

G Acute otitis media is most common in children with poor eustachian tube function during an upper respiratory illness. Purulence under pressure in the middle ear leads to spontaneous rupture of the tympanic membrane. Oral antibiotics must be directed against pneumococcus and *Haemophilus influenzae,* the latter being most common in children under age 5 years. Acute complications, usually seen before therapy, include serous labyrinthitis, meningitis, facial paralysis, and subdural abscess. Treatment may require intravenous antibiotics and mastoidectomy. A complication due to inadequate treatment or resistance is coalescent mastoiditis, usually diagnosed by noting persistent or recurrent otorrhea about 3 weeks after therapy for acute otitis media. Computed tomography scan shows dissolution of mastoid bony architecture. Treatment is intravenous antibiotics and simple mastoidectomy.

H Chronic otitis media is characterized by recurrent purulent otorrhea associated with tympanic perforation and conductive hearing loss. Contamination of the middle ear with water during bathing or swimming can exacerbate the problem. Chronic eustachian tube dysfunction prevents healing of the perforation. Edematous mucosal changes along with granulation disease and cholesterol granuloma ensue. Therapy includes water precautions, frequent suctioning, and topical antibiotic drops. Patients who respond may be candidates for tympanoplasty if the otorrhea is controlled for 3 or more months. Continued otorrhea despite medical management implies irreversible disease that requires tympanomastoidectomy. Computed tomography scan can confirm soft tissue changes in the middle ear and mastoid or point out bone destruction. It is also useful to predict or confirm complications, such as petrositis, sigmoid thrombophlebitis, extradural or brain abscess, suppurative labyrinthitis, or otitic hydrocephalus. These problems usually require advanced petrous bone dissections in addition to intravenous antibiotics.

I Cholesteatoma or keratoma is a form of chronic otitis media caused by invagination of keratinizing squamous epithelium in the middle ear or mastoid. Poor eustachian tube function predisposes to this process by providing negative pressure in the middle ear. This causes focal retraction or perforation of the tympanic membrane. Enzymatic resorption of bone by the cholesteatoma leads to complications that must be treated surgically in most cases.

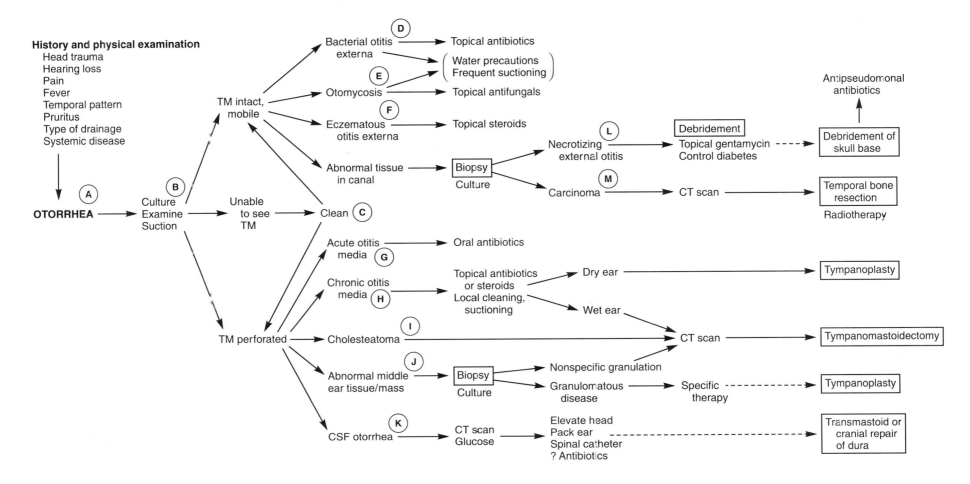

History and physical examination
- Head trauma
- Hearing loss
- Pain
- Fever
- Temporal pattern
- Pruritus
- Type of drainage
- Systemic disease

(J) Abnormal tissue in the middle ear may include chronic granulation disease, cholesteatoma, neoplasm, or a granuloma. Biopsy and culture usually determine the diagnosis. Granulomas such as tuberculosis or Wegener granulomatosis should be treated systemically. Tympanoplasty for correction of persistent perforation may be performed once the disease process is eradicated. Malignancy usually warrants temporal bone resection accompanied by radiation therapy.

(K) CSF otorrhea usually follows temporal bone trauma. Less commonly, advanced temporal bone malignancy can cause CSF otorrhea. Aural fluid placed on filter paper shows a clear halo around a serosanguinous center because CSF diffuses distally from blood and serum. Detection of glucose in the drainage is further evidence of CSF. Fracture or bony erosion leading to CSF leakage is best detected by computed tomography scanning. Subtle cases require scanning with technetium pertechnetate or spinal fluid injection with fluorescein dye. Infection of the CSF with resultant meningitis is a serious complication. There is controversy over the use of prophylactic antibiotic therapy to prevent this. Initial treatment of CSF leakage includes elevation of the head of the bed, sterile packing of the canal or mastoid, and reduction of CSF pressure by removal of fluid through a spinal catheter or repeated spinal taps. Transmastoid or cranial repair of the dura may be necessary if the leakage continues.

(L) Necrotizing (malignant) external otitis is usually seen in elderly diabetics. It is caused by *Pseudomonas aeruginosa* and characterized by the presence of granulation tissue at the junction of the cartilaginous and bony canal. It can lead to generalized skull base osteomyelitis and rapid death. Involvement of cranial nerves usually indicates a poor prognosis. Early treatment involves local debridement of granulations, topical gentamicin

Otorrhea (Continued)

drops, and control of diabetes. If resolution is not rapid, bony involvement should be assessed by technetium 99m pyrophosphate bone scan, baseline computed tomography, and gallium 67 scan. Debridement of the skull base to drain abscesses and remove sequestra is followed by 6 weeks of intravenous antibiotics directed at *P. aeruginosa.* A repeat gallium scan is obtained to ensure resolution of all soft tissue involvement before cessation of antibiotics.

(M) Malignancies of the canal include epidermoid carcinoma, basal cell carcinoma, and adeno-carcinoma of ceruminous glands. Location of these tumors rather than histology determines their propensity for recurrence. Foul otorrhea results from necrosis and infection. Persistent pain is a clue to diagnosis because otalgia is uncommon in uncomplicated chronic otitis. The threshold for biopsy should be low. Treatment involves temporal bone resection with postoperative radiation therapy. Advanced tumors can invade the middle ear and cranial cavity, giving rise to sensorineural or conductive hearing loss, facial paralysis and other cranial neuropathies, and meningismus. Distant metastases are common even after adequate local control.

REFERENCES

Cummings CW, Fredrickson JM, Harker LA, et al, eds. Otolaryngology—head and neck surgery. St. Louis: CV Mosby, 1986.

Paparella MM, Shumrick DA, eds. Otolaryngology. Vol II: head and neck. Philadelphia: WB Saunders, 1991.

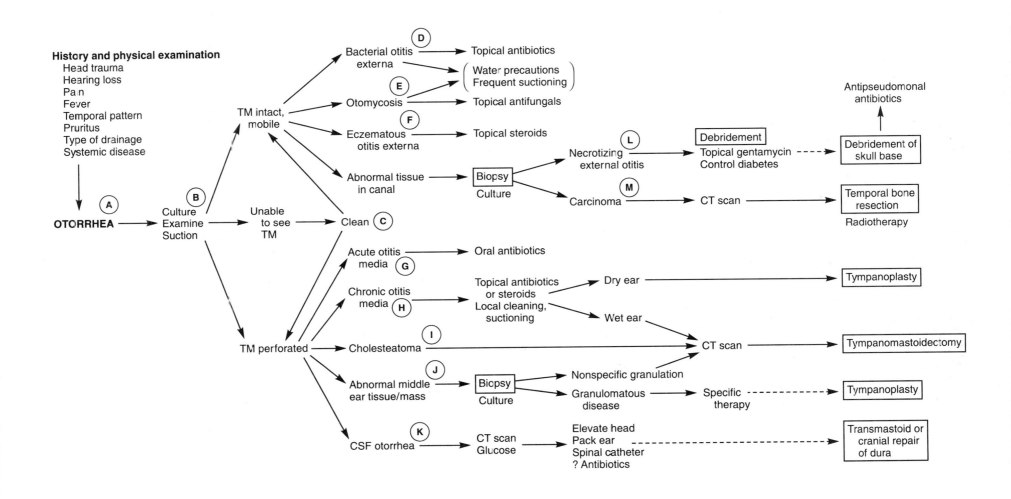

History and physical examination
  Head trauma
  Hearing loss
  Pain
  Fever
  Temporal pattern
  Pruritus
  Type of drainage
  Systemic disease

Epistaxis

Kenneth H. McCarley, M.D., and Bruce W. Jafek, M.D.

A. Causes of epistaxis are multiple and differ depending on the patient's age. The more common causes are trauma (inherent vulnerability of the vasculature due to lack of supporting stroma and thin mucosal lining), decreased humidity and subsequent drying of the mucosa (increased incidence of epistaxis in drier climates and during the winter months), inflammation (upper respiratory infections, allergic rhinitis, rheumatic fever), blood dyscrasias (leukemia, hemophilia, idiopathic thrombocytopenic purpura [ITP]), tumors and foreign bodies (polyps, juvenile nasopharyngeal angiofibroma, meningocele), and vascular anomalies (arteriosclerosis, aneurysm, hereditary hemorrhagic telangiectasia).

B. Look for other evidence of hemorrhage or mucosal or vascular anomalies. Identify the source of the bleeding. This requires equipment such as suction, nasal speculum, good lighting, local anesthesia, and proper protection for the physician. Most bleeding (90 percent) is anteroinferior along the septum (Kiesselbach area). The younger the patient, the more likely the bleeding site will be anterior.

C. Begin ambulatory treatment by applying gentle, constant pressure. Have the patient pinch the nose just distal to the bony cartilaginous junction for 15 to 20 minutes. Often this has failed at home and has prompted the visit to the emergency room.

D. Applying Gelfoam or Avitine to the site is recommended for patients with blood dyscrasias because these topical hemostatic agents do not have to be removed at a later time.

E. If a bleeding site is found, apply silver nitrate to cauterize the area. Dry the area with suction before attempting to cauterize. An important rule is to cauterize only one side of the septum to prevent a septal perforation.

F. If the above measures fail, pack the nose anteriorly. Use 0.5-inch impregnated gauze and apply in layers from the nasal floor to the nasal roof. This is effective in stopping bleeding in 90 percent of patients.

G. The patient may be sent home on antibiotics to return in 2 to 3 days for removal of the packing. If there is crusting and dryness of the nasal mucosa, saline rinses (1 pint of water with 1 teaspoon of salt and a pinch of baking soda) and application of an antibiotic ointment (Borofax, Neosporin) on an outpatient basis are helpful.

H. When ambulatory treatment fails, the patient is hospitalized. Correct a coagulopathy if present. If anterior packing has been placed properly and the bleeding persists, then posterior packing is required. This treatment is unpleasant for the patient. It requires intravenous antibiotics. For elderly patients, admission to the ICU is prudent since the posterior packing significantly lowers alveolar oxygenation and can cause hypercapnia. Those with marginal cardiopulmonary function may be pushed toward decompensation.

I. Posterior packing should be done by an otolaryngologist.

J. If packing fails, arterial ligation or embolization may be necessary. Because both the internal and the external carotid artery systems supply the nose, arteriographic study may be warranted before such therapy is initiated.

REFERENCES

Culbertson MC, Manning SC. Epistaxis. In Bluestone CD, Stool SE, eds. Pediatric Otolaryngology, 2nd ed. Philadelphia: WB Saunders, 1990:672–678.

Rosnagle R. Epistaxis. In: English GM, ed. Otolaryngology, Vol 2. Philadelphia: JB Lippincott, 1988:1–12.

Saunders WH. Epistaxis. In: Paparella MM, Shumrick DA, eds. Otolaryngology, 2nd ed. Philadelphia: WB Saunders, 1980:1994–2008.

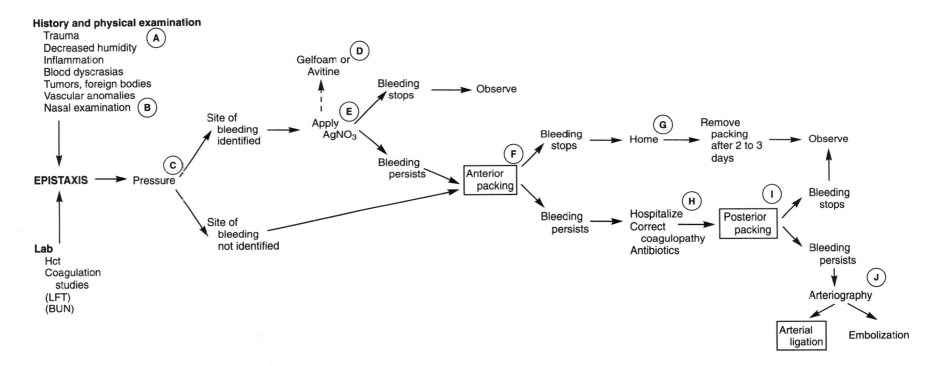

Maxillary Fractures

Scott Replogle, M.D.

(A) Significant force is required to fracture the maxilla because of its position and strength. Maxillary fractures are uncommon but are often associated with serious injuries such as cervical spine injuries and head injuries with cerebrospinal fluid leaks (25 percent in Le Fort II and III fractures). Epistaxis, scleral and periorbital hematoma, and infraorbital nerve injury are less serious findings.

(B) Malocclusion (commonly an anterior over-bite) in the absence of a mandibular fracture suggests a maxillary fracture. Palpable maxillary mobility is diagnostic.

(C) Clinical diagnosis is more important than x-ray findings. Of facial x-rays, the Waters view is the most helpful. Bone density computed to-mography scanning of the midface with reformations in different planes may be required to delineate the extent of maxillary fractures.

(D) Nondisplaced fractures with normal occlusion do not require fixation. Edentulous patients can accept some displacement by adjusting their dentures if the cosmetic alteration is not significant and the fractured segment is not mobile.

(E) Alveolar segment fractures can often be treated by monomaxillary fixation alone, using a single arch bar or other device. Larger segments may require reduction and intermaxillary fixation (IMF) to hold proper occlusion.

(F) Fractures above the alveolar segments that include the vault of the palate and the pter-ygoid processes constitute Le Fort I (Guerin) fractures.

(G) Fractures extending from the pterygoid plates through the zygomaticomaxillary junction and lateral wall of the maxilla, through the floor of the orbit, and across the nasofrontal junction constitute Le Fort II (pyramidal) fractures.

(H) Le Fort III fractures, or craniofacial dysjunc-tions, involve the entire maxilla as in the Le Fort II fracture but with lateral extension of the fracture line to include the zygoma.

(I) Maxillary fractures often do not fall into a pure Le Fort category but are mixed or include areas that are incomplete or nondisplaced. Treatment must be individualized with emphasis on occlusion and contour. Computed tomography scans are helpful in delineating details of mixed fractures. Open reduction–internal fixation is required. Bone grafts and occlusal splints are occa-sionally used. Maxillary sinus drainage is recom-mended in Le Fort fractures.

(J) Complex fractures involve severe comminu-tion, loss of bone, an associated orbital fissure or dural injury, or a concomitant mandibular frac-ture. Late or irreducible maxillary fractures are also more complex problems.

(K) Treatment of Le Fort I and II fractures in-volves closed reduction or disimpaction of the fractured segment and reestablishment of normal occlusion with arch bars and IMF, as for mandibular fractures.

(L) Pure Le Fort III fractures, like Le Fort I and II fractures, can be reduced with closed tech-niques, but fixation usually requires open reduction and interosseous wiring through a craniofacial ap-proach or individual external incisions as well as IMF.

(M) In addition to IMF, the maxillary fragments may be fixed to stable bone above the frac-ture. This involves wire suspension joining the stable bone to the arch bars or interosseous wiring. For Le Fort I–type fractures, the upper stabilization point is the pyriform margin above the fracture or the infraorbital rim.

(N) Le Fort II fractures may require superior stabilization by suspension over an uninjured zygoma or to the zygomaticofrontal rim. The wires are subsequently removed. Interosseous wiring of the nasofrontal, orbital rim, or lower maxillary buttress areas may be required.

(O) Stable suspension is usually to the frontal bone adjacent to the zygomaticofrontal frac-ture. Pull-out wires, as in N, are employed.

(P) External fixation currently is less commonly required as the principles of craniofacial sur-gery are better understood and direct reduction and interosseous wiring are employed. Dynamic traction from an external appliance is occasionally helpful.

(Q) An increasingly common choice for internal fixation of maxillary fractures is the use of rigid miniplate fixation. These plates are moldable, are usually made of titanium, and can be left in place. The relatively thin bone of the maxilla has been found to be thick enough to hold the screws for the plates. Use of this approach may require a somewhat wider exposure but avoids the need for wire suspension. Intermaxillary fixation is required only briefly or not at all.

(R) Complex fractures with marked comminution or bone loss have been treated successfully with primary bone grafting usually with appropriate interosseous wiring or rigid plate fixation.

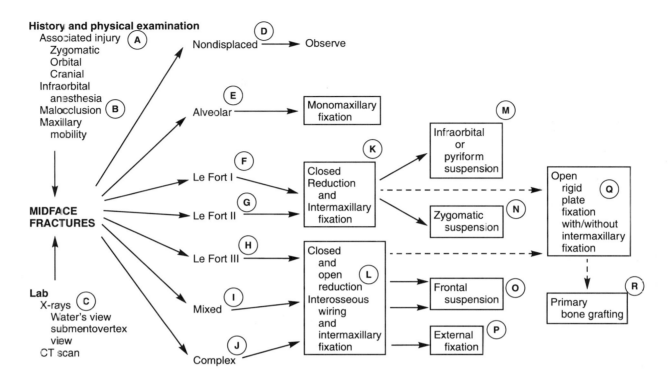

History and physical examination
Associated injury (A)
  Zygomatic
  Orbital
  Cranial
Infraorbital
  anesthesia
Malocclusion (B)
Maxillary
  mobility

**MIDFACE
FRACTURES**

Lab (C)
  X-rays
    Water's view
    submentovertex
    view
  CT scan

Nondisplaced (D) → Observe

Alveolar (E) → Monomaxillary fixation

Le Fort I (F)
Le Fort II (G)
→ Closed Reduction and Intermaxillary fixation (K)
→ Infraorbital or pyriform suspension (M)
→ Zygomatic suspension (N)

Le Fort III (H)
Mixed (I)
Complex (J)
→ Closed and open reduction Interosseous wiring and intermaxillary fixation (L)
→ Frontal suspension (O)
→ External fixation (P)

→ Open rigid plate fixation with/without intermaxillary fixation (Q)

→ Primary bone grafting (R)

REFERENCES

Archer WH. Oral and maxillary surgery. Philadelphia: WB Saunders, 1975.

Beals SP, Munro IR. The use of miniplates in craniomaxillofacial surgery. J Plast Reconstr Surg 1987; 79:33–38.

Dingman R, Natvig P. Surgery of facial fractures. Philadelphia: WB Saunders, 1964.

Foster CA, Sherman JE. Surgery of facial bone fractures. New York: Churchill Livingstone, 1987.

Habal Mutaz B, Ariyan S. Facial fractures. Philadelphia: BC Decker, 1989.

Kawamoto HK Jr, Wolfe SA, eds. Maxillofacial surgery. Clin Plast Surg 1982; 9:479–489.

Manson PN. Rigid fixation and bone grafts for craniofacial surgery. Clin Plast Surg 1989; 16:105–114.

Manson PN, Crawley WA, Yareinchuk MJ, et al. Midface fractures: advantages of immediate extended open reduction and bone grafting. J Plast Reconstr Surg 1985; 76:1–10.

Mathog RH. Maxillofacial trauma. Baltimore: Williams & Wilkins, 1984.

Rowe NL, Williams JLI. Maxillofacial injuries. Edinburgh: Churchill Livingstone, 1985.

Mandibular Fractures

Scott Replogle, M.D.

A Fifty percent of mandibular fractures are bilateral. Malocclusion (the failure of the first maxillary molar to interdigitate with the first mandibular molar on each side) is diagnostic if absent before injury. Trismus and temporomandibular joint pain are caused by displacement of the proximal segment and muscle injury. Body and parasymphyseal fractures cause injury to the mental nerve and an area of anesthesia. Intraoral laceration is common and should be treated with pericral rinses and systemic antibiotics effective against mouth organisms.

B X-rays are rarely needed to diagnose mandibular fracture but are essential to determine the number, location, and extent of fractures and the degree of displacement. The panoramic (Panorex) view of the mandible is the most helpful. Old fractures may be difficult to distinguish from new ones. Correlation with the history is essential.

C Fractures of the coronoid process are rare (2 percent) and usually result from a direct blow to the area. Because of splinting by surrounding tissues and few sequelae of inexact reduction, a soft diet and observation are often adequate treatment. If occlusion is lost during observation, fixation is required.

D Fractures of the condyle are frequent (36 percent) and are commonly bilateral. Intermaxillary fixation (IMF) is usually adequate treatment. In children a soft diet alone may suffice. Open reduction and internal fixation (ORIF) are required occasionally if the condylar head is displaced from the mandibular (or condylar) fossa.

E Ramus fractures are rare (3 percent).

F Fractures of the angle (20 percent) are often unstable because of distracting muscle pull on the fragments (class II fractures) and require ORIF.

G The body is involved in 21 percent of fractures. With a favorable angle of fracture and good teeth on both sides of the fracture, IMF may be adequate treatment. Unless obviously devitalized, loose, or diseased, a tooth in the line of the fracture should be retained to aid reduction. In such cases antibiotic coverage should be prolonged.

H Parasymphyseal fractures (14 percent) are notoriously difficult to stabilize and almost always require ORIF and lingual splints to prevent rotation of segments. Oblique fractures between the lingual and buccal cortexes are particularly difficult to reduce and maintain in occlusion. True symphyseal fractures are rarer and more stable.

I The rare (3 percent) alveolar fracture usually can be held with IMF or with monomandibular fixation if isolated.

J Favorable fractures have adequate, healthy teeth on both sides of the fracture (class I) and a fracture line that favors impaction rather than distraction by the pull of the muscles on the fragments. If the patient can tolerate IMF, treatment is intermaxillary wiring of opposed teeth.

K Unfavorable fractures are those with inadequate teeth, teeth on only one of either side of the fracture (class II or III), a fracture line that is distracted by the pull of the muscles on the fragments, and those that cannot be held in occlusion by IMF alone. Such fragments require ORIF to hold the teeth in occlusion.

L Complex fractures are usually comminuted or involve loss of bone segments and require external fixation until the missing bone can be safely replaced, although primary bone grafting can be successful.

M IMF splints the jaw by holding the teeth tightly together in the proper position (occlusion) during the healing of the fracture. Sixty percent of mandibular fractures can be treated in this closed manner. Erich arch bars or other supports are fixed to wires. The bars on the mandibular and maxillary teeth are then held together with wires or rubber bands to maintain occlusion. Other types of dental and interdental wiring are possible. Prefabricated occlusal or lingual splints are occasionally required. In the edentulous patient, dentures fixed to the bone can be used.

N ORIF either by an intraoral or external approach involves interosseous wiring or bone plating to stabilize the fragments followed by IMF. Lingual or occlusal splints are occasionally helpful.

O External fixation is required when other methods fail, when IMF is contraindicated, in some edentulous patients, and when there is severe comminution or bone loss. A Joe Hall Morris type of external appliance with large pin attachments can be constructed intraoperatively with pins, plastic tubing (eg, a chest tube) connecting the pins, and methylmethacrylate injected into the tubing to complete the fixation.

P An increasingly common choice for internal fixation of maxillary fractures is the use of a rigid miniplate or compression plate fixation. The mandible is usually thick enough to hold even compression plate screws and excellent fixation can be achieved, often minimizing or avoiding intermaxillary fixation. This is an excellent choice in the

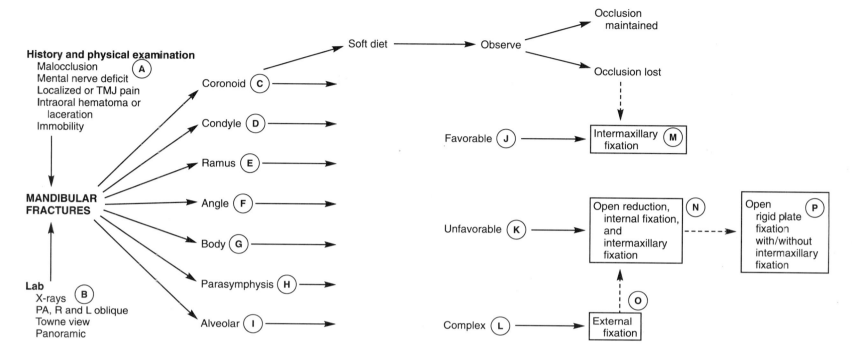

edentulous or uncooperative patient or when dentition is marginal for IMF or the stability of the fracture fixation is in question with interosseous wiring alone.

REFERENCES

Archer WH. Oral and maxillofacial surgery. Philadelphia: WB Saunders, 1975.

Busuito MJ, Smith DJ Jr, Robson MC. Mandibular fractures in the urban trauma center. J Trauma 1986; 26:8–16.

Dingman R, Natvig P. Surgery of facial fractures. Philadelphia: WB Saunders, 1964.

Ellis E 3rd, Moos KF, el-Attar A. Ten-years of mandibular fractures: an analysis of 2,137 cases. Oral Surg Oral Med Oral Pathol 1985; 59:120–129.

Foster CA, Sherman JE. Surgery of facial bone fractures. New York: Churchill Livingstone, 1987.

Habal MB, Ariyan S. Facial fractures. Philadelphia: BC Decker, 1989.

Jclewenimer AM, Greenberg AM. Management of mandibular trauma with rigid internal fixation. Oral Surg 1986; 62:630.

Kawamoto HK Jr, Wolfe SA, eds. Maxillofacial surgery. Clin Plast Surg 1982; 9:479–489.

Manson PN. Rigid fixation and bone grafting for craniofacial surgery. Clin Plast Surg 1989; 16:105–114.

Manson PN, Crawley WA, Yareinchuk MJ, et al. Midface fractures: advantages of immediate extended open reduction and bone grafting. J Plast Reconstr Surg 1985; 76:1–10.

Carcinoma of the Lip

Lawrence L. Ketch, M.D.

(A) Risk factors for lip carcinoma include lower lip, being a white male, tobacco or alcohol use, sun exposure, immunosuppression, and leukoplakia.

(B) About 7 to 8 percent of patients have palpable nodes when diagnosed. Adenopathy is on the basis of hyperplasia or inflammation in 30 to 50 percent of these patients.

(C) Lip cancer can spread along the mental nerve from its exit at the foramen of the mandible to the base of the skull. By the time this spread is detected by x-ray, the disease is highly advanced.

(D) Biopsy is usually performed under local anesthesia. Suspicious areas of ulceration or induration are excised. Lesions smaller than 1 cm are excised in toto. Larger lesions are shaved or sampled by a 2-mm dermal punch.

(E) Benign conditions that can simulate lip cancer include candida, herpes simplex, syphilis, erythema multiforme, sarcoid, and Crohn disease.

(F) Leukoplakia is considered premalignant. It is associated with cancer in 70 percent of cases. Multicentric invasive squamous cells are seen in 3 to 10 percent of such specimens. This rate closely parallels local recurrence rates in small tumors. Vermilionectomy is frequently performed with a V-shaped excision to ensure excision of cancer cells.

(G) Staging of the primary lesion (TMN classification) is by size:

T1, < 2 cm
T2, 2 to 4 cm
T3, > 4 cm

Frequency of recurrence depends on size (T grade) and histologic differentiation.

(H) Nodal metastasis correlates with size and histologic differentiation:

T1, 4 percent
T2, 35 percent
T3, 65 percent
Poorly differentiated, 60 percent

T2 lesions smaller than 3 cm have a lower risk than the T2 group as a whole. Fine-needle aspiration is helpful in accessing regional nodes.

(I) The frequency of local and regional relapse is directly proportional to primary size:

T1, 10 to 15 percent
T3, 50 to 70 percent

Relapse usually occurs within 2 years of treatment. Recurrence in the neck occurs in 43 percent of cases. Recurrence in the lip and in the neck occurs in 14 percent. Mean survival after lip recurrence is about 7 years; after neck recurrence it is about 2 years. In the presence of metastases 5-year survival is about 50 percent. Two-year disease-free survival after lip reexcision is 70 percent.

(J) Distant metastasis is unusual except in the presence of persistent and extensive neck disease. It usually involves the lungs and is rapidly fatal.

(K) Cure rates (95 percent) are similar to surgery. Contraindications to radiation include recurrence after primary radiotherapy, extensive precancerous changes of the remaining lip, young age, and large lesions (T3) with palpable nodes or possible mandibular involvement. Radiation therapy should be administered postoperatively to patients with large lesions.

REFERENCES

American Joint Committee on Cancer. Manual for staging of cancer. 2nd ed. Philadelphia: JB Lippincott, 1983.

Ariyan S. Cancer of the head and neck. St. Louis: CV Mosby, 1987.

Bailey BJ. Management of carcinoma of the lip. Laryngoscope 1977; 87:250–260.

Brown RG, Poole MD, Calamel PM, et al. Advanced and recurrent squamous carcinoma of the lower lip. Am J Surg 1976;132:492–497.

Dickie WR, Colville J, Graham WJH. Recurrent carcinoma of the lip. Oral Surg 1967;24:449–454.

Hendricks JL, Mendelson BC, Woods JE. Invasive carcinoma of the lower lip. Surg Clin North Am 1977;57:837–844.

Knabel MR, Koranda FC, Panje WR, et al. Squamous cell carcinoma of the upper lip. J Dermatol Surg Oncol 1982; 8:487–491.

Luce EA. Carcinoma of the lower lip. Surg Clin North Am 1986;66:3–11.

Lund C. Epidermoid carcinoma of the lip: histological grading in the clinical evaluation. Acta Radiol [Ther] [Stockh] 1975;14:465–474.

Waldron CA, Shafer WG. Leukoplakia revisited: a clinicopathologic study of 3256 oral leukoplakias. Cancer 1975; 36:1386–1392.

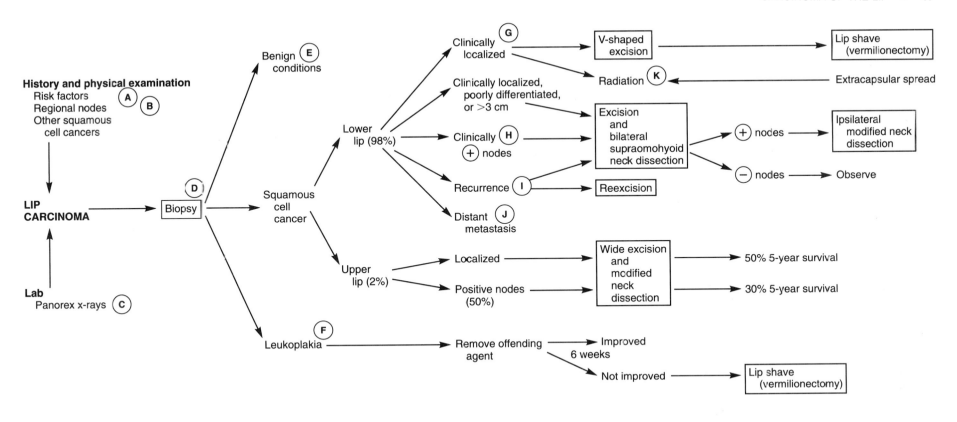

History and physical examination
Risk factors (A)
Regional nodes (B)
Other squamous
cell cancers

**LIP
CARCINOMA**

Lab
Panorex x-rays (C)

Biopsy (D)

Benign (E)
conditions

Squamous
cell
cancer

Leukoplakia (F)

Lower
lip (98%)

Upper
lip (2%)

Clinically (G)
localized

Clinically localized,
poorly differentiated,
or >3 cm

Clinically (H)
(+) nodes

Recurrence (I)

Distant (J)
metastasis

Localized

Positive nodes
(50%)

Remove offending
agent

V-shaped
excision

Radiation (K)

Excision
and
bilateral
supraomohyoid
neck dissection

Reexcision

Wide excision
and
modified
neck
dissection

Lip shave
(vermilionectomy)

Extracapsular spread

(+) nodes

(−) nodes

Ipsilateral
modified neck
dissection

Observe

50% 5-year survival

30% 5-year survival

Improved

6 weeks

Not improved

Lip shave
(vermilionectomy)

Carcinoma of the Oral Cavity

Stanley Coulthard, M.D.

A The patient with oral cavity carcinoma is usually in the fifth or sixth decade of life with a history of prolonged exposure to tobacco and alcohol. The patient who is both an alcoholic and a smoker has a 15 percent higher incidence of carcinoma of the oral cavity than the abstainer; the two irritants appear to act synergistically in causing oral carcinoma. Other irritants associated with oral cancer are betel nut (India) and products of dental disease. Head and neck examination usually reveals an oral ulcer, a submucosal mass, or an exophytic growing lesion. Early carcinoma of the oral cavity may present as erythroplasia or superficial hyperkeratosis. A neck mass, fixed or mobile, may be the first identifiable abnormality in primary head and neck cancer. It is mandatory that a thorough head and neck examination be performed in all patients with neck masses. Eighty percent of unilateral neck masses in adults are metastatic squamous cell carcinoma from head and neck cancers.

B Biopsy is performed when any intraoral lesion proves to be nonhealing and persistent. Tissue is obtained by either punch or incision techniques. Over 90 percent of oral cancers are squamous cell carcinomas.

C Fine-needle aspiration has proven to be valuable in the diagnosis and staging of squamous cell carcinoma. The reliability of the diagnosis is directly proportional to the experience of the cytologist reading the specimen. Further staging of the head and neck is possible using the imaging techniques of computed tomography and magnetic resonance imaging. These techniques now allow the identification of small nodes that may be undetectable clinically.

D To complete staging of oral cavity carcinoma in some patients, direct laryngoscopy, bronchoscopy, nasal pharyngoscopy, or esophagoscopy may be necessary. Synchronous head and neck cancers are found in 10 percent of cases.

E Carcinoma of the oral cavity 2 cm or less in diameter with no nodal involvement (stage I) can be treated effectively with either surgery or radiotherapy. Each modality has an equal chance of success and the choice of treatment is based on factors such as patient availability, acceptability, and functional results. Adequate operative excision includes removal of a cuff of 2 cm of normal tissue around the lesion. If the resulting defect would cause a functional problem, radiotherapy should be considered. Both external and interstitial radiation are available. For stage I intraoral carcinoma, an interstitial implant is all that is necessary.

F A stage II carcinoma of the oral cavity is a tumor that is 2 to 4 cm in greatest diameter with no evidence of neck node metastasis. If the neoplasm can be adequately excised without a significant functional defect, either surgery or radiotherapy can be offered. Because there is a higher incidence of neck node metastasis than in stage I disease, either radiotherapy to the neck or radical neck dissection is required. An indication of tumor aggressiveness can be obtained by observing the growth pattern of exophytic or ulcerative lesions and by determining histologic differentiation. The incidence of neck node involvement is much higher with an undifferentiated neoplasm.

G Stage III carcinoma of the floor of the mouth is a tumor larger than 4 cm in diameter with neck node involvement. Because this is advanced disease, neck nodes must be treated. Two or three courses of preoperative chemotherapy with cisplatin and 5-FU are sometimes advisable. After this, primary excision of the tumor and neck dissection must be accomplished. Radiotherapy may be given postoperatively. When the tumor is large, one must consider the patient's quality of life before beginning a resection that will leave significant functional and cosmetic defects.

H Stage IV carcinoma is 4 cm or larger and invades a contiguous structure. Neck nodes are positive. Preoperative chemotherapy with cisplatin and 5-FU is advisable. Resection is followed by radiotherapy. The final quality of life is important and the patient should be advised of what to expect after this treatment.

I A benefit of chemotherapy in terms of extending life expectancy has not been proven. Further study is necessary to confirm the significance of chemotherapy in combined modality treatment. Preoperative and preradiation therapy with chemotherapy results in reduced tumor bulk in many patients. This makes treatment easier.

J The overall cure rate of oral cavity carcinoma is 60 to 65 percent. Results are excellent in

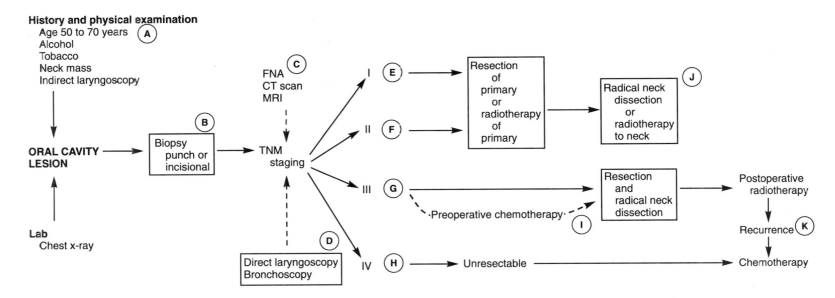

stage I and stage II cancers and disappointing in stage III and stage IV disease.

(K) Chemotherapy is a palliative treatment for advanced oral cavity cancer that cannot be resected without creating disabling functional defects. It is also used for recurrence of carcinoma after resection and irradiation.

REFERENCES

Applebaum EL, Callins WP, Bytell DE. Carcinoma of the floor of the mouth. Arch Otolaryngol 1980; 106:419–421.

Berktold RE: Carcinoma of the oral cavity: Selective Management according to site and stage. Otolaryngol Clin North Am 1985; 18(3):445–450.

Collins S, Spector GJ: Cancer of the oral cavity, oropharynx, and pharynx. In Ballenger JJ, ed. Diseases of the Nose, Throat, Ear, Head, and Neck, 13th ed. Philadelphia: Lea & Febiger, 1985, pp 603–691.

Edstrom S, Beran M, Ejnell H, et al. Aspects of treatment principles of tongue carcinomas. ORL 1981; 43:5–55.

Gelinas M, Blondeau F. Cancer of the oral cavity. J Otolaryngol 1981; 10:17–22.

Lore JM Jr. An atlas of head and neck surgery. Vol 2. Philadelphia: WB Saunders, 1973:487–520.

Silver CE, Nadler B, Croft CB. Oral and oropharyngeal carcinoma. Arch Otolaryngol 1978; 104:278–281.

Symposium on malignant disease of the oral cavity and related structures. Otolaryngol Clin North Am 1979; 12:3–255.

Parotid Tumor

John J. Coleman, III, M.D., and M. J. Jurkiewicz, M.D.

(A) A parotid neoplasm must be differentiated from diffuse enlargement due to systemic diseases such as

- Mumps
- Sjögren syndrome
- Alcoholism
- Sarcoidosis (6 percent)
- Lymphoma.

(B) Malignancy is suggested by a fixed hard mass with facial nerve deficit and palpable regional lymph nodes. Most malignant neoplasms, however, present as solitary, firm, asymptomatic nodules.

(C) Nerve weakness accompanies 8 to 33 percent of malignant parotid tumors. Pain occurs in 5.1 percent. Both are signs of poor prognosis.

(D) Parotid tumors of the deep lobe, particularly large pleomorphic adenomas, may present as oropharyngeal masses. Inspection and palpation of the oropharynx are important.

(E) Sialography may be helpful in detecting parotid stones.

(F) Warthin's tumor and oncocytoma concentrate technetium 99m.

(G) Fine-needle aspiration cytology may be useful in distinguishing between benign and malignant masses. In a recent series, 32 of 33 benign masses and 11 of 13 malignant masses were correctly predicted.

(H) Preoperative clinical evaluation is about 70 percent accurate in predicting benignity. About 80 percent of parotid tumors are benign,

and of these 75 percent are in the superficial lobe. Benign tumors include

Pleomorphic adenoma, 80 percent
Monomorphic adenoma, 1 to 4 percent
Warthin tumor, 10 percent
Oncocytoma, 1 percent.

(I) Eighty percent of malignant tumors are in the superficial lobe.

(J) Tumors of low-grade malignancy include

- Acinic cell adenocarcinoma
- Mucoepidermoid carcinoma, low or intermediate grade.

(K) Tumors of high-grade malignancy include

- Mucoepidermoid carcinoma, high grade
- Undifferentiated tumors
- Squamous cell carcinoma
- Malignant mixed tumors
- Adenocarcinoma, high grade
- Adenoid cystic carcinoma.

(L) Treatment for all benign tumors is parotidectomy with facial nerve preservation. Since 75 percent are in the superficial lobe of the parotid, superficial lobectomy is adequate in these. Conservative total parotidectomy should be performed for the 20 percent in the deep lobe. Simple enucleation is inadequate therapy because of the high incidence of recurrence. Superficial parotidectomy with facial nerve preservation is curative in 95 to 99 percent of cases of benign mixed tumors of the superficial lobe and is the first step in excision of questionably

malignant tumors. Frozen section has a high degree of accuracy in differentiating malignant from benign tumors. The risk of temporary damage to nerve VII is 20 percent; the risk of permanent injury is 2 percent. In temporary nerve damage, return of function is usually seen within 3 months.

(M) Treatment of low-grade malignant neoplasms is by conservative total parotidectomy or superficial parotidectomy if the tumor is localized to the superficial lobe and the frozen section shows clear margins.

(N) Operative treatment is total or conservative parotidectomy and cervical lymphadenectomy for all tumors except adenocarcinoma and adenoid cystic carcinoma, both of which commonly metastasize to the lung. High-grade tumors should receive adjuvant radiotherapy.

(O) Survival after recurrence is rare, but the course of the disease may be prolonged. Recurrence is usually manifested with both local and distant disease (80 percent). In the occasional patient who has a resectable local recurrence alone, operation and irradiation should be used. Radiation alone may be palliative but is rarely effective in curing recurrence.

(P) A benign tumor that recurs locally should be reexcised and confirmed with frozen and permanent sections. The facial nerve should be preserved when possible. Reexcision of all gross tumor has an 80 percent success rate.

(Q) Adjuvant radiotherapy of the parotid bed and skull base is important in the treatment of

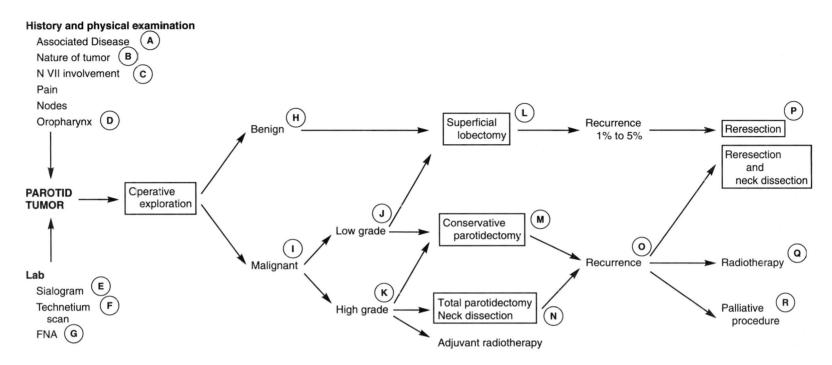

History and physical examination
Associated Disease (A)
Nature of tumor (B)
N VII involvement (C)
Pain
Nodes
Oropharynx (D)

PAROTID TUMOR

Lab
Sialogram (E)
Technetium scan (F)
FNA (G)

Benign (H)
Superficial lobectomy (L)
Recurrence 1% to 5%
Reresection (P)

Reresection and neck dissection

Operative exploration

Malignant (I)
Low grade (J)
Conservative parotidectomy (M)
Recurrence (O)
Radiotherapy (Q)

High grade (K)
Total parotidectomy Neck dissection (N)
Palliative procedure (R)

Adjuvant radiotherapy

adenoid cystic carcinoma because of the high incidence of perineural invasion. The negligible survival rate associated with recurrent parotid neoplasms recommends adjuvant radiotherapy in all adenoid cystic, undifferentiated, adenocarcinoma, and high-grade mucoepidermoid tumors. Histologic evidence of perineural invasion, facial nerve weakness, and cervical metastases are indications for adjuvant radiotherapy, although no well-controlled prospective trials have been carried out. Radiotherapy as a definitive treatment for parotid neoplasms is not usually employed.

(R) Invasion of the base of the skull with concomitant pain may be treated by trigeminal nerve section and tarsorrhaphy for exposure keratitis.

Although an occasional parotid neoplasm responds to chemotherapy, the inexorable course of the recurrent disease makes significant palliation unlikely. At present there is no good indication for chemotherapy.

REFERENCES

Batsakis JG. Tumors of the head and neck, clinical and pathological consideration. 2nd ed. Baltimore: Williams & Wilkins, 1979:1–76.

Conley J, Clairmont AA. Facial nerve in recurrent benign pleomorphic adenoma. Arch Otolaryngol 1979;105:247–251.

Conley J, Hamaker RC. Prognosis of malignant tumors of the parotid gland with facial paralysis. Arch Otolaryngol 1975;101:39–41.

Eneroth CM, Hanberger CA. Principles of treatment of different types of parotid tumors. Laryngoscope 1974;84:1732.

Hodgkinson DJ, Woods JE. The influence of facial nerve sacrifice in surgery of malignant parotid tumors. J Surg Oncol 1976;8:325–432.

Johns ME. Parotid cancer: a rational basis for treatment. Head Neck Surg 1980;3:132–144.

Kagan AR, Nussbaum H, Handler S, et al. Recurrences from malignant parotid salivary gland tumors. Cancer 1976; 37:2600–2604.

Perzik SL, Fisher B. The place of neck dissection in the management of parotid tumors. Am J Surg 1970;120:355–358.

Rankow RM, Polayes IM. Diseases of the salivary glands. Philadelphia: WB Saunders, 1976:343–355.

Rodriguez HP, Silver EC, Masa II, et al. Fine needle aspiration of parotid tumors. Am J Surg 1989;158:341–344.

Neck Mass

Thomas Eyen, M.D., and Arlen Meyers, M.B.A., M.D.

(A) A persistent firm lump in the neck is usually metastatic cancer and originates from a primary tumor above the clavicle.

(B) Excision of neoplastic parotid lesions is often recommended regardless of preoperative cytologic determination of malignancy. Parotid fine-needle aspiration can be used effectively for diagnosis and treatment planning and is recommended preoperatively. Experienced pathologists can diagnosis cancer with sensitivities and specificities of greater than 90 percent.

(C) In 5 to 8 percent of patients with squamous cell cancer in a neck node, no primary tumor site is found. Treatment (neck dissection vs. waiting for a primary to appear) remains controversial.

(D) A tender neck mass strongly suggests infection. The primary site should be drained and cultures obtained. If the mass persists for 4 weeks despite antibiotic treatment, it should be excised.

(E) Most midline neck masses that occur in children are congenital and benign. They include

- Thyroglossal duct cyst
- Pyramidal lobe of thyroid
- Dermoid cyst
- Sebaceous cyst.

(F) Submental and submaxillary nodes are frequently palpable in normal people as a result of chronic facial infections. Clinical judgment is required to differentiate an inflammatory from a metastatic node in patients with carcinoma of the lip, buccal mucosa, or floor of mouth.

(G) Supraclavicular nodes are usually either lymphoma or metastases from cancer of the breast, lung, pancreas, or stomach (Virchow node). Biopsy is indicated if the primary is not evident.

(H) Preference for node excision or aspiration biopsy vs. random biopsy of the nasopharynx, tongue, and pyriform sinus is controversial. If a node is excised, the skin incision should be placed so that it will fall within the specimen of a subsequent neck node dissection.

(I) Evaluation of a neck mass gives a reliable diagnosis in only 30 percent of patients. Needle aspiration biopsy is 90 to 95 percent accurate if cells are examined by an experienced pathologist. Fine-needle aspiration is rapidly replacing excisional biopsy as a first-line procedure in the diagnosis of lumps. Fine-needle aspiration can be done under local anesthesia on an ambulatory basis.

(J) Metastatic squamous cell carcinoma frequently responds to both radiation and chemotherapy for palliation. Lymphoma often responds to radiation.

(K) When the primary cancer is in the neck and the mass is a local metastasis, excision of the primary tumor with en bloc resection of the regional nodes can be curative. Adjunctive radiation or chemotherapy is usually advisable.

REFERENCES

Feldman PS, Kaplan MJ, Johns ME. Fine needle aspiration in squamous cell carcinoma of the head and neck. Arch Otolaryngol 1983; 109:735–742.

Frable MA, Frable WJ. Fine needle aspiration biopsy revisited. Laryngoscope 1982; 92:1414–1418.

Frakle WJ, Frable MA. Thin needle aspiration biopsy in the diagnosis of head and neck tumors. Laryngoscope 1974; 84:1069–1077.

Lindberg RD. Distribution of cervical lymph node metastases from squamous cell carcinoma of upper respiratory and digestive tracts. Cancer 1972; 29:1446–1454.

MacComb WS. Metastatic cervical nodes of unknown primary origin. Cancer 1974; 24:229–232.

Winegar LK, Griffin W. The occult primary tumor. Arch Otolaryngol 1973; 98:159–163.

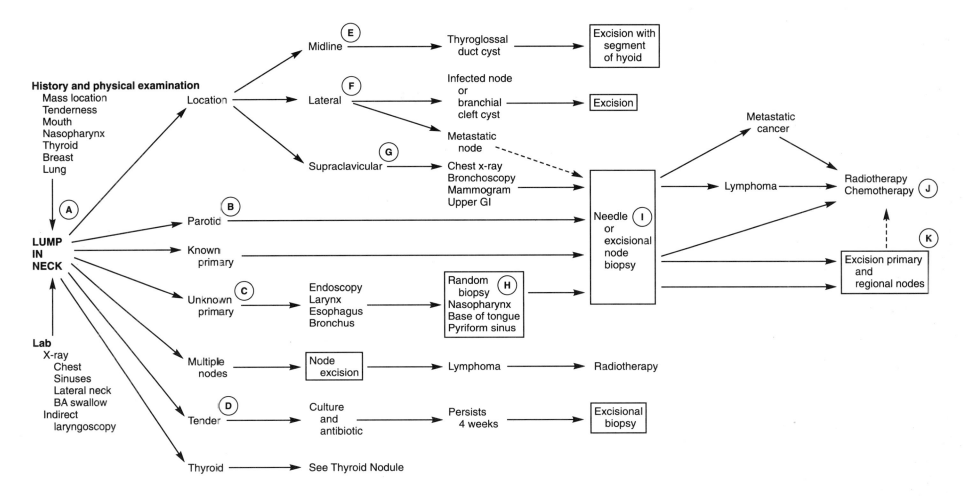

History and physical examination
Mass location
Tenderness
Mouth
Nasopharynx
Thyroid
Breast
Lung

(A)

**LUMP
IN
NECK**

Lab
X-ray
Chest
Sinuses
Lateral neck
BA swallow
Indirect
laryngoscopy

Location

Midline (E) → Thyroglossal duct cyst → Excision with segment of hyoid

Lateral (F) → Infected node or branchial cleft cyst → Excision

→ Metastatic node

Supraclavicular (G) → Chest x-ray Bronchoscopy Mammogram Upper GI

Parotid (B)

Known primary

Unknown primary (C) → Endoscopy Larynx Esophagus Bronchus → Random biopsy Nasopharynx Base of tongue Pyriform sinus (H)

Multiple nodes → Node excision → Lymphoma → Radiotherapy

Tender (D) → Culture and antibiotic → Persists 4 weeks → Excisional biopsy

Thyroid → See Thyroid Nodule

Needle or excisional node biopsy (I) → Metastatic cancer → Radiotherapy Chemotherapy (J)

→ Lymphoma →

Excision primary and regional nodes (K)

Carcinoma of the Larynx

Nathan W. Pearlman, M.D.

(A) The goal of treatment of laryngeal cancer is control or cure with preservation of as much voice as possible. Because surgery is often used to salvage radiation failures and total laryngectomy is used for failures of lesser resections, many patients live long enough to develop a second head and neck primary tumor. For this reason, results of a given approach are often expressed in terms of eventual control at the treated site. Cure of the patient at 5 years means something else. This explains the use of the terms "control" and "cure" in the paragraphs that follow.

(B) Cancer of the vocal cords arises in a smaller space than supraglottic cancer and tends to cause symptoms (hoarseness) earlier than the latter, which often remains symptomless until it spreads to the pharynx (otalgia), base of tongue (dysphagia), or neck nodes.

(C) Proper staging requires knowledge of vocal cord mobility. This is best determined by examining the awake patient either with a mirror or a fiberoptic laryngoscope.

(D) Computed tomography and magnetic resonance imaging detect cartilage and soft tissue invasion better than laryngograms or tomograms and, to a large extent, have supplanted the latter.

(E) CO_2 laser ablation or excision controls 90 to 95 percent of in situ and superficially invasive carcinomas limited to the midportion of the vocal cord. Treatment is outpatient, preserves the voice, and can be used more than once should the patient develop a second head and neck cancer (20 to 30 percent chance). Morbidity and mortality are essentially rare. Approximate cost for surgery, anesthesia, and use of the laser and operating/recovery room is currently $3000.

(F) Radiotherapy can be used for all stages of vocal cord cancer. Surgery is reserved for treatment failure. Radiotherapy preserves normal or near-normal voice in most patients. Control rates are 90 to 100 percent for Tis and T1NO lesions, 70 percent for T2NO disease, and 50 to 60 percent for T3NO cancers. Control falls off to a range of 20 to 40 percent when the anterior commissure or thyroid cartilage is invaded. Treatment is outpatient, lasts 6 to 7 weeks, and requires a reliable patient. It has a mortality of essentially zero. The major morbidity is acute or chronic pharyngitis, which is poorly tolerated by chronic alcoholics and persistent smokers and causes some to stop treatment before completion. The approximate cost of radiotherapy, treatment planning, and simulation and facility charges is currently $7500 to $8500.

(G) Vertical partial laryngectomy is suitable for tumors involving one cord, adjacent cartilage, the anterior commissure, and up to 20 to 30 percent of the contralateral cord. Control rates are about 90 percent for T1NO lesions, 80 percent for T2NO disease, and 60 percent for T3NO cancers; recurrences require total laryngectomy. The voice after partial laryngectomy is coarse, breathy, and inferior to that after radiotherapy. Inpatient treatment time is 10 to 14 days. Mortality is 1 to 2 percent. The major morbidity is chronic aspiration (15 to 20 percent), which is poorly tolerated by elderly patients and those with chronic lung disease or neurologic disorders. Such patients are poor candidates for the procedure. The approximate cost for surgery, anesthesia, operating/recovery room, and postoperative hospitalization is currently $11,000.

(H) Total laryngectomy can be used for all stages of laryngeal cancer but at the cost of voice loss. It is usually reserved for tumors too advanced for partial laryngectomy or irradiation and for failures of the latter. Control rates are 60 to 70 percent for T3NO lesions and 40 to 50 percent for T4NO disease. Recurrences require extensive surgery plus irradiation. Mortality is 2 to 3 percent. Morbidity (10 to 30 percent) includes fistulae, pneumonia, cardiac complications, and central nervous system problems. Treatment time is 2 to 3 weeks as an inpatient. The approximate cost is currently $14,000 to $15,000.

(I) Neck dissection is recommended for clinically negative (NO) necks that have more than a 20 percent chance of harboring occult metastases (T3-4 vocal cord cancers, T2-4 supraglottic tumors) and for all clinically positive (N+) necks. Cure, as opposed to control, is reduced to 40 to 50 percent when histologic micrometastases are found, regardless of primary size, and 30 to 35 percent when macrometastases are present. Neck dissection has less than 1 percent mortality and 10 percent morbidity (flap separation, infection) when combined with laryngectomy; it adds about $1000 to the cost of treatment.

(J) Horizontal (subtotal) partial laryngectomy is suitable for lesions of the epiglottis, aryepiglottic folds, false cords, and portions of the pyriform sinus. Control rates are about 80 percent for T1-T2NO lesions. Larger tumors require total laryngectomy. A voice is preserved, but it is coarser than that after radiotherapy. Aspiration is a greater problem than after vertical hemilaryngectomy. It may require total laryngectomy for control, thus limiting indications for the procedure. Mortality is 2 percent, and morbidity (aspiration, fistulae) is 30 to 40 percent. Treatment time and cost are somewhat greater than for total laryngectomy.

(K) As with vocal cord tumors, radiotherapy can be used for all stages of supraglottic cancer. A voice can be preserved in many patients. Surgery is reserved for treatment failure. Control rates are 70 to 90 percent for T1-T2NO lesions, 50 to 60 percent for T3NO tumors, and 30 percent for T4NO disease. Radiotherapy can be used in lieu of surgery for treatment of the neck. Control rates are about 95 percent for negative necks and 70

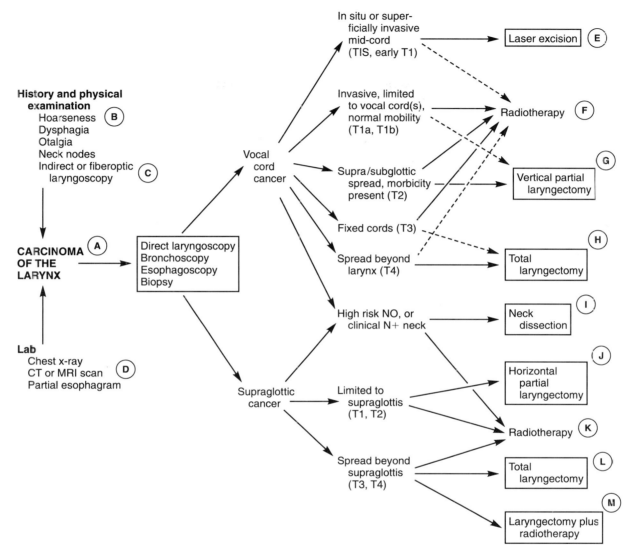

In situ or super-
ficially invasive
mid-cord
(TIS, early T1) → Laser excision Ⓔ

Invasive, limited
to vocal cord(s),
normal mobility
(T1a, T1b) → Radiotherapy Ⓕ

History and physical
examination Ⓑ
Hoarseness
Dysphagia
Otalgia
Neck nodes
Indirect or fiberoptic
laryngoscopy Ⓒ

Vocal
cord
cancer

Supra/subglottic
spread, morbidity
present (T2)

Vertical partial
laryngectomy Ⓖ

CARCINOMA Ⓐ
OF THE
LARYNX

Direct laryngoscopy
Bronchoscopy
Esophagoscopy
Biopsy

Fixed cords (T3)

Spread beyond
larynx (T4) → Total
laryngectomy Ⓗ

High risk NO, or
clinical N+ neck → Neck
dissection Ⓘ

Lab
Chest x-ray
CT or MRI scan Ⓓ
Partial esophagram

Supraglottic
cancer

Limited to
supraglottis
(T1, T2) → Horizontal
partial
laryngectomy Ⓙ

Radiotherapy Ⓚ

Spread beyond
supraglottis
(T3, T4) → Total
laryngectomy Ⓛ

Laryngectomy plus
radiotherapy Ⓜ

percent for positive disease if nodes are less than 3 cm. Bulkier disease requires a neck dissection. Treatment time and costs are similar to those for radiation for vocal cord cancer.

Ⓛ Total laryngectomy of supraglottic cancer is usually limited to advanced disease. Control rates are 50 to 60 percent for T3NO lesion and 20 to 30 percent for T4NO disease. Treatment time, costs, and morbidity and mortality are similar to those of total laryngectomy for vocal cord cancer.

Ⓜ Because results of surgery and radiotherapy alone are poor for advanced laryngeal cancer, both modalities are usually combined for such disease. Using this approach, cure rates improve to about 50 percent for stage IV disease (T4 NX, TX N2-3). Treatment time and cost nearly double with combined therapy, but morbidity and mortality are not much greater than with single modality treatment.

REFERENCES

McQuarrie DG, Adams GL, Shons AR, Browne GA. Head and neck cancer: clinical decisions and management principles. Chicago: Year Book Medical Publishers, 1986.
Mendenhall WM, Parsons JT, Stringer SP, et al. The role of radiation therapy in laryngeal cancer. CA 1990; 43:150–165.
Million RR, Cassisi NJ. Management of head and neck cancer: multidisciplinary approach. Philadelphia: JB Lippincott, 1984.
Rice DH, Spiro RH. Current concepts in head and neck cancer. American Cancer Society, 1989.
Silver CE, Moisa II. The role of surgery in the treatment of laryngeal cancer. CA 1990; 40:134–149.

Cardiopulmonary

Chest Injury

Alan Hopeman, M.D.

(A) Unless cervical spine injury can be excluded with certainty, nasotracheal intubation should be used to avoid cord injury by neck motion.

(B) At least two large-bore intravenous catheters must be inserted in a patient with serious injury to the chest. One should be a central line (internal jugular or subclavian) to permit monitoring of central venous pressure.

(C) Chest tubes are inserted for radiographic or physical evidence of hemothorax or pneumothorax. One or more size 36 to 40 French tubes are placed through the fifth or sixth intercostal space in the midaxillary line after finger inspection confirms that the pleural space and not the abdomen has been entered. After blunt injury, tubes should be inserted bilaterally if no breath sounds can be heard.

(D) Cardiorespiratory arrest after chest trauma is best treated by open cardiac massage performed through a left anterior thoracotomy. Access to the heart is gained by incising the pericardium vertically anterior to the phrenic nerve. Thoracotomy can be extended across the sternum to increase exposure. Injuries to the heart are controlled by finger pressure, clamps, balloon catheters, or sutures.

(E) Cardiac tamponade is characterized by shock, distended neck veins, and elevated central venous pressure. Pericardiocentesis is performed by aiming a large-bore needle from the left paraxiphoid area toward the left shoulder. If fluid is aspirated from the pericardium and the patient improves, operation through a median sternotomy is done promptly to repair a cardiac wound. If no improvement occurs, immediate left thoracotomy or subxiphoid pericardiotomy is performed. The presence of tamponade improves survival after a penetrating heart wound.

(F) Severe flail chest may require ventilation for several days. Oxygen and pain relief by intercostal nerve blocks or narcotics are sufficient for mild flail chest. Serial blood gas values are used to determine the need for ventilation or occasional operative stabilization of the chest wall.

(G) Clinical diagnosis of a ruptured diaphragm is difficult, especially with associated intrathoracic injury. Chest radiography is the best initial imaging tool but is normal in 20 to 50 percent of patients. Once herniation of abdominal contents occurs, x-rays should demonstrate the presence of stomach or small bowel in the chest. Barium enema should be done if this study is negative. Delayed presentation of a ruptured diaphragm is common. Diagnostic peritoneal lavage is positive in most cases, dictating laparotomy with examination of the entire diaphragmatic surface.

(H) Hemoptysis, pneumothorax with a large air leak, and mediastinal emphysema suggest tracheal or bronchial rupture. The rent usually is within 1 to 2 cm of the carina. A long cuffed endotracheal tube of the smallest acceptable size allows the normal lung to be ventilated while the damaged bronchus is sutured. Exposure of the proximal bronchus of both the right and left lungs is best done through a right thoracotomy.

(I) The usual site of aortic rupture is at the aortic isthmus. Other sites are the base of the innominate artery and the descending aorta. Mediastinal widening, multiple fractures of upper ribs on the left, an apical cap on the left lung, and deviation of the esophagus to the right are signs of rupture of the isthmus. An aortogram is done if bleeding is not life threatening. Contrast computed tomographic scanning is less sensitive and specific than aortography but is apt to be more available. Intraarterial digital subtraction angiography is faster than conventional aortography. It requires less contrast and smaller catheters.

(J) Pulmonary lacerations usually stop bleeding if the pleural space is drained adequately and the lung expands to the chest wall. Hemostasis is aided by low pulmonary blood pressure and large amounts of thromboplastin in lung tissue. Continued arterial bleeding may be from intercostal or internal mammary vessels. A rare source of bleeding from chest tubes is intraabdominal injury with a ruptured diaphragm.

(K) A small esophageal tear detected early may be sutured successfully. Pleural space drainage is mandatory. Tenuous closures in the distal esophagus can be protected with a gastric wrap. Temporary cervical esophagostomy prevents continued soiling from an esophageal leak until healing occurs.

(L) Cardiac contusion is suggested by electrocardiographic changes showing pericarditis or ischemia. A sensitive, noninvasive means of determining the extent of contusion is first-pass biventricular radionuclide angiography. This assesses ventricular segmental wall motion. Patients with large contusions need Swan-Ganz catheter monitoring of left ventricular filling pressure to prevent overloading during resuscitation. Treatment is largely passive and includes bed rest, monitoring, and fluid restriction.

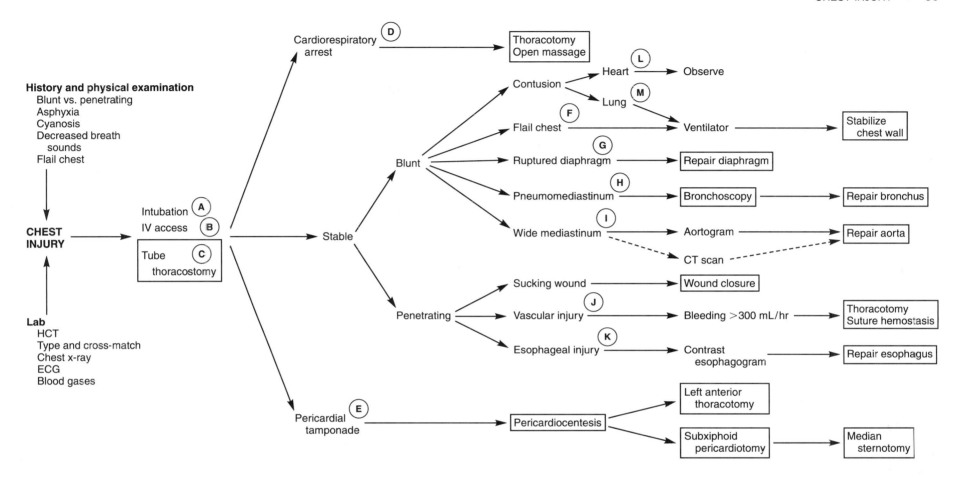

History and physical examination
Blunt vs. penetrating
Asphyxia
Cyanosis
Decreased breath
sounds
Flail chest

CHEST
INJURY

Lab
HCT
Type and cross-match
Chest x-ray
ECG
Blood gases

Intubation (A)
IV access (B)
Tube (C)
thoracostomy

Cardiorespiratory arrest — (D) — Thoracotomy Open massage

Stable

Blunt
Contusion — Heart — (L) — Observe
Contusion — Lung — (M)
Flail chest — (F) — Ventilator — Stabilize chest wall
Ruptured diaphragm — (G) — Repair diaphragm
Pneumomediastinum — (H) — Bronchoscopy — Repair bronchus
Wide mediastinum — (I) — Aortogram — Repair aorta
Wide mediastinum --- CT scan --- Repair aorta

Penetrating
Sucking wound — Wound closure
Vascular injury — (J) — Bleeding >300 mL/hr — Thoracotomy Suture hemostasis
Esophageal injury — (K) — Contrast esophagogram — Repair esophagus

Pericardial tamponade — (E) — Pericardiocentesis
Pericardiocentesis — Left anterior thoracotomy
Pericardiocentesis — Subxiphoid pericardiotomy — Median sternotomy

(M) Pulmonary contusion often can be managed with oxygen and fluid restriction. A ventilator is used if serial blood gas determinations indicate hypoxia or hypercarbia.

REFERENCES

Beall A, Gasior R, Bricker D: Gunshot wounds of the heart—changing patterns of surgical management. Ann Thorac Surg 1971; 11:523–531.

Bladergroen MR, Lowe JE, Postlethwait RW: Diagnosis and recommended management of esophageal perforation and rupture. Ann Thorac Surg 1986; 42:235–239.

Harley D, Mena I, Narahara K, et al: Traumatic myocardial dysfunction. J Thorac Cardiovasc Surg 1984; 87:336–393.

Menguy R: Near total esophageal exclusion by cervical esophagostomy and tube gastrostomy in the management of massive esophageal perforation. Ann Surg 1971; 173:613–616.

Moreno C, Moore E, Majure J, et al: Pericardial tamponade—a critical determinant for survival following penetrating cardiac wounds. J Trauma 1986; 26:821–825.

Morgan A, Flancbaum L, Esposito T, et al: Blunt injury to the diaphragm: an analysis of 44 patients. J Trauma 1986; 26:565–568.

Saber W, Moore E, Hopeman A, et al. Delayed presentation of traumatic diaphragmatic hernia. J Emerg Med 1986; 4:1–7.

Trinkle J, Toon R, Franz J, et al: Affairs of the wounded heart: penetrating cardiac wounds. J Trauma 1979; 19:467–472.

Turney S, Rodriguez A, Cowley R: Management of cardiothoracic trauma. Baltimore: Williams & Wilkins, 1990.

Pulmonary Embolism

W. Randolph Chitwood, Jr., M.D., and David C. Sabiston, Jr., M.D.

(A) Most clinically significant pulmonary emboli originate from either iliac or femoral deep venous thrombosis. Although fibrinogen scanning, plethysmography, and venous Doppler studies are valuable screening tests for deep venous thrombosis, the definitive diagnosis is established by venography. Major predisposing factors for deep venous thrombosis and pulmonary emboli include congestive heart failure, malignancy, prolonged bed rest, trauma, oral contraceptives, advanced age, previous pelvic or lower extremity surgery, previous thrombophlebitis or pulmonary embolism, pregnancy, and obesity.

(B) The most frequent presenting symptoms include dyspnea (75 percent), chest pain (65 percent), hemoptysis (25 percent), and altered mental status (20 percent). Common physical findings include tachycardia (60 percent), fever (45 percent), rales (40 percent), and tachypnea (40 percent).

(C) Pulmonary embolism occurs frequently after surgery. Both operative mortality and hospital costs are altered greatly by this complication. The expense of hospitalization may be more than doubled by a major thromboembolic event. In many hospitals, pulmonary embolism adds more than $10,000 to the charges of a major surgical procedure. Effective prophylaxis and rapid diagnosis and treatment are important for both patient and cost benefit.

(D) Chest x-ray ($100) is often nondiagnostic. It may demonstrate diminished pulmonary vascularity. Segmental or lobar parenchymal disease precludes the use of radioactive scanning techniques for diagnosis. With a clear chest x-ray, pulmonary scanning is often the first definitive

assessment. Only 10 to 20 percent of patients show electrocardiographic changes suggestive of pulmonary embolism. The electrocardiogram ($45) may show rhythm disturbances, T wave and ST segment changes, and P wave enlargement. It is often unhelpful. Arterial blood gases ($55) usually show a low PAO_2 and are helpful in establishing the diagnosis (90 percent). In 10 to 15 percent of patients with a pulmonary embolus, PAO_2 values exceed 80 mmHg.

(E) Unstable hemodynamics imply cardiovascular collapse.

(F) A normal ventilation–perfusion lung scan ($750) performed within 48 hours of symptoms usually excludes pulmonary embolism. A scan suggesting high probability of embolism is accurate in over 90 percent of patients. Segmental and lobar defects caused by pneumonia, neoplasm, and other infiltrates may obviate its use. Diffuse symmetric bilateral pulmonary disease does not preclude using radioactive lung scans for diagnosis.

(G) Vigorous medical monitoring and therapy are necessary to resuscitate patients who are hemodynamically unstable after a large embolus. Swan-Ganz pulmonary arterial monitoring is used ($300). β-Agonists including dopamine, dobutamine, and epinephrine are usually infused. A need for vasoactive alpha agents suggests profound hemodynamic collapse. Pulmonary arterial vasodilators are usually ineffective.

(H) Persistent and refractory hypotension despite maximal pharmacologic and respiratory support, in the presence of documented pulmonary emboli, is an indication for either acute pulmonary embolectomy or thrombolytic therapy. Support by

femorofemoral arteriovenous partial bypass may be helpful until definitive operation. Percutaneous cardiopulmonary bypass techniques can rapidly establish extracorporeal circulatory support before the patient reaches the operating room.

(I) Pulmonary angiography ($1400) is still considered the definitive test (over 95 percent accuracy) for elucidating pulmonary emboli. It should be done within 24 to 72 hours of onset of symptoms. Resolution of emboli begins early and extends to 21 days after the event. Elevation in mean pulmonary artery pressure and levels of hypoxemia correlate linearly with the degree of acute pulmonary embolic vascular obstruction.

(J) Patients with a demonstrable pulmonary embolus should be anticoagulated immediately with heparin (10,000-unit bolus followed by continuous drip therapy at a rate of 800 to 1200 U/hr). Activated partial thromboplastin times are used to regulate heparin. A therapeutic level is 2 to 2.5 times control level. A higher initial dose of heparin has been advocated. Intravenous heparin is maintained for 2 weeks, after which warfarin therapy is begun and continued for a minimum of 6 weeks. Throughout heparin therapy, bed rest with leg elevation above the atrial level is maintained. The cost of a 3-day ICU stay and the remaining care in a monitored hospital bed (11 days) currently adds approximately $7000 to charges.

(K) Bilateral pulmonary embolectomy requires cardiopulmonary bypass. Unilateral pulmonary arterial embolectomy can be done when extracorporeal circulation is not available. Survival of patients undergoing acute embolectomy is between 40 and 70 percent. The current cost of this procedure is approximately $25,000. Some advo-

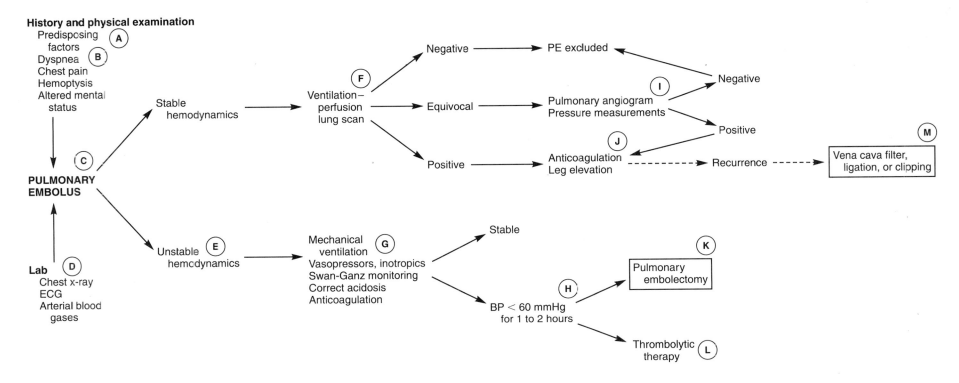

History and physical examination
Predisposing (A)
  factors
Dyspnea (B)
Chest pain
Hemoptysis
Altered mental
  status

(C)

**PULMONARY
EMBOLUS**

Lab (D)
Chest x-ray
ECG
Arterial blood
  gases

Stable
hemodynamics

Unstable (E)
hemodynamics

Ventilation–
perfusion
lung scan (F)

Mechanical (G)
ventilation
Vasopressors, inotropics
Swan-Ganz monitoring
Correct acidosis
Anticoagulation

Negative ⟶ PE excluded

Equivocal ⟶ Pulmonary angiogram
Pressure measurements

Positive ⟶ Anticoagulation
Leg elevation

(I) ⟶ Negative ⟶ PE excluded

Positive

(J)

Recurrence ⇢ Vena cava filter, (M)
ligation, or clipping

Stable

BP < 60 mmHg (H)
for 1 to 2 hours

Pulmonary (K)
embolectomy

Thrombolytic (L)
therapy

---

cate inferior vena cava interruption after an acute embolectomy.

(L) Unstable patients who are not selected as candidates for emergency embolectomy should be given thrombolytic agents systemically or by local catheter infusion. Streptokinase, urokinase, and recombinant tissue–type plasminogen can be used alone or in combination. Bleeding complications, recurrent emboli, and incomplete thrombolysis can pose problems. Costs for a loading dose and infusion of these thrombolytic agents for up to 6 hours are currently $130 (streptokinase) and $2300 (urokinase).

(M) Vena cava filter insertion may be required to prevent recurrent emboli. Newer filters can be positioned percutaneously under angiographic control. When anticoagulation is adequate, these devices are usually unnecessary. They are not uniformly successful because smaller emboli can

pass through them or emboli can propagate around the devices through collateral venous channels. Rarely, vena cava ligation or clipping is indicated. Specific indications for a filter or other caval procedure include recurrent emboli on adequate anticoagulation, heparin-induced thrombocytopenia or sensitivity, active peptic ulcer or other bleeding problems, septic emboli, pulmonary hypertension from recurrent chronic emboli, a recent neurosurgical procedure, and recent pulmonary embolectomy. A caval filtration device placed percutaneously currently adds approximately $2100 to hospital costs.

REFERENCES

Duranceau A, Jones RH, Sabiston DC Jr. The diagnosis of pulmonary embolism. Compr Ther 1976; 2:6–14.

Gray HH, Morgan JM, Paneth M, et al. Pulmonary embolectomy for acute massive pulmonary embolism: an analysis of 71 cases. Br Heart J 1988; 6:196–200.

Leeper KV, Popovich J Jr, Less BA, et al. Treatment of massive acute pulmonary embolism: the use of low doses of intrapulmonary arterial streptokinase combined with full doses of systemic heparin. Chest 1988; 93:234–240.

Lund O, Nielson TT, Rønne K, et al. Pulmonary embolism: long-term follow-up after treatment with full-dose heparin, streptokinase, or embolectomy. Acta Med Scand 1987; 221:61–71.

Maddox KL, Feldtman RW, Beall AC, et al. Pulmonary embolectomy for acute massive pulmonary embolism. Ann Surg 1982; 195:726–731.

Mills SR, Jackson DC, Older RA, et al. The incidence, etiologies, and avoidance of complications of pulmonary angiography in a large series. Radiology 1980; 136:295–299.

Newman GE, Sullivan DC, Gottschald A, et al. Scintigraphic perfusion patterns in patients with diffuse lung disease. Radiology 1982; 143:227–231.

Shawl FA, Domanski MJ, Wish MH, et al. Percutaneous cardiopulmonary bypass support in the catheterization laboratory: technique and complications. Am Heart J 1990; 120:195–203.

Silver D, Sabiston DC Jr. The role of vena caval interruption of the management of pulmonary embolism. Surgery 1975; 77:1–10.

Pleural Effusion and Empyema

Watts R. Webb, M.D.

(A) Fluid (serum, pus, blood, or chyle) in the pleural space is a sign of underlying pulmonary disease and is managed accordingly. A history of injury, thoracotomy, nonthoracic operation, thrombophlebitis, or infection may suggest the cause. Pulmonary involvement by tumor, primary or metastatic, usually produces a bloody effusion.

(B) Needle aspiration to determine whether the fluid contains blood, pus, bacteria, or tumor cells is performed if there is any doubt as to cause.

(C) Bronchoscopy is performed to exclude tumor and foreign body.

(D) Culture and smear determine the causative organism and its drug sensitivity in postpneumonic effusion and empyema.

(E) Because tuberculosis or fungal disease may produce serous pleural effusion without other evidence of disease, skin tests are performed with spontaneous effusion.

(F) Persistent postoperative drainage usually indicates incomplete lung expansion. Suction on chest tubes, physical therapy, coughing, endotracheal suctioning, and bronchoscopy expand the lung and obliterate the dead space.

(G) Postpneumonic empyema overall mortality rate is 9 to 21 percent; cure with antibiotics and thoracentesis is 15 to 20 percent.

(H) Spontaneous bloody pleural effusion suggests an embolus or malignant pleural neoplasm (usually metastatic).

(I) Tube thoracostomy allows lung reexpansion and obliteration of pleural dead space and thus avoids pleural infection (empyema). It alone is curative in 83 percent of patients with postinjury empyema.

(J) The cure rate for acute postpneumonic empyema treated with antibiotics and aspiration is about 20 percent in adults and may be as high as 85 percent in infants and children. It is 35 percent in adults who need tube drainage. If empyema is chronic (over 4 weeks in duration), 83 percent of patients need operation. Empyema after lung abscess is more difficult to treat and usually becomes chronic.

(K) The first indication of a bronchopleural fistula is coughing up serosanguineous fluid. Massive air leak and empyema may follow. Early bronchial leaks tend to correlate with technical error and late leaks with residual disease in the bronchial stump. Postthoracotomy empyema is most likely to follow resection for suppurative disease. The pleural cavity has tremendous resistance to even massive contamination unless the contamination is persistent, as with bronchial leak.

(L) Drugs for pleural symphysis (whether for malignancy, infection, or chyle) are most effective if all fluid can be completely and continuously evacuated. This usually requires tube drainage. Intrapleural talc is the most effective agent for achieving pleurodesis.

(M) Thoracoscopy can evaluate intrathoracic damage, determine the bleeding site, evacuate large clots, and allow cauterization of intercostal bleeding.

(N) Decortication releases the lung (usually completely normal) to refill the hemithorax by removing the clot with its encasing membrane (peel). Cure rate is 95 percent; mortality rate is 1 to 2 percent.

(O) Often bronchial stumps can be reclosed successfully, especially with muscle or musculoperiosteal flaps. The cure rate is 80 percent; the mortality rate is 0 to 10 percent.

(P) Postpneumonectomy empyema can be treated by dependent open drainage (rib resection and flaps), multiple daily irrigations of the cavity until clean (weeks to months), or tight closure of the cavity after instillation of a saline–antibiotic solution (cure rate, 90 to 95 percent). The addition of intrathoracic muscle transposition in resistant cases has achieved excellent results in 75 percent.

(Q) Thoracotomy to control bleeding is required in 1 to 5 percent of patients after injury.

(R) Rib resection with or without Eloesser flap is used for chronic undrained empyema. The cure rate is up to 100 percent; the mortality rate is 1 to 10 percent.

(S) Decortication or resection of empyema is preferred if significant lung tissue is trapped. This greatly reduces morbidity. The cure rate is 95 percent; the mortality rate is 5 percent.

(T) Various types of thoracoplasty close the residual space by removing overlying ribs and thickened pleura to allow the chest wall to fall in against the underlying lung. Thoracoplasty is usually of the Schede type, consisting of removal of the ribs and thick parietal pleura (cure rate, 15 percent).

(U) Resection for associated lung abscess is performed only for inadequate resolution with

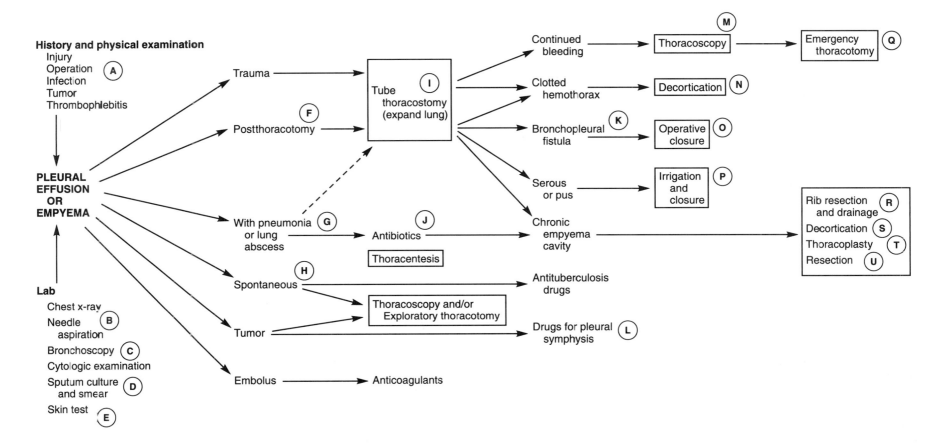

History and physical examination
Injury
Operation (A)
Infection
Tumor
Thrombophlebitis

PLEURAL EFFUSION OR EMPYEMA

Lab
Chest x-ray
Needle (B) aspiration
Bronchoscopy (C)
Cytologic examination
Sputum culture (D) and smear
Skin test (E)

Trauma

Postthoracotomy (F)

With pneumonia (G) or lung abscess

Spontaneous (H)

Tumor

Embolus

Tube thoracostomy (expand lung) (I)

Antibiotics (J)

Thoracentesis

Thoracoscopy and/or Exploratory thoracotomy

Anticoagulants

Continued bleeding

Clotted hemothorax

Bronchopleural (K) fistula

Serous or pus

Chronic empyema cavity

Antituberculosis drugs

Drugs for pleural (L) symphysis

Thoracoscopy (M)

Decortication (N)

Operative (O) closure

Irrigation and closure (P)

Emergency thoracotomy (Q)

Rib resection (R) and drainage
Decortication (S)
Thoracoplasty (T)
Resection (U)

medical therapy. The death rate, which ranges to 35 percent, is related to the pulmonary process.

REFERENCES

Arnold PG. Intrathoracic muscle flaps: a 10-year experience in the management of life threatening infections. Plast Reconstr Surg 1989; 84:92–98.

Benfield GFA. Recent trends in empyema thoracis. Br J Dis Chest 1981; 75:358–366.

Boutin JC, Velardocchio JM, Prudhomme A. Interet de la thoracoscopie. Presse Med 1984; 13:2635–2639.

Coon JL, Shuck JM. Failure of tube thoracostomy for post-traumatic empyema; an indication for early decortication. J Trauma 1975; 15:588–594.

Ferguson MK, Little AG, Skinner DB. Current concepts in the management of post-operative chylothorax. Ann Thorac Surg 1985; 40:542–545.

Hankins JR, Miller JE, Laughlin JS. The use of chest wall muscle flaps to close bronchopleural fistulas: experience with 21 patients. Ann Thorac Surg 1978; 25:491–499.

Jones JW, Kitahama A, Webb WR, et al. Emergency thoracoscopy: a logical approach to chest trauma management. J Trauma 1981; 21:280–284.

Kirby TJ, Ginsberg RJ. Role of open thoracotomy in undi-agnosed pleural diseases. In: Deslauriers J, Lacquet LK, eds. International trends in general thoracic surgery: surgical management of pleural diseases. Vol 6. St. Louis: CV Mosby, 1990:62–72.

Morrone N, Algranti E, Barreto E. Pleural biopsy with Cope and Abrams needles. Chest 1987; 92:1050–1052.

Stafford EG, Clagett OT. Postpneumonectomy empyema: neomycin instillation and definitive closure. J Thorac Cardiovasc Surg 1972; 60:771–775.

Webb WR, Ozmen V, Moulder PV, et al. Iodized talc pleurodesis for the treatment of pleural effusions. J Thorac Cardiovasc Surg 1992, in press.

Lung Abscess

Jeffrey S. Cross, M.D., and Michael R. Johnston, M.D.

A Before the middle of the 20th century, lung abscess was associated with a high mortality (30 to 70 percent) and was primarily treated surgically. With the introduction of effective antibiotics, lung abscess can now be treated nonsurgically. Medical therapy alone successfully treats 75 percent of patients, and overall mortality has decreased to 10 to 15 percent.

B Lung abscess occurs most frequently in middle-aged men with a male-to-female ratio of 3.5:1.

C A cavity with an air–fluid level seen on a standard chest x-ray is usually the first laboratory evidence of a lung abscess.

D A chest computed tomographic scan can more clearly define its extent, its relationship to the pleura, and whether other smaller cavities are present.

E For a single cavity, bronchoscopy is mandatory to exclude a bronchial obstruction. Bronchoscopy may give important information regarding endobronchial disease when multiple cavities are present.

F To best categorize lung abscesses a distinction must be made between *single* and *multiple* cavities. Aspiration of normal mouth flora and a subsequent necrotizing pneumonia are the most common cause of single lung abscesses. Predisposing factors include impaired neurologic status (alcoholism, seizure disorders, stroke, general anesthesia) and gingivodental disease. Other causes of a single abscess include obstruction from a foreign body or tumor, sequestration, and tuberculosis or fungal infections.

G Multiple cavities are most often a result of nonpulmonary disease processes. Examples include hematogenous seeding from septic thrombophlebitis, endocarditis, and intravenous drug abuse. Systemic vasculitides such as Wegener granulomatosis may also cause multiple abscesses.

H A needle aspiration biopsy may give both cytologic and bacteriologic information but risks the development of a pneumothorax and empyema.

I With multiple abscesses an *open biopsy* is often the most definitive and effective means of securing a diagnosis.

J If endocarditis is suspected, a cardiac echo should be performed. Either renal or sinus biopsies should be considered if vasculitis is suspected.

K If a foreign body is present in the airway, either endoscopic removal or open bronchotomy is necessary for resolution of the abscess.

L Treatment should be based on both the number of cavities and the bronchoscopic findings. A single cavity with no bronchial obstruction should respond to endobronchial drainage and appropriate intravenous antibiotics. Failure of a demonstrable clinical response within 2 weeks or development of a major complication should prompt exploration and resection of the involved lung.

M Tumor obstructions are diagnosed by bronchoscopy, then appropriately staged and considered for resection. With unresectable tumors, radiation therapy or laser ablation offers a good method of providing drainage and palliation.

N In treating multiple lung abscesses control of the underlying systemic disease is paramount. With effective therapy, sometimes including steroids and cytotoxic agents as well as parenteral antibiotics, the abscesses usually resolve.

O In high-risk patients, percutaneous drainage may be a reasonable approach for a large abscess but results in a more prolonged hospitalization and often incomplete resolution.

P Complications from lung abscess are similar with single or multiple cavities. An empyema occurs when an abscess ruptures into the pleural space. If the cavity communicates with a bronchus, a bronchopleural fistula will probably develop. Hemoptysis is common with lung abscess but massive hemoptysis is usually associated with an abscess caused by necrotizing pneumonia, fungal infection, or tuberculosis. Spill-over pneumonia occurs when purulent material is not effectively cleared from the bronchial tree and is aspirated into previously uninvolved lung. This is seen with very large abscesses and in patients who are either neurologically impaired or severely debilitated. It is an ominous sign. Full-blown sepsis can complicate any lung abscess and lead to multiorgan failure. Since a lung abscess is in direct vascular communication with the systemic circulation, metastatic abscesses can form in other organs, especially the brain. To avoid complications from lung abscesses, a vigorous diagnostic and treatment plan should be implemented that includes early surgical resection in immunocompromised patients and in those who do not rapidly improve with medical therapy.

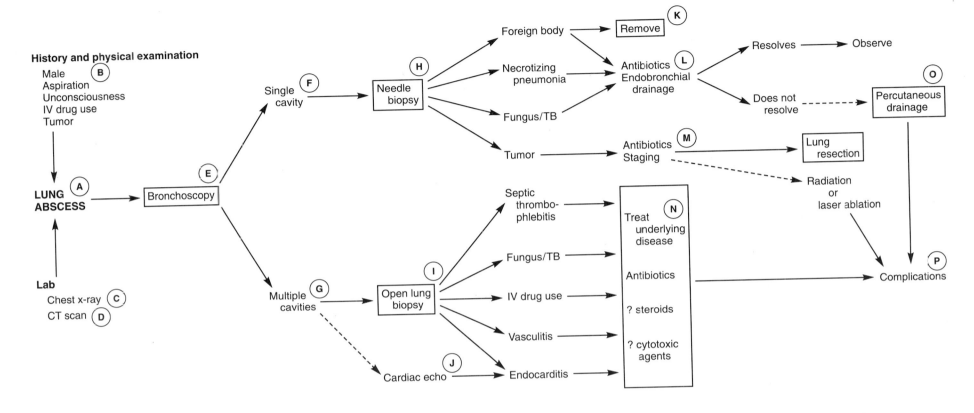

History and physical examination

Male (B)
Aspiration
Unconsciousness
IV drug use
Tumor

LUNG ABSCESS (A)

Lab

Chest x-ray (C)
CT scan (D)

Bronchoscopy (E)

Single cavity (F)

Multiple cavities (G)

Needle biopsy (H)

Open lung biopsy (I)

Cardiac echo (J)

Foreign body → Remove (K)

Necrotizing pneumonia

Fungus/TB

Tumor

Antibiotics Endobronchial drainage (L)

Resolves → Observe

Does not resolve

Antibiotics Staging (M)

Lung resection

Radiation or laser ablation

Percutaneous drainage (O)

Septic thrombophlebitis

Fungus/TB

IV drug use

Vasculitis

Endocarditis

Treat underlying disease (N)

Antibiotics

? steroids

? cytotoxic agents

Complications (P)

REFERENCES

Alexander JC, Wolfe WG. Lung abscess and empyema of the thorax. Surg Clin North Am 1980; 60:835.

Bartlett JG. Anaerobic bacterial infections of the lung. Chest 1987; 91:901–909.

Estrera SE, Platt MR, Lawrence JM, Shaw RR. Primary lung abscess. J Thorac Cardiovasc Surg 1980; 79:275–282.

Grinan NP, Lucena FM, Romero JV, et al. Yield of percutaneous needle lung aspiration in lung abscess. Chest 1990; 97:69–74.

Kaye M, Fox MJ, Bartlett JG, et al. The clinical spectrum of *Staphylococcus aureus* pulmonary infection. Chest 1990; 97:788–792.

Parker LA, Melton JW, Delany DJ, et al. Percutaneous small bore catheter drainage in the management of lung abscesses. Chest 1987; 92:213–217.

Rice TW, Ginsberg RJ, Todd TRJ. Tube drainage of lung abscesses. Ann Thorac Surg 1987; 44:356–359.

Schmitt GS, Ohar JM, Kanter KR, et al. Indwelling transbronchial catheter drainage of pulmonary abscess. Ann Thorac Surg 1988; 45:43–47.

Wilkens EW. Acute putrid abscess of the lung. Ann Thorac Surg 1987; 44:560–561.

Carcinoma of the Lung

Stephen J. Lahey, M.D.

(A) Any lung mass in a patient older than 60 years, especially one with a history of smoking, strongly favors a malignant diagnosis. In younger patients living in fungal (eg, histoplasmosis) endemic areas, further workup, such as skin testing, and careful observation are warranted.

(B) Obtaining either frequent sputum samples for cytologic screening or frequent screening chest x-rays in high-risk patients has no appreciable impact on prognosis or ultimate survival. A positive sputum cytology should prompt a diligent search for the primary lesion, since resection remains the most effective therapeutic modality for lung cancer.

(C) About 5 percent of all coin lesions less than 3 cm in size are malignant. The presence of associated symptoms (hemoptysis, pneumonic process distal to the lesion) increases the risk of malignancy incrementally.

(D) A lung mass larger than 3 cm has a high likelihood of malignancy. Efforts should be directed toward obtaining a tissue diagnosis and determining resectability.

(E) Findings on computed tomographic scan that contraindicate resection include bilaterality and major cardiac or pulmonary artery involvement.

(F) Conventional mediastinoscopy is recommended to sample all N2 nodes except those in the subaortic space, which may require the Chamberlain procedure.

(G) Although controversial, it is suggested by some that microscopic, intracapsular invasion of ipsilateral lower paratracheal (level 4) nodes with epidermoid carcinoma is not an absolute contraindication to definitive resection of the primary lung lesion.

REFERENCES

American Joint Committee on Cancer: Manual for staging of cancer. 3rd ed. Philadelphia: JB Lippincott, 1988:115–122.

Pearson FG, DeLarue NC, Ilves R, et al. Significance of positive superior mediastinal nodes identified at mediastinoscopy in patients with resectable cancer of the lung. J Thorac Cardiovasc Surg 1982; 83:1–11.

Shields TW: Carcinoma of the lung. In: Shields TW, ed. General thoracic surgery. 3rd ed. Philadelphia: Lea & Febiger, 1989:890–934.

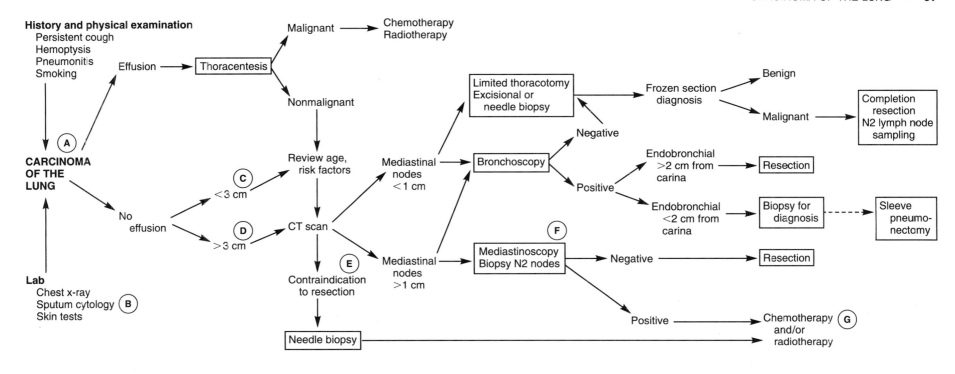

History and physical examination
Persistent cough
Hemoptysis
Pneumonitis
Smoking

CARCINOMA OF THE LUNG (A)

Lab
Chest x-ray
Sputum cytology (B)
Skin tests

Effusion → Thoracentesis → Malignant → Chemotherapy / Radiotherapy

Nonmalignant

No effusion → <3 cm (C) / >3 cm (D)

Review age, risk factors

CT scan

Contraindication to resection (E)

Mediastinal nodes <1 cm

Mediastinal nodes >1 cm

Needle biopsy

Limited thoracotomy / Excisional or needle biopsy

Bronchoscopy → Negative / Positive

Mediastinoscopy / Biopsy N2 nodes (F) → Negative / Positive

Frozen section diagnosis → Benign / Malignant

Completion resection N2 lymph node sampling

Endobronchial >2 cm from carina → Resection

Endobronchial <2 cm from carina → Biopsy for diagnosis --→ Sleeve pneumonectomy

Negative → Resection

Positive → Chemotherapy and/or radiotherapy (G)

Patent Ductus Arteriosus

Sidney Levitsky, M.D.

(A) Patent ductus arteriosus (PDA) is defined as a ductus that is patent in an infant older than 3 months. It occurs in 1 in 200 live births. Etiologic factors include maternal rubella, high-altitude environment, polygenic inheritance, prematurity, neonatal hypoxia, and respiratory distress of the newborn.

(B) A systolic thrill in the second left intercostal space or in the supersternal notch, a hyperdynamic cardiac impulse, bounding femoral pulses, and a continuous systolic–diastolic machinery murmur (the hallmark of this disease) are present. In premature infants, a systolic murmur is often heard. The intensity of this murmur varies with the state of hydration.

(C) Variations in radiologic findings depend on the magnitude of the shunt. Premature infants demonstrate increased vascular markings and mild cardiomegaly. Older children with large shunts show increased bilateral pulmonary vascular markings, enlargement of the pulmonary artery segment along the upper left cardiac border, enlargement of the left atrium and ventricle, and dilation of the aortic arch. Vigorous pulsations of the hilar vessels (hilar dance) are noted on fluoroscopy.

(D) With a small PDA, the electrocardiogram may be normal. In patients with large left-to-right shunts, there is evidence of left ventricular hypertrophy and P mitrale (left atrial enlargement).

(E) Two-dimensional echocardiography and pulsed-wave Doppler have replaced cardiac catheterization in the evaluation of PDA. Increases in left-atrial-to-aortic-root ratio are associated with a large shunt.

(F) In congenital heart disease, such as pulmonary atresia, critical pulmonary stenosis, hypoplastic right ventricle with an intact septum, interruption of the aortic arch, and hypoplastic left heart syndrome, patency of the PDA is necessary for survival. Differential diagnosis includes aortopulmonary septal defect, coronary AV fistula, pulmonary AV fistula, and a ventricular septal defect associated with aortic insufficiency.

(G) Prevention of PDA endocarditis (rarely seen in the postantibiotic era), avoidance of Eisenmenger syndrome, and congestive heart failure are major indications for operative intervention even when the patient is asymptomatic.

(H) Initial medical management includes fluid restriction, diuretics, and mechanical respiratory support. Indomethacin, a prostaglandin synthetase inhibitor, causes closure of a PDA in 75 percent of cases. The drug can be repeated after 48 hours if the ductus reopens. Contraindications to indomethacin include hepatic and renal dysfunction.

(I) Interruption of a PDA results in total cure and is associated with an operative mortality of less than 0.5 percent. For the infant less than 6 months old, ligation is preferred. For the older child, division is frequently used. Postoperative complications, including pneumothorax, bleeding, and chylous fistula, are rare.

REFERENCES

Ellison RC, Peckham GJ, Lang P, et al. Evaluation of the preterm infant for patent ductus arteriosus. Pediatrics 1983; 71:364–372.

Gersony WM, Peckham GJ, Ellison RC, et al. Effects of indomethacin in premature infants with patent ductus arteriosus: results of a national collaborative study. J Pediatr 1983; 102:895–906.

Gross RE, Hubbard JP. Surgical ligation of a patent ductus arteriosus. JAMA 1939; 112:729–731.

Keys A, Shapiro MJ. Patency of the ductus arteriosus in adults. Am Heart J 1983; 25:158–186.

Levitsky S, Fisher E, Vidyasagar D, et al. Interruption of patent ductus arteriosus in premature infants with respiratory distress syndrome. Ann Thorac Surg 1976; 22:131–137.

Mikhail M, Lee W, Toews W, et al. Surgical and medical experience with 734 premature infants with patent ductus arteriosus. J Thorac Cardiovasc Surg 1982; 83:349–357.

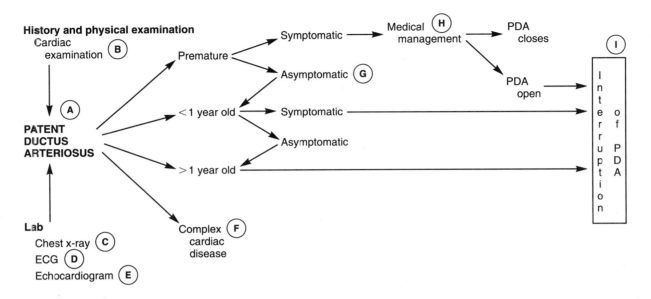

History and physical examination
  Cardiac
    examination (B)

(A)

**PATENT
DUCTUS
ARTERIOSUS**

Lab
  Chest x-ray (C)
  ECG (D)
  Echocardiogram (E)

Premature

Symptomatic → Medical (H) management → PDA closes

Asymptomatic (G)

PDA open →

<1 year old → Symptomatic

Asymptomatic

>1 year old

Complex (F) cardiac disease

Interruption of PDA (I)

Coarctation of the Aorta

James T. Anderson, M.D.

(A) Coarctation of the aorta (CA) has a 4:1 male-to-female ratio. It is a frequent accompaniment of Turner syndrome and other congenital cardiac anomalies but not of noncardiac anomalies. Symptoms in infancy usually are secondary to congestive heart failure. Patients who have no symptoms in infancy become symptomatic between ages 20 and 40 because of hypertension, endocarditis, heart failure, or stroke.

(B) Physical findings typically are a systolic murmur over the left chest, upper extremity hypertension, absence or weakening of pulses in the lower extremities, and a diagnostic pulse lag between the radial and femoral pulses.

(C) Chest x-ray at an early age is not diagnostic, showing only left ventricular hypertrophy and findings of other anomalies if present. At a later age, chest x-rays show typical rib notching secondary to developing collateral circulation. Barium swallow may show the inverted "3" sign.

(D) Noninvasive vascular studies can document diminished pulse pressures in the lower extremities.

(E) Medical therapy in infancy consists of digoxin and diuretics. If a good response is not obtained in 24 to 48 hours, right and left heart catheterization and aortography are performed before emergency surgical or angioplasty repair. An initially good response to drugs may later fail, manifested by growth retardation, chronic heart failure, or persistent severe upper body hypertension. This situation demands repair in infancy.

(F) Of infants requiring repair, 70 to 100 percent have other cardiac anomalies such as patent ductus arteriosus, 60 to 90 percent; ventricular septal defect, 50 percent; atrial septal defect, 9 to 12 percent; aortic stenosis, 4 to 9 percent; and other serious anomalies, 10 to 15 percent. Preductal coarctation occurs in most and is frequently associated with a large patent ductus arteriosus and a ventricular septal defect.

(G) Surgical repair of CA in infancy can be done by resection and end-to-end anastomosis or by subclavian flap angioplasty. Choice of technique is determined by the specific anatomy of each defect. Either technique can result in later restenosis (5 to 30 percent incidence) requiring reoperation or balloon angioplasty. Repair in infancy carries a 25 percent early mortality rate and a late mortality rate in years 1 to 5 of an additional 20 percent, primarily due to associated severe cardiac anomalies.

(H) Experience with balloon angioplasty for CA has been limited but does appear promising, especially in the high risk coarctation of early infancy. Recoarctation and late aneurysm formation may occur, but the overall risk may be less than for operation at this early age. In a few centers, balloon angioplasty is now the preferred primary approach. Longer follow-up is needed.

(I) When CA is repaired after infancy, there are fewer associated cardiac anomalies (25 to 40 percent) and they are more often mild (bicuspid aortic valve, 13 to 25 percent; patent ductus arteriosus, 3 to 10 percent; aortic arch anomalies; and subvalvular aortic stenosis). Complicated cardiac anomalies occur in only 10 to 15 percent of patients. The coarctation is usually postductal or juxtaductal.

(J) Elective repair of CA is usually done between ages 5 and 10 years, when the aortic size more nearly approaches adult size and permits good end-to-end anastomosis.

(K) Early results of elective repair of CA show an operative mortality rate of 2 to 4 percent. Morbidity results from hemorrhage in 8 to 16 percent (increasing with age because of the increasingly friable proximal aorta and collateral intercostal arteries), from mesenteric arteritis in 4 to 10 percent (heralded by abdominal pain, fever, and signs of peritonitis 2 to 4 days postoperatively, associated with hypertension, and believed to be due to the sudden exposure of a previously protected vascular bed to an elevated pulse pressure), and from paraplegia in 0.4 percent of patients. Routine use of shunts, bypass, or hypothermia does not appear to alter the incidence of paraplegia.

(L) Late complications of elective CA repair may be recoarctation, hypertension, premature cardiovascular disease, and early death. Residual or recoarctation follows 20 to 40 percent of repairs done at an early age but follows only 5 percent of those done at the usual age of elective repair. Persistent or recurrent hypertension is rare without restenosis after repair before age 20 years but occurs frequently (20 to 40 percent of patients) after repair in adults. Long-term follow-up reveals an increased incidence of cardiovascular disease, particularly in patients with persistent hypertension. The average age of death appears to be lower than in the general population.

(M) Patients with CA after infancy who do not undergo surgical repair die at an average age of 35 years of heart failure (18 to 22 percent), aortic rupture (22 percent), bacterial endocarditis (18 to 22 percent), intracranial hemorrhage (12 percent), and other related causes (25 percent).

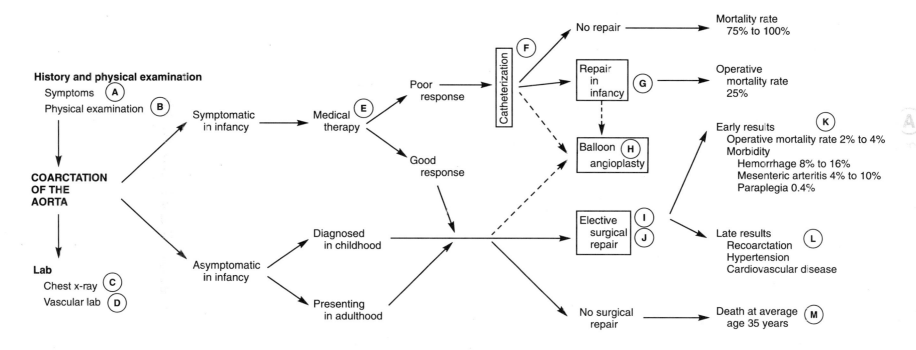

History and physical examination
Symptoms (A)
Physical examination (B)

COARCTATION OF THE AORTA

Lab
Chest x-ray (C)
Vascular lab (D)

Symptomatic in infancy → Medical therapy (E) → Poor response / Good response → Catheterization (F) → No repair → Mortality rate 75% to 100%

Repair in infancy (G) → Operative mortality rate 25%

Balloon angioplasty (H)

Asymptomatic in infancy → Diagnosed in childhood / Presenting in adulthood → Elective surgical repair (I) (J) → Early results (K): Operative mortality rate 2% to 4%, Morbidity: Hemorrhage 8% to 16%, Mesenteric arteritis 4% to 10%, Paraplegia 0.4%

Late results (L): Recoarctation, Hypertension, Cardiovascular disease

No surgical repair → Death at average age 35 years (M)

REFERENCES

Beermen LB, Neches WH, Patnode RE, et al. Coarctation of the aorta in children: late results after surgery. Am J Dis Child 1980; 134:464–466.

Brewer LA, Fosburg RG, Mulder GA, et al. Spinal cord complications following surgery for coarctation of the aorta. J Thorac Cardiovasc Surg 1972; 64:368–379.

Clarkson PM, Nicholson MR, Barratt-Boyes BG, et al. Results after repair of coarctation of the aorta beyond infancy: a 10 to 28 year follow-up with particular reference to late systemic hypertension. Am J Cardiol 1983; 51:1481–1488.

Fenchel G, Steil E, Seybold-Epting W, et al. Repair of symptomatic aortic coarctation in the first three months of life: early and late results after resection and end-to-end anastomosis and subclavian flap angioplasty. J Cardiovasc Surg 1988; 29:257–263.

Kamau P, Miles V, Toews W, et al. Surgical repair of coarctation of the aorta in infants less than six months of age. J Thorac Cardiovasc Surg 1981; 81:171–179.

Rao PS. Balloon angioplasty of aortic coarctation: a review. Clin Cardiol 1989; 12:618–628.

Trinquet F, Vouhe PR, Vernant F, et al. Coarctation of the aorta in infants: which operation? Ann Thorac Surg 1988; 45:186–191.

Tynan M, Finley JP, Fontes V, et al. Balloon angioplasty for the treatment of native coarctation: results of valvuloplasty and angioplasty of congenital anomalies registry. Am J Cardiol 1990; 65:790–792.

Ziemer G, Jonas RA, Perry SB, et al. Surgery for coarctation of the aorta in the neonate. Circulation 1986; 74 (suppl I):25–31.

Neonatal Cyanosis

David R. Clarke, M.D.

(A) A history of prenatal viral illness or drug use during the first trimester increases the likelihood of a serious congenital defect. Prematurity usually is not associated with an increased incidence of pathologic cyanosis. Exceptions are hyaline membrane disease and patent ductus arteriosus.

(B) Physiologic causes of cyanosis do not require treatment. Peripheral cyanosis results from vasomotor instability, temporal local venous congestion, or response to cold. Central cyanosis may be triggered by crying that causes increased pulmonary vascular resistance and right-to-left shunting through a patent foramen ovale.

(C) Bluish discoloration of the skin, nailbeds, or mucous membranes occurs when more than 3 g/100 mL of reduced hemoglobin is in the capillary blood.

(D) Important findings include collapse, effusion, cardiomegaly, and increased or decreased pulmonary vascularity.

(E) Normal arterial PO_2 at 5 minutes of age averages 19.5 mmHg. It rises to an average of 62 mmHg by 60 minutes of age.

(F) Suctioning the airway and placing the infant in a warm incubator with 100 percent oxygen differentiate most cardiac problems from most respiratory problems. The latter respond to 100 percent oxygen. Congenital anomalies such as tracheal stenosis and bilateral choanal atresia may require intubation.

(G) Persistent fetal circulation is characterized by a diffuse ground glass appearance of the chest x-ray without electrocardiographic or echocardiographic evidence of heart disease. A pulmonary vasodilator such as prostaglandin E_1 or tolazoline may be used and cardiac catheterization avoided.

(H) Signs of congestive heart failure include cardiomegaly, hepatomegaly, and pulmonary vascular congestion.

(I) Septal defects include patent ductus arteriosus, aorticopulmonary window, atrial septal defect, ventricular septal defect, and endocardial cushion defect.

(J) Diaphragmatic hernia in the neonate is seven times as frequent on the left side as on the right. The defect in the posterolateral diaphragm is an enlarged foramen of Bochdalek. Passage of a nasogastric tube before a chest roentgenogram identifies the stomach in the left hemithorax. Laying the infant on the affected side and decompressing the gastrointestinal tract facilitates ventilation. Ventilatory assistance with a mask should not be attempted. Endotracheal tube ventilation avoids further distention of the gastrointestinal tract. Metabolic acidosis must be corrected. Total body base deficit in milliequivalents can be determined by multiplying the body weight in kilograms times base excess times 0.3. Half of this deficit should be corrected with a single bolus of sodium bicarbonate.

(K) Congenital lobar emphysema is usually unilobar and is more often present on the right side. Lobectomy for congenital lobar emphysema in an infant is technically simple and can be accomplished with a mortality rate of 7 percent.

(L) Cystic adenomatoid malformation usually affects a single lobe. When the left lower lobe is affected, a diaphragmatic hernia should be excluded. Single lung cysts can produce cyanosis.

(M) Other conditions not requiring operative repair include hyaline membrane disease, meconium aspiration, pneumonia, pulmonary hemorrhage, hypoplasia or agenesis, systemic infection, primary hypoglycemia, adrenal insufficiency, central nervous system disease, polycythemia, myocarditis, arrhythmia, and methemoglobinemia.

(N) When the aortic arch is left sided, a right thoracotomy with an extrapleural approach is preferred for division of the fistula and single-layer end-to-end esophageal anastomosis. Depending on birth weight and the clinical condition of the patient, survival ranges from 38 to 92 percent.

(O) A transverse subcostal incision is preferred in the repair of diaphragmatic hernia. The abdominal approach allows inspection of the entire gastrointestinal tract, a gastrostomy, and insertion of a Silon chimney if necessary. The diaphragm is closed with a double row of nonabsorbable sutures. Care is taken to remove the hernia sac if one is present. Aggressive surgical therapy is associated with a 50 to 70 percent salvage rate when severe respiratory distress is present in the neonate.

(P) A No. 10 or 12 Argyle drainage tube is inserted anteriorly or laterally. Water seal drainage or 8 to 10 cm of suction can be applied to the thoracostomy tube. Hemothorax or chylothorax in the neonate can be managed similarly, although chylothorax may respond to simple aspiration of the fluid.

REFERENCES

Goetzman, BW, Sunshine P, Johnson JD, et al. Neonatal hypoxia and pulmonary vasospasm: response to tolazoline. J Pediatr 1976; 89:617–621.

Lees MH, Sunderland CO, Menashe VD. Differential diagnosis of cyanosis in the neonate. South Med J 1974; 67:611–615.

Redo SF. Principles of surgery in the first six months of life. Hagerstown, MD: Harper and Row, 1976.

Riemenschneider TA. Problems in family practice: evaluation of cyanosis in the newborn. J Fam Pract 1976; 3:201–204.

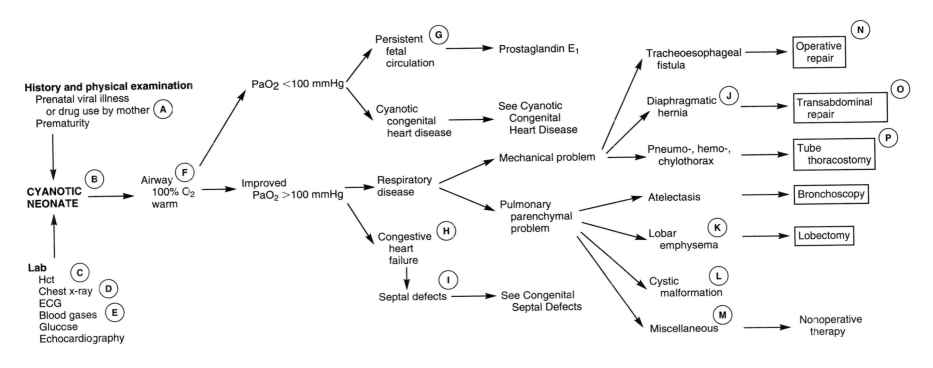

Cyanotic Congenital Heart Disease

David R. Clarke, M.D.

(A) Cyanosis in neonates may be episodic with agitation and often represents severe hypoxia (PaO$_2$ <30 mmHg).

(B) Anomalies that can produce signs and symptoms of congestive heart failure include total anomalous pulmonary venous drainage (TAPVD), transposition of the great arteries with ventricular septal defect (VSD), and truncus arteriosus.

(C) Findings on chest x-ray may include increased or decreased pulmonary vascularity, cardiomegaly, specific chamber enlargement, and lateralization of the aortic arch.

(D) Two-dimensional echocardiography is helpful before cardiac catheterization. If the infant or child is in stable condition and is neither acidotic nor in heart failure, heart catheterization may be unnecessary provided that two-dimensional echocardiography reveals anatomy compatible with long-term survival.

(E) Catheterization is urgent in the cyanotic neonate or infant with severe hypoxia (PaO$_2$ <30 mmHg), significant acidosis, heart failure, the need for balloon atrial septostomy (transposition of great arteries), or uncertain diagnosis. Catheterization, including saturation and pressure measurements in all cardiac chambers and appropriate cineradiography, provides accurate anatomic diagnosis in 95 percent of cases.

(F) Evidence of increased pulmonary blood flow includes signs of congestive heart failure, an enlarged pulmonary artery, hypervascular lungs on chest x-ray, and pulmonary hypertension (pulmonary blood flow exceeding systemic flow) on catheterization.

(G) If cyanosis is severe and decreased pulmonary blood flow is suspected, immediate palliation is achieved by maintaining or increasing ductus arteriosus patency with intravenous infusion of prostaglandin E$_1$ (0.1 μg/kg/minute).

(H) Uncorrected total anomalous pulmonary venous drainage is fatal in 80 to 90 percent of patients within the first year of life.

(I) Without treatment, the mean survival with transposition is 3 months. Atrial septostomy allows survival of 78 percent of patients at 1 year. Only 10 percent of patients are alive at 3 years.

(J) Average longevity of neonates with untreated truncus is 5 weeks; 15 to 30 percent live a year. Pulmonary artery banding has such a high mortality rate (50 percent) that early conduit repair is usually considered. The mortality rate for early total repair is 12 to 30 percent.

(K) Less common anomalies marked by increased pulmonary blood flow include tricuspid atresia without pulmonic stenosis, single ventricle, and hypoplastic left heart syndrome. Pulmonary artery banding or more complex palliation is required. The modified Fontan procedure is definitive treatment.

(L) Pulmonary atresia occurs with or without a VSD. If the ventricular septum is intact, balloon atrial septostomy is sometimes required. Opening the atretic valve and inserting a shunt is palliative.

(M) Tricuspid atresia involves complete agenesis of the tricuspid valve, atrial septal defect (ASD), VSD, and right ventricular hypoplasia. Pulmonary blood flow is decreased in 85 percent of cases. Palliation is achieved with a Blalock-Taussig shunt.

(N) Tetralogy of Fallot consists of pulmonary outflow hypoplasia, large VSD, overriding aorta, and right ventricular hypertrophy. It constitutes 10 percent of congenital heart disease. Most infants are cyanotic. An arterial saturation value less than 70 percent is the most common indication for operation.

(O) Other defects that decrease pulmonary blood flow include single ventricle with pulmonic stenosis, transposition with VSD and left ventricular outflow obstruction, and pulmonary stenosis plus ASD. The Blalock-Taussig shunt is palliative for all three. Definitive repair is by the Fontan procedure, the Rastelli procedure, and pulmonary valvulotomy, respectively.

(P) Balloon atrial septostomy performed by catheter through the femoral vein allows mixing of oxygenated and unoxygenated blood at the atrial level. This procedure is sometimes palliative in TAPVD and is usually necessary when transposition of the great arteries is present.

(Q) Pulmonary artery banding is occasionally useful before closure of a large VSD or to prepare the left ventricle for the pressure load before an arterial switch operation.

(R) The Blalock-Taussig operation is anastomosis of the subclavian artery to the pulmonary artery on the side opposite the aortic arch. The resultant increase in pulmonary flow improves oxygenation and allows pulmonary artery growth.

(S) When pulmonary arteries are small or an anomalous left anterior descending coronary artery is present, the Blalock-Taussig shunt provides palliation until the child is large enough for definitive repair.

(T) The operative mortality rate for correction of TAPVD in infancy is 13 to 48 percent; the late mortality rate is 2 to 14 percent.

(U) The Mustard or Senning operation directs systemic venous blood into the pulmonary artery and oxygenated blood into the aorta. The

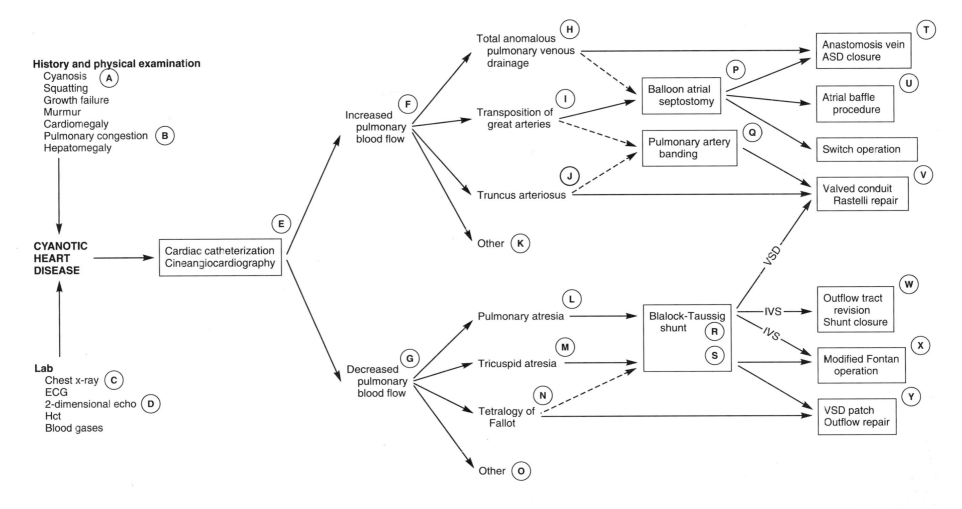

operative mortality rate is 0 to 9 percent. The late mortality rate is 10 to 20 percent.

(V) A Rastelli-type operation includes patch closure of the VSD and placement of a Dacron conduit containing a valve between the right ventricle and the distal main pulmonary artery.

(W) After palliation of pulmonary atresia with intact ventricular septum, growth of the right ventricle may permit definitive repair, consisting of revision of the pulmonary outflow with closure of the ASD and a surgical shunt. If the ventricle

remains small, a modified Fontan procedure is definitive. Not more than 70 percent of these children survive to adulthood.

(X) The Fontan operation connects the right atrium or vena cava directly or through a conduit to the right ventricle or pulmonary artery. A modified Fontan operation can be used in children aged 4 to 15 years if there is normal vascular resistance. The early mortality rate is 13 to 19 percent.

(Y) Definitive repair of tetralogy of Fallot can be done primarily in infancy with an operative

mortality rate of 8 percent. Mortality is less in older children. Previous shunts may deform pulmonary arteries and complicate total repair.

REFERENCES

Adams FH, Emmanouilides GC, eds. Moss' heart disease in infants, children, and adolescents. 3rd ed. Baltimore: Williams & Wilkins, 1983.

Keith JD, Rowe RD, Vlad P. Heart disease in infancy and childhood. 3rd ed. New York: Macmillan, 1978.

Stark J, de Leval M, eds. Surgery for congenital heart defects. New York: Grune & Stratton, 1983.

Congenital Obstructive Cardiac Anomalies

David N. Campbell, M.D.

(A) Indications for cardiac catheterization, pressure measurements, and cineangiography include systemic hypertension, dyspnea (suggesting congestive heart failure), and chest x-ray or electrocardiogram indicating increasing heart size. Investigation should be done before cardiac failure is irreversible or sudden death occurs.

(B) The most common anomalies include pulmonary atresia, tricuspid atresia, and hypoplastic left heart.

(C) Indications for repair of pulmonic stenosis include symptoms, severe right ventricular hypertrophy or strain, and systolic pressure gradient across the stenosis greater than 50 mmHg. Operative technique depends on the type of pulmonic stenosis.

(D) Isolated peripheral pulmonic stenosis is uncommon and difficult to manage. Repair techniques include patch enlargement of a proximal stenosis or balloon angioplasty if the stenosis occurs in the branches.

(E) Pure valvular pulmonary stenosis is best treated by balloon dilation at catheterization. Surgically, it can be treated by using 1 to 2 minutes of inflow occlusion, opening the main pulmonary artery, and splitting the fused commissures (valvulotomy). Valvectomy may be necessary if the valve tissue is unicuspid or the leaflets are severely thickened. The mortality rate is low (1 percent). Long-term results are excellent, although asymptomatic pulmonary insufficiency is common (50 percent).

(F) Indications for myectomy of concomitant subvalvular muscular infundibular hypertrophy include fixed scarred endothelial stenosis and right ventricular pressure greater than 200 mmHg.

(G) Indications for surgical intervention in aortic stenosis include symptoms, progressive left ventricular hypertrophy, and a measured gradient across the lesion greater than 50 to 60 mmHg.

(H) Rapid valvulotomy can be done safely in newborns using inflow occlusion. In older infants and children an open procedure with cardiopulmonary bypass is recommended. The mortality rate is low (less than 3 percent). Again, balloon dilation in the cath lab is used in many centers.

(I) Reoperation is necessary in 15 percent of cases because of either progressive aortic insufficiency or restenosis. Most patients require a valve replacement at that time. In a child with a small aortic annulus, a Konno aortoventriculoplasty may be used to place an adult-sized valve. Mechanical valves are used for replacement of left-sided valves in these Konno procedures. The operation of choice, however, is an allograft aortic root replacement with a human valve.

(J) Recurrence rate is 20 percent. Many patients require valve replacement when progressive aortic insufficiency occurs and the gradient cannot be relieved without splitting open the left ventricular outflow tract with a Konno procedure.

(K) Operation for congenital mitral stenosis should be delayed as long as possible. Medical management is preferable unless cardiac decompensation occurs. Results of mitral valvuloplasty are generally poor even for those with fused commissures. Valve replacement is often required, particularly for parachute valves and those with short chordae. The mortality rate for mitral valve replacement in children is 30 to 35 percent. The 5-year survival rate is only 50 percent.

(L) Coarctations may present in the newborn as shock. Immediate operation is no longer necessary since prostaglandin E_1 opens the ductus and allows the child's condition to be stabilized and repair to be performed with an operative risk of less than 5 percent.

(M) In infants the recurrence rate when the subclavian artery flap aortoplasty is used is low (5 to 10 percent). The recurrence rate after resection plus end-to-end anastomosis is now similar. Patch aortoplasty should be used only to treat recurrence. As an initial operation, synthetic patch aortoplasty has an unacceptably high rate of aneurysm formation on the wall opposite the stiff patch. Balloon angioplasty is the procedure of choice for recoarctation.

(N) Most children with interrupted aortic arch develop symptoms in the first 6 weeks of life because the ductus closes and there is no flow to the lower body. Operation is often emergent but prostaglandin E_1 allows time for preoperative preparation. Controversy exists as to the best method of repair, eg, end-to-end anastomosis, graft interposition, or Blalock-Park procedure.

REFERENCES

Ankeney JL, Tzeng TS, Liebman J. Surgical therapy for congenital aortic valvular stenosis: a 23 year experience. J Thorac Cardiovasc Surg 1983; 85:41–48.

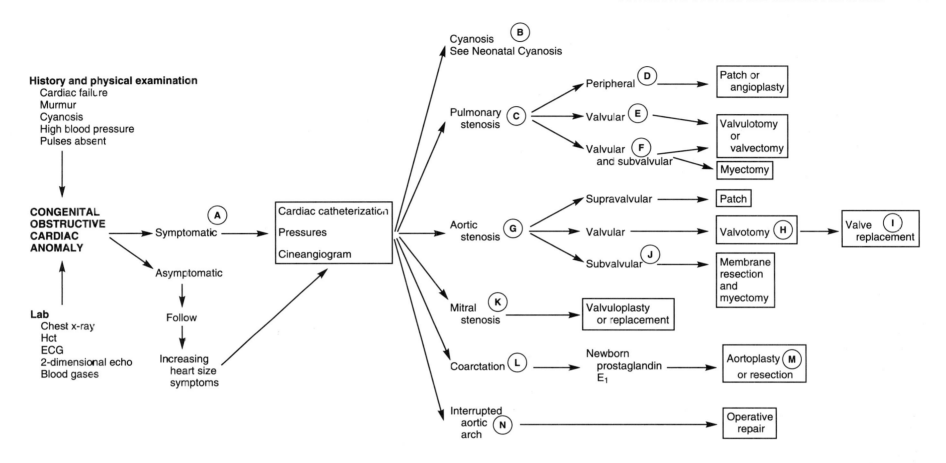

History and physical examination
Cardiac failure
Murmur
Cyanosis
High blood pressure
Pulses absent

CONGENITAL OBSTRUCTIVE CARDIAC ANOMALY

Lab
Chest x-ray
Hct
ECG
2-dimensional echo
Blood gases

Symptomatic (A)

Asymptomatic

Follow

Increasing heart size symptoms

Cardiac catheterization
Pressures
Cineangiogram

Cyanosis (B)
See Neonatal Cyanosis

Pulmonary stenosis (C)
→ Peripheral (D) → Patch or angioplasty
→ Valvular (E) → Valvulotomy or valvectomy
→ Valvular and subvalvular (F) → Myectomy

Aortic stenosis (G)
→ Supravalvular → Patch
→ Valvular → Valvotomy (H) → Valve replacement (I)
→ Subvalvular (J) → Membrane resection and myectomy

Mitral stenosis (K) → Valvuloplasty or replacement

Coarctation (L) → Newborn prostaglandin E₁ → Aortoplasty (M) or resection

Interrupted aortic arch (N) → Operative repair

Awariefe SO, Clarke DR, Pappas G. Surgical approach to critical pulmonary valve stenosis in infants less than six months of age. J Thorac Cardiovasc Surg 1983; 85:375–387.

Bergdahl L, Ljunquist A. Long-term results after repair of coarctation of the aorta by patch grafting. J Thorac Cardiovasc Surg 1980; 80:177–181.

Cain T, Campbell D, Paton B, et al. Operation for discrete subvalvular aortic stenosis. J Thorac Cariovasc Surg 1984; 87:366–370.

Griffith BP, Hardesty RL, Siewers RD, et al. Pulmonary valvulotomy alone for pulmonary stenosis: results in children with and without muscular infundibular hypertrophy. J Thorac Cardiovasc Surg 1982; 83:577–583.

Kirklin JW, Barratt-Boyes BG. Cardiac surgery. New York: Churchill Livingstone, 1988.

Lock JE, Castaneda-Zuniga WR, Fuhrman BP, et al. Balloon dilation angioplasty of hypoplastic and stenotic pulmonary arteries. Circulation 1983; 67:962–967.

Spencer F. Congenital heart disease. In: Schwartz S, ed. Schwartz's principles of surgery. New York: McGraw-Hill, 1969, pp 553–626.

Williams WG, Pollock JC, Geiss DM, et al. Experience with aortic and mitral valve replacement in children. J Thorac Cardiovasc Surg 1981; 81:326–333.

Congenital Septal Defects

David N. Campbell, M.D.

(A) Fewer than 5 percent of infants with septal defects have associated syndromes, the most common being Down and Turner syndromes.

(B) A loud pulmonic closure sound (P_2) suggests pulmonary hypertension.

(C) Chest x-ray may show a change in the silhouette of the heart and great vessels and an increase or decrease in pulmonary vasculature.

(D) Most septal defects are diagnosed by clinical examination, routine laboratory studies, and two-dimensional echocardiogram. Cardiac catheterization confirms the diagnosis but is used only when something out of the ordinary is suspected.

(E) Common symptomatic septal defects in infants include aortopulmonary window, truncus arteriosus, large ventricular septal defect (VSD), and large complete atrioventricular septal defect (CAV defect).

(F) Aortopulmonary window so frequently leads to pulmonary hypertension and early pulmonary vascular obstructive disease that it warrants immediate catheter confirmation and early repair.

(G) A ductus arteriosus patient after 2 months of age has only a 12 percent probability of closure. Since the risk of complications such as arteritis with even a hemodynamically insignificant lesion is greater than the risk of repair, any ductus remaining patent beyond that time should be studied and closed. Between 5 and 20 percent are associated with other anomalies.

(H) About 30 percent of hemodynamically significant atrial septal defects (ASDs) remain asymptomatic.

(I) One fifth of VSDs, usually small membranous or muscular, close spontaneously. Children with moderate to large VSDs should be studied by catheterization at 18 months to detect a significant shunt because pulmonary hypertension is seldom reversible after 2 years.

(J) Complete AV septal defects are always repaired. Operative risk is decreased from 17 percent to 7 percent after age 2 years.

(K) Important findings during catheterization of septal defects are pressures and oxygen saturations in all four chambers and great vessels and the left-to-right shunt ($Q_p:Q_s$), which is the ratio of pulmonary blood flow to systemic blood flow.

(L) Indications for repair of ASDs include presence of symptoms, left-to-right shunt ($Q_p:Q_s$) greater than 1.5:1, and pulmonary hypertension.

(M) Secundum-type ASDs are most common (80 percent). Primary repair with suture closure is possible in 80 percent. Long-term prognosis is excellent, hemodynamic cure expectancy is 93 percent, and hospital mortality rate is 1 percent.

(N) Ostium primum atrial septal defects account for 5 percent of all ASDs and are a forme fruste of CAV septal defects except that no VSD is present. Eighty-eight percent of patients have a deformed mitral valve. The mitral valve is usually repaired by closing the cleft in the septal leaflet. A pericardial patch closes the ASD. Operative mortality rate is less than 10 percent. If reoperation is required for residual shunt or if there is mitral valve dysfunction, valve replacement is often (80 percent) necessary. Late survival rate is excellent.

(O) Fifteen percent of ASDs have associated partial anomalous pulmonary venous drainage. Operation to divert the pulmonary venous drainage through the ASD to the left atrium most commonly uses a pericardial patch to direct the entry of the pulmonary veins through the ASD.

(P) Indications for operation for VSD include presence of symptoms, $Q_p:Q_s$ greater than 2:1, aortic insufficiency, and pulmonary hypertension. In infants, the operative mortality rate is 8 percent for complete correction using deep hypothermia and circulatory arrest. This obviates initial banding and a later corrective repair.

(Q) Small membranous VSDs are often closed primarily through the right atrium with interrupted sutures. Moderate and large defects require a prosthetic patch. Repair in children over 1 year old with mild to moderate pulmonary vascular disease can be accomplished with a mortality rate less than 5 percent. Long-term results are dependent on the degree of pulmonary vascular disease and its regression. If repair is carried out before age 2 years, long-term survival is over 90 percent. After 2 years of age, moderate to severe pulmonary vascular disease is likely to persist and lead to death within 10 years.

(R) Muscular VSDs may be difficult to find through thick right ventricular trabeculations. In infants with complete defects, palliation with banding is considered. Correction is easier when the child is older. Some defects close spontaneously.

(S) In CAV septal defect there is a left-to-right shunt at both the atrial and ventricular levels and the atrioventricular valves are not distinct. Because of the complexity of the repair, operation under 1 year of age is undertaken only when symptoms develop. The ventricular septum is closed with a prosthetic patch, the common leaflets are separated, and the septal leaflets of the mitral

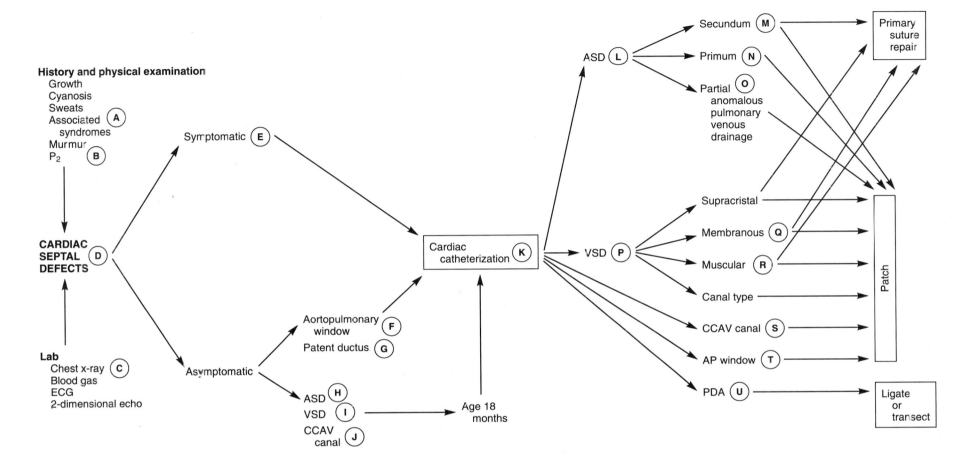

valve are fused by closing the cleft and suspending it from the VSD patch. The atrial septum is then closed. The operative mortality rate for elective closure is 7 percent. Mitral regurgitation after repair is common but usually mild; if severe, prosthetic valve replacement may be necessary.

(T) Aortopulmonary window closure is performed on cardiopulmonary bypass (deep hypothermia in infants) through the aorta using a Dacron patch to complete the septum. Mortality rate is 0 to 5 percent and long-term outcome is excellent when the defect is repaired in infancy before pulmonary vascular disease develops.

(U) Most cases of patent ductus arteriosus can be closed with simple ligation. If larger than 1.5 cm in diameter or calcified, patent ductus arteriosus may require transection or use of cardiopulmonary bypass. Mortality rate is less than 1 percent and prognosis is excellent. New occlusion devices are being studied to evaluate closure transvenously during cardiac catheterization. They are experimental at this time.

REFERENCES

Clarke CP, Richardson JP. The management of aortopulmonary window—advantages of transaortic closure with Dacron patch. J Thorac Cardiovasc Surg 1976; 72:48–51.

Clarke DR. Atrial septal defects. In: Eiseman B, ed. Prognosis of surgical disease. Philadelphia: WB Saunders, 1980.

DuShane JW, Kirklin JW. Late results of repair of ventricular septal defect on pulmonary vascular disease. In: Kirklin JW, ed. Advances in cardiovascular surgery. New York: Grune & Stratton, 1973.

Feldt RH. Atrioventricular canal defects. Philadelphia: WB Saunders, 1976.

Keith JD, Rowe RD, Vlad P. Heart disease in infancy and childhood. New York: Macmillan, 1978.

Kirklin JW, Barratt-Boyes BG. Cardiac surgery. New York: Churchill Livingstone, 1988.

Spencer F. Atrial septal defect, anomalous pulmonary veins, and atrioventricular canal. In: Sabiston D, Spencer F, eds. Gibbon's surgery of the chest. 4th ed. Philadelphia: WB Saunders, 1983.

Wright JS, Newman DC. Ligation of the patent ductus arteriosus—technical considerations at different ages. J Thorac Cardiovasc Surg 1978; 75:695–698.

Acute Myocardial Infarct

Aubrey C. Galloway, M.D., Frederick Feit, M.D.,
and Ben Eiseman, M.D.

(A) Acute myocardial infarct (AMI) occurs in nearly 1.5 million people annually in the United States and accounts for 25 percent of the nation's deaths.

(B) Identifiable risk factors include male gender, smoking, hypertension, hypercholesterolemia, obesity, diabetes, type A personality, and a sedentary lifestyle.

(C) Electrocardiographic abnormalities include ST segment elevation of 0.2 mV or 25 percent height of R wave with hyperacute T waves. ST segment depression or T wave inversion may occur. Progression to Q waves suggests transmural infarction. Lack of Q waves suggests subendocardial damage. Five percent of AMI have nonspecific or absent electrocardiographic changes.

(D) Peripheral blood myocardial creatine phosphokinase-MB (CPK-MB) isoenzymes peak in 5 to 24 hours and are measured every 6 hours for 1 day. Lactic dehydrogenase (LDH) enzymes rise after 24 to 48 hours and peak at 3 to 6 days. Any level of CPK-MB isoenzyme or a ratio of LDH_1/LDH_2 greater than 0.75 is 90 percent sensitive and specific for AMI.

(E) Portable chest x-ray can demonstrate cardiac enlargement or pulmonary congestion.

(F) Echocardiography documents mechanical complications and cardiac function.

(G) Prompt treatment is indicated to minimize early deaths, 60 percent of which occur within 1 hour after onset of AMI. Arrhythmia is often fatal and occurs in 75 to 95 percent of patients. Arrhythmias due to electrical instability include premature ventricular contractions, ventricular tachycardia, junctional tachycardia, or ventricular fibrillation. Those caused by pump failure include sinus tachycardia, supraventricular tachycardia, or atrial fibrillation/flutter. Those caused by conduction disturbances include sinus bradycardia and atrioventricular or intraventricular heart block.

(H) Coronary care unit management includes electrocardiogram monitoring, oxygen, morphine for pain, intravenous lidocaine, and aspirin. β-blockers are used for tachycardia or hypertension. Intravenous nitroglycerin or calcium channel blockers are used for recurrent pain or ischemia.

(I) Cardiogenic shock occurs in 10 to 15 percent of all patients with AMI and in 5 percent after thrombolytic therapy. Treatment includes Swan-Ganz catheter monitoring, arterial blood gas and pressure monitoring, inotropic support, intraaortic balloon pump, and emergency cardiac catheterization. Angioplasty or emergency bypass operation is usually required.

(J) A stress test is performed 8 to 10 days after patient stabilization, and cardiac catheterization is performed if this is positive.

(K) Thrombolysis with streptokinase, anistreplase, or tissue plasminogen activator is used within the first 4 to 6 hours of AMI onset in those under 76 years of age who do not have other contraindications such as cerebrovascular disease or recent operation. Currently only 20 percent of AMI patients receive thrombolytic therapy.

(L) With thrombolytic therapy 60 to 80 percent of patients lyse their clots with immediate pain relief and electrocardiogram normalization, often accompanied by reperfusion arrhythmias.

There is a 0.5 percent risk of intracranial hemorrhage or bleeding from other sites. Thrombolysis reduces immediate mortality from AMI by approximately 35 percent.

(M) Indications for cardiac catheterization after AMI include hemodynamic instability, recurrent ischemia, absence of reperfusion after thrombolytic therapy, a positive stress test, or poor ventricular function. About half of such patients are treated medically and the other half require angioplasty or operation.

(N) Long-term medical therapy after AMI includes risk factor modification, β-blockers, and aspirin. Calcium channel blockers and nitrates are also used for diffuse disease or recurrent ischemia. One-year survival after AMI exceeds 90 percent if thrombolysis and interventional therapy are used compared with 80 to 85 percent using conventional therapy.

(O) Angioplasty is used for ischemia associated with severe or recent total occlusion. It is successful in about 90 percent of patients and carries a mortality risk of 1 percent. About 8 percent of those undergoing angioplasty require operative bypass within a year.

(P) Emergency operation is indicated for unsuccessful angioplasty, left main coronary artery disease, severe triple vessel disease, and mechanical defects (ventricular septal defect, mitral insufficiency, ventricular rupture). Emergency bypass has a risk of 2 to 3 percent in hemodynamically stable patients, whereas operative risk is 15 to 20 percent in those in cardiogenic shock or with mechanical defects.

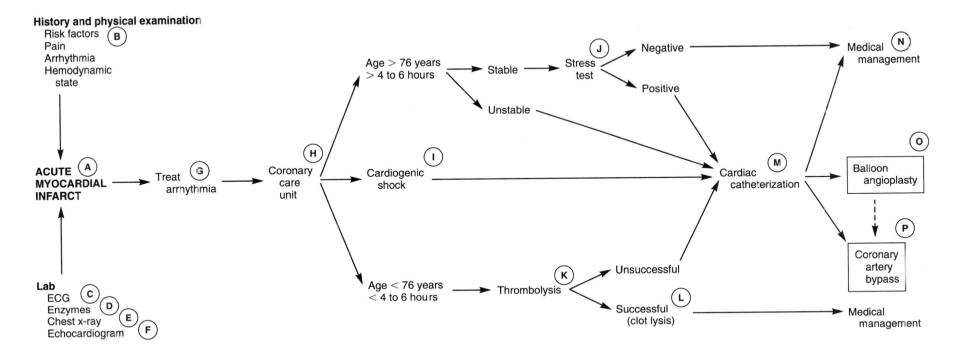

History and physical examination
Risk factors   (B)
Pain
Arrhythmia
Hemodynamic
  state

ACUTE (A)
MYOCARDIAL
INFARCT

Treat (G)
arrhythmia

Coronary (H)
care
unit

Age > 76 years
> 4 to 6 hours → Stable → Stress test (J) → Negative → Medical management (N)
→ Positive

Unstable → Cardiac catheterization (M)

Cardiogenic shock (I)

Age < 76 years
< 4 to 6 hours → Thrombolysis (K) → Unsuccessful
→ Successful (clot lysis) (L) → Medical management

Cardiac catheterization (M) → Balloon angioplasty (O) ⇢ Coronary artery bypass (P)

Lab
ECG   (C)   (D)
Enzymes   (E)
Chest x-ray   (F)
Echocardiogram

REFERENCES

The AIMS Trial Study Group. Effects of intravenous APSAC on mortality after acute myocardial infarction. Lancet 1988; 1:545–549.

ISIS-2 Collaborative Group. Randomized trial of intravenous streptokinase, oral aspirin, both, or neither among 17,187 cases of suspected acute myocardial infarction: ISIS-2. Lancet 1988; 2:349.

Pasternack RC, Braunwald E, Sobel BE. Acute myocardial infarction. In: Braunwald E, ed. Heart disease. Philadelphia: WB Saunders, 1988: 1222–1313.

The TIMI Study Group. Comparison of invasive and conservative strategies after treatment with intravenous tissue plasminogen activator in acute myocardial infarction: results of the thrombolysis in myocardial infarction (TIMI) phase II trial. N Engl J Med 1989; 320: 618.

Coronary Artery Disease

Jack G. Copeland, M.D.

(A) Coronary artery disease is the major cause of death in the United States, killing about 650,000 people each year. The incidence among men over age 65 is approximately 25 percent.

(B) Asymptomatic patients with coronary artery disease are difficult to identify. Screening low-risk populations is expensive, time consuming, and inaccurate. Screening those with previous myocardial infarction (MI) and known risk factors, using exercise to elicit ischemic changes, identifies groups at high risk for left main coronary disease (ST depression >2 mm on exercise treadmill) and other degrees of disease (ST depression >1 mm).

(C) Symptomatic patients whose angina is stable and controlled by nitrates, β-blockers, or calcium channel blockers are followed. Exercise stress testing is helpful in stratifying symptomatic patients. A markedly positive exercise tolerance test requires further evaluation by cardiac catheterization. As angina becomes more frequent and severe (unstable), patients are increasingly disabled and more likely to have an MI. Catheterization and operative intervention are indicated. Most patients with unstable angina can be cooled down with intravenous nitroglycerin or intraaortic balloon pumping before bypass surgery. This lowers the risk of operation.

(D) For 20 to 25 percent of patients, the first evidence of MI is sudden death. Ten to fifteen percent of those reaching a hospital die. Thrombolysis, percutaneous transluminal angioplasty, or coronary bypass surgery, undertaken in an attempt to reverse myocardial damage, must be accomplished within 2 hours of the onset of infarction to be beneficial. Complications of MI that might necessitate emergency operation are ruptured interventricular septum and ruptured papillary muscle of the mitral valve. Another complication is ventricular arrhythmia. This can be studied electrophysiologically and treated with medications or an automatic implantable defibrillator. Patients with left ventricular aneurysm and recurrent ventricular arrhythmia can be treated by resection of the aneurysm. Scar tissue resulting from transmural infarction can stretch with time, creating a symptomatic ventricular aneurysm that requires resection. MI can also cause ischemic cardiomyopathy that leads to heart failure and consideration for cardiac transplantation.

(E) Factors contributing to high risk are a family history of coronary artery disease, hyperlipidemia, previous MI, diabetes, hypertension, and heavy smoking.

(F) Coronary artery bypass grafting (CABG) is performed in about 300,000 patients annually in the United States alone. A common technique is anastomosis of one internal mammary artery to a major left-sided coronary artery, usually the left anterior descending. Saphenous vein grafts are used for other bypasses. In most patients, three or more coronary vessels are bypassed. Graft patency is optimal (92 percent at 1 year for internal mammary artery and vein grafts) if aspirin, 325 mg, is given through a nasogastric tube 6 hours postoperatively and orally once a day thereafter. Longitudinal follow-up shows gradual deterioration of vein grafts beginning between 5 and 7 years after operation. This results in a 50 to 60 percent patency rate at 12 years. Internal mammary artery grafts appear to have better patency rates.

CABG is the treatment of choice in chronically stable patients with left main coronary narrowing (50 percent narrowing on an angiogram equals 70 percent narrowing of the vessel lumen) and multiple vessel disease, if one of the vessels is the proximal left anterior descending. CABG is better than medical therapy in patients with multivessel disease and impaired ventricular function (ejection fraction <0.5). In unstable patients the operation is indicated if any coronary artery is narrowed significantly. Operative mortality for elective CABG is 1 to 3 percent.

REFERENCES

Barner HB, Standeven JW, Reese J, et al. Twelve-year experience with internal mammary artery for coronary artery bypass. J Thorac Cardiovasc Surg 1985; 90: 668–675.

Braunwald E. Coronary artery surgery at the crossroads (editorial). N Engl J Med 1977; 297: 661–663.

Campeau L, Enjalbert M, Lesperance J, et al. Atherosclerosis and late closure of aortocoronary saphenous vein grafts: sequential angiographic studies at 2 weeks, 1 year, 5 to 7 years, and 10 to 12 years after surgery. Circulation 1983; 68:II1–II6.

Chesebro JH, Clements IP, Fuster V, et al. A platelet-inhibitor-drug trial in coronary-artery bypass operations; benefit of perioperative dipyridamole and aspirin therapy on early postoperative vein-graft patency. N Engl J Med 1982; 307:6.

Goldman S, Copeland J, Moritz T, et al. Improvement in early saphenous vein graft patency after coronary artery bypass surgery with antiplatelet therapy: results of a Veterans Administration cooperative study. Circulation 1988; 77:1324–1332.

Loop FD, Lytle BW, Cosgrove DM, et al. Influence of the internal mammary artery graft on 10-year survival and other cardiac events. N Engl J Med 1986; 314:1–6.

Murphy ML, Hultgren HN, Detre K, et al. Treatment of chronic stable angina; a preliminary report of survival data of the randomized Veterans Administration cooperative study. N Engl J Med 1977; 297:621–627.

Myers WO, Davis K, Foster ED, et al. Surgical survival in the coronary artery surgery study (CASS) registry. Ann Thorac Surg 1985; 40:245–260.

History and physical examination
Chest pain
Family history of CAD
Hypertension
Diabetes
Smoking
Obesity

Lab
ECG
Lipid profiles
Chest x-ray

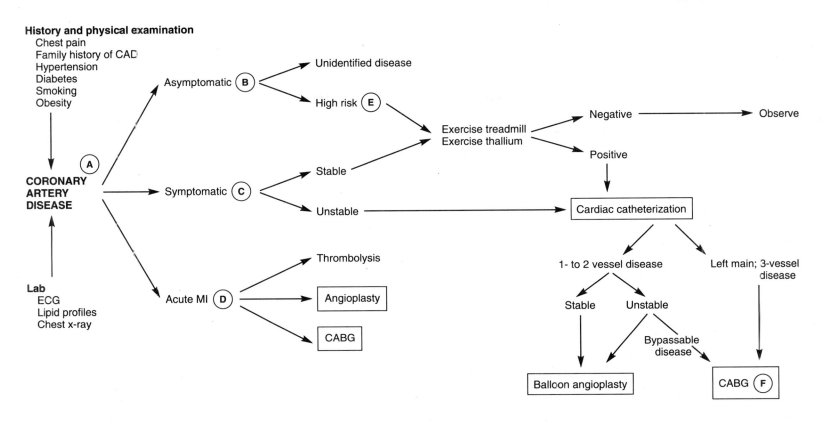

Aortic Valve Stenosis

Bruce C. Paton, M.D., F.R.C.S. (Ed.), F.R.C.P. (Ed.)

(A) A history of a murmur since childhood suggests congenital, not acquired, disease. Rheumatic heart disease accounts for 20 percent of acquired aortic stenosis (AS). Cardinal symptoms are angina, exertional syncope, and dyspnea on exertion. Onset of symptoms is crucial. Untreated, most patients die within 4 years of developing symptoms.

(B) Cardinal signs include a thrill over the upper end of the sternum, a harsh ejection systolic murmur in the second right interspace, and a prominent left ventricular impulse.

(C) The aortic valve is significantly stenosed when a transvalvular gradient greater than 50 mmHg is present, or when the cross-sectional area of the valve is less than 0.5 cm/m. Congenitally deformed bicuspid valves, with or without calcification, are the most common cause of AS under the age of 65 years (60 percent). Over 65 years of age, senile calcific degeneration is common.

(D) Left ventricular enlargement is moderate without associated aortic or mitral regurgitation. Left ventricular hypertrophy may not be radiologically apparent.

(E) Electrocardiography confirms left ventricular hypertrophy.

(F) Echo Doppler is as accurate as cardiac catheterization for determining a transvalvular gradient. Cardiac catheterization is necessary in patients over 40 years of age to assess coronary disease and in patients with angina or associated cardiac lesions. Without angina, severe coronary disease is unlikely. Half the patients with angina will be found to have coronary artery disease.

(G) If the gradient is less than 50 mmHg and the patient has neither symptoms nor coronary disease, observation is justified until there is an increase in gradient (measured by Doppler), changes of progressive hypertrophy in the electrocardiogram, or symptoms. Restudy is then indicated. Operation may be necessary.

(H) If the gradient is greater than 50 mmHg but lower than 70 mmHg, observation may be justified if symptoms and coronary disease are absent. As soon as symptoms develop operation is strongly indicated. Operation is indicated in all patients with a gradient greater than 70 mmHg. There is a 3 percent risk of sudden death in patients with a gradient greater than 50 mmHg.

(I) The most urgent indications for operation are a gradient greater than 55 mmHg or progressive symptoms.

(J) Coronary artery disease coexisting with AS should be corrected by simultaneous aortic valve replacement and coronary bypass. Operative mortality for the combined procedure is 4 to 6 percent.

(K) Valve replacement is almost always the operation of choice.

(L) Operative debridement and valvuloplasty are occasionally effective, but there is a high rate of restenosis within 5 years. Balloon valvuloplasty may be palliative, making later operation safer, or be sufficient alone in the sick older patient. Restenosis occurs in 40 percent of patients within 6 months.

(M) Excellent long-term results have been obtained with freeze-dried allografts. Procurement is difficult. Degeneration is a risk but is less with freeze-drying than with other types of preservation.

(N) Prosthetic valves, available in ball and tilting disc designs, are durable but require lifetime anticoagulation to prevent thromboembolism. Operative mortality is 3 to 5 percent for aortic valve replacement alone and as high as 25 percent for multiple valve replacement. Left ventricular function is the most important determinant of operative mortality.

(O) Porcine biprotheses are durable with few complications for 5 years. Beyond 5 years, there is an increasing incidence of degeneration and need for replacement. Xenografts are not advised in patients under 35 years of age because of a high rate of calcification. They are best used in patients over 60 years of age.

(P) The best event-free postoperative course is obtained with a freeze-dried allograft without the need for anticoagulants (90 percent event-free at 10 years). Survival after aortic valve replacement is 60 to 70 percent at 10 years, depending more on cardiac than valve function. Late complications include thromboembolism (including valve thrombosis), complications of anticoagulation, paravalvar

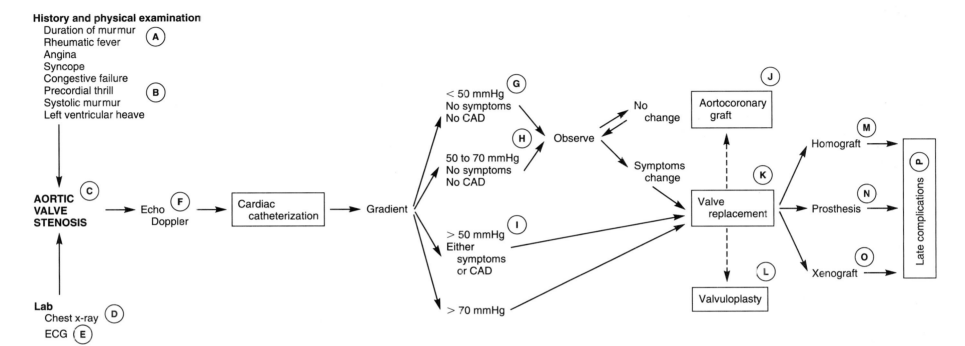

History and physical examination
Duration of murmur
Rheumatic fever (A)
Angina
Syncope
Congestive failure
Precordial thrill (B)
Systolic murmur
Left ventricular heave

AORTIC VALVE STENOSIS (C) → Echo Doppler (F) → Cardiac catheterization → Gradient

Lab
Chest x-ray (D)
ECG (E)

< 50 mmHg No symptoms No CAD (G)
50 to 70 mmHg No symptoms No CAD (H) → Observe → No change / Symptoms change
> 50 mmHg Either symptoms or CAD (I)
> 70 mmHg

Aortocoronary graft (J)
Valve replacement (K) → Homograft (M) / Prosthesis (N) / Xenograft (O) → Late complications (P)
Valvuloplasty (L)

leak, prosthetic endocarditis, mechanical failure (strut fracture, disc wear), and progress of cardiac disease.

REFERENCES

Ardehali A. Comparison of indications for aortic valve replacement in 1978 and 1988. Am J Cardiol 1990; 66:1016–1018.

Chobadi R, Wurzel M, Teplitsky I, et al. Coronary artery disease in patients 35 years of age or older with valvular aortic stenosis. Am J Cardiol 1989; 64:811–812.

Cosgrove DM, Ratleff NB, Schaff HV. Aortic valve decalcification: history repeated with a new result. Ann Thorac Surg 1990; 49:689–690.

Lund O, Pilegaard HK, Magnussen K, et al. Long-term prosthesis related and sudden cardiac related complications after valve replacement for aortic stenosis. Ann Thorac Surg 1990; 50:396–406.

Lytle B, Cosgrove DM, Taylor PC, et al. Primary isolated aortic valve replacement: early and late results. J Thorac Cardiovasc Surg 1989; 97:675–694.

Miller FA. Aortic stenosis: most cases no longer require invasive hemodynamic study. J Am Coll Cardiol 1989; 13:551–553.

O'Brien MF, Stafford G, Gardner M. The viable cryopreserved allograft aortic valve. J Cardiac Surg 1987; 1:153–157.

O'Neill W. Predictors of long-term survival after percutaneous aortic valvuloplasty: report of the Mansfield Scientific Balloon Aortic Valvuloplasty Registry. J Am Coll Cardiol 1991; 17:193–198.

Pellika PA, Nishimura RA, Bailey KR, et al. The natural history of adults with asymptomatic, hemodynamically significant aortic stenosis. J Am Coll Cardiol 1990; 15:1012–1017.

Mitral Stenosis

Glenn J.R. Whitman, M.D.

(A) Most patients with mitral stenosis have a history of rheumatic fever. Two thirds of these patients are women. Twenty-five percent of patients have pure stenosis. Dyspnea after exertion is the principal symptom. This is the result of an increase in cardiac output that raises left atrial pressure, leading to shortness of breath and, in some cases, frank pulmonary edema. Thromboembolism is also an important historical feature of mitral stenosis. Without surgical therapy, 20 percent of patients develop systemic embolization with an associated 10 to 15 percent mortality.

(B) Severe mitral stenosis can be associated with so-called mitral facies, ie, pinkish-purple patches on the cheeks. Occasionally, severe left atrial enlargement that impinges on the left recurrent laryngeal nerve causes a hoarse voice. Auscultation reveals accentuation of S_1 if the anterior leaflet is mobile, an opening snap, and a loud P_2 with a narrowly split S_2. The diastolic murmur begins after the opening snap and is low pitched. Its duration is proportional to the severity of the stenosis. Atrial fibrillation is common.

(C) In over 90 percent of patients with moderate to severe mitral stenosis who are in sinus rhythm, the electrocardiogram shows left atrial enlargement. Right ventricular hypertrophy is often seen in patients with pulmonary systolic pressure greater than 70 mmHg. A posteroanterior x-ray of the chest may show pulmonary artery enlargement. A lateral view is useful to show left atrial enlargement. Two-dimensional echocardiography is crucial not only to determine the severity of stenosis and the presence of left atrial thrombus, but to provide information regarding the pliability of the valve leaflets and the degree of fusion and distortion of the subvalvular apparatus. These factors are important to assess reparability of the valve.

(D) Symptomatic improvement depends on decreasing left atrial pressure and pulmonary venous congestion. Avoidance of exercise and diuretics are helpful. With atrial fibrillation, digitalis and β-blockers are used to slow the heart rate, increase the duration of diastole, and thereby decrease left atrial pressure. If atrial fibrillation is of recent onset, procainamide or quinidine may be administered to convert to sinus rhythm. If cardioversion is contemplated, 3 or 4 weeks of anticoagulation is recommended to decrease the risk of systemic embolization. Atrial fibrillation and heart failure are indications for long-term anticoagulation.

(E) Once symptoms from mitral stenosis progress, survival is improved by surgical therapy. Mitral valve orifice size less than $1.0\ cm^2/m^2$ is an indication for surgery.

(F) Cardiac catheterization is performed to determine the presence of coronary disease and other valvular lesions that are difficult to assess by echocardiography in the presence of mitral stenosis.

(G) When the mitral valve leaflets are thick, immobile, and calcified with subvalvular chordal fusion, commissurotomy is not indicated. Such valves should be replaced with or without associated aortic valve replacement or coronary bypass.

(H) In patients with pliable leaflets, minimal calcification, and only mild to moderate chordal shortening and fusion, open commissurotomy is the procedure of choice. Mortality is less than 1 percent, and recurrence rates are approximately 2 to 3 percent per year. Intraoperative transesophageal echo is useful in evaluating the results and in assessing any degree of resultant mitral regurgitation, a finding that might necessitate the performance of a concomitant mitral annuloplasty. The finding of coronary artery disease necessitates myocardial revascularization. If aortic valvular disease that requires replacement is also present, the performance of a mitral commissurotomy should be carefully considered. If there is any doubt as to its effectiveness and long-term anticoagulation is anticipated, a mitral valve replacement with chordal preservation should be performed in an effort to decrease the development of recurrent symptoms and the necessity for reoperation.

REFERENCES

Bonchek LI. Indications for surgery of the mitral valve. Am J Cardiol 1980; 46:155–158.

David TE, Uden DE, Strauss HD, et al. The importance of the mitral apparatus in left ventricular function after connection of mitral regurgitation. Circulation 1983; 68 (suppl II):II–76–82.

Gross RJ, Cunningham JN Jr, Snively SS, et al. Long-term results of open radical mitral commissurotomy: ten-year follow-up study of 202 patients. Am J Cardiol 1981; 47:821–825.

Scott WC, Miller DC, Haverick A, et al. Operative risk of mitral valve replacement: discriminant analysis of 1329 procedures. Circulation 1985; 72(suppl II):108–119.

Seltzer A, Cohen KE. Natural history of mitral stenosis: a review. Circulation 1972; 45:878–890.

Spencer FC. A plea for early, open mitral commissurotomy. Am Heart J 1978; 95:668–670.

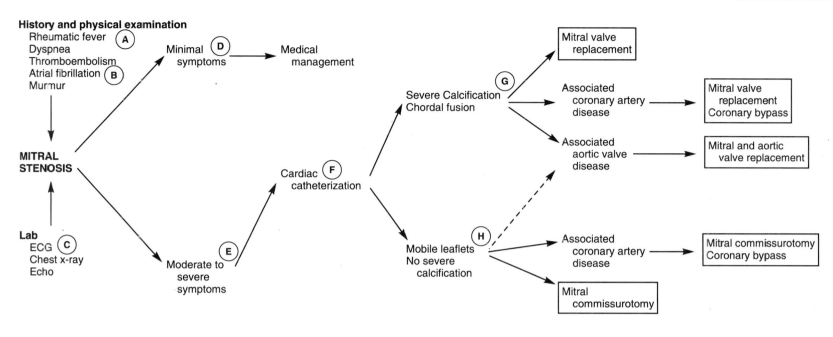

History and physical examination
Rheumatic fever (A)
Dyspnea
Thromboembolism
Atrial fibrillation (B)
Murmur

MITRAL STENOSIS

Lab
ECG (C)
Chest x-ray
Echo

Minimal (D) symptoms → Medical management

Moderate to severe symptoms (E)

Cardiac catheterization (F)

Severe Calcification Chordal fusion (G)

Mobile leaflets No severe calcification (H)

Mitral valve replacement

Associated coronary artery disease → Mitral valve replacement Coronary bypass

Associated aortic valve disease → Mitral and aortic valve replacement

Associated coronary artery disease → Mitral commissurotomy Coronary bypass

Mitral commissurotomy

Gastrointestinal

Blunt Abdominal Trauma

James M. Brown, M.D., and Ernest E. Moore, M.D.

(A) Unrecognized intraabdominal injury is a frequent cause of preventable death. Symptoms and signs of such injury are notoriously unreliable and are often masked by head injury, major fractures, or intoxication with alcohol or other toxins. About one third of patients who require emergent laparotomy have a benign abdominal examination. In contrast to penetrating trauma, the decision to perform laparotomy for blunt trauma is complex because structural injury is less obvious and associated multisystem injuries may demand more urgent attention.

(B) Severity of trauma is related to the force and duration of impact as well as to the mass of the patient contact area. In deceleration injury, organs move forward at the terminal velocity on impact tearing sites of attachment. Lap-belts can cause sudden elevation in intraabdominal pressure and produce hollow visceral rupture. Ecchymoses and abrasions are clues to internal hemorrhage. Pressure over the lower ribs helps establish whether or not ribs are fractured. Lower rib fractures can be associated with hepatic or splenic injury. Contour of the abdomen should be appraised before superficial and deep palpation.

(C) Although laboratory values are rarely helpful immediately, trends in comparison to baseline are important. Declining hematocrit, persistent leukocytosis, or hyperamylasemia indicates need for further evaluation. Hematuria in the setting of pelvic fracture prompts intravenous pyelography in addition to cystography and urethrography. Blood should be typed and crossmatched in patients with shock. Coagulation parameters are measured in the presence of liver disease.

(D) Lateral cervical spine films may show fractures that need attention during resuscitation. A chest film may demonstrate occult thoracic trauma (rib fractures, hemopneumothorax, pulmonary contusion, or torn aorta) or overt abdominal trauma (free air, ruptured diaphragm). Pelvic x-rays are important to identify occult fractures.

(E) The primary survey is a rapid assessment of the relative threat as well as the nature and degree of injuries. It is done simultaneously with initial resuscitation, placement of large-bore intravenous lines, and insertion of a Foley catheter. The intravenous lines allow rapid administration of crystalloid solution and blood, whereas the catheter provides decompression of the bladder before peritoneal lavage.

(F) The secondary survey consists of systematic reassessment and detailed physical examination from head to toe. Neurologic, chest, abdominal, vascular, orthopedic, and soft tissue examinations should be carefully recorded. Blood in the nasogastric return suggests a duodenal injury.

(G) Hemodynamic instability with overt peritonitis or massive hemoperitoneum precludes further diagnostic testing. The patient is taken promptly to the operating room for laparotomy.

(H) A stable patient presenting in a delayed fashion should have the diagnostic workup directed toward the primary complaint. Abdominal computed tomography scanning is ideally suited for this setting.

(I) Risk to the patient correlates directly with energy imparted. High-speed automobile impacts, falls from greater than 25 feet, and auto—pedestrian and industrial accidents are high-energy transfer injuries.

(J) Lower energy transfer accidents usually cause limited damage. In an alert stable patient abdominal computed tomography scanning effectively excludes immediate life-threatening injuries. Most minor splenic injuries and some hepatic lesions can be managed nonoperatively.

(K) After high-energy impact or severe head injury (Glasgow Coma Scale <8), critical abdominal injuries can be excluded rapidly with diagnostic peritoneal lavage. A catheter is inserted into the abdominal cavity below the umbilicus using local anesthetic. If aspiration shows no gross blood, 1 L of saline is infused and allowed to drain back. Return of over 10 mL of gross blood or red blood cell counts greater than $100,000/mm^3$ and amylase greater than 20 IU/L with an alkaline phosphatase greater than 3 IU/L indicate need for operation. A white cell count greater than $500/mm^3$ is considered a relative indication for operation. The false-negative rate for diagnostic peritoneal lavage is 2 percent. Most frequently overlooked injuries are isolated tears of the diaphragm, bladder, or small bowel perforation and contained pancreatic transection.

(L) Despite newer generation scanners with high resolution, computed tomography scanning is complementary to rather than competitive with diagnostic peritoneal lavage. An advantage of computed tomography scanning is the ability to grade injuries to the spleen, liver, and kidneys. The amount of intraperitoneal blood can also be estimated.

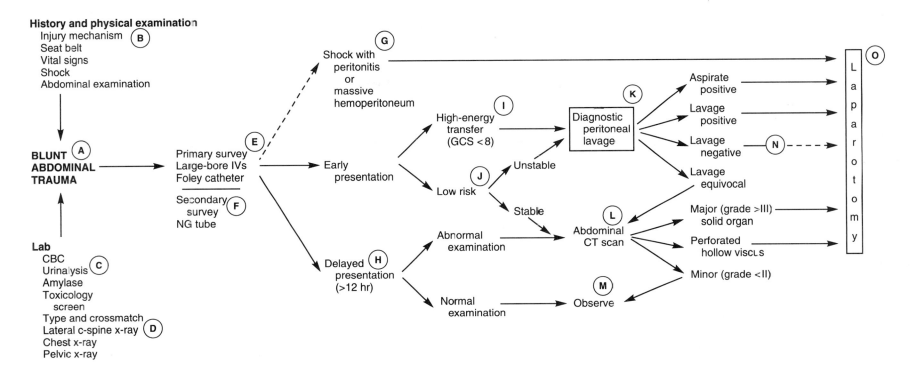

History and physical examination
Injury mechanism (B)
Seat belt
Vital signs
Shock
Abdominal examination

BLUNT (A)
ABDOMINAL
TRAUMA

Lab
CBC
Urinalysis (C)
Amylase
Toxicology screen
Type and crossmatch
Lateral c-spine x-ray (D)
Chest x-ray
Pelvic x-ray

(M) Observation requires repeated abdominal examination, monitoring of vital signs, and serial laboratory testing.

(N) A high-speed, head-on auto impact in which the nonrestrained driver is thrust into the steering wheel can rupture the duodenum. Evaluation by thin barium swallow screens for this possibility.

(O) Laparotomy is required to diagnose and safely manage most intraabdominal injuries. A midline incision is recommended because it can be done rapidly and extended for additional exposure. Control of hemorrhage is the first goal and should be followed by an orderly evaluation of abdominal contents. The retroperitoneum must be opened to evaluate the pancreas and distal duodenum. The bowel must be inspected systematically from stomach to rectum. The diaphragm should be examined.

REFERENCES

Cox EF. Blunt abdominal trauma: a 5-year analysis of 870 patients requiring celiotomy. Ann Surg 1984; 199:467–474.

Davis JJ, Cohen I, Nance FC. Diagnosis and management of blunt abdominal trauma. Ann Surg 1976; 183:672–678.

Fabian TC, Mangiante EC, White TJ, et al. Computed tomography in blunt abdominal trauma. J Trauma 1986; 26:602–608.

Henneman PL, Marx JA, Moore EE, et al. Diagnostic peritoneal lavage: accuracy in predicting necessary laparotomy following blunt and penetrating trauma. J Trauma 1990; 30:1345–1355.

Klein S, Johs S, Fujitani R, et al. Hematuria following blunt abdominal trauma: the utility of intravenous pyelography. Arch Surg 1988; 123:1171–1177.

Marx JA, Moore EE, Bar-Or D. Peritoneal lavage in small bowel colon injuries: the value of enzyme determinations. Ann Emerg Med 1990; 12:68–70.

Marx JA, Moore EE, Jorden RC, et al. Limitations of computed tomography in the evaluation of acute abdominal trauma: a prospective comparison with diagnostic peritoneal lavage. J Trauma 1985; 25:933–937.

McAnena OJ, Moore EE, Marx JA. Initial evaluation of the patient with blunt abdominal trauma. Surg Clin North Am 1990; 70:495–515.

Moore JB, Moore EE, Markovchick V, et al. Diagnostic peritoneal lavage for abdominal trauma—superiority of the open technique at the infraumbilical ring. J Trauma 1981; 21:570–572.

Penetrating Abdominal Trauma

David V. Feliciano, M.D.

(A) The extent of resuscitation and evaluation in patients with penetrating abdominal wounds depends on whether or not peritoneal penetration has occurred. A stable asymptomatic patient with an anterior abdominal stab wound does not need a chest x-ray, urinalysis, or intravenous pyelogram until peritoneal penetration is confirmed.

(B) X-ray evidence of pneumothorax or hemothorax in a patient with abdominal penetration documents that a thoracoabdominal wound with injury to the diaphragm is present.

(C) An abdominal x-ray showing extensive free air is strongly suggestive of gastrointestinal perforation. When an abdominal x-ray shows a missile on the side of the abdomen opposite from an entrance wound, laparotomy is mandatory because 96 to 98 percent of such patients have visceral or vascular injury.

(D) Microscopic or gross hematuria, evident after spontaneous voiding or nontraumatic passage of a bladder catheter, is diagnostic of abdominal penetration and proves injury to the kidney, ureter, or bladder. An intravenous pyelogram can identify the site of such injury in many patients.

(E) In the hypotensive patient, insertion of large-bore (7.5 French or 14 gauge) intravenous catheters is attempted in the upper extremities or at the thoracic inlet because compression or clamping of the inferior vena cava may be required during the subsequent laparotomy.

(F) A nasogastric tube decompresses the stomach and permits easier examination of the patient. It is mandatory before diagnostic peritoneal lavage is performed. The rapid return of bloody contents through the nasogastric tube confirms penetration of the peritoneum and perforation of the stomach.

(G) When laparotomy is required, preoperative use of one or more antibiotics with aerobic and anaerobic coverage lowers the incidence of postoperative intraabdominal abscess and wound infection.

(H) Signs of intraabdominal injury mandating laparotomy are present in 55 to 60 percent of patients with abdominal stab wounds and in 75 to 90 percent of patients with abdominal gunshot wounds. Shock, peritonitis, and major evisceration are easily recognized signs.

(I) There are three means of evaluating an asymptomatic patient who has a possible penetrating stab wound of the anterior abdominal wall. The first is local wound exploration for peritoneal penetration followed by diagnostic peritoneal tap (positive, 20 mL blood, foreign body, gastrointestinal or biliary contents) or lavage (positive, $>100,000$ RBC/mm^3, >500 WBC/mm^3, foreign body, gastrointestinal or biliary contents). A positive tap or lavage (diagnostic peritoneal lavage) is an indication for laparotomy. This combined technique has an accuracy of 95 to 96 percent and rarely misses significant intraabdominal injuries. The second approach is double contrast computed tomography. In early evaluation it has an accuracy of 75 to 80 percent. As with blunt trauma, a major concern is computed tomography accuracy when small perforations of the gastrointestinal tract are present. Observation with serial physical examinations for a period of 24 to 48 hours is the third option. It has an accuracy rate of 95 to 97 percent and is suitable when a small number of patients with penetrating wounds are encountered.

(J) There are also options in the evaluation and management of the asymptomatic patient with a stab or gunshot wound in the posterior abdomen or flank. Observation by serial physical examinations is accurate in 95 percent of patients. Computed tomography scanning with either double (intravenous or oral) or triple contrast (add Gastrografin enema) has an accuracy rate of 92 to 97 percent.

(K) Options for management of the asymptomatic patient with a gunshot wound proximal to the abdomen include either diagnostic peritoneal tap and lavage or observation. A positive diagnostic peritoneal tap (20 mL of blood, foreign body, gastrointestinal or biliary contents) mandates laparotomy. A negative tap is followed by a diagnostic peritoneal lavage. Because penetration of the peritoneal cavity by a bullet causes visceral or vascular injury in 96 to 98 percent of patients, return of as few as 5000 RBC/mm^3 is considered a positive lavage. Observation by serial physical examinations can be used when it is impossible to verify that a missile penetrated the peritoneum as it passed through the anterior abdominal wall of an obese patient.

(L) Any patient admitted after a negative diagnostic peritoneal lavage or initial physical examination is observed for 24 to 48 hours. Laparotomy is indicated if hypotension or signs of peritonitis develop during this period.

(M) Laparotomy is performed through a midline incision. Hemorrhage from viscera or vascular structures is controlled first. Before opening a stable hematoma, gastrointestinal perforations are rapidly closed in a transverse fashion using sutures or noncrushing clamps.

(N) The survival rate of patients with abdominal stab wounds that cause visceral or vascular injury is 98 percent. Most deaths are caused by

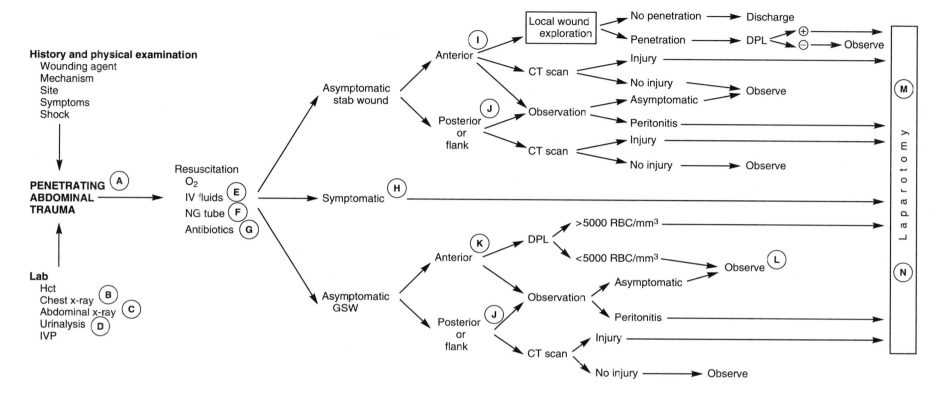

History and physical examination
Wounding agent
Mechanism
Site
Symptoms
Shock

PENETRATING (A)
ABDOMINAL ──→
TRAUMA

Resuscitation
O_2
IV fluids (E)
NG tube (F)
Antibiotics (G)

Lab
Hct
Chest x-ray (B)
Abdominal x-ray (C)
Urinalysis (D)
IVP

Asymptomatic stab wound

Anterior (I) ──→ Local wound exploration ──→ No penetration ──→ Discharge
                                          ──→ Penetration ──→ DPL ⟨+ ──→ ／ − ──→ Observe
                  ──→ CT scan ──→ Injury
                              ──→ No injury ──→ Observe

Posterior or flank (J) ──→ Observation ──→ Asymptomatic ──→ Observe
                                        ──→ Peritonitis
                       ──→ CT scan ──→ Injury
                                   ──→ No injury ──→ Observe

Symptomatic (H)

Asymptomatic GSW

Anterior (K) ──→ DPL ──→ >5000 RBC/mm³
                     ──→ <5000 RBC/mm³ ──→ Observe (L)
             ──→ Observation ──→ Asymptomatic
                             ──→ Peritonitis

Posterior or flank (J) ──→ CT scan ──→ Injury
                                    ──→ No injury ──→ Observe

Laparotomy (M) (N)

shock during the first 24 hours after laparotomy. The survival rate of patients with abdominal gunshot wounds that cause visceral or vascular injury is 88 percent. If patients with abdominal vascular injuries are excluded, the survival rate is 97 percent.

REFERENCES

Demetriades D, Rabinowitz B. Indications for operation in abdominal stab wounds: a prospective study of 651 patients. Ann Surg 1987; 205:129–132.

Demetriades D, Rabinowitz B, Sofianos C, et al. The management of penetrating injuries of the back: a prospective study of 230 patients. Ann Surg 1988; 207:72–74.

Feliciano DV. Abdominal trauma. In: Schwartz SI, Ellis H, eds. Maingot's abdominal operations. East Norwalk, CT: Appleton & Lange, 1989; 457–512.

Feliciano DV, Bitondo CG, Steed G, et al. Five hundred open taps or lavages in patients with abdominal stab wounds. Am J Surg 1984; 148:772–777.

Feliciano DV, Burch JM, Spjut-Patrinely V, et al. Abdominal gunshot wounds: an urban trauma center's experience with 300 consecutive patients. Ann Surg 1988; 208:362–370.

Meyer DM, Thal ER, Weigelt JA, et al. The role of abdominal CT in the evaluation of stab wounds to the back. J Trauma 1989; 29:1226–1229.

Moore EE, Moore JB, Van Duzer-Moore S, et al. Mandatory laparotomy for gunshot wounds penetrating the abdomen. Am J Surg 1980; 140:847–851.

Phillips T, Sclafani SJA, Goldstein A, et al. Use of the contrast-enhanced CT enema in the management of penetrating trauma to the flank and back. J Trauma 1986; 26:593–601.

Rehm CG, Sherman R, Hinz TW. The role of CT scan in evaluation for laparotomy in patients with stab wounds of the abdomen. J Trauma 1989; 29:446–450.

Duodenal Injury

R. Russell Martin, M.D., and Kenneth L. Mattox, M.D.

(A) Early preoperative diagnosis of duodenal injury is difficult because of the retroperitoneal location of the duodenum.

(B) Abdominal radiographs occasionally show free air and fluid.

(C) Contrast studies occasionally show duodenal extravasation.

(D) Complete inspection of the duodenum is necessary when injury is suspected. This requires a Kocher maneuver and sometimes takedown of the ligament of Treitz.

(E) Adequate debridement of compromised tissue is necessary. Sutures must be placed in viable tissue. If there is significant narrowing after closure, a technically questionable closure, or pancreatic injury, pyloric exclusion is advisable (pyloric closure plus gastrojejunostomy).

(F) When suture repair produces tension, a Roux-en-Y loop anastomosis to the duodenum is preferable to serosal or pedicle bowel flaps.

(G) Injuries at the ampulla are rare. Pancreaticoduodenectomy is indicated only if all duct structures are injured.

(H) Hematoma seen at laparotomy requires evacuation to avoid obstruction and to detect duodenal or pancreatic injury.

(I) Duodenal obstruction from a hematoma can occur as late as 1 to 3 weeks after injury. The obstruction is relieved spontaneously in many patients during a period of observation. Support by nasogastric suction and total parenteral nutrition is required. Obstruction by a hematoma should raise the suspicion of associated injuries.

REFERENCES

Jordan GL. Injury to the pancreas and duodenum. In: Mattox KI, Moore EE, Feliciano DV, eds. Trauma. Norwalk, CT: Appleton & Lange, 1988:473–494.

Martin TD, Feliciano DV, Mattox KL, Jordan GL Jr. Severe duodenal injuries. Arch Surg 1983; 118:631–635.

Stone HH, Fabian TC. Management of duodenal wounds. J Trauma 1979; 19:334–339.

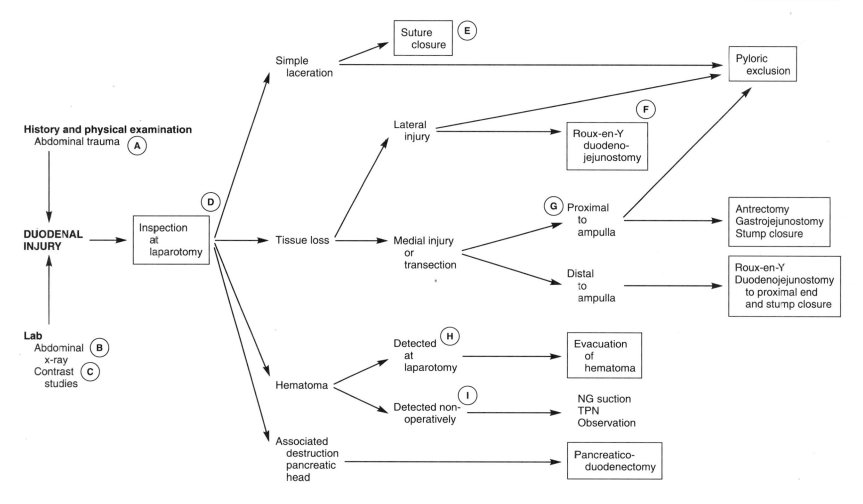

History and physical examination
Abdominal trauma (A)

DUODENAL INJURY

Lab
Abdominal (B)
x-ray
Contrast (C)
studies

Inspection at laparotomy (D)

Simple laceration

Suture closure (E)

Pyloric exclusion

Tissue loss

Lateral injury (F)

Roux-en-Y duodeno-jejunostomy

Medial injury or transection

Proximal to ampulla (G)

Antrectomy
Gastrojejunostomy
Stump closure

Distal to ampulla

Roux-en-Y
Duodenojejunostomy
to proximal end
and stump closure

Hematoma

Detected at laparotomy (H)

Evacuation of hematoma

Detected non-operatively (I)

NG suction
TPN
Observation

Associated destruction pancreatic head

Pancreatico-duodenectomy

Pancreatic Injury

R. Russell Martin, M.D., and Kenneth L. Mattox, M.D.

(A) Diagnosis of pancreatic injury is usually made during laparotomy performed for associated injuries.

(B) Computed tomography scanning is the most sensitive and specific imaging test preoperatively.

(C) Serum amylase is elevated in only 65 percent of patients with complete transection.

(D) Peritoneal lavage is not sensitive for retroperitoneal injury.

(E) Preoperative and intraoperative pancreatography in injured patients wastes valuable time. Equivalent data can be obtained by inspection at laparotomy.

(F) All pancreatic injuries require drainage and debridement of devitalized tissue. In an unstable patient, hemostasis and drainage alone may be advisable even though a pancreatic fistula is anticipated. Most fistulas close spontaneously; somatastatin can hasten closure.

(G) Pancreaticoduodenectomy, with its problematic anastomoses, is advisable only when the head of the pancreas, bile duct, and duodenum are extensively injured. If possible, injuries to the pancreas and duodenum should be treated separately.

(H) Pyloric exclusion (closure of the pylorus and gastrojejunostomy) is a safe and expedient method of treatment for combined pancreatic and duodenal injuries.

(I) If debridement requires resecting 80 percent or more (>12 cm) of the pancreas and the patient is stable, a Roux-en-Y limb to the pancreatic tail can be constructed to avoid diabetes mellitus.

Exocrine insufficiency after extensive resection is rare.

(J) Although pancreatic resections do not require splenectomy, splenic salvage does not justify a prolonged operation in a severely injured patient.

REFERENCES

Graham JM, Mattox KL, Jordan GL Jr. Traumatic injuries of the pancreas. Am J Surg 1978; 136:744–748.

Jones RC. Management of pancreatic trauma. Am J Surg 1985; 150:698–704.

Pederzoli P, Bassi C, Falconi M, et al. Conservative treatment of external pancreatic fistulas with parenteral nutrition alone or in combination with continuous intravenous infusion of somatostatin, glucagon, or calcitonin. Surg Gynecol Obstet 1986; 163:428–432.

Vaughn GD III, Frazier OH, Graham DY, et al. The use of pyloric exclusion in the management of severe duodenal injuries. Am J Surg 1977; 134:785–790.

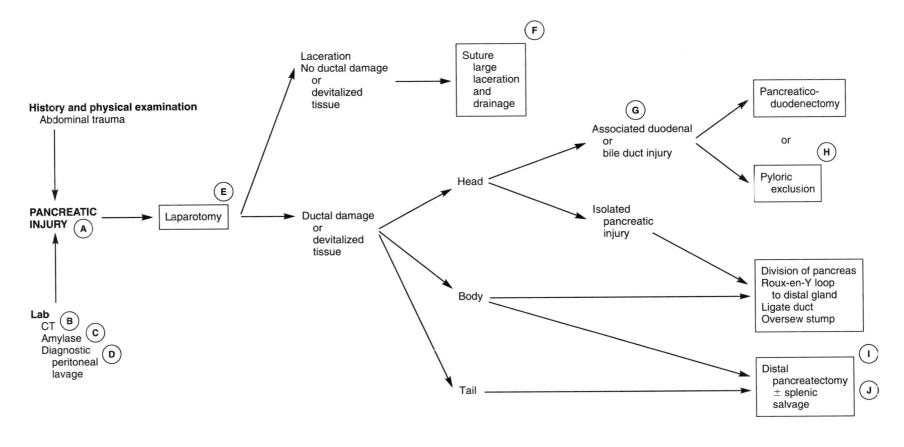

History and physical examination
Abdominal trauma

PANCREATIC
INJURY (A)

Lab (B)
CT
Amylase (C)
Diagnostic (D)
peritoneal
lavage

Laparotomy (E)

Laceration
No ductal damage
or
devitalized
tissue

Suture
large
laceration
and
drainage (F)

Ductal damage
or
devitalized
tissue

Head

Body

Tail

Associated duodenal
or
bile duct injury (G)

Isolated
pancreatic
injury

Pancreatico-
duodenectomy

or

Pyloric
exclusion (H)

Division of pancreas
Roux-en-Y loop
to distal gland
Ligate duct
Oversew stump

Distal
pancreatectomy
± splenic
salvage (I) (J)

Penetrating Injury of the Colon

Philip T. Neff, M.D., and Ernest E. Moore, M.D.

(A) The time and mechanism of injury as well as the patient's prehospital status are important factors in determining operative management. Paramedics often provide this information. Fresh blood found on rectal examination or sigmodoscopy is presumptive evidence of colon injury unless an alternative source of bleeding can be identified.

(B) The penalty for delay in treating colon injury is severe. Wounds in proximity to the retroperitoneal colon or rectum warrant laparotomy despite the absence of abdominal signs, unless diagnostic studies are unequivocally normal.

(C) Associated solid visceral or vascular injury is frequent with penetrating abdominal wounds and can be a source of major blood loss. If hypotension exists, blood is typed and crossmatched and serial hematocrits are obtained.

(D) Diagnosis of colon injury is based on suspicion of significant visceral or vascular injury rather than on specific findings of colon involvement. Initial evaluation follows that employed for penetrating trauma. Gunshot wounds of the abdomen mandate laparotomy if the bullet violates the peritoneal cavity. Plain abdominal x-rays (anteroposterior and lateral views) are used to assess missile trajectory. An intravenous pyelogram is done preoperatively for hematuria or when the missile trajectory is near the ureter. Stab wounds warrant local wound exploration followed by diagnostic peritoneal lavage if there are no signs of peritoneal irritation or shock. Retroperitoneal colon injury must be considered with penetrating back or flank wounds. Triple-contrast computed tomography scan may detect such injury in the asymptomatic patient.

(E) Prophylactic antibiotics are effective when given before the abdominal incision. The antibiotics should provide activity against anaerobic and aerobic bacteria. Broad-spectrum antibiotic coverage with a single agent, such as a third-generation cephalosporin or an extended-spectrum penicillin, is effective.

(F) A long midline abdominal incision rapidly provides wide exposure of the peritoneal cavity. Overt colon perforations are closed with intestinal clamps while abdominal exploration is completed, vascular control is accomplished, and the patient is resuscitated.

(G) Management of low-energy colon injury is based on hemodynamic stability, colon injury severity (CIS), associated trauma index (ATI), and time delay from injury. The splanchnic circulation is uniquely sensitive to shock, and vasoconstriction often persists despite adequate restoration of oxygen delivery.

(H) Severity of injury can be graded anatomically by the CIS index.

Grade I: serosal injury
Grade II: single wall injury
Grade III: <50 percent involvement
Grade IV: >50 percent involvement
Grade V: colon wall and adjacent blood supply injury.

Lower grade injuries are amenable to primary suture repair (with meticulous colon wound debridement), but more extensive wounds and larger grade injuries usually require segmental colon resection.

(I) The ATI is a means to quantify the magnitude of associated intraabdominal injury.

Organ 1: risk factor × injury estimate = score 1
Organ 2: risk factor × injury estimate = score 2
Organ 3: risk factor × injury estimate = score 3
Organ X: risk factor × injury estimate = score X
Total = ATI score

The complication–risk designation for each organ is based on the reported incidence of postoperative morbidity associated with the respective injury. Colon and pancreas are assigned a weight factor of 5; liver, duodenum, and major vascular—4; spleen, kidney, and extrahepatic biliary—3; small bowel, stomach, and ureter—2; and bladder, soft tissue, and minor vascular—1. The severity of injury to each organ system is estimated as follows: 1, minimal; 2, minor; 3, moderate; 4, major; and 5, maximum. The sum of the individual organ injury scores comprises the final ATI.

(J) Suture repair is performed in the low-risk patient after careful debridement of the colon wound. Optimal candidates have a low-energy gunshot wound or stab wound that involves less than 50 percent of the colonic circumference (CIS grade I to III) remote from the mesenteric surface. When the ATI is less than 25, the colon may be safely returned to the abdominal cavity. Left- and right-sided colon injuries are managed in the same way.

(K) When the ATI exceeds 25 or the patient has sustained protracted shock, the safest policy is to exteriorize the primary repair. Exteriorization of the repaired colon is a compromise between colostomy and primary suturing. Success of exteriorization depends on adequate mobilization of the injured segment to prevent obstruction and tension on the suture line and maintenance of a moist environment for the repair. The intact exteriorized repair is returned to the peritoneal cavity on the 10th postoperative day under light general anesthesia.

(L) Patients who have persistent shock, severe head injury, or associated injuries from which a protracted convalescence is anticipated should undergo colostomy. Colostomy is also preferred for patients presenting more than 6 hours after

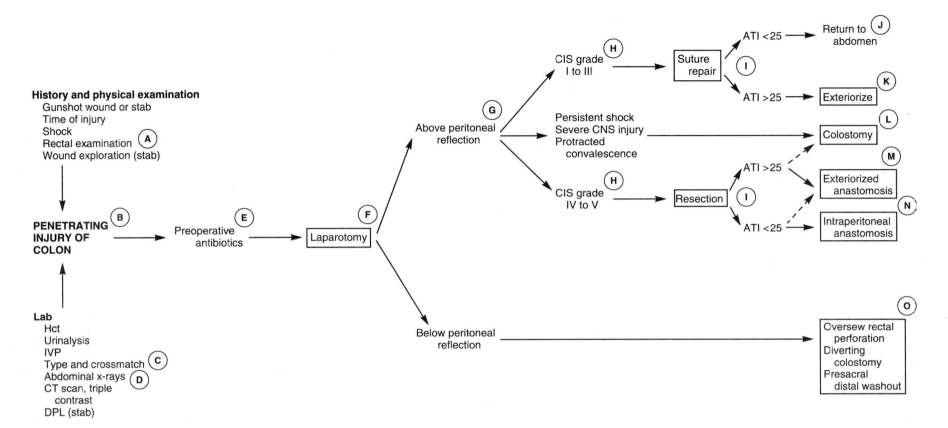

injury with fecal contamination and for patients with extensive associated abdominal injuries (ATI >25). Colostomy is done by stapling the mucous fistula and anchoring it adjacent to the end colostomy within the peritoneal cavity. Use of an intracolonic bypass conduit that prevents fecal flow and intestinal secretions from coming in contact with the intraluminal anastomotic site may obviate need for colostomy. Prograde colonic lavage is not helpful. The morbidity rate for colostomy closure is high because of dense peritoneal adhesions and loss of bowel related to initial injury. Delaying closure more than 6 weeks does not lessen the risk of complications. Preoperative barium studies are done to exclude a residual colonic fistula or stricture if an injury has been repaired distal to the colostomy. Standard bowel preparation is essential. The skin is closed over a double suction drain.

(M) In a patient at risk for intraperitoneal sepsis, the safest approach is to exteriorize the reanastomosed colon. Approximately 20 percent of exteriorized colons require conversion to colostomy.

(N) In the case of extensive bowel wall disruption or compromised blood supply, the involved bowel segment should be resected. The mesentery should be preserved to the edge of the colon, confirmed by active arterial bleeding. In hemodynamically stable patients with an ATI less than 25, the anastomosis can be returned to the abdomen.

(O) The fat-containing, poorly vascularized supralevator spaces tolerate infection poorly. Diversion of the fecal stream and wide pelvic drainage are critical. Primary suturing of rectal injury is desirable but not always feasible with low-lying perforations. Distal washout is best achieved in the operating room, but may be done postoperatively as well. Associated urologic trauma is frequent; resulting urinary fistulas increase the risk of pelvic sepsis. In rare instances high-energy, widely de-

Penetrating Injury of the Colon (Continued)

structive wounds of the pelvis may necessitate abdominoperineal resection.

REFERENCES

Baker LW, Thomson SR, Chadwich SJD. Colon wound management and prograde colonic lavage in large bowel trauma. Br J Surg 1990; 77:872–875.

Borlase BC, Moore EE, Moore FA. The abdominal trauma index—a critical reassessment and validation. J Trauma 1990; 30:1340–1344.

Kirkpatrick JR, Rajpal SG. The injured colon—therapeutic considerations. Am J Surg 1975; 129:187–191.

Moore FA, Moore EE, Ammons L, et al. Presumptive antibiotics for penetrating abdominal wounds. Surg Gynecol Obstet 1989; 169:99–103.

Ravo B, Ger R. A preliminary report on the intracolonic bypass as an alternative to a temporary colostomy. Surg Gynecol Obstet 1989; 159:541–545.

Shannon FL, Moore EE. Primary repair of the colon—when is it a safe alternative? Surgery 1985; 98:851–859.

Shannon FL, Moore EE, Moore FA, et al. Value of distal colon washout in civilian rectal trauma—reducing gut bacterial translocation. J Trauma 1985; 28:989–994.

Thompson JS, Moore EE. Factors affecting the outcome of exteriorized colon repairs. J Trauma 1988; 22:403–406.

Thompson JS, Moore EE, Moore JB. Comparison of penetrating injuries of the right and left colon. Ann Surg 1981; 193:414–418.

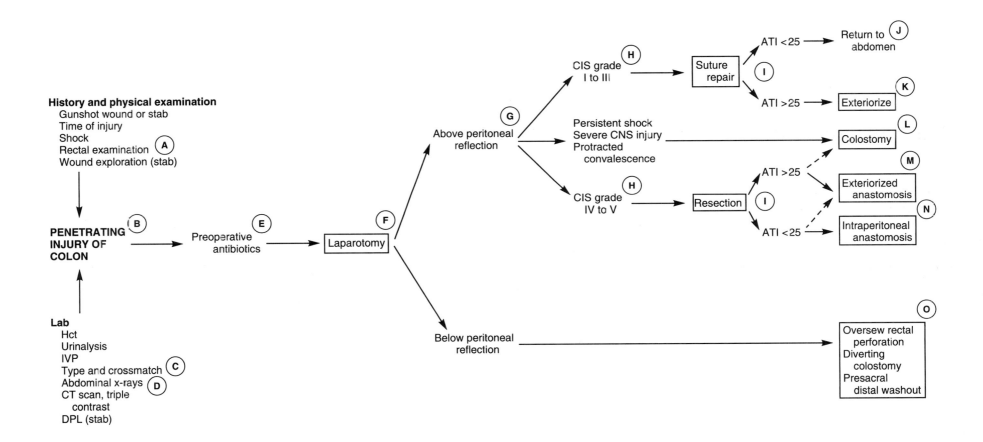

History and physical examination
  Gunshot wound or stab
  Time of injury
  Shock
  Rectal examination (A)
  Wound exploration (stab)

PENETRATING (B)
INJURY OF
COLON

Lab
  Hct
  Urinalysis
  IVP
  Type and crossmatch (C)
  Abdominal x-rays (D)
  CT scan, triple
    contrast
  DPL (stab)

Preoperative (E)
antibiotics

Laparotomy (F)

Above peritoneal (G)
reflection

Below peritoneal
reflection

CIS grade (H)
I to III

Persistent shock
Severe CNS injury
Protracted
  convalescence

CIS grade (H)
IV to V

Suture
repair

ATI <25 → Return to (J)
            abdomen

(I)

ATI >25 → Exteriorize (K)

Colostomy (L)

Resection (I)

ATI >25 → Exteriorized (M)
            anastomosis

ATI <25 → Intraperitoneal (N)
            anastomosis

Oversew rectal (O)
  perforation
Diverting
  colostomy
Presacral
  distal washout

Achalasia

Alex G. Little, M.D.

(A) Achalasia means failure of chalasia (Greek) or relaxation. Involved in the pathophysiology is loss of vagal innervation of the esophageal body and the lower esophageal sphincter (LES). Neural degeneration within the visceromotor axis, which extends from the dorsal motor nucleus of the vagus to the myenteric plexus in the esophageal wall, is documented. Diffuse esophageal spasm is similar to achalasia because patients have frequent simultaneous contractions. It differs in that the LES is usually normal and occasional peristalsis is seen. This is a rare disorder that does not usually require surgical intervention. Chagas' disease is found in South America and is caused by a parasite called *Trypanosoma cruzi*, which destroys the myenteric plexus. Clinically this disorder is indistinguishable from achalasia.

(B) The age of onset is variable but most commonly achalasia occurs in the third or fourth decade. Symptoms include dysphagia in all patients, regurgitation with or without aspiration in most, and chest pain in occasional patients.

(C) Barium swallow shows proximal esophageal dilation with distal beaklike narrowing.

(D) Esophagoscopy shows esophageal dilation with retained food. The esophageal mucosa may demonstrate retention esophagitis.

(E) Manometry is the diagnostic test for achalasia. It documents incomplete or absent LES relaxation and an absence of peristalsis due to simultaneous rather than sequential contractions. Contractions are usually weak. Vigorous achalasia is the diagnostic term used for the patient with stronger esophageal contractions and chest pain.

Manometric studies involve a brief outpatient procedure using a three- or four-lumen tube with multiple pressure sensors.

(F) The incidence of esophageal cancer is increased in achalasia, and this risk is unaffected by therapy.

(G) Calcium channel blocking agents and long-acting nitrates may be slightly effective for a short period of time but are rarely sufficient.

(H) It is impossible to restore normal function to the disordered esophageal body. The aim of therapy is to decrease the functional obstruction created by the inadequately relaxing LES. The two available options are forceful pneumatic dilation and open surgical myotomy. The wide variation in reported results for both methods of treatment are related to technique and operator experience.

	Relief of Dysphagia	Reflux	Perforations	Mortality Rate
	(%)	(%)	(%)	(%)
Forceful dilation	65–90	1–20	1–5	0–0.8
Esophagomyotomy	80–95	3–50	0–4	0–1.4

(I) The advantages of forceful pneumatic dilation are the avoidance of thoracotomy and the relatively low complication rate. The disadvantages include a 5 percent risk of perforation and less consistent long-term relief of dysphagia. Dilation is relatively contraindicated in patients with vigorous achalasia, those with marked esophageal tortuosity, and in patients with associated gastroesophageal reflux.

(J) Principles of esophagomyotomy are (1) left thoracotomy for ideal exposure and full mobilization of the esophageal hiatus, (2) single myotomy from the inferior pulmonary vein extending unequivocally onto the gastric wall, and (3) reconstruction with a modified Belsey fundoplication to prevent iatrogenic reflux.

The concern with esophageal myotomy alone without an antireflux procedure is achieving the perfect myotomy. If a myotomy is insufficient, the patient will not have relief of dysphagia. If the myotomy is excessive, severe reflux will result. A combination of full gastroesophageal mobilization, an unequivocally sufficient myotomy, and a Belsey fundoplication result in relief of dysphagia, prevention of reflux, and excellent results.

REFERENCES

Carter R, Brewer LA. Achalasia and esophageal carcinoma. Am J Surg 1975; 130:114–120.

Ellis FH, Crozier RE, Watkins E. Operation for esophageal achalasia. J Thorac Cardiovasc Surg 1984; 88:344–351.

Heimlich HJ, O'Connor TW, Flores DC. The case for pneumatic dilation in achalasia. Ann Otol 1978; 87:519–522.

Little AG, Soriano A, Ferguson MK, et al. Surgical treatment of achalasia: results with esophageal myotomy and Belsey repair. Ann Thorac Surg 1980; 45:489–494.

Sauer L, Pellegrini CA, Wade LW. The treatment of achalasia. Arch Surg 1989; 124:929–932.

Slater G, Sicular AA. Esophageal perforations after forceful dilation in achalasia. Ann Surg 1982; 195:186–188.

Traube M, Hongo M, Magyar L, et al. Effects of nifedipine in achalasia and in patients with high-amplitude peristaltic esophageal contractions. JAMA 1984; 252:1733–1766.

Vantrappen G, Hellemans J, Deloof W, et al. Treatment of achalasia with pneumatic dilations. Gut 1971; 12:268–275.

Vantrappen G, Janssens J, Hellemans J, et al. Achalasia, diffuse esophageal spasm, and related motility disorders. Gastroenterology 1979; 76:450–457.

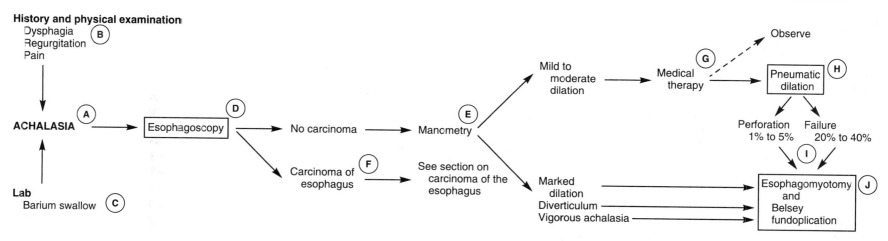

Carcinoma of the Esophagus

Manson Fok, M.B., B.S. (H.K.), F.R.C.S. (Ed.),
and John Wong, Ph.D. (Syd.), F.R.A.C.S.

(A) Dysphagia occurs when at least half the lumen of the esophagus is obstructed. Other symptoms include regurgitation, weight loss, and hoarseness. The last-named is due to palsy of the laryngeal nerve, usually the left.

(B) Heavy consumption of tobacco and alcohol, mineral deficiency in the diet, and food contaminated with nitrosamines are risk factors. Increased incidence is seen in Barrett esophagus and lye stricture and with other aerodigestive malignancies.

(C) Chest x-ray examination may show a hilar mass, tracheal compression and deviation, aspiration pneumonia, or pulmonary metastasis. Features important in assessing operability are pulmonary emphysema and evidence of tuberculosis. Mucosal irregularity and shouldering on the barium study are diagnostic and indicate the level and length of the tumor. Radiographic features suggestive of advanced disease include angulation, sinus formation, and fistulization.

(D) Mass screening in areas of high incidence using balloon exfoliative cytology enables the detection of early esophageal cancer. Early detection and treatment are associated with good prognosis. The accuracy of this method of screening is 97 percent.

(E) Endoscopic examination enables histologic confirmation by biopsy or cytology. Accuracy is enhanced by vital staining and endoscopic ultrasound. Endoscopic ultrasound is possible only in nonobstructing lesions. Accuracy of endoscopic ultrasound is 80 to 90 percent compared with accuracy of computed tomography scan or magnetic resonance imaging scan of 45 and 75 percent, respectively. Detection of submucosal secondaries helps determine the level of esophageal transection. The stomach should also be examined for concurrent gastric pathology.

(F) Flexible bronchoscopy is performed to detect tracheobronchial tumor involvement. Signs may include a widened carina, external compression, tumor infiltration, and fistulization. The last two signs are contraindications to resection.

(G) Additional investigations may offer more precise preoperative staging.

(H) Parenteral nutrition is used if weight loss exceeds 15 percent of ideal body weight and if albumin or transferrin are low. Cell-mediated immunity is impaired by malnutrition.

(I) Pulmonary assessment is important in deciding for transthoracic resection, transhiatal resection (less stressful), or a bypass operation. About 25 percent of patients are considered inoperable because of advanced disease with limited cardiopulmonary reserve.

(J) Endoscopic insertion of a prosthesis or thermocoagulation using a neodymium:yttrium-aluminum-garnet laser or bicap probe have comparable effects on short-term palliation. They may be performed alone or in combination with external radiotherapy. There is a 10 to 15 percent morbidity, including aspiration, fistulization, and perforation of the esophagus. Photodynamic therapy is of limited value.

(K) Radiotherapy is palliative but the survival rate is poor. As primary treatment for all stages of esophageal carcinoma, radiotherapy alone has a 5-year survival of only 5 percent.

(L) Some tumor regression follows chemotherapy, but the response is at best transient. There is no evidence that it prolongs survival.

(M) Chemotherapy–radiation therapy combinations used as preoperative adjunctive therapy are of some advantage. Complete or partial response is seen in 40 to 60 percent of patients, but there is no proof they improve survival. Chemoradiotherapy significantly increases pulmonary complications of surgery. Radiotherapy alone confers no benefits.

(N) There is no proven benefit of brachytherapy, immunotherapy, or hyperthermia either alone or in combinations, when used preoperatively.

(O) For operable patients, resection offers the best palliation of symptoms and a chance of cure. The 5-year survival for curative resection is 30 percent, for palliative resection 5 percent, and 0 percent for patients with bypass.

(P) At laparotomy, 5 percent of patients may be found to be unresectable and unsuitable for bypass. Postoperatively, endoscopic intubation or laser may be offered for palliation.

(Q) For those unsuitable for resection, a gastric or colonic bypass affords good palliation. The substitute organ is placed retrosternally or subcutaneously with the anastomosis in the neck to avoid a thoracotomy. Operative morbidity is high and patients with advanced disease and limited pulmonary reserve are better treated by intubation or laser.

(R) Pharyngolaryngoesophagectomy is the operation of choice for cervical esophageal cancer using a pharyngogastric anastomosis and a terminal tracheostome. For high cervical lesions, a free jejunal graft or a tubed pectoralis major myocutaneous flap can be used for reconstruction. Postoperative radiotherapy is given if a neck dissection

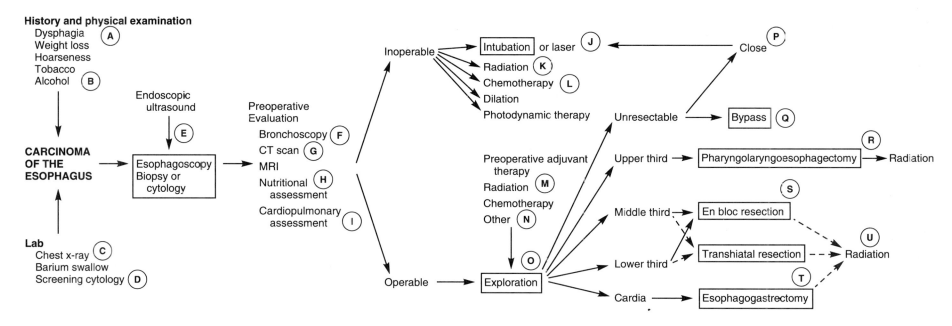

was not done. For lesions in the superior mediastinal segment, a split sternum approach offers adequate exposure.

(S) For middle and lower third esophageal cancers, resection is performed using an abdominal and right-thoracic approach. This permits en bloc resection of the tumor, lymph nodes, and thoracic duct. Left-sided thoracotomy limits exposure for lesions around the aortic arch. For patients with limited pulmonary reserve unsuitable for thoracotomy, transhiatal resection is an alternative, but is associated with 15 to 25 percent operative morbidity, including excessive bleeding, tumor rupture, tracheal perforation, or recurrent laryngeal nerve injury, especially for tumors of the middle third.

Survival after transhiatal resection also may be less than with transthoracic resection because of a less radical tumor clearance.

(T) For lesions involving the cardia, esophagogastrectomy is performed using an abdominal and right-thoracic approach or a transhiatal approach. Total gastrectomy may be necessary if the tumor involves more than a third of the stomach. Colon or small bowel can be used for reconstruction.

(U) There is no evidence that postoperative radiotherapy or chemotherapy improves survival. Radiotherapy may control local recurrence with known residual disease.

REFERENCES

DeMeester TR, Barlow AP. Surgery and current management for cancer of the esophagus and cardia. In: Ravitch MM, ed. Current problems in surgery. Vol 25. Chicago: Year Book, 1988:477–605.

Earlam R, Cunha-Melo JR. Oesophageal squamous cell carcinoma: II. A critical review of radiotherapy. Br J Surg 1980; 67:457–461.

Kelsen DP. Preoperative chemotherapy in esophageal carcinoma. World J Surg 1987; 11:433–438.

Orringer MB. Transhiatal esophagectomy without thoracotomy for carcinoma of the thoracic esophagus. Ann Surg 1984; 200:282–288.

Wong J. Stapled esophagogastric anastomosis in the apex of the right chest after subtotal esophagectomy for carcinoma. Surg Gynecol Obstet 1987; 164:568–572.

Wong J, Cheung HC, Lui R, et al. Esophagogastric anastomosis performed with a stapler: the occurrence of leakage and stricture. Surgery 1987; 101:408–415.

Gastroesophageal Reflux

Joseph LoCicero, III, M.D.

(A) Symptomatic gastroesophageal reflux (heartburn) occurs occasionally in as many as one in three people. It is common (25 percent) during pregnancy. Gastroesophageal reflux may present with pulmonary complaints or masquerade as atypical chest pain. Pathogenesis is a combination of failure of defense mechanisms, eg, inadequate lower esophageal sphincter pressure, and aggressive factors in the refluxed material.

(B) An upper gastrointestinal series rules out other diagnoses such as ulcer, cancer, or stricture. These abnormalities require evaluation by endoscopy. A sliding hiatal hernia is seen in more than half of patients over age 50. A causal relationship between hiatal hernia and reflux may exist. Fluoroscopy or cineradiography after gastric loading with barium assesses gastroesophageal reflux. Normal findings do not rule it out.

(C) Initial management (phase 1) includes elevation of the head of the bed; early evening meal; and avoidance of fat, chocolate, alcohol, tobacco, harmful medications, and antacids. Alginic acid (Gaviscon) may decrease symptoms. Weight loss in obese patients is helpful.

(D) A pH electrode is positioned 5 cm above the lower esophageal sphincter and a reference lead is placed on the arm. The pH probe is monitored to detect drops below pH 4. Correlation with reflux symptoms determines a positive test (sensitivity, 88 percent; specificity, 98 percent).

(E) Esophageal motility is studied manometrically using an infused catheter. Because of great variation in individual lower esophageal sphincter pressures, a single pressure reading has no value. A reflux patient usually has a pressure of 6 mmHg or less. Despite repeat measurements and slow or rapid pullthrough, manometry has poor sensitivity (58 percent).

(F) Endoscopy is the most common method of diagnosing esophagitis, although classification of the degree of inflammation is not well defined. When erythema, edema, and friability are considered to be esophagitis, the sensitivity of endoscopy is high (95 percent) but the specificity is low (41 percent). A biopsy should always be obtained.

(G) Phase 2 medical treatment in patients with confirmed gastroesophageal reflux is an H_2 receptor blocking agent (cimetidine), which improves symptoms and decreases need for antacids. Other H_2 blockers are ranitidine and famotidine. Both are effective but more expensive than cimetidine.

(H) About 10 percent of patients with gastroesophageal reflux who have a documented hypotensive lower esophageal sphincter and acid reflux require an antireflux operation. The Nissen transabdominal fundoplication and the Belsey transthoracic fundoplication each increase the resting pressure of the lower esophageal sphincter and improve chronic reflux in about 90 percent of patients. The transabdominal procedures allow evaluation of the stomach, biliary system, and pancreas. Mortality rate after any of these procedures is 0.1 to 1.6 percent. Complications are infrequent but can be significant. The gas-bloat syndrome, occurring most often after the Nissen fundoplication, is the inability to belch or vomit. Symptoms persist or recur in 10 percent of patients.

REFERENCES

Boesby S. Relationship between gastroesophageal acid reflux, basal gastroesophageal sphincter pressure and gastric acid secretion. Scand J Gastroenterol 1977; 12:547–551.

Brand DL, Eastwood IR, Martin D, et al. Esophageal symptoms, manometry and histology before and after antireflux surgery: a long-term follow-up study. Gastroenterology 1979; 76:1393–1401.

DeMeester TR, Wang C, Wessly JA, et al. Technique, indications and clinical use of 24-hour esophageal pH monitoring. J Thorac Cardiovasc Surg 1980; 79:656–700.

Ellis FH Jr, Crozier RE. Reflux control by fundoplication: a clinical and manometric assessment of the Nissen operation. Ann Thorac Surg 1984; 38:387–392.

Johnson LF, DeMeester TR. Evaluation of elevation of the head of the bed, bethanechol and antacid foam tablets on gastroesophageal reflux. Dig Dis Sci 1981; 26:673–680.

Orringer M, Sinner D, Belsey R. Long term results of the Mark IV operation for hiatal hernia and analyses of recurrences and their treatment. J Thorac Cardiovasc Surg 1972; 63:25–33.

Richter JE, Castell DO. Gastroesophageal reflux. Ann Intern Med 1982; 97:93–103.

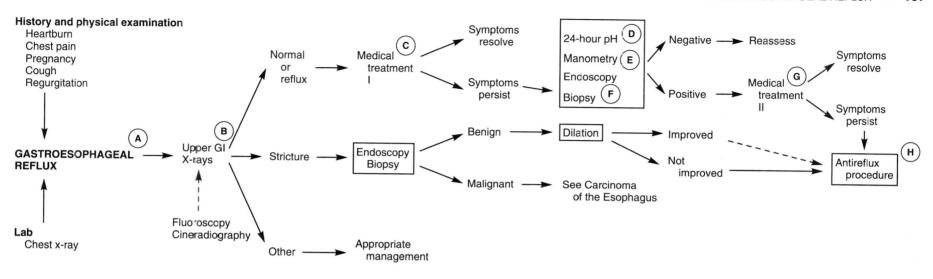

History and physical examination
Heartburn
Chest pain
Pregnancy
Cough
Regurgitation

Lab
Chest x-ray

GASTROESOPHAGEAL REFLUX

Gastric Ulcer

Sean J. Mulvihill, M.D., and Haile T. Debas, M.D.

(A) The classic history of epigastric pain relieved by food or antacids is present in most patients with gastric ulcers. Studies using endoscopy to screen for gastric ulcers indicate that about 15 percent of patients have active ulcers without symptoms.

(B) Vomiting may be due to gastric outlet obstruction from prepyloric ulcers or ulcerating antral carcinoma. The incidence of bleeding from stress ulceration has declined significantly. Bleeding from type I gastric ulcer, particularly in the elderly, remains a life-threatening problem.

(C) Weight loss is suggestive of malignancy but can occur in chronic gastric outlet obstruction.

(D) Gastric cancer may have only signs and symptoms of anemia.

(E) Medications such as aspirin, nonsteroidal antiinflammatory agents, and steroids can cause acute gastric ulcers or erosions.

(F) The detection of guaiac-positive stools on rectal examination is an important clue to the presence of gastric pathology. An anterior rectal mass (Blumer shelf) suggests metastatic gastric cancer.

(G) Most gastric ulcers arise within 2 cm of the junction between the antral and fundic mucosa on the lesser curvature. This locus minoris resistantiae is sensitive to ulceration for reasons that are unknown. Unlike duodenal ulcer, the pathogenesis of gastric ulcer appears more related to decreased mucosal resistance than to increased acid–peptic activity.

(H) Plain films of the abdomen are necessary only when perforation is suspected. Free air is seen in about 70 percent of cases. A chest x-ray may demonstrate pulmonary metastases and inoperability of a gastric cancer.

(I) Achlorhydria is associated with gastric malignancy.

(J) Perforation of a gastric ulcer has a mortality rate of 10 to 40 percent, dependent mainly on the presence of associated illness and the duration of perforation. Optimal management includes excision of the ulcer, usually by distal gastrectomy. In unstable patients, simple excision of the ulcer with closure or four-quadrant biopsy with omental closure may be performed. Recurrence rates approximate 40 to 90 percent, however. The addition of truncal vagotomy and pyloroplasty reduces this rate significantly.

(K) Medical therapy is the initial management for benign gastric ulcers. Although the benefits of antacids are unproved, blockage of acid secretion with histamine H_2-receptor antagonists significantly increases healing rates over placebo. Misoprostol, a prostaglandin analogue, appears particularly beneficial in ulcers induced by nonsteroidal antiinflammatory agents. Sucralfate and colloidal bismuth are also superior to placebo in healing benign gastric ulcers. Repeat endoscopy with biopsy is indicated to exclude underlying malignancy in patients who remain symptomatic after 12 weeks of therapy. The main indications for operation in patients with benign gastric ulcer are nonhealing after a trial of medical therapy, multiply-recurrent ulceration, and inability to exclude malignancy. Prolonged courses of medical therapy without appropriate endoscopic evaluation should be discouraged.

(L) After resuscitation, initial management of bleeding gastric ulcer includes endoscopy for diagnosis and biopsy. Occasionally bleeding can be controlled endoscopically by cauterization. Inhibition of acid secretion with histamine H_2-receptor antagonists, titration of secreted acid with antacids, and mucosal protection with agents such as sucralfate all are of intuitive but unproved value in aiding cessation of bleeding. For the rare patient with massive bleeding from diffuse gastritis, selective left gastric embolization is indicated.

(M) The most sensitive diagnostic tool for gastric ulcer is upper gastrointestinal endoscopy. Biopsy and brushing of all chronic gastric ulcers is mandatory to exclude malignancy. The likelihood of a false-negative biopsy of a malignant gastric ulcer is directly related to the number of specimens sampled. The brush cytology is occasionally positive when the biopsy is negative. Upper gastrointestinal contrast studies are complementary to upper gastrointestinal endoscopy in the assessment of gastric ulcers. Radiating mucosal folds and small size (<3 cm in diameter) correlate with but do not prove benignancy.

(N) The most common type of gastric ulcer (55 to 60 percent of patients) is corporeal, or type I. The optimal operation for these patients is distal gastrectomy, incorporating the ulcer, with gastroduodenal anastomosis. The addition of truncal vagotomy does not appreciably alter long-term recurrence rates. In the elective setting, gastrectomy has a mortality rate of 2 percent and a long-term recurrence rate of 2 percent in patients with type I gastric ulcer. Proximal gastric vagotomy with ulcer excision has an advantage in terms of lower mortality and morbidity rates, but ulcer recurrence occurs in 8 to 25 percent of patients.

(O) Csendes and associates (1987) proposed a new class of gastric ulcers arising at the gastroesophageal junction. In the United States ulcers at this location are uncommon, but in Chile they represent 27 percent of all benign gastric ulcers. It is not clear that these ulcers are significantly different from type I ulcers. As with more distal ulcers, resection has the lowest long-term recurrence rate. To encompass the ulcer, the resection must be carried as a tongue high on the lesser curvature.

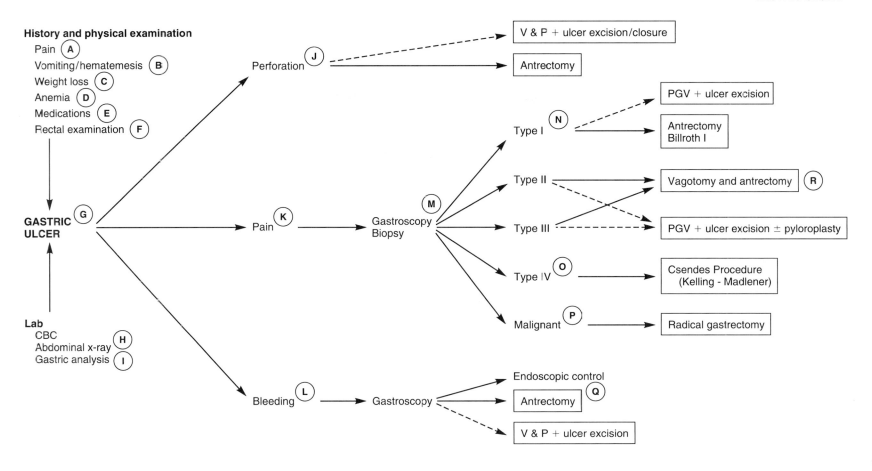

History and physical examination
- Pain (A)
- Vomiting/hematemesis (B)
- Weight loss (C)
- Anemia (D)
- Medications (E)
- Rectal examination (F)

GASTRIC ULCER (G)

Lab
- CBC
- Abdominal x-ray (H)
- Gastric analysis (I)

Perforation (J)
→ V & P + ulcer excision/closure
→ Antrectomy

Pain (K) → Gastroscopy Biopsy (M)
- Type I (N) → PGV + ulcer excision
- Type I → Antrectomy Billroth I
- Type II → Vagotomy and antrectomy (R)
- Type III → PGV + ulcer excision ± pyloroplasty
- Type IV (O) → Csendes Procedure (Kelling - Madlener)
- Malignant (P) → Radical gastrectomy

Bleeding (L) → Gastroscopy
- → Endoscopic control (Q)
- → Antrectomy
- → V & P + ulcer excision

To avoid narrowing the gastric inlet, reconstruction with a Roux-en-Y esophagogastrojejunostomy (Csendes procedure) is recommended for patients with type IV gastric ulcers within 2 cm of the gastroesophageal junction.

(P) The presence of pulmonary metastases and ascites indicates inoperability in patients with malignant gastric ulcers. When resection for cure appears possible, a radical subtotal gastrectomy with antecolic Billroth II reconstruction is preferred.

(Q) Indications for operation for continued bleeding from a benign gastric ulcer include:

1. Exsanguinating bleeding with shock
2. Persistent bleeding for over 24 hours requiring more than a 4-unit transfusion
3. Rebleeding during the same hospitalization

The optimal operation is resection of the ulcer by distal gastrectomy with Billroth I anastomosis. A second acceptable option is ulcer excision with vagotomy and pyloroplasty in selected patients. In the unstable patient, simple ulcer excision or oversewing of the ulcer is the most expedient operation, but long-term recurrences are common. For the rare patient with massive bleeding from diffuse gastritis, total gastrectomy is indicated if all other nonoperative measures fail to control the hemorrhage.

(R) Types II and III gastric ulcers are those that occur in the presence of duodenal ulcer or in the prepyloric location, respectively. These types

Gastric Ulcer (Continued)

each comprise 20 to 25 percent of patients with benign gastric ulcer. Treatment of these patients is directed at the underlying increased acid secretion. Truncal vagotomy with antrectomy, incorporating the ulcer in the resection, is the treatment of choice. Proximal gastric vagotomy with ulcer excision is an acceptable alternative but has higher recurrence rates than truncal vagotomy and antrectomy. Data suggest that the addition of pyloroplasty to proximal gastric vagotomy to increase gastric emptying reduces recurrence rates.

REFERENCES

Buckner JW III, Austin JC, Steinberg JB, et al. Factors predicting failure of medical therapy for gastric ulcers. Am J Surg 1989; 158:570–573.

Csendes A, Braghetto I, Smok G. Type IV gastric ulcer: a new hypothesis. Surgery 1987; 101:361–366.

Hodnett RM, Gonzalez F, Lee WC, et al. The need for definitive therapy in the management of perforated gastric ulcers: review of 202 cases. Ann Surg 1989; 209:36–39.

Isenberg JI, Peterson WL, Elashoff JD, et al. Healing of benign gastric ulcer with low-dose antacid or cimetidine: a double-blind, randomized, placebo-controlled trial. N Engl J Med 1983; 308:1319–1324.

Oi M, Oshida K, Sugimura S. The location of gastric ulcer. Gastroenterology 1959; 36:45–56.

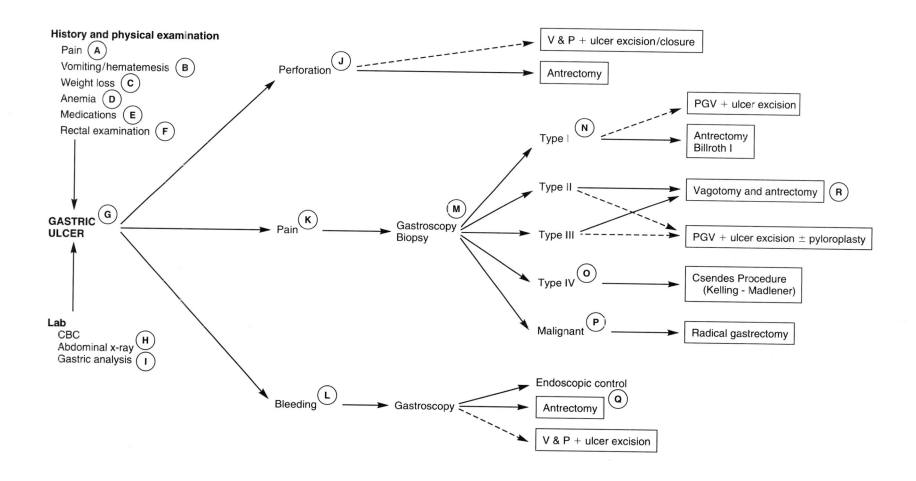

Duodenal Ulcer

Max M. Cohen, M.D.

(A) Endoscopy and upper gastrointestinal x-rays complement each other in the diagnosis of duodenal ulcer. Endoscopy is clearly superior in the presence of bleeding.

(B) Medical management achieves ulcer healing within 6 weeks in up to 90 percent of patients (virtually 100 percent with omeprazole). Up to 90 percent of patients develop a recurrence within 1 year of stopping treatment and approximately one third recur even on maintenance therapy. Dietary management alone is ineffective. Cessation of smoking promotes ulcer healing. Hospitalization for uncomplicated duodenal ulcer is never necessary. The standard for medical treatment is an H_2-receptor antagonist. Intractability and confirmed presence of *Helicobacter pylori* might warrant a trial with supplemental antibiotic therapy. Ulceration associated with the use of aspirin or other nonsteroidal antiinflammatory drugs is an indication for treatment with misoprostol (synthetic prostaglandin E_1 analogue).

(C) A definitive ulcer operation is reserved for low-risk patients seen within 12 hours of perforation, who have a good history of chronic duodenal ulcer. After a Graham closure, approximately one third of such patients require a definitive ulcer operation. All should be on treatment with an H_2 blocker.

(D) Most patients' (80 percent) bleeding from a duodenal ulcer stops within 24 hours with only supportive therapy, including intravenous fluids, H_2 blockers, and transfusion. Such patients may be refed promptly. Emergency surgery to control bleeding carries an operative mortality of up to 10 percent. The risk is increased by delaying surgery, particularly in elderly and high-risk patients. Repeated attempts to control bleeding by nonsurgical means in these patients is hazardous.

(E) Serum gastrin (fasting) should be measured on several occasions if a gastrinoma (Zollinger-Ellison syndrome) is suspected on clinical grounds (eg, massive hypersecretion, prominent gastric rugae, distal location of ulcer, multiple ulcers, diarrhea, frequent recurrence) and in all patients who develop recurrent ulceration after surgery. The upper limit of normal plasma gastrin is 50 pg/mL. It should be noted that plasma gastrin is mildly elevated in patients taking antisecretory drugs. Most patients with gastrinoma have a plasma gastrin of more than 200 pg/mL. The most reliable biochemical provocative test is the secretin stimulation test.

(F) Endoscopic control of bleeding duodenal ulcers has been achieved with lasers, electrocautery, and injection of agents such as alcohol. The modality of choice is probably bicapsular coagulation. Multiple endoscopic attempts to control bleeding only delay the necessary operation and increase operative mortality.

(G) More than 90 percent of patients who have a high-grade obstruction and a chronic ulcer history require definitive surgery within a year. Endoscopy is the best measure of the degree of obstruction. Patients with significant obstruction persisting for more than a few days should have surgical treatment with either vagotomy and antrectomy or vagotomy and drainage.

(H) Once the diagnosis of gastrinoma is made, gastric acid hypersecretion is controlled medically. The current drug of choice is omeprazole, which, if given in sufficient dosage and at proper intervals, is virtually always effective.

(I) Each surgical option has its risks and benefits. Vagotomy and antrectomy is the operation most likely to cure the ulcer (98 percent) but it carries an operative mortality of 1 to 3 percent and significant long-term sequelae in up to 15 percent of patients. Vagotomy and a drainage procedure (either pyloroplasty or gastrojejunostomy) are safer (1 percent mortality) with less morbidity (10 to 12 percent sequelae) but are associated with a higher recurrence rate (6 to 12 percent). Highly selective vagotomy is the safest operation (mortality less than 0.5 percent) but it has an ulcer recurrence rate of up to 30 percent (as high as 40 percent in patients resistant to therapy with H_2 blockers).

REFERENCES

Brearley S, Keighley MRB. Selection of patients for surgery following peptic ulcer hemorrhage. Br J Surg 1987; 74:893–896.

Cohen MM. Surgical treatment of duodenal ulcer: risks and benefits. Ann Roy Coll Phys Surg Can 1986; 19:357–361.

Crofts TJ, Park KGM, Steele RJC, et al. A randomized trial of nonoperative treatment for perforated peptic ulcer. N Engl J Med 1989; 321:970–973.

Freston JW. Overview of medical therapy of peptic ulcer disease. Gastroenterol Clin North Am 1990; 19:121–140.

Hoffmann J, Olesen A, Jensen HE. Prospective 14 to 18 year follow up study after parietal cell vagotomy. Br J Surg 1987; 74:1056–1059.

Jaffin BW, Kaye MD. The prognosis of gastric outlet obstruction. Ann Surg 1985; 201:176–179.

Kurata JH, Corbay ED. Current peptic ulcer time trends. J Clin Gastroenterol 1988; 10:259–268.

Laine L. Multipolar electrocoagulation in the treatment of peptic ulcers with nonbleeding visible vessels: a prospective controlled trial. Ann Intern Med 1989; 110:510–514.

Mulholland MW, Debas HT. Chronic duodenal and gastric ulcer. Surg Clin North Am 1987; 67:489–507.

Peterson WL. Bleeding peptic ulcer epidemiology and nonsurgical management. Gastroenterol Clin North Am 1990; 19:155–170.

Tytgat GNJ, Rauws EAJ. *Campylobacter pylori* and its role in peptic ulcer disease. Gastroenterol Clin North Am 1990; 19:183–196.

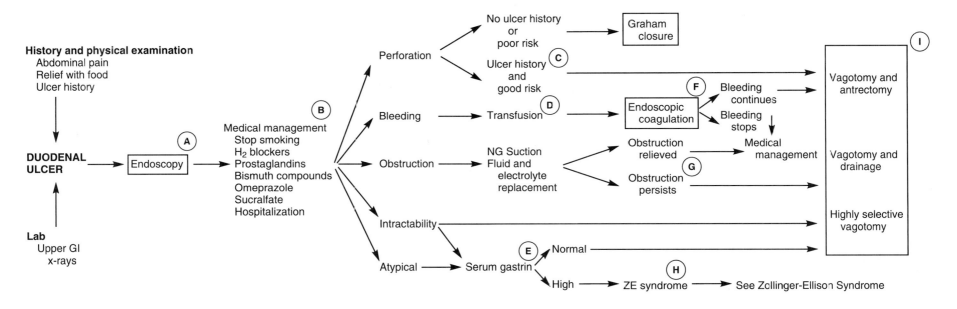

Postgastrectomy Syndrome

Bruce E. Stabile, M.D., Edward Passaro, Jr., M.D.,
and Philip C. Watt, M.D.

(A) Postprandial epigastric pain, nausea, and bilious vomiting suggest alkaline reflux gastritis. Pain is unrelieved by antacids or food but may subside after vomiting bile. Weight loss and anemia are frequent. Diagnosis rests on symptoms, endoscopic demonstration of bile reflux, mucosal erythema and erosions, and biopsy evidence of gastritis. Correlation between histologic findings and symptoms is poor.

(B) Diarrhea is common after truncal vagotomy but is persistent and disabling in only 5 percent of patients. The mechanism is not known.

(C) Dumping results from unregulated gastric emptying caused by resection, ablation, or bypass of the pyloric sphincter. Symptoms include colic, distention, nausea, emesis, diarrhea, flatulence, borborygmi, weakness, dizziness, diaphoresis, flushing, palpitations, and occasional syncope, all occurring shortly after eating. Provocative testing with oral hypertonic glucose reproduces symptoms and correlates with decreases in plasma volume and increases in gastric emptying rate and blood glucose. Symptoms of late hypoglycemia are those of an epinephrine response, including diaphoresis, palpitations, tremulousness, and weakness. This occurs 2 to 4 hours after eating.

(D) Afferent loop obstruction after Billroth II gastrectomy presents as postprandial right upper quadrant pain and fullness relieved by sudden projectile vomiting of bile unmixed with food. Ultrasonography may show a dilated duodenum and afferent jejunal limb.

(E) The blind loop syndrome results from stasis and bacterial proliferation that cause bile salt deconjugation, impaired lipolysis, diarrhea, weight loss, and malabsorption of fat-soluble vitamins and B_{12}. A 72-hour stool collection for fecal fat confirms steatorrhea and the carbon 14–cholate breath test documents bacterial overgrowth.

(F) Malabsorption may involve fat, protein, fat-soluble vitamins, B_{12} folate, iron, calcium, and a variety of trace elements. Manifestations include weight loss, steatorrhea, anemia, and metabolic bone disease. Fecal fat and serum iron, calcium, and vitamin levels are measured. A Schilling test and a small bowel biopsy are often useful.

(G) Recurrent ulcer is least frequent (1 to 2 percent) after vagotomy and antrectomy. The most common cause is inadequate vagotomy. Other causes are inadequate gastric resection, incomplete gastric outlet obstruction, and poor antral drainage. Work-up includes upper gastrointestinal series, endoscopy, acid secretory studies, and serum calcium and gastrin levels.

(H) Most postoperative gastric bezoars are phytobezoars. Causes include inadequate mastication, hypoacidity, decreased proteolysis, and impaired gastric emptying. Bezoars may cause early satiety, foul breath, epigastric fullness, nausea, vomiting, and, occasionally, gastric obstruction.

(I) The risk of developing gastric cancer after gastrectomy for benign gastroduodenal lesions is slight. Most cancers occur after 10 years.

(J) Cholestyramine is poorly tolerated. Metoclopramide promotes gastric emptying and diminishes reflux. Results with these drugs are inconsistent in mild cases and poor in severe cases. Cisapride may be of benefit if other drugs fail.

(K) Dietary changes include withholding fluids during meals, avoiding lactose and excessive fat, and adding bran. Kaolin-pectate, diphenoxylate, paregoric, and codeine are usually helpful.

(L) A high-protein, high-fat, low-carbohydrate diet and recumbency after meals reduce the emptying rate and the osmolarity of gastric contents. Multiple small feedings and avoidance of liquids with meals also help. For treatment of late hypoglycemia, the diet should be low in sugar and high in protein and fat.

(M) Antibiotics and pancreatic enzymes control bacterial overgrowth and decrease steatorrhea over the short term. Decompression of the blind loop is necessary for permanent correction.

(N) Gastric lavage and cellulytic, proteolytic, and mucolytic enzymes successfully dissolve most bezoars. Operative removal is rare.

(O) Roux-en-Y gastrojejunostomy using a 40-cm jejunal limb prevents reflux of alkaline contents into the gastric remnant. Vagotomy is required. Results are excellent in 75 to 95 percent of patients.

(P) Operation is rarely indicated for unremitting diarrhea unassociated with dumping. Somatostatin can be tried in these cases to alleviate diarrhea and dumping before any remedial surgery. Results of reversing a 10-cm segment of jejunum approximately 100 cm distal to the ligament of Treitz are disappointing. For dumping, a 10-cm segment of proximal jejunum is interposed between the gastric remnant and the duodenum. An antiperistaltic loop is generally preferred and gives

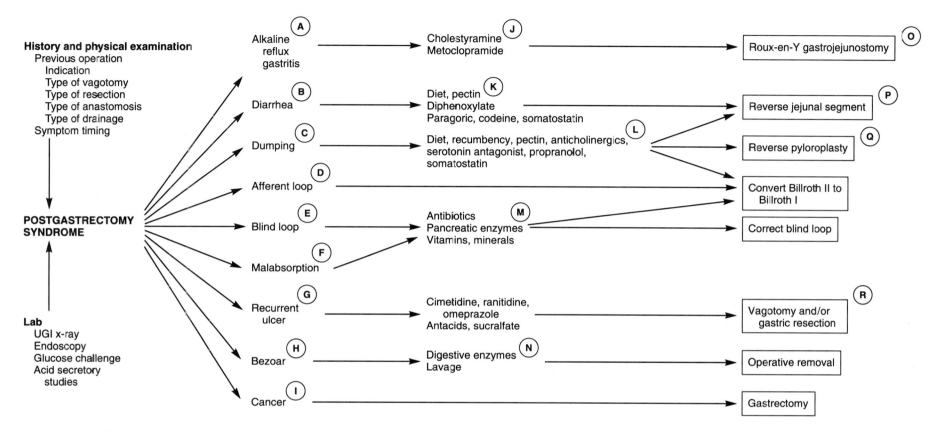

History and physical examination
Previous operation
  Indication
  Type of vagotomy
  Type of resection
  Type of anastomosis
  Type of drainage
  Symptom timing

**POSTGASTRECTOMY
SYNDROME**

Lab
UGI x-ray
Endoscopy
Glucose challenge
Acid secretory
  studies

good results in 90 percent of patients. Vagotomy prevents jejunal ulcer formation.

(Q) Pyloric reconstruction after Heineke-Mikulicz pyloroplasty is simple and effective in about 75 percent of cases.

(R) Vagotomy plus antrectomy is usually indicated for recurrent ulcer. A solitary gastrinoma is excised.

REFERENCES

Clark CG. Medical complications of gastric surgery for peptic ulcer. Compr Ther 1981; 8:26–32.

Kaushik SP, Ralphs DNL, Hobsley M, et al. Use of a provocation test for objective assessment of dumping syndrome in patients undergoing surgery for duodenal ulcer. Am J Gastroenterol 1980; 74:251–257.

Kelly KA, Becker JM, van Heerden JA. Reconstructive gastric surgery. Br J Surg 1981; 68:687–691.

McCallum RW. Cisapride: a new class of prokinetic agent. Am J Gastroenterol 1991; 86:135–149.

Sawyers JL. Management of postgastrectomy syndromes. Am J Surg 1990; 159:8–14.

Stabile BE, Passaro E Jr. Recurrent peptic ulcer. Gastroenterology 1976; 70:123–135.

Storer EH. Postvagotomy diarrhea. Surg Clin North Am 1976; 56:1461–1468.

Wiznitzer T, Shapira N, Staler J, et al. Late hypoglycemia in patients following vagotomy and pyloroplasty. Int Surg 1974; 59:229–232.

Woodward ER, Hocking MP. Postgastrectomy syndromes. Surg Clin North Am 1987; 67:509–520.

Upper Gastrointestinal Bleeding

Lawrence W. Norton, M.D.

(A) Common causes of upper gastrointestinal bleeding are peptic ulcer disease, drug- or alcohol-induced gastritis, and esophageal varices. Recent trauma or sepsis suggests the possibility of stress ulcer. Retching can tear gastric or esophageal mucosa (Mallory-Weiss tear). Gastric cancer, esophagitis, and hemobilia are rare causes of bleeding.

(B) Crystalloid fluid is infused intravenously. A nasogastric tube (32 to 36 Fr) is passed to determine if bleeding is active. Absence of blood in the stomach does not exclude bleeding distal to the pylorus. Blood is transfused in the presence of ongoing hemorrhage if more than 1 L of blood is estimated to have been lost.

(C) Medical treatment begins with saline gastric lavage. The histamine H_2-receptor antagonist famotidine is given intravenously (20 mg q 12 hours). An antacid such as magnesium aluminum hydroxide buffer (30 to 120 mL/h) can raise gastric pH but is useful only for slow bleeding.

(D) Some patients bleed massively and require surgical control before medical treatment and endoscopy can be accomplished.

(E) Endoscopy is performed if the patient is not bleeding massively. A bleeding site is identified in 90 percent of patients. One third have two or more sites of bleeding. Despite its diagnostic usefulness, endoscopy has not reduced the mortality of upper gastrointestinal bleeding (10 percent).

(F) When operation is required before the source of hemorrhage is identified, a longitudinal pylorotomy is made to inspect the distal stomach and proximal duodenum. If no bleeder is found, the pylorotomy is closed transversely and the proximal gastric mucosa is examined through a transverse gastrotomy.

(G) Endoscopic control of bleeders in the stomach and duodenum is possible by either electrocoagulation laser phototherapy, heater probe therapy, or local injection of ethanol, epinephrine, or sclerosants. Electrocoagulation is as effective as laser therapy and less expensive. It is more effective treatment for diffuse bleeding than sclerotherapy. Ethanol, epinephrine, and sclerosants such as 1% sodium tetradecyl sulfate or 5% ethanolamine oleate can be injected directly around bleeding vessels in ulcer craters.

(H) If endoscopic cauterization fails to stop bleeding from drug- or alcohol-induced gastritis, stress ulcer, or Mallory-Weiss tear, arterial embolization can be tried. With the use of Gelfoam or clot, this technique controls bleeding in about 70 percent of patients. An alternative therapy is infusion of vasopressin intravenously (0.2 to 0.4 pressor units/minute). Bleeding stops in 50 percent of patients. Vasopressin infused selectively into the left gastric artery controls bleeding in 50 to 84 percent of patients.

(I) About 10 percent of patients with upper gastrointestinal bleeding require operation. The operative mortality and recurrent bleeding rates are each 10 percent. Operation is indicated when bleeding exceeds 2500 to 3000 mL during the first 24 hours of treatment or 1500 mL during the second 24 hours, or when bleeding recurs during treatment.

(J) The mortality rate after operation for a bleeding duodenal ulcer is higher among patients over age 65 years who have associated diseases. Vagotomy and pyloroplasty is recommended for these patients. Others may undergo the more definitive (and morbid) operation of vagotomy and antrectomy.

(K) The mortality rate of emergency operation for gastric ulcer bleeding (15 percent) is higher than that for duodenal ulcer (5 to 10 percent). An ulcer at the cardia can be managed by oversewing the bleeding vessel and performing vagotomy and pyloroplasty. Occasionally a proximal ulcer can be excised. A distal gastric ulcer is excised locally or removed by hemigastrectomy.

(L) Stress ulcer bleeding can be resistant to vagotomy and require near-total gastrectomy. Because of associated severe disease, stress ulcer hemorrhage causes death in 30 percent of patients.

REFERENCES

Cutler JA, Mendeloff AL. Upper gastrointestinal bleeding: nature and magnitude of the problem in the U.S. Dig Dis Sci 1981; 26(suppl):90–96.

Dempsey DT, Burke DR, Reilly RS, et al. Angiography in poor-risk patients with massive nonvariceal upper gastrointestinal bleeding. Am J Surg 1990; 159:282–286.

Dronfield MW, Langman MJ, Atkinson M, et al. Outcome of endoscopy and barium radiography for acute upper gastrointestinal bleeding: controlled trial in 1037 patients. Br Med J 1982; 284:545–548.

Elerding SC, Moore EE, Wolz JR, et al. Outcome of operations for upper gastrointestinal tract bleeding: an update. Arch Surg 1980; 115:1473–1477.

Kim B, Wright HK, Bordan D, et al. Risks of surgery for upper gastrointestinal hemorrhage: 1972 vs 1982. Am J Surg 1985; 149:474–476.

Larson DE, Farnell MB. Upper gastrointestinal hemorrhage. Mayo Clin Proc 1983; 58:371–378.

Larson G, Schmidt T, Gott J, et al. Upper gastrointestinal bleeding: predictors of outcome. Surgery 1986; 100:765–772.

Papp JP. Endoscopic electrocoagulation of actively bleeding arterial upper gastrointestinal lesions. Am J Gastroenterol 1979; 71:516–521.

Sugawa C, Fujita Y, Ikeda T, et al. Endoscopic hemostasis of bleeding of the upper gastrointestinal tract by local injection of ninety-eight percent dehydrated ethanol. Surg Gynecol Obstet 1986; 162:159–163.

Vellacott KD, Dronfield MW, Atkinson M, et al. Comparison of surgical and medical management of bleeding peptic ulcers. Br Med J 1982; 284:548–550.

History and physical examination
Peptic ulcer disease
Alcoholism
Sepsis (A)
Drugs
Vomiting

UPPER GI BLEEDING

IV fluids (B)
NG tube
(transfusion)

Saline (C)
lavage
IV famotidine
(antacids)

Lab
Hct
Type and
crossmatch
LFT

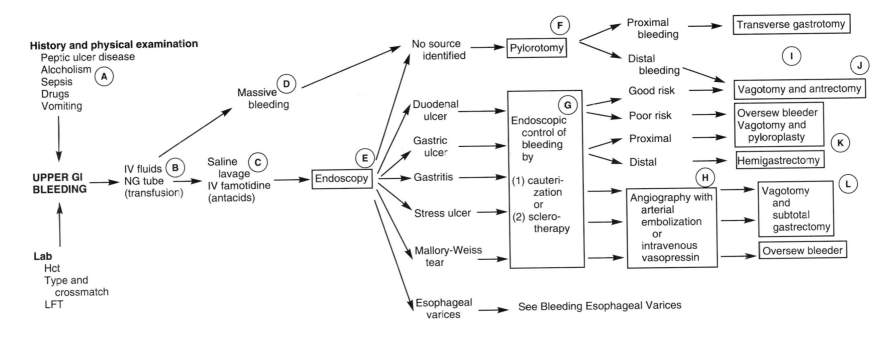

Massive (D)
bleeding

Endoscopy (E)

No source
identified → Pylorotomy (F) → Proximal bleeding → Transverse gastrotomy

Distal bleeding → Vagotomy and antrectomy (I) (J)

Duodenal ulcer
Gastric ulcer
Gastritis
Stress ulcer
Mallory-Weiss tear → Endoscopic control of bleeding by (G)
(1) cauterization
or
(2) sclero-therapy

Good risk → Vagotomy and antrectomy
Poor risk → Oversew bleeder, Vagotomy and pyloroplasty (K)
Proximal → Hemigastrectomy
Distal

Angiography with arterial embolization or intravenous vasopressin (H) → Vagotomy and subtotal gastrectomy (L)
→ Oversew bleeder

Esophageal varices → See Bleeding Esophageal Varices

Bleeding Esophageal Varices

Greg Van Stiegmann, M.D.

A Prognosis of bleeding esophageal varices depends primarily on the status of liver function. Mortality by 1 year after bleeding approaches 60 percent in patients with advanced cirrhosis.

B Endoscopy is performed when hemodynamic stabilization is achieved. Presence of varices and no other potential bleeding site is adequate evidence that bleeding was from varices. Up to 25 percent of patients with varices and bleeding have a nonvariceal source (eg, Mallory-Weiss tear, gastritis) of hemorrhage.

C Flexible endoscopic sclerotherapy or elastic band ligation should be instituted as soon as a variceal source of bleeding is confirmed. Active variceal bleeding can be controlled in 90 to 95 percent of cases using these techniques. Sclerotherapy with rigid endoscopes is no more effective than that done with flexible instruments.

D Intravenous vasopressin (0.4 to 0.8 U/min) stops variceal bleeding in up to 65 percent of patients. Recurrent bleeding occurs in half of cases.

E Balloon tamponade temporarily halts bleeding in 80 to 90 percent of patients. Sixty percent rebleed, however. There is significant morbidity associated with this therapy, including aspiration and perforation.

F Liver transplantation is the best treatment for patients with advanced cirrhosis and bleeding varices. Patients at lower risk (Child A and Child B) may be maintained using endoscopic therapy until deterioration of liver function occurs.

G Sclerotherapy or endoscopic ligation are repeated at 1- to 2-week intervals until varices are small or eradicated, usually after 4 to 6 sessions. Both treatments decrease the incidence of recurrent bleeding and appear to result in improved survival with optimal preservation of liver function. Repeated sclerotherapy is associated with complication rates of 20 to 40 percent. Endoscopic ligation appears to be safer, with overall complications of about 5 percent. Both procedures are performed in an outpatient setting on awake and sedated patients.

H Elective shunt operation may be indicated for patients who have good liver function or those who live in geographically remote areas. Portocaval shunts should be avoided in liver transplant candidates. The optimal shunt operation appears to be the selective splenorenal shunt, although this remains controversial.

I Nonelective shunt operations are generally central portocaval anastomoses with or without use of a prosthetic graft. Operative transection/devascularization of the stomach and distal esophagus combined with splenectomy is better suited for the patient who is a liver transplant candidate. Patients who undergo the latter operation require endoscopic surveillance and institution of endoscopic therapy if varices recur.

J Radiologic embolization of varices either by a percutaneous transhepatic approach or using a mini laparotomy with the surgeon catheterizing the splanchnic venous system through a venous branch of the small bowel mesentery is best suited for the high-risk patient. Angiographic occlusion of the splenic artery may help control bleeding temporarily. All patients treated this way require endoscopic follow-up to detect recurrent varices.

K Definitions for failure of endoscopic therapy vary. The author believes that patients who experience two or more portal hypertension-related bleeds after initiation of endoscopic therapy should be considered for operative treatment or transplantation.

L Surveillance endoscopy is performed at 3- or 6-month intervals to detect and treat any varices that recur.

REFERENCES

Bornman PC, Kahn D, Terblanche J, et al. Rigid versus fiberoptic endoscopic injection sclerotherapy: a prospective randomized controlled trial in patients with bleeding esophageal varices. Ann Surg 1988; 208:175–178.

Del Guercio LRM, Kinkhabwalla NN, Berman HL. Current concepts in portal hypertension. Bull NY Acad Sci 1985; 61:753–762.

Infante-Rivard C, Esnaola S, Villeneuve JP. Role of endoscopic variceal sclerotherapy in the long-term management of variceal bleeding: a meta-analysis. Gastroenterology 1990; 96:1087–1092.

Orozoo H, Juarez F, Uribe M, et al. Sugiura procedure outside Japan: the Mexican experience. Am J Surg 1986; 152:539–542.

Stiegmann GV, Goff JS, Sun JH, et al. Endoscopic ligation of esophageal varices. Am J Surg 1990; 159:21–26.

Terblanche J, Burroughs AK, Hobbs KEF. Controversies in the management of bleeding esophageal varices. N Engl J Med 1989; 320:1469–1475.

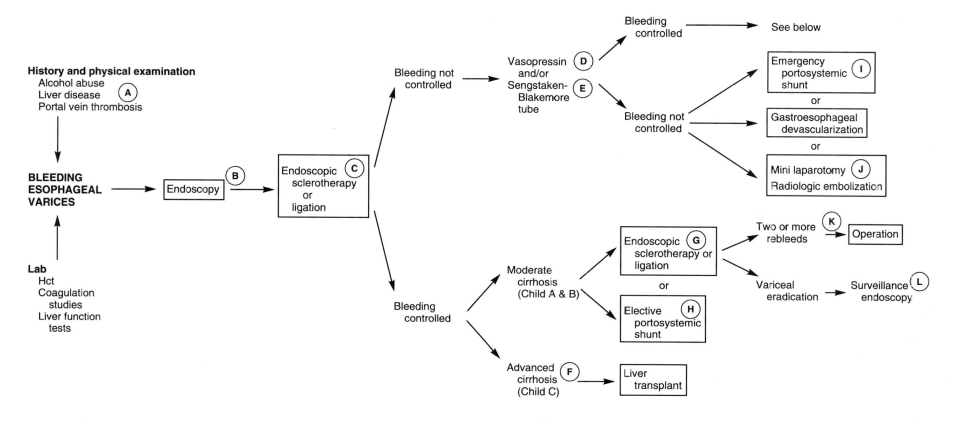

Jaundice: Diagnostic Workup

John Marek, M.D., and Greg Van Stiegmann, M.D.

(A) Diagnosis of jaundice can be made in about 80 percent of patients on the basis of history and physical examination alone. Laboratory studies are done primarily to confirm or deny clinical suspicion. Test sequencing depends on probabilities of suspected diagnoses.

(B) Liver function tests include aspartate transaminase (serum glutamic oxaloacetic transaminase) and alanine transaminase (serum glutamic pyruvic transaminase); bilirubin, direct and indirect; alkaline phosphatase; albumin; and prothrombin time. These should help differentiate obstructive from nonobstructive jaundice. Abnormalities such as low albumin or elevated prothrombin time suggest underlying liver dysfunction.

(C) Chest x-ray is to detect metastases.

(D) Abnormal abdominal x-ray may demonstrate calcified stones or a mass.

(E) Hemolysis screening tests include complete blood count, peripheral blood smear, lactate dehydrogenase, and haptoglobulin determinations. Hemolysis alone is unlikely to elevate total bilirubin over 5 mg/dL in the absence of liver disease.

(F) Ultrasonography and abdominal computed tomography both have a 90 to 95 percent sensitivity in demonstrating a dilated biliary tree suggestive of obstructive jaundice. Ultrasound is cheaper and avoids radiation; computed tomography is effective in obese patients and in the presence of intestinal gas.

(G) Ultrasound demonstration of diffuse common bile duct dilation and gallstones is sufficient for diagnosis in the absence of other pathology.

(H) CA 19-9 is a tumor-associated antigen useful in preoperative staging and postoperative prognosis and follow-up of pancreatic cancer. Tumor markers occasionally help differentiate benign from malignant pancreatic disease.

(I) Percutaneous needle aspiration biopsy can be used to diagnose either a palpable mass or one identified by ultrasound. It may be useful for patients who are not candidates for surgical palliation.

(J) Endoscopic retrograde cholangiopancreatographic (ERCP) demonstration of obstruction of both biliary and pancreatic ducts (double duct sign) is highly specific for pancreatic cancer. Endoscopic biopsy or cytology may be diagnostic. Biliary stents can be placed endoscopically for palliation or for operative preparation.

(K) Immunoglobulin-M acute phase antibody against hepatitis A (IgM anti-HAV) proves recent A virus infection. Immunoglobulin-G antibody against hepatitis A indicates remote infection.

(L) Hepatitis B surface antigen (HBsAg) identifies acute or chronic hepatitis B or the B carrier state.

(M) Serologic tests for mononucleosis, cytomegalovirus, or herpes are sometimes performed to diagnose less common causes of viral hepatitis.

(N) The genome of a non-A non-B hepatitis virus has been identified as hepatitis C; an antibody to hepatitis C virus is available. It appears to be a common cause of community-acquired and transfusion-associated non-A non-B hepatitis.

(O) Positive antibody to hepatitis B core antigen (anti-HBc) indicates convalescent B infection. Positive antibody to hepatitis B surface antigen (anti-HBs) indicates remote B virus infection.

(P) Liver biopsy remains the backup method for diagnosing hepatocellular diseases of unclear cause, such as those due to drugs, toxins, or other viruses.

(Q) Klatskin tumor obstruction at the proximal end of the bile duct is best identified by percutaneous transhepatic cholangiography. Ampullary tumors are directly visualized during ERCP.

(R) Hepatocellular diseases include Wilson disease and hemochromatosis.

REFERENCES

Chopra S, Griffin PH. Laboratory tests and diagnostic procedures in evaluation of liver disease. Am J Med 1985; 79:221–230.

Frank BB. Clinical evaluation of jaundice: a guideline of the patient care committee of the American Gastroenterological Association. JAMA 1989; 262:3031–3034.

Hoofnagle JH. Type A and type B hepatitis. Lab Med 1983; 14:705–716.

Schmiegel W. Tumor markers in pancreatic cancer—current concepts. Hepatogastroenterology 1989; 36:446–449.

Stevens CE, Taylor PE, Pindyck J, et al. Epidemiology of hepatitis C virus: a preliminary study in volunteer blood donors. JAMA 1990; 263:49–53.

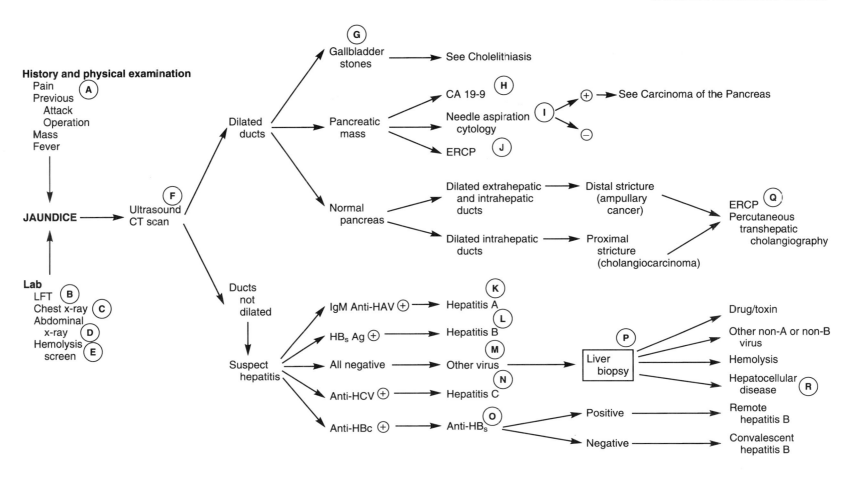

History and physical examination
Pain (A)
Previous
  Attack
  Operation
Mass
Fever

JAUNDICE → Ultrasound (F) CT scan

Lab
LFT (B)
Chest x-ray (C)
Abdominal
  x-ray (D)
Hemolysis
  screen (E)

Dilated ducts →
- Gallbladder stones (G) → See Cholelithiasis
- Pancreatic mass →
  - CA 19-9 (H)
  - Needle aspiration cytology (I) → (+) → See Carcinoma of the Pancreas / (−)
  - ERCP (J)
- Normal pancreas →
  - Dilated extrahepatic and intrahepatic ducts → Distal stricture (ampullary cancer)
  - Dilated intrahepatic ducts → Proximal stricture (cholangiocarcinoma)
  → ERCP (Q) Percutaneous transhepatic cholangiography

Ducts not dilated →
Suspect hepatitis →
- IgM Anti-HAV (+) → Hepatitis A (K)
- HB$_s$ Ag (+) → Hepatitis B (L)
- All negative → Other virus (M) → Liver biopsy (P) →
  - Drug/toxin
  - Other non-A or non-B virus
  - Hemolysis
  - Hepatocellular disease (R)
- Anti-HCV (+) → Hepatitis C (N)
- Anti-HBc (+) → Anti-HB$_s$ (O) →
  - Positive → Remote hepatitis B
  - Negative → Convalescent hepatitis B

Obstructive Jaundice: Interventional Options

John Marek, M.D., and Greg Van Stiegmann, M.D.

(A) The term obstructive jaundice implies mechanical obstruction.

(B) Preoperative nutritional supplementation is sometimes helpful. If bilirubin is greater than 15 mg/dL, patients can benefit by temporary biliary tract drainage using endoscopic retrograde cholangiopancreatography (ERCP) sphincterotomy or stent before definitive treatment.

(C) Dilation of the entire biliary tree in the absence of stones suggests the presence of an ampullary tumor and can best be evaluated by a combination of ERCP and duodenotomy.

(D) Bile duct carcinoma at the confluence of the bile ducts (Klatskin tumor) is best diagnosed by percutaneous transhepatic visualization of the proximal biliary tree. This slow-growing tumor can be treated palliatively by either stent placement through the tumor or biliary bypass and curatively by resection followed by hepaticojejunostomy.

(E) Percutaneous or endoscopic dilation of strictures has variable success but is prudent in high-risk patients before operative repair is attempted.

(F) ERCP sphincterotomy and stone removal are advisable in patients with suppurative cholangitis as a temporary measure to manage septic shock. Common bile duct stone removal through ERCP is successful in about 90 percent of cases.

(G) Approximately 90 percent of retained common bile duct stones can be removed endoscopically. Cholecystectomy is necessary in about 20 percent of patients in whom symptoms of cholecystitis develop.

(H) Lithotripsy is most valuable in fragmenting gallbladder stones but can be used for common duct stone dissolution as well.

(I) Radiologic extraction of stones can be accomplished through T tube or percutaneous transhepatic routes.

(J) Tissue specimen biopsy is obtained by percutaneous needle aspiration, brush biopsy cytology, or direct biopsy at ERCP. Stent placement at the time of endoscopic examination provides palliation.

(K) The success of operative repair depends on meticulous mucosa-to-mucosa anastomosis of the biliary structure to a Roux limb of jejunum or mobilized duodenum.

(L) Choledochoscopy is indicated when the common duct is widely dilated and contains multiple small stones.

(M) If tissue diagnosis of tumor cannot be obtained despite all preoperative studies and intraoperative biopsies and the differential diagnosis is pancreatitis vs. cancer, some surgeons advocate resection for cure because of the probability that tumor has been missed by biopsy techniques.

(N) Cholecystectomy can be performed either by formal laparotomy or endoscopically through multiple limited access incisions. Comparative risks and indications are evolving. The primary advantage of laparoscopic cholecystectomy is limited morbidity and cost.

(O) Operative bypass of the biliary or gastrointestinal tract obviates incipient or actual obstruction. Because of the poor prognosis of pancreatic cancer, some surgeons advocate bypass even when the tumor appears to be resectable.

(P) Procedures for curative resection include total pancreaticoduodenectomy, pylorus-preserving pancreaticoduodenectomy, and various types of partial pancreatectomies.

REFERENCES

Buice WS, Walker LG. The role of intra-operative biopsy in the treatment of resectable neoplasms of the pancreas and periampullary region. Am Surg 1989; 55:307–310.

Funovics JM, Karner J, Pratschner TH, et al. Current trends in the management of carcinoma of the pancreatic head. Hepatogastroenterolology 1989; 36:450–455.

Harbin WP, Mueller PR, Ferrucci JT Jr. Transhepatic cholangiography: complications and use patterns of the fine-needle technique. Radiology 1980; 135:15–22.

Vogt DP, Hermann RE. Choledochoduodenostomy, choledochojejunostomy or sphincteroplasty for biliary and pancreatic disease. Ann Surg 1981; 193:161–168.

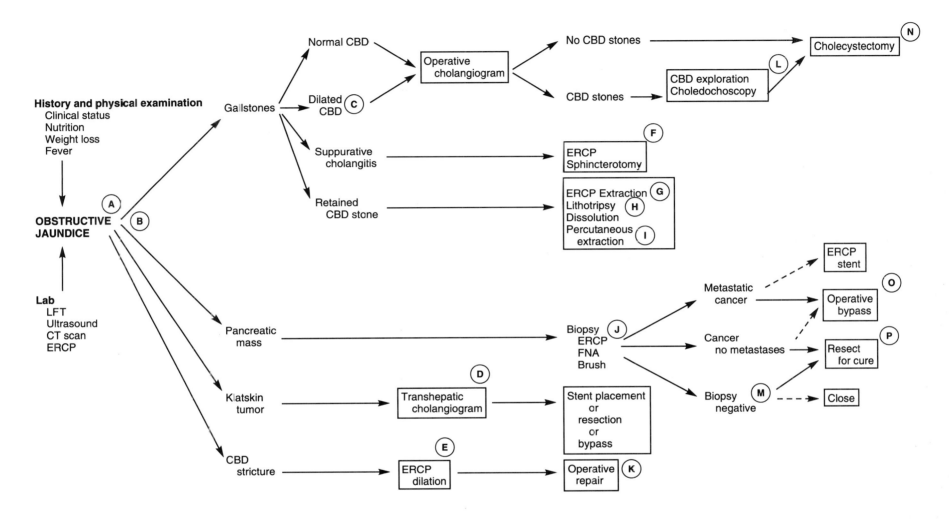

Cholelithiasis

Lawrence W. Norton, M.D.

(A) Gallstones are diagnosed in over 600,000 Americans each year. About 300,000 persons undergo cholecystectomy annually. The incidence of gallstones increases with age. Most gallstones (75 percent) are composed of a mixture of bile pigments and cholesterol. Pure gallstones are rare. Pigmented stones (10 percent) can be caused by hemolytic anemia. The cause of mixed stones is a combination of factors, including supersaturation of bile with cholesterol, gallbladder stasis, and altered nucleation.

(B) Ultrasound accurately detects gallstones in 90 to 95 percent of patients. The technique is rapid and can be used in the presence of jaundice. It provides information in regard to biliary duct dilation. Oral cholecystography is slightly more accurate but requires more time to perform and cannot be used in jaundiced patients.

(C) Radionuclide scans using technetium 99m-labeled derivatives of iminodiacetic acid (DIP-IDA, HIDA, etc.) can image the bile ducts and gallbladder in circumstances of suspected cholecystitis. Failure of the radionuclide to enter the gallbladder suggests cholecystitis. Accuracy of the technique is about 90 percent. False positive tests can be caused by alcohol ingestion, a recent meal, and other conditions.

(D) Between 20 and 40 percent of patients with asymptomatic gallstones will develop symptoms within 10 years and require cholecystectomy. Another 5 to 18 percent will undergo emergency cholecystectomy for a complication of gallstones. Whether or not these risks justify prophylactic cholecystectomy is controversial.

(E) Chronic cholecystitis implies symptoms (usually intermittent, postprandial, right upper quadrant abdominal pain) due to gallstones. About half of such patients will need emergency cholecystectomy or hospitalization without operation for complications of gallstones within 10 years. Because of this risk, cholecystectomy is recommended.

(F) Acute cholecystitis is characterized by moderate to severe upper abdominal pain, nausea or vomiting, fever, and leukocytosis. Jaundice may or may not be apparent. Immediate treatment is nonoperative. Antibiotics are given to patients with evidence of sepsis or severe cholecystitis. When symptoms disappear and gallstones are confirmed, cholecystectomy is recommended. Acalculous cholecystitis (5 percent) is often a complication of severe illness and is sometimes interpreted as a component of multiple organ failure. A risk of acute cholecystitis with or without stones is gallbladder perforation.

(G) Serum amylase levels are frequently elevated in patients with acute cholecystitis. Values return to normal rapidly in most instances. In a few patients, passage of a common bile duct stone causes clinical pancreatitis.

(H) Elective cholecystectomy can be performed by either an open or a laparoscopic technique. The latter represents a significant advance in terms of decreased morbidity and convalescence time. The most worrisome complication of laparoscopic cholecystectomy is injury to the common bile duct (up to 1 percent). Open cholecystectomy is advised when exploration of the common bile duct seems likely. Intraoperative cholangiography is justified in most patients (the exception is when a single stone is obstructing the ampulla) and can be performed during either open or laparoscopic cholecystectomy. If cholangiography performed during laparoscopic cholecystectomy shows common bile duct stones, endoscopic retrograde cholangiopancreatography and sphincterotomy can be performed postoperatively with 90 percent expectation of stone passage.

(I) Most patients respond to treatment rapidly with disappearance of pain, fever, and leukocytosis within 2 to 3 days. Patients whose symptoms and signs progress during treatment, particularly elderly men who are at risk for early perforation, require emergency operation.

(J) Emergency cholecystectomy increases risk considerably. Mortality rates approach 10 percent in patients over 60 years of age.

(K) In patients with significant comorbidities (eg, cardiac or pulmonary disease), a lengthy operation is unwise. Drainage of the gallbladder and removal of stones by cholecystostomy is advisable. The procedure can be performed under local anesthesia but general anesthesia is often preferable. Mortality (6 to 13 percent) and morbidity (35 percent) rates are high despite limited operating time. Interval cholecystectomy is recommended after cholecystostomy, although about one third of patients remain asymptomatic after resolution of cholecystitis and removal of the tube.

(L) Electrohydraulic extracorporeal shock-wave lithotripsy can fragment gallstones in over 90 percent of patients. Only half of these patients are stone-free at 2 years, however, either because some stone fragments are retained or because new stones form. Oral medication is mandatory to foster

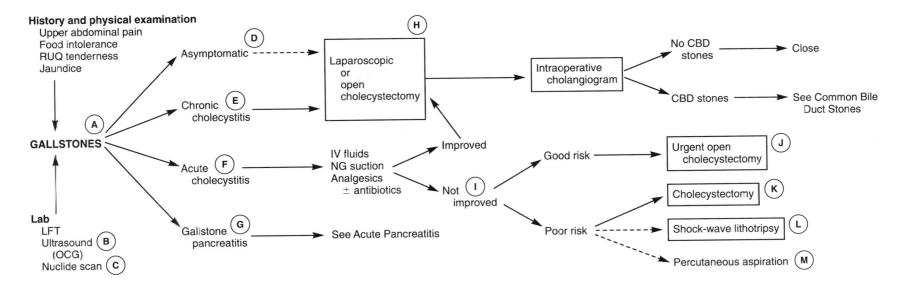

History and physical examination
Upper abdominal pain
Food intolerance
RUQ tenderness
Jaundice

(A) GALLSTONES

Lab
LFT
Ultrasound (B)
(OCG)
Nuclide scan (C)

(D) Asymptomatic

(E) Chronic cholecystitis

(F) Acute cholecystitis

(G) Gallstone pancreatitis

(H) Laparoscopic or open cholecystectomy

IV fluids
NG suction
Analgesics
± antibiotics

Improved

(I) Not improved

See Acute Pancreatitis

Intraoperative cholangiogram

No CBD stones → Close

CBD stones → See Common Bile Duct Stones

Good risk → (J) Urgent open cholecystectomy

Poor risk → (K) Cholecystectomy

(L) Shock-wave lithotripsy

(M) Percutaneous aspiration

dissolution of fragments and to prevent new stone formation.

(M) In high-risk patients, percutaneous aspiration of the gallbladder under computed tomography or ultrasound control can be performed. Aspiration of bile and instillation of agents to dissolve gallstones have been attempted in patients with cholelithiasis on an elective basis. Results are variable and data are insufficient to recommend these procedures.

REFERENCES

Acosta JM, Rossi R, Gali DMR, et al. Early surgery for acute gallstone pancreatitis: evaluation of a systematic approach. Surgery 1978; 83:367–370.

Berk RN, Leopold GR. The present status of imaging of the gallbladder. Invest Radiol 1978; 13:477–489.

Howard RJ. Acute acalculous cholecystitis. Am J Surg 1981; 141:194–198.

Jarvinev JH, Hastbacka J. Early cholecystectomy for acute cholecystitis: a prospective randomized study. Ann Surg 1980; 191:501–505.

Lund J. Surgical indications in cholelithiasis: prophylactic cholecystectomy elucidated on the basis of long term follow-up on 526 non-operated cases. Ann Surg 1960; 151:153–162.

Peters JH, Ellison C, Innes JT, et al. Safety and efficacy of laparoscopic cholecystectomy. Ann Surg 1991; 213:3–12.

Reddick EJ, Olsen DO. Outpatient laparoscopic laser cholecystectomy. Am J Surg 1990; 160:485–489.

Sackman M, Delius M, Sauerbruch T, et al. Shock-wave lithotripsy of gallbladder stones: the first 175 patients. N Engl J Med 1988; 318:393.

Trowbridge PE. A randomized study of cholecystectomy with and without drainage. Surg Gynecol Obstet 1982; 155:171–176.

Common Bile Duct Stones

Philippe Gertsch, M.D., and Leslie Blumgart, M.D.

(A) Common bile duct (CBD) stones may be residual after cholecystectomy or primary (ie, formed in intrahepatic bile ducts as a result of liver disease or in the CBD after cholecystectomy).

(B) After cholecystectomy there is a 1 to 8 percent probability of residual CBD stones. Stones are unsuspected in 7 percent of cases, which emphasizes the need for routine operative cholangiography. The rate of retained stones is reduced to 1 percent by intraoperative choledochoscopy and cholangiography.

(C) Although leaving a single small (<5 mm diameter) CBD stone visualized by operative cholangiography in a small duct is debatable, the high probability of spontaneous passage outweighs the anticipated morbidity of duct exploration. Not every physician agrees, and the duct might be explored.

(D) Residual CBD stones can be treated nonoperatively for 6 weeks to see whether they will pass and to permit maturation of the T tube tract for radiologically directed extraction. Most stones smaller than 5 mm pass spontaneously.

(E) Mono-octanoin infusion (±7 days) effectively dissolves approximately half the residual CBD stones or diminishes their size so that they pass.

(F) Radiologically directed removal of CBD stones using a Dormia basket has a success rate of 95 percent and morbidity of 5 percent. About 30 percent of patients require more than one attempt.

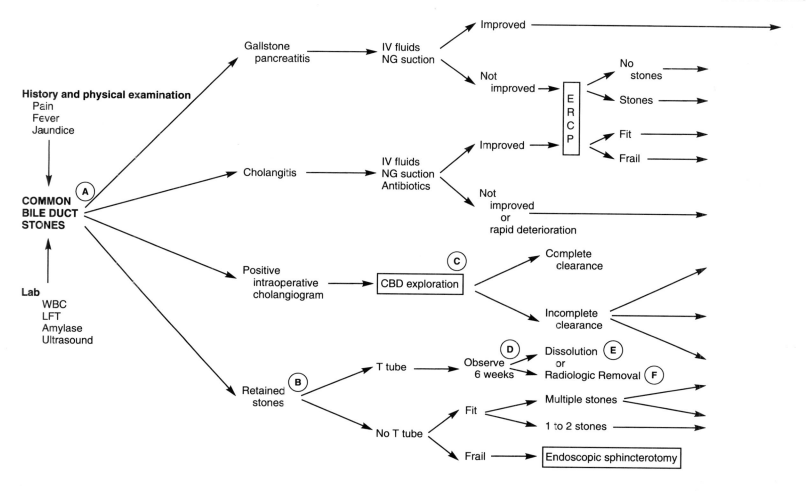

History and physical examination
Pain
Fever
Jaundice

COMMON
BILE DUCT (A)
STONES

Lab
WBC
LFT
Amylase
Ultrasound

Gallstone pancreatitis → IV fluids NG suction → Improved

Not improved → ERCP → No stones / Stones

Cholangitis → IV fluids NG suction Antibiotics → Improved → ERCP → Fit / Frail

Not improved or rapid deterioration

Positive intraoperative cholangiogram → CBD exploration (C) → Complete clearance / Incomplete clearance

Retained stones (B) → T tube → Observe 6 weeks (D) → Dissolution (E) or Radiologic Removal (F)

No T tube → Fit → Multiple stones / 1 to 2 stones

Frail → Endoscopic sphincterotomy

Common Bile Duct Stones (Continued)

(G) In most cases stones pass spontaneously. Cholecystectomy may be performed by laparoscopy when absence of CBD stones has been documented. This indication is not yet established, however, and studies should be undertaken.

(H) The immediate risks of surgery and endoscopy are comparable. The potential long-term effects of endoscopic sphincterotomy are still unclear.

(I) Surgery is associated with high mortality. Percutaneous transhepatic biliary drainage may be the best initial management.

(J) For multiple stones, especially primary stones with debris, in a large duct (>15 mm) and in the elderly, choledochoduodenostomy is advised. It is also useful during reoperation when an anastomosis of 2 to 5 cm in diameter can be made. A stone impacted at the terminal portion of the common bile duct requires transduodenal sphincteroplasty.

(K) The classic indications for anastomosis of the cut end of the common duct to a Roux-en-Y loop of jejunum include gross CBD dilation where a 2 to 5 cm anastomosis is possible, multiple stones, intrahepatic stones, and a young patient. Typically these indications occur in patients with cholangiohepatitis.

(L) With one or two residual stones, CBD exploration plus choledochoscopy or postexploratory cholangiography is the procedure of choice. The hospital mortality rate is 1 to 2 percent and morbidity is 5 to 8 percent. With a stone impacted at the ampulla, operative sphincteroplasty is required.

(M) The minimum operation is CBD exploration, removal of stones, and T tube placement. When the gallbladder is present and the patient is unstable, removal of stones from the gallbladder and cholecystostomy may be adequate. Choledochoduodenostomy may be preferred to T tube drainage provided the bile duct is at least 2 cm in diameter.

REFERENCES

Burhenne HJ. Percutaneous extraction of retained biliary tract stones in 661 patients. Am J Roentgenol 1980; 134:889–898.

Girard RM, Gegros G. Stones in the common bile duct—surgical approaches. In: Blumgart LH, ed. Surgery of the liver and biliary tract. New York: Churchill Livingstone, 1988:577–585.

Hawes RH, Cotton PB, Vallon AG. Follow-up 6 to 11 years after duodenoscopic sphincterotomy for stones in patients with prior cholecystectomy. Gastroenterology 1990; 98:1008–1012.

Miller BM, Kozarek RA, Ryan JA, et al. Surgical versus endoscopic management of common bile duct stones. Ann Surg 1988; 207:135–141.

Pessa ME, Hawkins IF, Vogel SB. The treatment of acute cholangitis. Percutaneous transhepatic biliary drainage before definitive therapy. Ann Surg 1987; 205:389–393.

Saharia PC, Cameron JL. Clinical management of cholangitis. Surg Gynecol Obstet 1976; 142:369–372.

Way LW, Motson RW. Dissolution of retained common bile duct stones. In: Longmire WP Jr (ed). Advances in surgery. Vol 10. Chicago: Year Book, 1976:112–114.

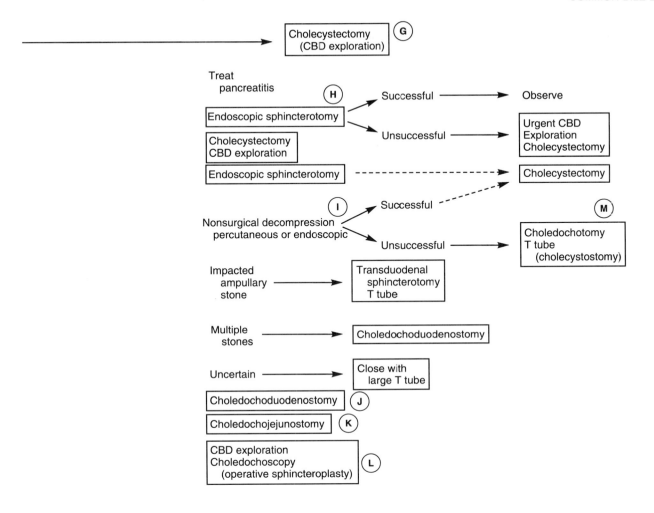

Liver Tumor

John Terblanche, Ch.M., F.C.S. (S.A.), F.R.C.S. (Eng.)

(A) Early liver lesions are asymptomatic and may be found incidentally by imaging or at laparotomy. Surgical resection offers the only chance of cure.

(B) Unexplained hepatomegaly requires full investigation. Weight loss and pain are signs of late malignancy. Sudden deterioration in a cirrhotic patient suggests malignancy.

(C) α-Fetoprotein and ultrasound are used to screen cirrhotic patients for primary tumor. A solid lesion on ultrasound or computed tomography scan suggests tumor. Angiography or enhanced computed tomography scans are 95 percent accurate in detecting primary malignant and benign tumors and provide the most cost-effective means of diagnosis. Tagged red cell scan is valuable for diagnosing hemangioma. Needle biopsy or fine-needle aspiration cytology provides definitive diagnosis but should be avoided in resectable lesions abutting the surface of the liver.

(D) Preoperative screening for metastases is essential. Computed tomography scan is more accurate than chest x-ray. It is important despite higher cost.

(E) Small benign lesions can be mistaken for metastases at laparotomy. Biopsy may be required. Hemangiomas, which usually have a typical appearance, should not be biopsied.

(F) Fewer than 10 percent of patients have locally removable colorectal carcinoma and hepatic metastases suitable for resection. A single metastasis is ideal for resection, but up to three lesions in one lobe can be removed.

(G) Metastatic neuroendocrine tumors should be considered for curative or palliative resection. Selective arterial embolization is occasionally of value.

(H) Resection is contraindicated in most other metastatic tumors. Some childhood tumors, including Wilms tumor, are exceptions.

(I) Small hepatocellular carcinomas in low-risk cirrhotic patients occasionally can be detected by screening (under 55 percent). Carcinoma is usually a terminal manifestation of end-stage cirrhosis. Hepatocellular carcinoma without cirrhosis is usually multifocal, but occasionally (less than 5 percent) a single resectable lesion is present.

(J) Cholangiocarcinoma is rare (10 percent). Treatment is resection, but 5-year survival is unusual.

(K) Cystadenocarcinoma of the liver is rare but worth resecting. Hepatoblastoma in children has over 30 percent 5-year survival after resection. Angiosarcoma is rare and usually inoperable.

(L) The most common lesion is hemangioma (2 to 4 percent of patients). Diagnosis is confirmed by imaging. Treatment is expectant. Less than 1 percent are both symptomatic and large. Only these require resection. Spontaneous rupture and hemorrhage are exceedingly rare.

(M) Both lesions, particularly hepatic adenoma, are associated with a history of oral contraceptives and a risk of hemorrhage. Resection is indicated for hemorrhage, pain, or large size. Oral contraceptives should be discontinued. Imaging and biopsy are required for diagnosis.

(N) Stop oral contraceptives after diagnosis and follow the patient with liver imaging. Lesions that do not regress should be resected or have hepatic artery embolization.

(O) Although formal hepatic lobectomy is frequently performed, smaller resections, including subsegmental resections with a 1-cm tumor-free margin, can be adequate. Operative mortality is near zero when patients are treated by experienced surgeons. Intraoperative ultrasound is useful to plan resection. Total inflow occlusion of the porta hepatis allows for virtually bloodless resection. Kelly clamp or finger fracture techniques are as effective as using expensive lasers and other devices. Total resections and liver transplantation are contraindicated in metastatic tumors and primary hepatic carcinoma. Adjuvant chemotherapy is of no proven value.

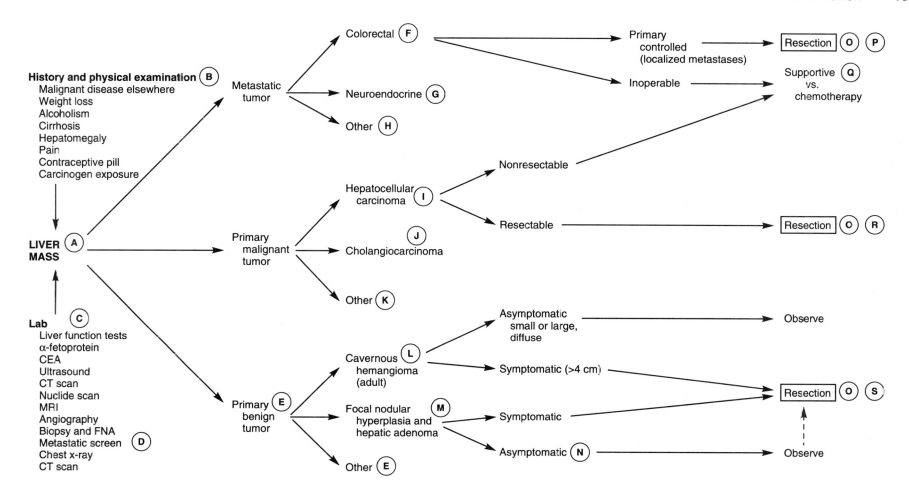

History and physical examination (B)
Malignant disease elsewhere
Weight loss
Alcoholism
Cirrhosis
Hepatomegaly
Pain
Contraceptive pill
Carcinogen exposure

LIVER MASS (A)

Lab (C)
Liver function tests
α-fetoprotein
CEA
Ultrasound
CT scan
Nuclide scan
MRI
Angiography
Biopsy and FNA
Metastatic screen (D)
Chest x-ray
CT scan

Metastatic tumor
→ Colorectal (F)
→ Neuroendocrine (G)
→ Other (H)

Colorectal (F)
→ Primary controlled (localized metastases) → Resection (O) (P)
→ Inoperable → Supportive vs. chemotherapy (Q)

Primary malignant tumor
→ Hepatocellular carcinoma (I)
→ Cholangiocarcinoma (J)
→ Other (K)

Hepatocellular carcinoma (I)
→ Nonresectable → Supportive vs. chemotherapy
→ Resectable → Resection (O) (R)

Primary benign tumor (E)
→ Cavernous hemangioma (adult) (L)
→ Focal nodular hyperplasia and hepatic adenoma (M)
→ Other (E)

Cavernous hemangioma (adult) (L)
→ Asymptomatic small or large, diffuse → Observe
→ Symptomatic (>4 cm) → Resection (O) (S)

Focal nodular hyperplasia and hepatic adenoma (M)
→ Symptomatic → Resection (O) (S)
→ Asymptomatic (N) → Observe

(P) Fifteen to forty percent 5-year survival is achieved with one to three metastases and no extrahepatic spread. Carcinoembryonic antigen is useful to screen for recurrence after resection of colorectal carcinoma.

(Q) Systemic or regional chemotherapy is of little value in primary or metastatic tumors. Treatment is largely supportive. New chemotherapy regimens are under review.

(R) Small encapsulated hepatocellular carcinoma in a cirrhotic liver should be resected locally if the patient is Child grade A. The mortality is near zero whereas 5-year survival is over 50 percent. Isolated hepatocellular carcinoma without cirrhosis has a 30 to 40 percent 5-year survival after resection. The rare fibrolamellar variant has over 50 percent 5-year survival.

(S) Large lesions may require resection for symptoms. Resection of benign tumors should be undertaken only by expert liver surgeons. Resection is also indicated for complications. Operative mortality should be zero.

REFERENCES

Bornman PC, Terblanche J, Blumgart RL, et al. Giant hepatic hemangiomas: diagnostic and therapeutic dilemmas. Surgery 1987; 191:445–449.

Fortner JG. Recurrence of colorectal cancer after hepatic resection. Am J Surg 1988; 155:378–382.

Hughes KS, Rosenstein RB, Songhorabodi S, et al. Resection of the liver for colorectal carcinoma metastases: a multi-institutional study of long-term survivors. Dis Colon Rectum 1988; 31:1–4.

Ohnishi K, Tanabe Y, Ryu M, et al. Prognosis of hepatocellular carcinoma smaller than 5 cm in relation to treatment study of 100 patients. Hepatology 1987; 7:1285–1290.

Terblanche J. Surgery of liver tumors. HPB Surg 1989; 1:173–184.

Acute Pancreatitis

Alexander S. Rosemurgy, M.D., and Larry C. Carey, M.D.

(A) The diagnosis of acute pancreatitis includes a constellation of symptoms and signs, generally with hyperamylasemia/hyperlipasemia. Abdominal pain and pancreatic enzyme elevation alone are not enough to make the diagnosis because there are extrapancreaticobiliary causes of abdominal pain and hyperamylasemia.

(B) Few patients with acute pancreatitis fail to demonstrate an elevation in amylase. Isoenzyme determinations are helpful in excluding acute pancreatitis when amylase and lipase levels are marginally elevated. Abdominal pain and marginal elevations in amylase and lipase are seen with extrapancreatic processes.

(C) Acute pancreatitis is usually due to alcoholism or biliary stone disease. Ultrasound of the right upper quadrant reveals the presence or absence of gallstones, choledocholithiasis, common bile duct dilation, pancreatic enlargement, and peripancreatic fluid.

(D) The initial therapy of acute pancreatitis consists of stopping oral intake, rehydration, and pain relief. Nasogastric intubation is useful in the presence of ileus but does not affect the outcome of mild pancreatitis. The use of antibiotics is controversial. No prophylactic value of antibiotics is recognized.

(E) Ranson has identified 11 signs to predict and identify the severity of acute pancreatitis. The signs are:

At Admission	During Initial 48 Hours of Therapy
Age over 55 years	HCT fall by 10
WBC over 16,000/mm³	BUN rise by 5 mg/dL
Blood glucose over 200 mg/dL	Calcium below 8 mg/dL
LDH over 350 IU/L	Base deficit greater than 4 mEq/L
SGOT over 250 SFU/dL	Fluid sequestration of >600 mL
	PO₂ below 60 mmHg

Patients with less than 3 signs suffer mild pancreatitis whereas those with more than 3 signs have severe pancreatitis.

(F) Mild pancreatitis, usually a self-limiting disease, requires fluids, analgesia, monitoring, and nutrition.

(G) Severe pancreatitis, a life-threatening disease, usually requires mechanical ventilation, hemodynamic support, and early nutritional support.

(H) Computed tomographic scanning delineates anatomy and complications. The finding of peripancreatic fluid collections, pseudocysts, or peripancreatic necrosis is not an absolute indication for surgical treatment. Instead, in the absence of deterioration and sepsis, observation is in order because many abnormalities seen on computed tomography resolve with time. Persistent abnormalities may require elective surgical treatment after the acute illness has passed. If patients deteriorate, ventilatory and hemodynamic support should be instituted early. Dynamic contrast-enhanced computed tomography should be used in this setting to identify pancreatic necrosis.

(I) In patients suffering biliary pancreatitis, cholecystectomy should be undertaken during the initial hospitalization. The advent of laparoscopic cholecystectomy has changed the approach to patients with gallstone pancreatitis. If a preoperative ultrasound documents choledocholithiasis or if choledocholithiasis is suspected, an endoscopic retrograde cholangiopancreatography may be undertaken. If common bile duct stones are found, sphincterotomy with or without stone retrieval is useful. After sphincterotomy and stone retrieval, laparoscopic cholecystectomy can be undertaken avoiding conventional celiotomy and common bile duct exploration. If endoscopic retrograde cholangiopancreatography is not undertaken preoperatively, operative cholangiography is a must.

(J) Computed tomography-guided fine-needle aspiration should be used to detect infection of the peripancreatic necrosis. Documented infection should lead quickly to operative debridement. Differentiation between inflammation and infection is critical.

(K) The role of peritoneal lavage in this setting is controversial. At best, peritoneal lavage improves early-phase systemic circulatory and respiratory effects mediated by toxins in the ascitic fluid. Lavage does not modify the underlying pancreatitis and thus may not alter the outcome. At worst, lavage may increase the risk of peritoneal sepsis. The usefulness of adding antiproteases to the lavage fluid remains hopeful, though unestablished.

(L) Mortality in patients with very severe peripancreatic necrosis can be reduced from 40 percent to 10 percent by aggressive surgical treatment. There is no role for percutaneous drainage of infected peripancreatic necrosis. Results with open vs. closed drainage after operative debride-

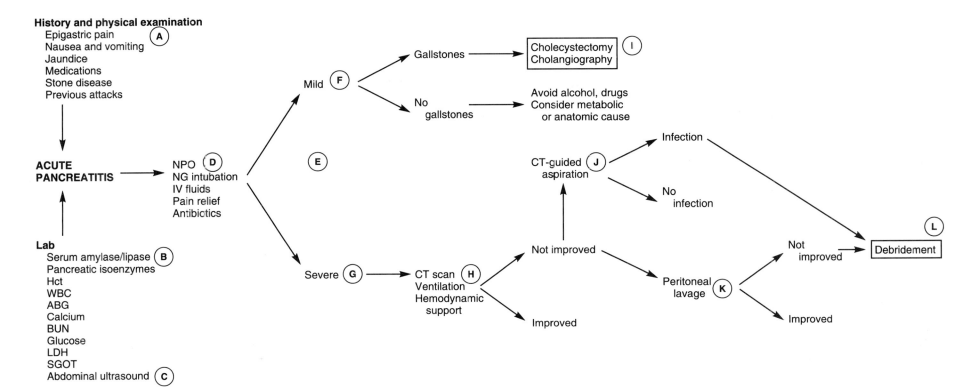

History and physical examination
Epigastric pain (A)
Nausea and vomiting
Jaundice
Medications
Stone disease
Previous attacks

ACUTE PANCREATITIS

NPO (D)
NG intubation
IV fluids
Pain relief
Antibiotics

Lab
Serum amylase/lipase (B)
Pancreatic isoenzymes
Hct
WBC
ABG
Calcium
BUN
Glucose
LDH
SGOT
Abdominal ultrasound (C)

Mild (F)
Gallstones → Cholecystectomy Cholangiography (I)
No gallstones → Avoid alcohol, drugs Consider metabolic or anatomic cause

(E)

Severe (G) → CT scan (H) Ventilation Hemodynamic support

Not improved
Improved

CT-guided aspiration (J)
Infection
No infection

Peritoneal lavage (K)
Not improved
Improved

Debridement (L)

ment are comparable. For patients with very severe peripancreatic necrosis, there may be a role for debridement with marsupialization. Pancreatotomy is rarely, if ever, necessary in the treatment of severe pancreatitis.

REFERENCES

Acosta JM, Ledesma CL. Gallstone migration as a cause of acute pancreatitis. N Engl J Med 1974: 290:484–487.

Bradley EL. Management of infected pancreatic necrosis by open drainage. Ann Surg 1987; 206:542–548.

Carey LC. The etiology of pancreatitis. In: Moody FG, Carey LC, Jones RS, et al., eds. Surgical treatment of digestive disease. Chicago, Year Book 1990:459–469.

Choi TK, Mok F, Zhan WH, et al. Somatostasin in the treatment of acute pancreatitis: a prospective randomized controlled trial. Gut 1989; 30:223–227.

Kelly TR. Gallstones pancreatitis: the timing of surgery. Surgery 1980; 88:345–349.

Mayer AD, McMahon MJ, Corfield AP, et al. Controlled clinical trial of peritoneal lavage for the treatment of severe acute pancreatitis. N Engl J Med 1985; 312:399–404.

Ranson JHC, Rifkind KM, Roses DF, et al. Prognostic signs and the role of operative management in acute pancreatitis. Surg Gynecol Obstet 1974; 139:69–81.

Weaver DW, Bouwman DL, Walt AJ, et al. Correlation between clinical pancreatitis and isoenzyme patterns of amylase. Surgery 1982; 92:576–580.

Wilson C, Imrie CW. Effective intraperitoneal antiprotease therapy for taurocholate-induced pancreatitis in rats. Br J Surg 1990; 77:1252–1255.

Chronic Pancreatitis

Charles F. Frey, M.D.

(A) Chronic pancreatitis is progressive, inflammatory, fibrotic destruction of the pancreas. Two types of chronic pancreatitis are recognized. Chronic calcific pancreatitis is spotty and lobular with multiple intraductal strictures and calcifications. Not all patients show calcification initially, but with time calcification will result. Alcohol abuse is the most frequent cause of chronic pancreatitis of this type, although hyperparathyroidism, heredity, and tropical pancreatitis account for a few patients. Chronic obstructive pancreatitis is characterized by more uniform distribution of lesions throughout the gland behind an obstruction of the major pancreatic ductal system. It is often the result of tumor, trauma, or necrotic pseudocyst after necrotizing pancreatitis.

(B) Pain associated with chronic pancreatitis can be severe and disabling and lead to narcotic addiction. Pain is often due to ductal hypertension. Scarring and inflammation around the nerve endings can be another source of pain.

(C) Complications of pancreatitis, aside from exocrine and endocrine insufficiency, result from fibrosis and inflammation of the parenchyma, stricturing of the ducts, compression by pseudocysts and retention cysts, or thrombosis of major vascular structures. They include pseudocysts, common bile duct or duodenal obstruction, ascites, pleural effusion, pericardial tamponade, portal or splenic vein thrombosis, partial or left-sided portal hypertension, or hemoductal hemorrhage from pseudoaneurysms.

(D) In a patient whose only complaint is pain, objective evidence of pancreatic disease should be sought. Hyperamylasemia during exacerbation of pain in chronic calcific pancreatitis is sometimes present. Cholecystokinin and secretin stimulation tests to assess pancreatic exocrine secretions are time consuming and abnormal only in advanced disease. Structural abnormalities of the pancreas and the major pancreatic duct are best assessed by computed tomography and endoscopic retrograde cholangiography. The biliary tract is best evaluated by ultrasonography. Angiography may be helpful in differentiating carcinoma of the pancreas from chronic pancreatitis as well as identifying any unusual anatomy.

(E) Chronic pancreatitis may be difficult to distinguish from pancreatic carcinoma. Absence of a history of alcoholism and onset of symptoms in patients in their 60s and 70s raises the suspicion of carcinoma. Celiac and superior mesenteric artery angiography helps rule out cancer.

(F) Pancreatic ascites and pancreatic pleural fistulas result from disruption of the pancreatic duct usually in association with obstruction of the proximal duct. Some fistulas resolve spontaneously after a trial of total parenteral nutrition with or without somatostatin. Should a fistula fail to close, a Roux-en-Y limb is anastomosed to the fistula on the surface of the pancreas.

(G) Pseudoaneurysms most frequently involve the splenic artery and are best treated by angiographic embolization as a definitive procedure. If this is not possible, resection of the involved pancreas (distal pancreatectomy if the splenic artery is involved) or pancreaticoduodenectomy (if gastroduodenal or pancreaticoduodenal vessels are involved) is indicated. Sometimes control of the pseudoaneurysm can be obtained by proximal ligation of the feeding vessel. Least desirable and least effective is direct ligation of the bleeding pseudoaneurysm within the pseudocyst.

(H) One of the principal indications for operation is the relief of pain and the avoidance of narcotic addiction. Narcotics are not indicated in the management of chronic pain. The hope that the patient's pain may subside over time as a result of burnout of the exocrine tissue due to scarring and atrophy is only applicable to patients with mild pancreatitis, not requiring narcotics. Not all patients with chronic pancreatitis have pain but may seek a physician's help because of steatorrhea or diabetes.

(I) Significant common bile duct obstruction occurs in about 20 percent of patients and is dealt with by choledochojejunostomy or choledochoduodenostomy if the patient has no pancreatic pain. If the patient has pain plus common bile duct obstruction, then the Frey or Beger procedure should be employed to provide pain relief by main pancreatic ductal decompression and common bile duct decompression.

(J) Duodenal obstruction is treated by gastrojejunostomy in the absence of pain. If pain is present, then either the Frey or Beger procedure, sometimes in conjunction with gastrojejunostomy, or pancreaticoduodenectomy alone may be necessary.

(K) Splenic vein thrombosis with left-sided portal hypertension and bleeding varices is best treated by splenectomy.

(L) Medical treatment for chronic pancreatitis consists of improving the patient's nutrition and putting the pancreas at rest by reducing pancreatic exocrine secretion and involving the patient in a program to reduce alcohol consumption (eg, Alcoholics Anonymous). Stopping alcohol does not prevent the progression of exocrine and endocrine deterioration. Pancreatic enzyme supplements and H_2 blockers facilitate fat, carbohydrate, and protein absorption. Proteolytic enzymes inhibit cholecystokinin stimulation of the pancreas by slowing cholecystokinin release in the duodenum.

(M) Should pain persist or recur frequently and be sufficiently severe to require narcotics for

History and physical examination

Pain (B)
Steatorrhea
Diabetes
Alcoholism
Narcotic addiction (C)
CBD obstruction
Duodenal obstruction
Pancreatic fistula
Ascites
Splenic vein thrombosis

CHRONIC PANCREATITIS (A)

Lab
FBS
Fecal fat
Secretion tests (D)
LFT
US biliary tract
CT scan pancreas
and liver
ERCP
Celiac and SMA (E)
angiogram

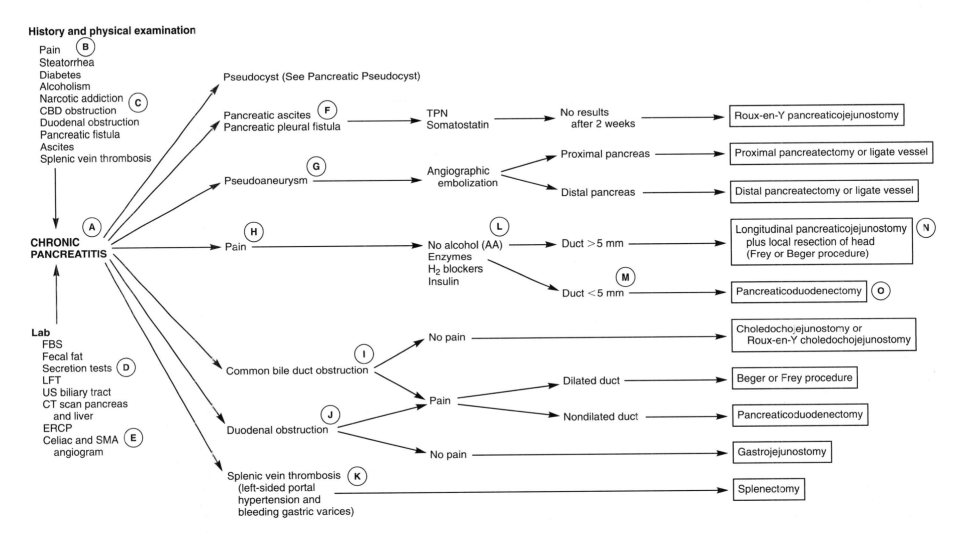

Pseudocyst (See Pancreatic Pseudocyst)

Pancreatic ascites (F)
Pancreatic pleural fistula → TPN / Somatostatin → No results after 2 weeks → Roux-en-Y pancreaticojejunostomy

Pseudoaneurysm (G) → Angiographic embolization → Proximal pancreas → Proximal pancreatectomy or ligate vessel
→ Distal pancreas → Distal pancreatectomy or ligate vessel

Pain (H) → No alcohol (AA) (L) / Enzymes / H₂ blockers / Insulin → Duct >5 mm → Longitudinal pancreaticojejunostomy plus local resection of head (Frey or Beger procedure) (N)
→ Duct <5 mm (M) → Pancreaticoduodenectomy (O)

Common bile duct obstruction (I) → No pain → Choledochojejunostomy or Roux-en-Y choledochojejunostomy
→ Pain

Duodenal obstruction (J) → Pain → Dilated duct → Beger or Frey procedure
→ Nondilated duct → Pancreaticoduodenectomy
→ No pain → Gastrojejunostomy

Splenic vein thrombosis (K) (left-sided portal hypertension and bleeding gastric varices) → Splenectomy

---

relief, then operation is indicated. Factors affecting the choice of operation include the size of the major pancreatic duct, the number and location of retention cysts, the site of ductal strictures (whether in the proximal or distal pancreas), anomalies of the pancreatic ductal system such as pancreas divisum, the site of fistulas of the major pancreatic duct, and the presence of a pancreatic mass that may require resection of tumor.

(N) Longitudinal pancreaticojejunostomy is the operation of choice when the major pancreatic duct is 5 mm or greater in diameter. The jejunum is sewn to the capsule of the pancreas, not to the mucosa. The incision must be carried from the tail of the pancreas to the duodenum. When the head of the pancreas is thickened, it is essential that local resection of the head be carried out (Frey or Beger procedure) to drain the ducts

of Wirsung and Santorini and the uncinate ducts along with their tributary ducts and associated retention cysts. In the absence of local resection of the head of the pancreas, pain relief initially present in 90 percent of patients drops to 50 percent by 3 to 5 years. With local resection, preliminary data indicate 80 percent pain relief at 5 years.

(O) If the main pancreatic duct is less than 5 mm in diameter, pancreaticoduodenectomy is in-

Chronic Pancreatitis (Continued)

dicated in patients in whom there is disease of the proximal pancreas or main pancreatic duct. Pain relief occurs in 85 to 90 percent of patients at 5 years. When there is evidence of disease in the distal pancreas and none in the proximal pancreas, distal pancreatectomy gives good results, with 80 percent pain relief at 5 years. If pancreaticoduodenectomy is impossible in a patient with a small major pancreatic duct, the body and tail of the pancreas can undergo autotransplantation to the pelvis. Total pancreatectomy is only occasionally necessary in patients with chronic pancreatitis. Postoperatively, all patients should be maintained on pancreatic enzymes and H_2 blocker therapy.

REFERENCES

Ammann RW, Akovbiantz A, Largiades F, et al. Course and outcome of chronic pancreatitis: longitudinal study of mixed medical-surgical series of 24 patients. Gastroenterology 1984; 86:820–828.

Beger HG, Krantzberger W, Bittner R, et al. Duodenum-preserving resection of the head of the pancreas in patients with severe chronic pancreatitis. Surgery 1985; 97:467–473.

Frey CF, Smith GJ. Description and rationale of a new operation for chronic pancreatitis. Pancreas 1987; 2:701–707.

Frey CF, Suzuki M, Isaji S, et al. Pancreatic resection for chronic pancreatitis. Surg Clin North Am 1989; 69:499–528.

Taylor RH, Bagley FH, Braasch JW, et al. Ductal drainage or resection for chronic pancreatitis. Am J Surg 1981; 141:28–33.

History and physical examination

Pain (B)
Steatorrhea
Diabetes
Alcoholism
Narcotic addiction (C)
CBD obstruction
Duodenal obstruction
Pancreatic fistula
Ascites
Splenic vein thrombosis

CHRONIC PANCREATITIS (A)

Lab
FBS
Fecal fat
Secretion tests (D)
LFT
US biliary tract
CT scan pancreas
and liver
ERCP
Celiac and SMA (E)
angiogram

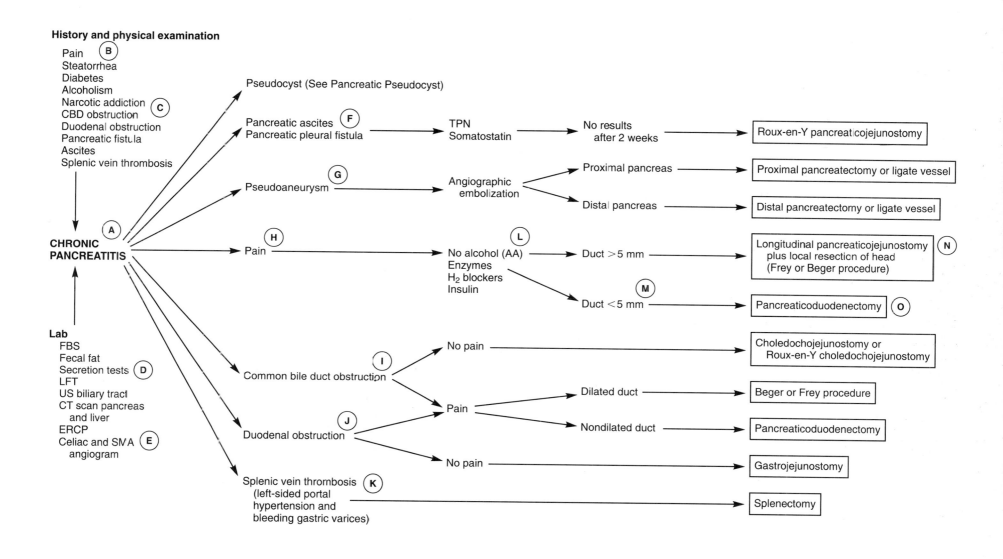

Pseudocyst (See Pancreatic Pseudocyst)

Pancreatic ascites (F)
Pancreatic pleural fistula → TPN / Somatostatin → No results after 2 weeks → Roux-en-Y pancreaticojejunostomy

Pseudoaneurysm (G) → Angiographic embolization → Proximal pancreas → Proximal pancreatectomy or ligate vessel
→ Distal pancreas → Distal pancreatectomy or ligate vessel

Pain (H) → No alcohol (AA) (L) / Enzymes / H₂ blockers / Insulin → Duct >5 mm → Longitudinal pancreaticojejunostomy plus local resection of head (Frey or Beger procedure) (N)
→ Duct <5 mm (M) → Pancreaticoduodenectomy (O)

Common bile duct obstruction (I) → No pain → Choledochojejunostomy or Roux-en-Y choledochojejunostomy
→ Pain → Dilated duct → Beger or Frey procedure
→ Nondilated duct → Pancreaticoduodenectomy

Duodenal obstruction (J) → No pain → Gastrojejunostomy

Splenic vein thrombosis (K) (left-sided portal hypertension and bleeding gastric varices) → Splenectomy

Pancreatic Pseudocyst

Edward L. Bradley, III, M.D.

(A) Clinical suspicion of pancreatic pseudocyst is aroused in any patient with pancreatitis who fails to improve after a week of therapy. Pseudocyst is usually associated with an abdominal mass and persistent pain. In the absence of documented pancreatitis, or when evidence of alcoholism or biliary tract disease is lacking, all pseudocysts should be regarded as cystic pancreatic neoplasms, making biopsy mandatory.

(B) The behavior of pancreatic pseudocysts is time dependent. Pseudocysts that are less than 6 weeks old and arise in conjunction with an episode of acute pancreatitis are called acute pseudocysts. Spontaneous resolution of acute pseudocysts is relatively common (30 to 50 percent). One third persist to become chronic pseudocysts. Complications occur in only 10 to 15 percent. Chronic pseudocysts are defined either as pseudocysts that are associated with chronic pancreatitis or acute pseudocysts that have reached 6 weeks of age. Chronic pseudocysts rarely undergo spontaneous resolution (10 percent). They are more commonly associated with complications (30 to 40 percent) when not definitively treated. Chronic pseudocysts should therefore be drained when recognized.

(C) Each commonly employed pancreatic imaging procedure has advantages and disadvantages. Sonography and computed tomography involve no risk. Sonography ($200) is less expensive than computed tomography ($700) or endoscopic retrograde cholangiopancreatography ($1200). Endoscopic pancreatography is reserved for complicated pseudocysts, recurrences, and when pancreatic duct obstruction or common duct stenosis is suspected.

(D) Uncomplicated acute pseudocysts, being dynamic structures, require only serial monitoring. Weekly sonographic studies are necessary to determine their eventual course.

(E) Drainage for chronic pseudocysts is controversial. Internal drainage remains the standard therapy against which competitive therapies are measured. Careful evaluation of alternative approaches is required.

(F) Small asymptomatic pseudocysts (<5 cm) and pseudocysts that decrease in size during serial monitoring may be safely followed.

(G) Acute pseudocysts (>5 cm) that persist after 6 weeks become, by definition, chronic pseudocysts and are treated as such.

(H) Acute pseudocysts that increase in size during the monitoring period should undergo external drainage to prevent rupture.

(I) Secondary infection of a pancreatic pseudocyst must be differentiated from infected pancreatic necrosis. An infected pseudocyst has thick, well-defined walls and purulent content. Treatment by external drainage is highly effective. In infected necrosis, friable walls surround necrotic tissue and scant amounts of dishwater-colored fluid. For infected necrosis, extensive surgical debridement and drainage with open packing are often required.

(J) Rupture is usually manifested as a pancreatic fistula into the peritoneal cavity (pancreatic ascites) or into the chest (pancreatic hydrothorax). If a fluid collection has not resolved after 2 weeks of hyperalimentation, pancreatography and operative resection of the fistula or Roux-en-Y drainage is indicated.

(K) Although uncommon, hemorrhage accounts for more than 75 percent of deaths from complicated pseudocysts. Preexploration angiography is extremely useful, both to localize the site of bleeding and to plan the appropriate procedure. Ligation of the affected artery, usually the splenic, or pancreatic resection may be required. Packing and external drainage may be the only way to control torrential bleeding. Angiographic embolization of pseudoaneurysms might be useful in a high-risk patient.

(L) Persistent obstruction of the gastrointestinal tract by a pseudocyst is unusual. This possibility should be kept in mind, however, particularly when the common duct seems to be involved. Ampullary stenosis or chronic pancreatic cholangiopathy due to enveloping fibrosis must also be considered and sought at surgery.

(M) External drainage of pancreatic pseudocysts can be performed by surgical or percutaneous means. Because of the demonstrated safety and lower cost of transcutaneous drainage, there is little reason to perform elective surgical external drainage. Percutaneous drainage works best when performed as continuous drainage rather than as simple aspiration (80 percent success rate vs. 30 percent). Caution must be exercised in using percutaneous drainage, however, since 15 percent of "pseudocysts" are in fact cystic neoplasms. Percutaneous drainage precludes the use of biopsy to sample the pseudocyst wall. The finding of mucoid viscous fluid or the failure of the pseudocyst to promptly collapse suggests cystic neoplasm and calls for surgical excision. An insufficient number of chronic pseudocysts have been treated by percutaneous drainage to permit meaningful comparison with surgical internal drainage. Advantages of percutaneous drainage are lower cost (almost 50 percent less) and better patient acceptance. Disadvantages include uncertain mortality risk, unknown morbidity (secondary infections, hemorrhagic complications, persistent pancreatic fistulas), absence of long-term follow-up, and risk of inappropriate treatment of potentially malignant cystic neoplasms. Until such objections have been overcome, percutaneous drainage should be reserved for the

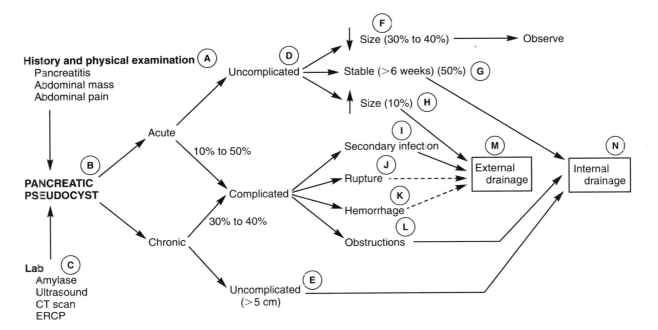

urgent treatment of complicated acute pseudocysts (rapid expansion or secondary infection) and for use in poor-risk patients.

(N) Internal drainage can be accomplished by surgical cystenteric anastomosis (cystoduodenostomy, cystogastrostomy, or cystojejunostomy Roux-en-Y). Since the risk and effectiveness of the three procedures are equal (mortality rate, 3 to 5 percent), choice of an elective surgical procedure is determined primarily by location of the pseudocyst and its adherence to surrounding structures. Transgastric cystogastrostomy and transduodenal cystoduodenostomy are anastomoses performed without sutures, except as needed for hemostasis.

They depend on inflammatory adherence of adjacent structures to prevent a leak. If the wall of the pseudocyst is not adherent to either the stomach or duodenum, cystojejunostomy (Roux-en-Y) is the procedure of choice. A prohibitive mortality rate (10 to 15 percent) attends routine excision of pseudocysts. Frozen-section biopsy of the pseudocyst wall should be done to exclude cystic malignancy. Recurrence rates after cystenteric anastomoses approximate 10 percent.

Limited experience with transenteric transendoscopic drainage using electrocautery or laser has been reported. In the absence of sutures, this technique depends on inflammatory adherence of the pseudocyst to the adjacent intestine, a feature absent in 42 percent of the author's 138 surgical cases. Accordingly, an endoscopic approach to internal drainage cannot be recommended at this time.

REFERENCES

Aranha GV, Prinz RA, Esquerra AC, et al. The nature and course of cystic pancreatic lesions diagnosed by ultrasound. Arch Surg 1983; 118:486–492.

Bradley EL III. Pseudocysts: complications of pancreatitis. Philadelphia: WB Saunders, 1982.

Walt AJ, Bouwman DZ, Weaver DW, et al. The impact of technology on the management of pancreatic pseudocysts. Arch Surg 1990; 125:759–763.

Carcinoma of the Pancreas

Carlos Fernández-del Castillo, M.D., and Andrew L. Warshaw, M.D.

(A) The only established risk factor for carcinoma of the pancreas is cigarette smoking. In over 90 percent of patients, jaundice and pain are present at the moment of diagnosis.

(B) CA 19-9 is the most extensively studied serum marker for this neoplasm. Its sensitivity can reach 89 percent. It is frequently positive in other gastrointestinal tumors.

(C) Computed tomography and ultrasound demonstrate a tumor in most patients and, by evidencing metastases or gross peripancreatic extension, give all the information that is needed for staging.

(D) If no metastases are demonstrated and jaundice is present, endoscopic retrograde cholangiopancreatography is indicated. It is the most sensitive test for the diagnosis of pancreatic cancer and the mainstay for the differentiation of periampullary tumors. Percutaneous transhepatic cholangiography may also demonstrate the site of obstruction but is usually reserved for patients in whom endoscopic retrograde cholangiopancreatography cannot be practiced. Biliary drainage by placement of an internal stent is possible by either means and may be desirable to reduce symptoms before definitive surgery. Preoperative biliary decompression has not been shown to reduce operative morbidity or mortality.

(E) More than 40 percent of patients with no obvious metastases demonstrable by computed tomography have small (1 to 2 mm) liver, peritoneal, and omental nodules. This incidence rises to 65 percent with tumors in the body or tail. Laparoscopy can readily detect these lesions and thus avoid unnecessary surgery in some patients. Cytologic examination of peritoneal washings obtained at laparoscopy is positive for cancer cells in about 30 percent of cases and appears to be an additional useful index for staging.

(F) Histologic confirmation of cancer should be obtained in unresectable patients and can be done percutaneously. The authors do not favor this approach in potentially resectable patients because of the risk of tumor seeding.

(G) Intraoperative radiation therapy improves quality of life by providing substantial relief of pain and can also increase survival time.

(H) Pancreatic cancer comprises 85 percent of the tumors of the pancreatobiliary junction. Resectability and survival rates for ampullary and duodenal carcinomas are far better than for pancreatic cancer and, in the absence of demonstrated metastases, should be surgically explored.

(I) Angiography is carried out both to exclude involvement of major vessels (superior mesenteric and portal veins in particular), which if present contraindicates resection in most cases, and to delineate the vascular anatomy, which has anomalies in up to 24 percent of patients. If computed tomography, laparoscopy, and angiography are negative, 78 percent of tumors are resectable.

(J) To minimize dissemination of viable tumor cells during surgical manipulation, the authors currently use low-dose (10 Gy) external beam irradiation preoperatively.

(K) Use of large-bore stenting tubes placed endoscopically or percutaneously provides excellent palliation for biliary obstruction, equivalent to surgical bypass in durability and without the need for an operation. Patients with duodenal obstruction require gastrojejunostomy and therefore should have their biliary obstruction treated surgically at the same time.

(L) Surgical resection of pancreatic cancer provides the only possibility of cure. Five-year survival rates if no tumor is left behind can be up to 36 percent. Mortality for pancreatoduodenectomy is now less than 5 percent in many institutions. There seem to be no major differences in survival with different techniques. Complication rates are also similar although total pancreatectomy produces a diabetic state that may be difficult to control. Cancers in the body or tail of the pancreas are rarely resectable and probably incurable.

REFERENCES

Fernández-del Castillo C, Warshaw AL. Diagnosis and preoperative evaluation of pancreatic cancer with implications for management. Gastroenterol Clin North Am, 1990; 19:915–933.

Fontham ETH, Correa P. Epidemiology of pancreatic cancer. Surg Clin North Am 1989; 69:551–567.

Freeney PC, Marks WM, Ryan JA, et al. Pancreatic ductal adenocarcinoma: diagnosis and staging with dynamic CT. Radiology 1988; 166:125–133.

Grace PA, Pitt HA, Longmire WP. Pylorus preserving pancreatoduodenectomy: an overview. Br J Surg 1990; 77:986–974.

Pleskow DK, Berger HJ, Gyves J, et al. Evaluation of a serologic marker, CA 19-9, in the diagnosis of pancreatic cancer. Ann Intern Med 1989; 110:704–709.

Trede M, Schwall G, Saeger HD. Survival after pancreatoduodenectomy. Ann Surg 1990; 211:447–458.

Warshaw AL. Implications of peritoneal cytology for staging of early pancreatic cancer. Am J Surg 1991; 161:26–30.

Warshaw AL, Gu Z-Y, Wittenberg J, Waltman AC. Preoperative staging and assessment of resectability of pancreatic cancer. Arch Surg 1990; 125:230–233.

Warshaw AL, Swanson RS. Pancreatic cancer in 1988: possibilities and probabilities. Ann Surg 1988; 208:541–553.

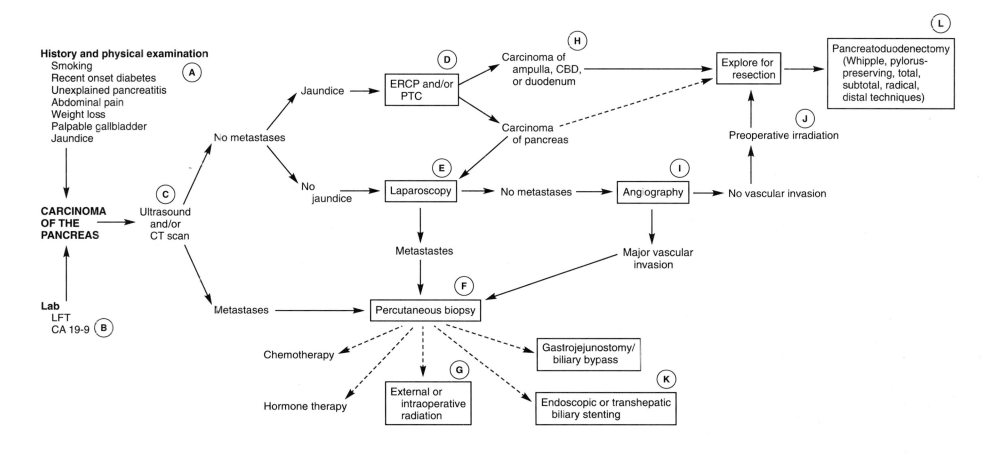

History and physical examination (A)
- Smoking
- Recent onset diabetes
- Unexplained pancreatitis
- Abdominal pain
- Weight loss
- Palpable gallbladder
- Jaundice

Lab (B)
- LFT
- CA 19-9

CARCINOMA OF THE PANCREAS

Ultrasound and/or CT scan (C)

No metastases

Metastases

Jaundice → ERCP and/or PTC (D)

→ Carcinoma of ampulla, CBD, or duodenum (H)

→ Carcinoma of pancreas

No jaundice → Laparoscopy (E) → No metastases → Angiography (I) → No vascular invasion

Metastastes

Major vascular invasion

Percutaneous biopsy (F)

Chemotherapy

Hormone therapy

External or intraoperative radiation (G)

Gastrojejunostomy/ biliary bypass

Endoscopic or transhepatic biliary stenting (K)

Explore for resection

Preoperative irradiation (J)

Pancreatoduodenectomy (Whipple, pylorus-preserving, total, subtotal, radical, distal techniques) (L)

Small Bowel Obstruction

Ian McColl, M.S.

(A) Abdominal x-ray studies include an upright view of the chest and upright and supine views of the abdomen. Characteristically, loops of small bowel are distended and show air—fluid levels. This appearance may be absent even when the bowel is gangrenous.

(B) Otherwise unexplained acidosis and abdominal pain, especially severe, continuous pain, may be the earliest signs of dead bowel from arterial occlusion. A marked increase in the white cell count is often associated.

(C) Vomiting and sequestration of fluid in the bowel lead to dehydration and acidosis. Continuous pain or abdominal or rectal tenderness is an indication for early laparotomy. The patient with possible small bowel obstruction should be examined hourly.

(D) After induction of anesthesia, a hernia may reduce spontaneously, especially in children. Operative repair should continue, however. It is rarely necessary to perform laparotomy to check bowel viability under these circumstances.

(E) Tumors may obstruct small bowel intraluminally or extraluminally. Resection of a segment of intestine is usually required in either instance.

(F) Causes of mesenteric vascular disease include arterial embolism, arterial or venous throm-

bosis, and low cardiac output. The clinical picture is one of severe continuous abdominal pain with few signs except pallor. Obvious abdominal signs usually indicate dead bowel, which only rarely can be resurrected by embolectomy or reconstructive procedures.

(G) It may be prudent on occasion to bring out the two ends of bowel rather than perform a primary anastomosis. Occasionally, so much bowel must be resected that insufficient gut remains for anything but parenteral nutrition. This characteristically occurs in elderly patients with superior mesenteric artery occlusion and dead gut from the proximal jejunum to the midtransverse colon. There are times when no resection should be done because the patient will survive only 1 or 2 days.

(H) For gallstone ileus, enterotomy and removal of the stone are all that is required.

(I) Treatment may require appendectomy, drainage of pus, exteriorization of perforated colon, or simply antibiotics.

(J) Because of the frequency of recurrent bowel ischemia, a second-look operation is sometimes indicated, particularly when skip areas of ischemia were identified during the first operation.

(K) Intubation of the entire small intestine by means of a Baker tube inserted orally or

through a gastrostomy is one means of stenting the bowel to avoid recurrent obstruction. The tube must remain 1 to 2 weeks to be of benefit.

(L) Plication of intestinal loops to the anterior abdominal wall by suturing (Noble procedure) is seldom indicated. Passing a suture through the mesentery to hold the bowel in position has also been employed.

REFERENCES

DeCosse JJ, Rhodes RS, Wentz WB, et al. The natural history and management of radiation induced injury of the gastrointestinal tract. Ann Surg 1969; 170:369–384.

Ebert PA, Zuidema GD. Primary tumors of the small intestine. Arch Surg 1965; 91:452–455.

Frazee RC, Mucha P, Farnell MB, et al. Volvulus of the small intestine. Ann Surg 1988; 208:565–568.

Golladay ES, Byrne WJ. Intestinal pseudo-obstruction. Surg Gynecol Obstet 1982; 153:257–273.

Hofstetter SR. Acute adhesive obstruction of the small intestine. Surg Gynecol Obstet 1981; 152:141.

Kirsner JB. The local and systemic complications of inflammatory bowel disease. JAMA 1979; 242:1177–1183.

McMillin RD, Bivins BA, Griffen WO Jr. Intraluminal stenting in the management of recurrent intestinal obstruction. Am Surg 1981; 47:74–77.

Weigelt JA, Snyder WH III, Normal JL. Complications and results of 160 Baker tube plications. Am J Surg 1980; 140:810–815.

History and physical examination
    Previous laparotomy
    Hernia
    Bowel neoplasm
    Abdominal pain
    Abdominal distention
    Obstipation
    Vomiting
    Hyperactive bowel sounds

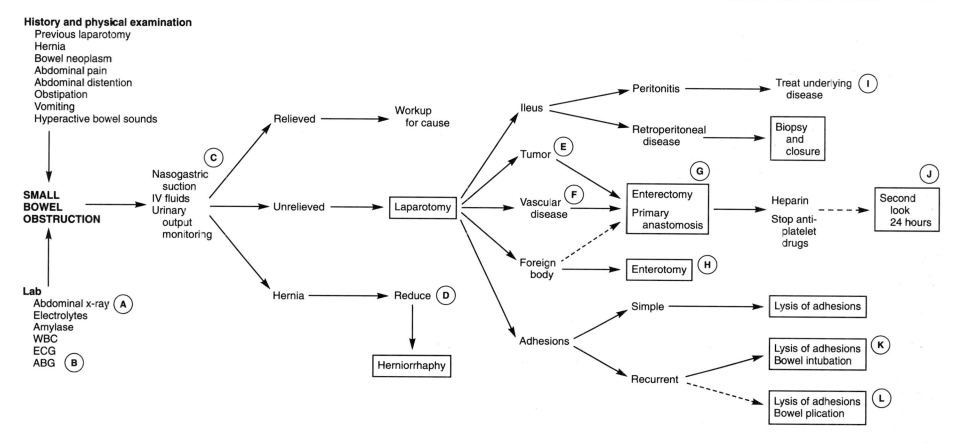

SMALL BOWEL OBSTRUCTION

Lab
    Abdominal x-ray (A)
    Electrolytes
    Amylase
    WBC
    ECG
    ABG (B)

Acute Mesenteric Vascular Occlusion

B. Timothy Baxter, M.D., and William H. Pearce, M.D.

(A) Acute mesenteric vascular occlusion (AMVO) causes death in 65 to 90 percent of patients largely because of delay in diagnosis. Nonspecific early symptoms and the lack of any reliable non-invasive diagnostic tests make early diagnosis difficult.

(B) Risk factors include older age, associated atherosclerotic vascular disease, coronary artery disease (especially a recent myocardial infarction or arrhythmia), cardiogenic shock with pressor support or intraaortic balloon assistance, and a known hypercoagulable state (malignancy or clotting inhibitory deficiency).

(C) Characteristically, there is sudden onset of severe abdominal pain associated with bowel evacuation. Physical findings are few. Hypotension in the absence of myocardial infarction is highly suggestive of intestinal ischemia.

(D) An electrocardiogram can detect myocardial infarction or arrhythmia. An echocardiogram can determine wall motion and the presence of an atrial or ventricular clot.

(E) Arterial blood gas determinations demonstrate metabolic acidosis in only 50 percent of patients with intestinal ischemia. Acidosis is generally considered to be a late finding of transmural infarction or shock. Hyperamylasemia, hemoconcentration, elevations of creatinine phosphokinase and lactic dehydrogenase, and hyperphosphatemia are associated with intestinal ischemia but are neither sensitive nor specific.

(F) Abdominal x-rays may differentiate AMVO from nonvascular diseases. Plain radiographic findings of AMVO include thickening of the bowel wall or air within the bowel wall or portal vein.

(G) Clotting profiles (prothrombin time, partial thromboplastin time, protein C and S, platelet count, and antithrombin III) identify known hypercoagulable states. Usually these tests require several days to complete and play no role in the early diagnosis of AMVO. The results become important once an accurate diagnosis has been made (ie, venous thrombosis).

(H) Restoring blood volume improves perfusion of still viable gut. Swan-Ganz catheter monitoring is essential.

(I) Strangulated small bowel and ischemic volvulus can mimic AMVO in the elderly. Each can cause few clinical symptoms.

(J) Mesenteric angiography is the best diagnostic test in AMVO. A lateral aortogram demonstrates the orifices of the major visceral vessels. In selected patients, the catheter is left in place for subsequent intraarterial infusions.

(K) Intense mesenteric vasoconstriction occurs with severe cardiac failure after massive myocardial infarction, sepsis, postcoronary artery bypass, intraaortic balloon pump assistance, or the use of high-dose pressors. Mesenteric angiography shows pruning of the mesenteric arcades and allows direct infusion of papaverine into the superior mesenteric artery (SMA).

(L) In patients with nonocclusive mesenteric ischemia, peritoneal signs mandate laparotomy. Necrotic bowel is resected. Postoperatively, intraarterial papaverine infusion is continued along with attempts to improve cardiac function.

(M) Venous thrombosis is an uncommon cause (5 percent) of acute intestinal ischemia. Causes include portal hypertension, pancreatitis, trauma (particularly splenectomy), and hypercoagulable states. The venous phase of selective SMA angiography may fail to opacify the superior mesenteric vein. Infusion computed tomography scanning can be diagnostic. Thirty-eight percent of patients develop peritonitis. Overall mortality is 12 percent but exceeds 40 percent in those who develop necrotic bowel. Long-term anticoagulation is required for patients with an identifiable coagulopathy.

(N) Embolic and thrombotic occlusions of the SMA occur with nearly equal frequency. SMA occlusion occurs at the origin with thrombotic occlusion and at some distal branch with emboli. Sparing of the proximal SMA branches limits ischemia to the distal small bowel and proximal colon. With thrombosis, the transverse colon and proximal jejunum are ischemic. In 40 to 80 percent of patients, the ascending colon is involved.

(O) Proximal SMA embolectomy is possible in 90 percent of patients. With small emboli (rare), bowel infarction is limited and embolectomy is unwarranted. Survival is significantly improved when operation is performed within 24 hours of the initial symptoms (80 percent vs. zero). Long-term anticoagulation is necessary since the incidence of recurrent embolism is high.

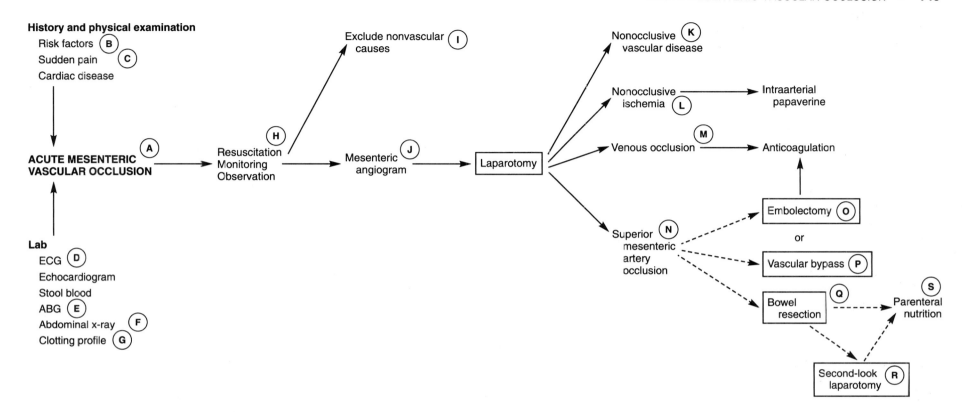

History and physical examination
Risk factors (B)
Sudden pain (C)
Cardiac disease

ACUTE MESENTERIC VASCULAR OCCLUSION (A)

Lab
ECG (D)
Echocardiogram
Stool blood
ABG (E)
Abdominal x-ray (F)
Clotting profile (G)

Resuscitation Monitoring Observation (H)

Exclude nonvascular causes (I)

Mesenteric angiogram (J)

Laparotomy

Nonocclusive vascular disease (K)

Nonocclusive ischemia (L) → Intraarterial papaverine

Venous occlusion (M) → Anticoagulation

Superior mesenteric artery occlusion (N)

Embolectomy (O)
or
Vascular bypass (P)

Bowel resection (Q)

Parenteral nutrition (S)

Second-look laparotomy (R)

(P) A vascular bypass from the aorta to visceral vessels is possible only in 20 to 40 percent of patients.

(Q) Unfortunately, in 60 to 70 percent of patients there are frank gangrenous changes in all or part of the small bowel. If most of the bowel is necrotic, revascularization is unprofitable, and a decision is made to resect most of the remaining bowel or simply to close. Survival is limited to hours. Severity of coexisting diseases and the expected quality of life are important considerations. Revascularization may be indicated to preserve bowel length to avoid hyperalimentation. Roughly 3 feet of small intestine and some portion of the colon is the minimum length of bowel for survival without total parenteral nutrition.

(R) A second-look operation is planned when marginally viable bowel is not resected in the hope of preserving length. Once the decision is made to reexplore, improvement in clinical parameters should not alter the plan.

(S) Justification for home hyperalimentation depends on the remaining length of bowel. If total parenteral nutrition is required as a total calorie and fluid source, the average daily cost currently varies between $300 and $400. The annual cost is $110,000 to $145,000, excluding catheter placement and maintenance.

REFERENCES

Bergan JJ, Flinn WR, McCarthy WJ, et al. Acute mesenteric ischemia. In: Bergan JJ, Yao JST, eds. Vascular surgical emergencies. Orlando: Grune & Stratton, 1987; 401–413.

Bergan JJ, McCarthy WJ, Flinn WR, et al. Nontraumatic mesenteric vascular emergencies. J Vasc Surg 1987; 5:903–909.

Boley SJ, Borden EB. Acute mesenteric vascular disease. In: Wilson S, Veith F, Hobson R, Williams R, eds. Vascular surgery: principles and practice. New York: McGraw-Hill, 1987; 559–672.

Harward TR, Green D, Bergan JJ, et al. Mesenteric venous thrombosis. J Vasc Surg 1989; 9:328–333.

Rogers DM, Thompson JE, Garrett WV, et al. Mesenteric vascular problems—a 26-year experience. Ann Surg 1982; 195:554.

Short Bowel Syndrome

Leslie Wise, M.D., and Ronald E. Greenberg, M.D.

(A) The short bowel syndrome (SBS) occurs when extensive small bowel resection, bypass, or disease causes profound loss of absorptive capacity resulting in malabsorption of water, electrolytes, protein, carbohydrate, fat, trace elements, and vitamins. SBS usually results when more than 50 percent of the small bowel is resected or bypassed. Severity is determined by site of resection (eg, jejunum vs. ileum), degree of postresection adaptation, hepatic and pancreatic functional reserve, and, importantly, whether the ileocecal valve and colon remain intact. The ileocecal valve retards intestinal transit, allowing for increased absorption of nutrients, and prevents reflux of colonic contents, which promotes small bowel bacterial overgrowth.

(B) SBS leads to diarrhea, steatorrhea, weight loss, dehydration, perianal excoriation, and metabolic acidosis, as well as symptoms due to electrolyte (mainly potassium, calcium, and sodium) and vitamin (B_{12}, A, D, E, K) deficiencies. Causes of SBS include mesenteric vascular disease (superior mesenteric artery embolus, thrombosis, low flow state; superior mesenteric vein thrombosis), midgut volvulus, strangulated hernia, Crohn's disease, trauma, radiation enteritis, jejunoileal bypass, neoplasm, congenital jejunoileal atresia, and neonatal necrotizing enterocolitis.

(C) The goals of treatment are to maintain an adequate fluid and electrolyte balance, to ensure adequate nutrition (including trace minerals and vitamins), to palliate symptoms, and to treat complications. Acute phase management necessitates keeping the patient NPO for 10 to 14 days, initiating total parenteral nutrition (TPN), and supplementing additional fluid and electrolytes. H_2 receptor antagonists are infused continuously to counter gastric acid hypersecretion (seen after massive small bowel resection) and to prevent stress ulcer. Diarrhea is treated symptomatically with either Lomotil, loperamide, paregoric, or codeine. Perianal excoriation is treated with aluminum paste, zinc oxide, or coraya. During the acute phase, the patient requires frequent recording of input and output and repetitive measurement of electrolytes (especially calcium and magnesium), blood urea nitrogen, glucose, and zinc. Insertion of a central venous catheter is helpful.

(D) After massive small bowel resection, adaptation occurs over several weeks to months. Epithelial hyperplasia leads to an increase in caliber and absorptive surface of the remaining intestinal segment. Because luminal nutrients stimulate this adaptive phase, oral feedings should be started early. A lactose-free solution of glucose polymer and protein hydrolysate is introduced gradually through a soft nasoenteral or gastrostomy tube. TPN is gradually tapered and may be cycled as a supplement to tube feedings.

(E) Long-term management depends on the length of residual small bowel. For patients with more than 60 to 80 cm of bowel (50 cm if the ileocecal valve is intact), feeding can progress until a normal or modified oral diet is tolerated. Patients are instructed to eat dry solids 1 hour apart from isotonic liquids. A low-oxalate, lactose-free diet, often divided between five and six feedings per day, should achieve adequate caloric intake (32 absorbed kcal/kg, or approximately 1.5 to 2 times usual intake). Previously, a low-fat, high-carbohydrate diet with medium-chain triglyceride supplementation was advocated. Data suggest that fat restriction may not be required, because net caloric absorption is higher and volume output is unchanged on a high-fat compared with a high-carbohydrate diet. Patients may suffer an exacerbation of diarrhea on a high-fat diet. This can be alleviated by feeding less than 40 g of fat per day. Oral supplements of Ca^{2+}, Mg^{2+}, zinc, and fat-soluble vitamins are required (in addition to periodic B_{12} injections) to prevent deficiency states.

(F) After extensive small bowel resection, oral feedings may not be tolerated. Nasoenteral feedings providing an undiluted low-fiber, lactose-free enteral formula by continuous infusion can be tried at home. Motivated patients are able to insert a fine-bore nasoenteral feeding tube on a nightly basis. Elemental diets have no advantage over polymeric diets, which are less expensive and less likely to exacerbate diarrhea. The cost of home enteral nutrition is about $30 per day.

(G) Diarrhea is treated with standard symptomatic therapy. The long-acting somatostatin analogue sandostatin slows transit time, reduces intestinal output, and decreases diarrhea but does not obviate the need for TPN in dependent patients. Diarrhea due to bile salt malabsorption can be treated with cholestyramine resin, but this may exacerbate steatorrhea by further depleting the residual bile salt pool. Small bowel bacterial overgrowth, common after resection of the ileocecal valve, can be treated with oral antibiotics (eg, tetracycline, metronidazole). Repeated attacks of dyspnea and drowsiness due to D-lactic acidosis respond to antibacterial therapy. Parenteral vitamin B_{12} (200 µg/month) is given to patients after terminal ileal resection for the rest of their lives. Patients with SBS are at increased risk for calcium oxalate renal stones and cholesterol gallstones. Secondary pancreatic insufficiency may contribute

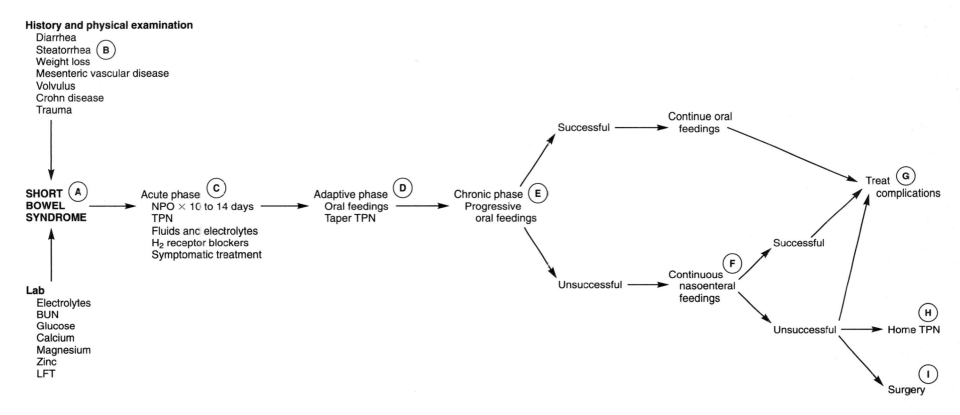

History and physical examination
Diarrhea
Steatorrhea (B)
Weight loss
Mesenteric vascular disease
Volvulus
Crohn disease
Trauma

**SHORT (A)
BOWEL
SYNDROME**

Lab
Electrolytes
BUN
Glucose
Calcium
Magnesium
Zinc
LFT

Acute phase (C)
NPO × 10 to 14 days
TPN
Fluids and electrolytes
H₂ receptor blockers
Symptomatic treatment

Adaptive phase (D)
Oral feedings
Taper TPN

Chronic phase (E)
Progressive
oral feedings

Successful → Continue oral feedings

Unsuccessful → Continuous nasoenteral feedings (F)

Successful

Unsuccessful → Home TPN (H)

Treat (G)
complications

Surgery (I)

---

to steatorrhea and can be treated by pancreatic enzyme supplements.

Manifestations of K^+, Ca^{2+}, Mg^{2+}, Fe^{2+}, and zinc deficiency (eg, weakness, Chvostek or Trousseau sign, anemia, rash) as well as deficiency of the fat-soluble vitamins A, D, K, and E (eg, night blindness, hypocalcemia and metabolic bone disease, bleeding diathesis, and neurologic symptoms) mandate routine monitoring and supplementation. Patients on maintenance TPN need serial liver function tests to detect cholestatic liver disease and, possibly, cirrhosis. Permanent indwelling, intravascular catheters for TPN can cause infection.

(H) If oral or continuous nasoenteral feedings fail, home TPN may be necessary. Patients who have a net positive secretory response to oral feedings require long-term TPN to avoid fluid def-

icits. The cost of home TPN (3000 calories daily) is approximately $400 per day.

(I) Surgery is rarely indicated to increase small bowel absorption and should not be tried for at least 6 months after the initial intestinal resection. Procedures include reverse intestinal segment, recirculating loop, colonic interposition, artificial ileocecal valve, growing intestinal neomucosa, small bowel tapering and lengthening procedures, retrograde electrical pacing, and small bowel transplantation.

REFERENCES

Allard JP, Jeejeebhoy KN. Nutritional support and therapy in the short bowel syndrome. Gastroenterol Clin North Am 1989; 589–601.

Devine RM, Kelly KA. Surgical therapy of the short bowel syndrome. Gastroenterol Clin North Am 1989; 18:603–618.

Heymsfield SB, Smith-Andrews JL, Hersh T. Home nasoenteric feeding for malabsorption and weight loss refractory to conventional therapy. Ann Intern Med 1983; 98:168–170.

Ladefoged K, Christensen KC, Hegnhoj J, et al. Effect of a long acting somatostatin analogue SMS 201–995 on jejunostomy effluent in patients with severe short bowel syndrome. Gut 1989; 30:943–949.

McIntyre PB, Fitchew M, Lennard-Jones JE. Patients with a high jejunostomy do not need a special diet. Gastroenterology 1986; 91:25–33.

Nightingale JMD, Lennard-Jones JE, Walker ER, et al. Jejunal reflux in short bowel syndrome. Lancet 1990; 336:765–768.

Thompson JS, Rikkens LF. Surgical alternatives for the short bowel syndrome. Am J Gastroenterol 1987; 82:97–106.

Wise L. Short bowel syndrome. In Najarian JS, Delaney JP, eds. Advances in Gastrointestinal Surgery. Chicago: Year Book Medical Publishers, 1989; 360–369.

Woolf GM, Miller C, Kurian R, et al. Diet for patients with a short bowel: high fat or high carbohydrate? Gastroenterology 1983; 84:823–828.

Enterocutaneous Fistula

Josef Fischer, M.D.

(A) Enterocutaneous fistula continues to carry a 20 percent mortality rate, although in some studies mortality has been as low as 6 percent. Satisfactory results require both judgment and meticulous care. Death is usually due to sepsis now that malnutrition and electrolyte imbalance are preventable. Adequate nutrition of patients with established sepsis remains difficult to achieve.

(B) A sinogram of every sinus tract (No. 5 pediatric feeding tube), using water-soluble contrast media, delineates the source and extent of the tract and associated abscesses. Barium studies rarely are required and, if performed, often do not reveal the fistula(s).

(C) Bowel function and healing are impaired by abnormal colloid oncotic pressure due to low serum albumin levels. Liberal albumin administration may restore albumin to 3.3 g/dL, a level at which healing is promoted.

(D) Needle aspiration of an obvious pointing abscess can be followed by a Hypaque sinogram to delineate the extent of the abscess and its origin from the bowel before drainage.

(E) A subclavian cannula is inserted for total parenteral nutrition. Patients should be hydrated with crystalloid to ensure safe cannulation of large veins.

(F) Antibiotics are required when a patient is frankly septic. An average of eight to nine antibiotics are ultimately required during the total course of therapy for a patient with a fistula.

(G) An abscess adjacent to the fistula keeps the tract open.

(H) Fistulas arising from irrevocably damaged bowel do not heal.

(I) Nasogastric suction does not decrease fistula output and may produce reflux esophagitis and subsequent stricture.

(J) Enteral nutrition may be attempted with special easily absorbable supplements such as amino acids. It is usually wise to maintain parenteral nutrition for 5 to 10 days after starting feedings since the gut at rest does not resume effective absorption immediately. About 4 feet of normal gut is needed for enteral nutrition.

(K) Mortality after an operation to repair a fistula should be 2 percent or less. A complication rate of 12 percent or less is expected.

(L) If the fistula has not closed after 4 to 5 weeks without sepsis, an operation is usually necessary. Preoperative nutritional status can be evaluated by measuring short half-life proteins (transferrin, retinol-binding protein, and thyroxine-binding prealbumin). When albumin increases spontaneously, hepatic protein synthesis is adequate. Principles of operative management include incision through healthy skin, relief of all distal obstruction, excision of marginally competent bowel, reanastomosis of all small intestinal blind loops, gastrostomy (which may be used for drainage and later feeding), and postoperative parenteral nutrition.

(M) Histamine H_2 antagonists may cut down drainage from enterocutaneous fistulas. Somatostatin or the octareotide analogue has not proved helpful in closing enterocutaneous fistulas. Somatostatin or its analogues may be helpful in closing pancreatic fistulas, however. In several large series using contemporary treatment, a spontaneous closure rate of 33 to 45 percent is reported. Spontaneous closure may be followed by return of a fistula if there is diseased bowel or distal obstruction.

REFERENCES

Aguirre A, Fischer JE, Welch CE. The role of surgery and hyperalimentation in therapy of gastrointestinal-cutaneous fistulae. Ann Surg 1974; 180:393–400.

Edmunds LH, Williams GM, Welch CE. External fistulas arising from the gastrointestinal tract. Ann Surg 1960; 152:445–471.

Fischer JE. The management of high-output intestinal fistulas. Adv Surg 1975; 9:139–179.

Fischer JE. The pathophysiology of enterocutaneous fistulas. World J Surg 1983; 7:446–450.

McPhayden VB Jr, Dudrick SJ. Management for gastrointestinal fistulas with parenteral hyperalimentation. Surgery 1973; 74:100–105.

Reber MA, Robert C, Way LW, Dunphy JE. Management of external gastrointestinal fistulas. Ann Surg 1978; 188:460–467.

Soeters PB, Ebeid AM, Fischer JE. Review of 404 patients with gastrointestinal fistulas: impact of parenteral nutrition. Ann Surg 1979; 190:189–202.

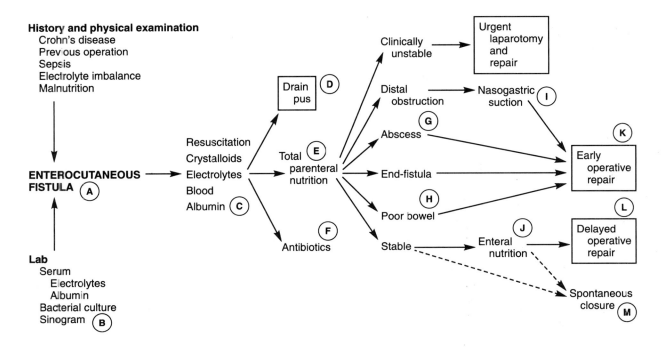

History and physical examination
Crohn's disease
Previous operation
Sepsis
Electrolyte imbalance
Malnutrition

ENTEROCUTANEOUS FISTULA (A)

Lab
Serum
Electrolytes
Albumin
Bacterial culture
Sinogram (B)

Resuscitation
Crystalloids
Electrolytes
Blood
Albumin (C)

Drain pus (D)

Total parenteral nutrition (E)

Antibiotics (F)

Clinically unstable → Urgent laparotomy and repair

Distal obstruction → Nasogastric suction (I)

Abscess (G)

End-fistula

Poor bowel (H)

Stable

Enteral nutrition (J)

Early operative repair (K)

Delayed operative repair (L)

Spontaneous closure (M)

Gastrointestinal Lymphoma

Robert T. Osteen, M.D., William Cody, M.D., and Ben Eiseman, M.D.

(A) Fever, night sweats, and weight loss are typically associated with advanced-stage, bulky tumors or gastrointestinal perforation.

(B) Waldeyer's ring is locally involved in approximately 20 percent of patients with gastrointestinal lymphoma.

(C) Characteristic radiologic findings include the following: (1) stomach—thickened rugal folds, mass, ulcer; and (2) small bowel—localized thickened folds, submucosal nodules.

(D) Endoscopic biopsy is diagnostic for gastric lymphoma in less than half of patients. Misdiagnoses of carcinoma or undifferentiated neoplasm are common.

(E) Computed tomography scans can image enlarged retroperitoneal and mesenteric nodes. Chest computed tomography scan may demonstrate mediastinal disease or pericardial involvement.

(F) Lymphangiography can show architectural distortions of lymph nodes that are not enlarged by computed tomography scan. Only retroperitoneal lymph nodes adjacent to the iliac vessels, vena cava, and aorta can be imaged reliably. Lymphangiography is indicated before surgical staging to localize potentially involved lymph nodes for biopsy.

(G) Gallium 67 scanning is most useful for evaluation of diffuse histiocytic lymphoma in extraabdominal sites.

(H) Bone scan is indicated in the patient with bone pain.

(I) Bone marrow biopsy is frequently positive in patients with poorly differentiated lymphoma. The marrow is negative in 47 percent of all patients. It is less likely to be positive in men although the 5-year survival rate of men (35 percent) is lower than for women (55 percent).

(J) Stage I: Involvement of a single lymph node region (I) or a single extralymphatic organ or site (Ie); further subdivision into stage Ie with no serosal involvement (Ie$_1$) or with serosal involvement or perforation (Ie$_2$). Gastrointestinal lymphomas are transmural and frequently ulcerate. Bleeding and perforation can complicate large ulcerated lesions. The mass is over 10 cm in diameter in 6 percent of stage I patients.

(K) Stage II: Involvement of two or more lymph node groups on the same side of the diaphragm or with involvement of a contiguous extra lymphatic organ (IIe). Only 20 percent of patients present with stage I or II disease. Low-grade lymphomas are localized in less than 10 percent of cases. Intermediate-grade lymphomas are localized in approximately 35 percent of cases.

(L) Stage III: Involvement of lymph nodes on both sides of diaphragm. Stage IV: Multiple or disseminated foci of involvement of one or more extralymphatic organs or tissues with or without lymphatic involvement.

(M) Complete resection of stage Ie disease is advisable but such limited disease is uncommon.

(N) Five-year survival of stage I patients is 61 percent.

(O) Five-year survival of stage II patients is 47 percent.

(P) Five-year survival of stage III patients is 48 percent and that of stage IV patients is 36 percent. Limited surgical resection may be indicated for deep ulceration, bleeding, or perforation. Resections performed routinely to prevent complications or to enhance the effectiveness of chemotherapy or radiotherapy are controversial except in patients with low-grade lymphoma and limited extent of disease. Most patients receive combination chemotherapy.

REFERENCES

Brooks JJ, Entline HT. Primary gastric lymphomas: a clinicopathologic study of 58 cases with long-term follow-up and literature review. Cancer 1983; 51:701–711.

Fisher RI, Hubbard SM, DeVita VT, et al. Factors predicting long-term survival in diffuse mixed, histiocytic and undifferentiated lymphoma. Blood 1981; 58:45–51.

Fleming ID, Mitchell S, Dilawari RA. The role of surgery in the management of gastric lymphoma. Cancer 1982; 49:1135–1141.

Maor MH, Maddux B, Osborne B, et al. Stages IE and IIE non-Hodgkin's lymphomas of the stomach: comparison of treatment modalities. Cancer 1984; 54:2330–2337.

Mentzer SJ, Osteen RT, Pappas TN, et al. Surgical therapy of localized abdominal non-Hodgkin's lymphomas. Surgery 1988; 103:609–614.

Shepard FA, Evans WK, Kutas G, et al. Chemotherapy following surgery for Stages IE and IIE non-Hodgkin's lymphoma of the gastrointestinal tract. J Clin Oncol 1988; 6:253–260.

Taal BG, Jager DH, Burgers JMV, et al. Primary non-Hodgkin's lymphoma of the stomach: changing aspects and therapeutic choices. Eur J Cancer Clin Oncol 1989; 25:439–450.

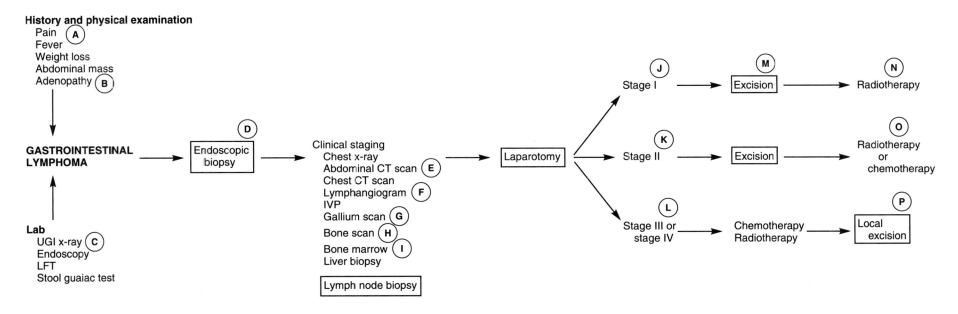

History and physical examination
Pain (A)
Fever
Weight loss
Abdominal mass
Adenopathy (B)

GASTROINTESTINAL LYMPHOMA

Lab
UGI x-ray (C)
Endoscopy
LFT
Stool guaiac test

Endoscopic biopsy (D)

Clinical staging
Chest x-ray
Abdominal CT scan (E)
Chest CT scan
Lymphangiogram (F)
IVP
Gallium scan (G)
Bone scan (H)
Bone marrow (I)
Liver biopsy

Lymph node biopsy

Laparotomy

Stage I (J) → Excision (M) → Radiotherapy (N)

Stage II (K) → Excision → Radiotherapy or chemotherapy (O)

Stage III or stage IV (L) → Chemotherapy Radiotherapy → Local excision (P)

Crohn's Disease of the Small Bowel

Victor W. Fazio, M.D., F.R.A.C.S.

(A) The cause of Crohn's disease is unknown. Neither medical nor surgical treatment is curative. The aim of management is to foster the patient's longevity and quality of life and not simply to deal with a present problem.

(B) An affected patient will present with one or several of the following: abdominal pain, diarrhea, fever, weight loss, fatigue, or anal pain.

(C) Upper and lower intestinal contrast x-rays as well as colonoscopy confirm that the disease process is limited to the small bowel.

(D) Acute ileitis can mimic an acute flareup of Crohn's disease. The bowel wall is spongy, edematous, and violaceous. The lumen is not narrowed and the cecum is normal. Should appendectomy be done, fistulization from the appendiceal stump or diseased ileum is rare, in contrast with appendectomy associated with Crohn's ileitis.

(E) Medical treatment of Crohn's disease aims to alleviate symptoms, to restore nutrition, and to provide emotional support. Steroids are required frequently. Azathioprine exerts a steroid-sparing effect but is used infrequently because of side effects. Failure of medical treatment is an indication for operative management.

(F) Bowel obstruction, internal fistula or abscess, and perianal disease are the most common indications for operation in patients with ileitis and ileocolitis. Anorectal and anovaginal fistulas are treated conservatively. If recurrent and symptomatic, advancement rectal flap repair is done where the rectum appears normal. Fistula cure then approximates 75 percent.

(G) Resection of diseased small bowel is favored over bypass procedures in almost all patients with intractable disease or obstruction. Recurrence rates are no higher if resection of normal-appearing bowel proximal to disease is limited to 2 to 4 inches. At 15 years, recurrence rates for ileocolitis and ileitis are 50 percent and 38 percent, respectively. Operative mortality rates are 2 to 4 percent compared with a 6 percent overall mortality rate for Crohn's disease.

(H) Vagotomy and gastrojejunostomy are used for failed medical treatment of gastroduodenal Crohn's disease. Revision rates approach 50 percent at 10 years.

(I) The decision to perform an anastomosis or to divert the intestine after resection is made on the basis of the patient's condition in regard to residual sepsis, malnutrition, and other factors that favor dehiscence. Preoperative total parenteral nutrition in the debilitated patient decreases the risk of primary anastomotic dehiscence.

(J) Strictureplasty is used after resection of distal ileal disease to treat rates of proximal obstructing skip lesions (20 percent of patients). Post-strictureplasty of abdominal sepsis (7 percent), re-stricture (2 percent), and new stricture (9 percent) at 5 years compare favorably with resection and with the added gain of intestinal preservation. Exclusion bypass (end of ileum to side of transverse colon) can be used for ileocecal Crohn's disease in the few instances in which resection is deemed hazardous (20 percent of patients). The bypassed segment is resected at a second stage.

REFERENCES

Farmer RG, Hawk WA, Turnbull RB Jr. Clinical patterns in Crohn's diseases: a statistical study of 614 cases. Gastroenterology 1975; 69:627–635.

Farmer RG, Whelan G, Fazio VW. Long-term follow-up of patients with Crohn's disease: relationship between the clinic pattern and prognosis. Gastroenterology 1985; 88:1818–1825.

Fazio VW. Regional enteritis (Crohn's disease): indications for surgery and operative strategy. Surg Clin North Am 1983; 63:27–48.

Fazio VW, Galandiuk S, Jagelman DG, Lavery IC. Strictureplasty in Crohn's disease. Ann Surg 1989; 210:621–625.

Goligher JC. Crohn's disease (granulomatous enteritis). In: Goligher JC, ed. Surgery of the anus, rectum and colon. 4th ed. London: Balliere-Tindall, 1980.

Hellers G. Crohn's disease in Stockholm County 1955–1974: a study of epidemiology results of surgical treatment and long-term prognosis. Acta Chir Scand (Suppl)1979; 490.

Higgens CW, Allan RN. Crohn's disease of the distal ileum. Gut 1980; 21:933–940.

Jones IT, Fazio VW, Jagelman DG. The use of transanal rectal advancement flaps in the management of fistulas involving the anorectum. Dis Colon Rectum 1987; 30:919–923.

Lock MR, Fazio VW, Farmer RG, et al. Recurrence and reoperation for Crohn's disease. N Engl J Med 1981; 304:1586–1588.

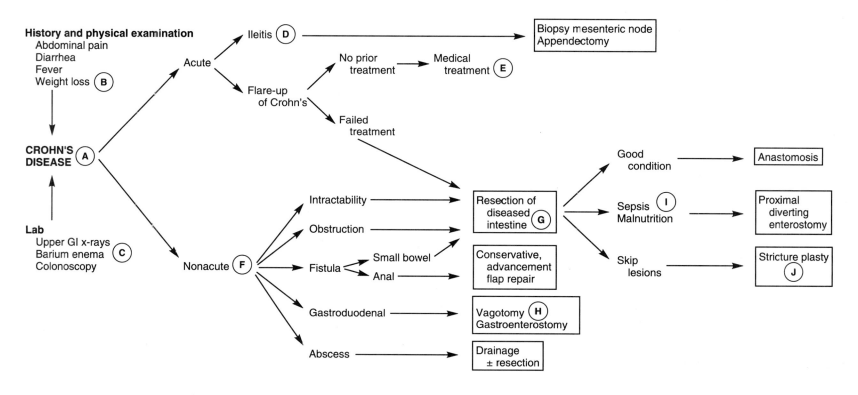

Acute Right Lower Quadrant Pain

Richard G. Fiddian-Green, B.M., B.Ch., F.R.C.S.

(A) In most cases of acute right lower quadrant pain, the diagnosis may be confidently made from the history alone. Especially important in the history are the character of the pain, especially its relationship to coughing and movements, the duration of the symptoms, previous history, loss of appetite, and other organ-specific symptoms. Physical examination confirms the diagnosis in most cases and is especially important in determining whether or not peritonitis is present. Reexamination after tensing the abdominal musculature can determine whether the source of the problem is intraabdominal or extraabdominal.

(B) Resuscitation should aim to eliminate all occult evidence of compensated shock in addition to eliminating all evidence of overt hypotensive shock. Costs may be greatly reduced by avoiding diagnostic tests that do not alter management and by avoiding admission of patients who do not require operative intervention.

(C) In those patients in whom the working diagnosis is uncertain, the diagnosis can usually be made by repeating the history and physical examination 1 or 2 hours later and considering the results of diagnostic tests. Repeated examinations are of greatest value if performed by the same clinician. Examples of conditions that can cause right lower quadrant pain but do not require immediate laparotomy are acute pancreatitis, diverticulitis, acute ileitis, Crohn disease, psoas abscess, omental torsion, intussusception, mesenteric adenitis, liver abscess, carcinoma of the cecum, and tropical diseases such as amebiasis, ascariasis, and typhoid fever. A Spigelian hernia is an uncommon cause of acute right lower quadrant pain. Examination while the abdomen is tensed is of value in making this diagnosis but exploration is usually required to confirm it.

(D) Preoperative tests include electrolytes, electrocardiogram, and chest x-ray. Blood may also be taken for type and cross-match.

(E) Some conditions can cause right lower quadrant pain but are recognized readily as nonsurgical problems. They include musculoskeletal disease, rectus hematoma, salpingitis, epididymitis, ureteral stone, ruptured ovarian cyst, bleeding graafian follicle, gastroenteritis, and giardiasis.

(F) Patients with the diagnosis of leaking aneurysm should be admitted directly to the operating room.

(G) The diagnosis of an acute mesenteric occlusion is based on history alone. Delay in obtaining angiographic studies increases the likelihood of gut infarction. Angiographic studies, however, may neither establish nor exclude the diagnosis. These patients are best admitted directly to the operating room. Embolectomy or resection may be necessary.

(H) An effort should be made to resolve the problem without sacrificing the fallopian tube.

(I) Antibiotics should be administered preoperatively to patients with a diagnosis of peritonitis. The wound is best left open after drainage of an intraabdominal abscess.

REFERENCES

Bailey H. Demonstrations of physical signs of clinical surgery. Bristol: John Write & Sons, Ltd., 1960.

Fiddian-Green RG. Should measurements of tissue pH and PO_2 be included in the routine monitoring of ICU patients? Crit Care Med 1991; 19(2):141–143.

Silen W (ed). Cope's early diagnosis of the acute abdominal abdomen. 16th ed. New York: Oxford University Press, 1983.

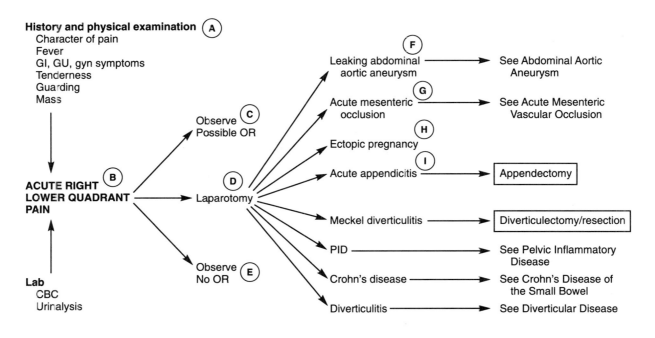

History and physical examination (A)
  Character of pain
  Fever
  GI, GU, gyn symptoms
  Tenderness
  Guarding
  Mass

ACUTE RIGHT (B)
LOWER QUADRANT
PAIN

Lab
  CBC
  Urinalysis

Observe (C)
Possible OR

Laparotomy (D)

Observe (E)
No OR

Leaking abdominal (F)
aortic aneurysm → See Abdominal Aortic
                     Aneurysm

Acute mesenteric (G)
occlusion → See Acute Mesenteric
              Vascular Occlusion

Ectopic pregnancy (H)

Acute appendicitis (I) → Appendectomy

Meckel diverticulitis → Diverticulectomy/resection

PID → See Pelvic Inflammatory
        Disease

Crohn's disease → See Crohn's Disease of
                    the Small Bowel

Diverticulitis → See Diverticular Disease

Volvulus

Hugo V. Villar, M.D.

(A) Volvulus, a folding of bowel upon itself, causes 1 percent of all bowel obstructions and 10 percent of colonic obstructions. Sigmoid volvulus is most common (80 percent), followed by cecal volvulus (15 percent).

(B) Volvulus of either small or large intestine causes abdominal pain, constipation, distention, and vomiting in most patients. Sigmoid volvulus often affects older men with a history of chronic brain syndrome and chronic constipation.

(C) Abdominal x-rays differentiate types of volvulus in most instances. A dilated loop of colon in the right upper quadrant with an "omega" or "inner tube" configuration suggests sigmoid volvulus. A dilated loop of colon with central density in the left upper quadrant is a clue to cecal volvulus. Pseudo-obstruction of the right colon (Ogilvie's syndrome) and acute gastric dilation can be mistaken for volvulus radiographically. The combination of plain abdominal films ($120) and barium enema ($200) should make the differential diagnosis in almost 100 percent of the cases.

(D) Barium enema is necessary only if the diagnosis of cecal volvulus is questionable.

(E) Operation for small bowel obstruction caused by volvulus is begun when the patient is rehydrated and vital organ function is satisfactory. Resection of bowel with end-to-end anastomosis is required more often than simple lysis of adhesions.

(F) Placing the patient in a jackknife position for proctoscopy can untwist the colon spontaneously. Proctoscopy provides more adequate decompression than colonoscopy. Proctosigmoidoscopy should provide satisfactory decompression of sigmoid volvulus in about 90 percent of patients. Risk of perforation is less than 1 percent. Decompression by the flexible colonoscope has a higher risk of perforation.

(G) After decompression, elective resection of the sigmoid is recommended for good-risk patients. The risk of recurrent volvulus is 50 to 90 percent.

(H) If proctoscopy fails to decompress the sigmoid or if peritoneal signs appear, the patient should be operated on urgently. Depending upon the degree of risk, either end sigmoid colostomy with a Hartmann pouch or sigmoid resection with primary anastomosis should be performed.

(I) In older patients, detorsion, cecopexy, and cecostomy should be performed. Resection is necessary in the presence of cecal necrosis.

(J) Cecal volvulus occurs because of incomplete fusion of the cecum and ascending colon to the posterior peritoneum. This allows clockwise rotation. If the ileocecal valve is competent, a closed loop obstruction occurs. A second danger is perforation when the transverse diameter of the cecum exceeds 9 cm. In young, healthy individuals, right colectomy should be done to prevent recurrence. The mortality rate of a right colectomy is less than 2 percent and the complication rate is about 5 percent. The average hospital stay is 8 to 10 days because of the usually prolonged preoperative period. The total hospital bill including physician's charges is about $20,000.

(K) Patients with sigmoid volvulus often have complications, and the mortality rate for the first episode is about 30 percent because of associated pulmonary, cardiovascular, or renal disease. If a patient requires emergency operation, the average hospital stay is about 10 to 15 days. The surgical fee for colon resection is $1,625. The anesthesia fee is $860. Hospital fees including hospital stay and operating room charges total $25,000.

REFERENCES

Di Felice G. Sigmoid volvulus treated by colonoscopy. Gastrointest Endosc 1986; 32:244–245.

Friedman JD, Odland MD, Burbrick MP. Experience with colonic volvulus. Dis Colon Rectum 1989; 32:409–416.

Gibney EJ. Sigmoid volvulus in rural Ghana. Br J Surg 1989; 75:737.

Jones IT, Fazio VW. Clonic volvulus: etiology and management. Dig Dis 1989; 7:203–209.

Kukura JS, Dent TL. Colonoscopic decompression of massive nonobstructive cecal dilation. Arch Surg 1977; 112:512–517.

Lowman RM, David L. An evaluation of cecal size in impending perforation of the cecum. Surg Gynecol Obstet 1956; 103:711–718.

Mangiante ED, Croce MA, Fabian TC, et al. Sigmoid volvulus: a four-decade experience. Am Surg 1989; 55:41–44.

Mashiah A, Mashiah T. Surgical treatment of recurrent sigmoid volvulus under local anesthesia. J Am Gastroenterol Soc 1988; 36:648–649.

History and physical examination

Pain
Obstipation
Chronic brain syndrome
Chronic constipation
Dehydration
Distention

Lab

Abdominal x-rays
Barium enema

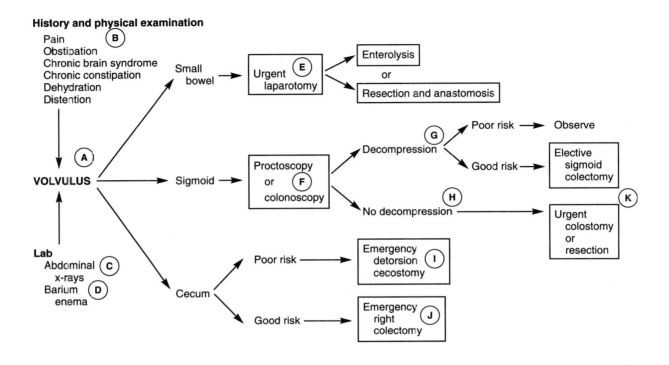

Diverticular Disease

Gilbert Hermann, M.D., and Charles Abernathy, M.D.

(A) Colonic diverticula are common in the elderly (30 percent by age 60). Diverticulitis with perforation can occur from the third decade on. Perforation of cecal diverticula is seen with increasing frequency, particularly in younger patients. Two thirds of patients with demonstrated diverticula remain asymptomatic.

(B) Barium enema demonstrates diverticula in virtually every patient with the disease. It can localize the site of inflammation in some patients and occasionally show perforation, obstruction, and fistula. Endoscopy is less helpful except in the appraisal of colonic obstruction and, sometimes, bleeding.

(C) Computed tomography scanning can detect pericolic abscess resulting from perforation of an inflamed diverticulum. In a patient with acute left lower quadrant abdominal pain and tenderness, computed tomography scanning with colonic contrast can establish simultaneously the diagnosis of diverticula and abscess. Ultrasonography can detect a diverticular abscess but with less accuracy.

(D) Obstruction of the left colon or sigmoid colon due to perforation of a diverticulum is sometimes difficult to differentiate from carcinoma. Mucosal biopsy cannot be relied on to rule out carcinoma.

(E) Bleeding complicates diverticular disease in as many as 25 percent of patients. Ninety percent of these patients stop bleeding spontaneously.

(F) An inflamed diverticulum tends to perforate into mesenteric fat, creating a contained abscess. Free perforation into the intraperitoneal space is unusual. It occurs more often in immunocompromised patients. A mesenteric abscess can perforate secondarily into the peritoneum, causing localized or generalized peritonitis. The severity of acute diverticulitis is graded on the basis of such possibilities.

(G) Intermittent, mild to moderate pain and tenderness in the left lower quadrant of the abdomen is often attributed to diverticular disease. The cause of transient pain presumably is inflammation of an obstructed diverticulum. A high-fiber diet that reduces colonic intraluminal pressure is effective in reducing the frequency and severity of symptoms in many patients.

(H) A fistula may involve the bladder, presenting as pneumaturia, or the small bowel. A fistula to the skin is rare. A diverting colostomy is usually the first step in treatment, but with a satisfactory bowel preparation, primary repair often can be done in one stage.

(I) Free air in the peritoneum and generalized peritonitis in a patient suspected to have a perforated diverticulum are indications for immediate operation. A pericolic abscess requires operative excision if the patient is septic. Percutaneous catheter drainage of a diverticular abscess can be used only in a stable nonseptic patient. It has a low rate of success and usually delays operative treatment.

(J) A one-stage rather than a two-stage operative repair of a fistula is possible when primary anastomosis of colon is safe. This implies an absence of pus or significant inflammation at the site of the fistula.

(K) Resection of involved colon and pericolic abscess followed by primary anastomosis is accomplished by some surgeons with acceptable morbidity and mortality. The procedure is reserved for better risk patients who have minimal peritoneal contamination.

(L) The safest means to manage a perforated diverticulum and pericolic abscess in an acutely ill patient is resection of involved colon and the abscess, diverting colostomy, and closure of the end of the distal colon as a Hartmann pouch. This procedure requires later closure of the colostomy by colocolostomy to restore continuity of the lower gastrointestinal tract. Nevertheless, it is associated with the lowest rates of morbidity and mortality and is advised for most patients.

(M) Closure of the colostomy by colocolostomy is undertaken about 3 months after the initial operation. Ideally, all evidence of inflammation should be gone. Inflammation or pus can remain at the site of colectomy for several months and the timing of colostomy closure is difficult to judge. Colostomy closure for any reason is reported to cause complications in 20 to 30 percent and death in 1 percent of patients.

(N) Colectomy for diverticular disease presenting only as pain is performed rarely. The length of colon to be removed becomes an issue, unlike colectomy for either abscess or bleeding, where only the involved bowel is removed.

REFERENCES

Kourtesis GH, Williams RA, Wilson SE. Surgical options in acute diverticulitis: value of sigmoid resection in dealing with the septic focus. Aust NZ J Surg 1988; 58:955–958.

Krukowski ZH, Koruth NM, Matheson NA. Evolving practice in acute diverticulitis. Br J Surg 1985; 72:684–686.

Larson DM, Masters SS, Spiro HM. Medical and surgical therapy in diverticular disease: a comparative study. Gastroenterology 1976; 71:734–737.

Painter NS, Burkitt DP. Diverticular disease of the colon: a deficiency disease of Western civilization. Br Med J 1971; 2:450–454.

Schmit PJ, Bennion RS, Thompson JE Jr. Cecal diverticulitis: a continuing diagnostic dilemma. World J Surg 1991; 15:367–371.

Tyau ES, Prystowsky JB, Joehl RJ, et al. Acute diverticulitis: complicated problem in the immunocompromised patient. Arch Surg 1991; 126:855–859.

Wise L. Surgical management of ruptured diverticulitis. Am J Surg 1981; 14:122–127.

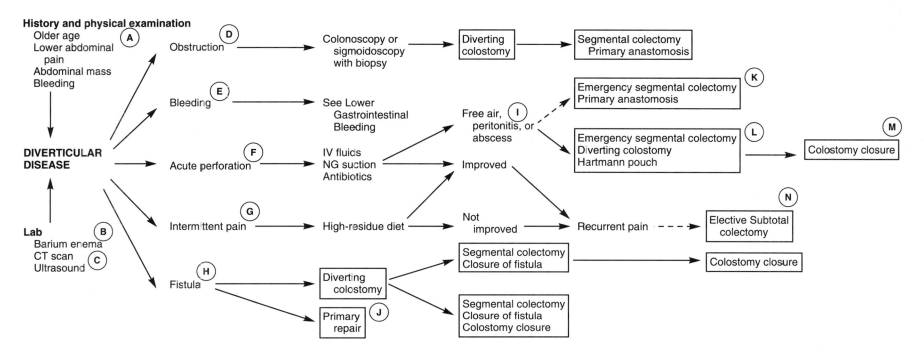

History and physical examination
  Older age (A)
  Lower abdominal
    pain
  Abdominal mass
  Bleeding

**DIVERTICULAR
DISEASE**

Lab (B)
  Barium enema
  CT scan (C)
  Ultrasound

(D) Obstruction → Colonoscopy or sigmoidoscopy with biopsy → Diverting colostomy → Segmental colectomy Primary anastomosis

(E) Bleeding → See Lower Gastrointestinal Bleeding

(F) Acute perforation → IV fluids NG suction Antibiotics → Free air, (I) peritonitis, or abscess → Emergency segmental colectomy Primary anastomosis (K)

→ Emergency segmental colectomy Diverting colostomy Hartmann pouch (L) → Colostomy closure (M)

IV fluids NG suction Antibiotics → Improved

(G) Intermittent pain → High-residue diet → Not improved → Recurrent pain ⇢ Elective Subtotal colectomy (N)

(H) Fistula → Diverting colostomy → Segmental colectomy Closure of fistula → Colostomy closure

Fistula → Primary repair (J) → Segmental colectomy Closure of fistula Colostomy closure

Lower Gastrointestinal Bleeding

Robert W. Beart, Jr., M.D.

(A) Bleeding from the rectum can result from any gastrointestinal source. The most frequent colonic causes are diverticular disease, angiodysplasia, and ischemic colitis. Coagulation disorders, local trauma, and irradiation colitis are increasingly common causes.

(B) Ninety percent of gastrointestinal bleeding proximal to the ligament of Treitz can be detected by nasogastric aspiration. If blood is recovered, gastroscopy usually identifies the source unless it is in the distal duodenum.

(C) Bright red blood passed on the surface of stools or dripping from the anus is due to anorectal disease (hemorrhoids or fissure) or distal rectal lesions such as carcinoma. Anoscopy and sigmoidoscopy are useful to exclude these problems.

(D) Persistent colonic hemorrhage is evaluated by radionuclide scanning using radiolabeled red blood cells. This test will identify at least 80 percent of patients bleeding more rapidly than 0.5 mL/min. If the scan is positive within 10 minutes, it usually suggests the site of bleeding. If the scan is negative, bleeding has ceased or the rate is very low. Further evaluation by colonoscopy should be done.

(E) If the red blood cell radionuclide scan is positive, selective angiography of the superior and inferior mesenteric arteries is performed. Extravasation of contrast medium into the lumen of the colon localizes the site of bleeding in 60 to 80 percent of patients. Vasopressin (0.2 U/min) may control bleeding if infused selectively. Bleeding stops with infusion in about 50 percent of patients. These patients can be observed with the expectation that 50 to 70 percent will rebleed or undergo elective resection.

(F) Colonoscopy is useful in patients who are not bleeding profusely. It is used to search for a source of hemorrhage in patients not requiring emergency operation. Success varies from 30 to 80 percent. If the lesion that clearly caused the bleeding is identified, segmental colectomy is performed.

(G) Lower gastrointestinal hemorrhage from an unknown site that requires transfusion of more than 3000 mL of whole blood within 24 hours must be treated by emergency operation. If no bleeding site is identified at surgery, total abdominal colectomy is performed.

REFERENCES

Baum S. Angiography and the gastrointestinal bleeder. Radiology 1981; 143:469–472.

Flickinger FW. Location of active lower GI bleeding by technetium-99m sulfur colloid scan. J Nucl Med 1981; 22:38–39.

Foster JH, Dunphy JE. Massive gastrointestinal hemorrhage. In: Hary JD, ed. Critical surgical illness. Philadelphia: WB Saunders, 1980:290–329.

Jensen DM, Machiacado GA, Tapia JI. Emergent colonoscopy in patients with severe hematochezia. Gastrointest Endosc 1983; 29:177.

McGuire HH, Hanes BW. Massive hemorrage from diverticulosis of the colon: guidelines for therapy based on bleeding patterns observed in fifty cases. Ann Surg 1972; 175:847–855.

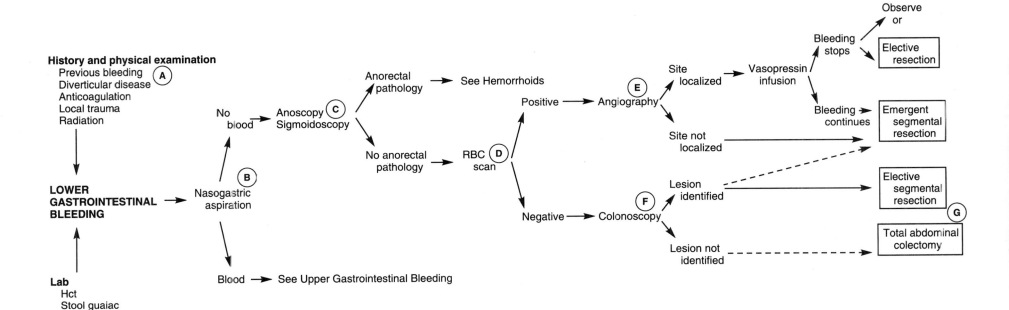

History and physical examination
  Previous bleeding (A)
  Diverticular disease
  Anticoagulation
  Local trauma
  Radiation

LOWER GASTROINTESTINAL BLEEDING

Lab
  Hct
  Stool guaiac

Ulcerative Colitis

Robert W. Beart, Jr., M.D.

(A) Ulcerative colitis usually presents with diarrhea, abdominal pain, and fever. Arthritis, uveitis, pyoderma, and hepatitis can be additional systemic manifestations.

(B) Sigmoidoscopy is the first step in diagnosis. The rectal mucosa appears edematous and friable. An abdominal x-ray shows colonic dilation (toxic megacolon) in 3 to 5 percent with negative stool cultures. It usually shows continuous involvement of the colon beginning at the anus.

(C) Massive hemorrhage is a rare complication of acute ulcerative colitis. If transfusion of more than 3000 mL of whole blood is required within 24 hours, emergency proctocolectomy is necessary. The rectum should be carefully examined preoperatively and removed only if necessary to control bleeding.

(D) Perforation of the colon occurs in only 3 percent of patients but causes more deaths than any other complication. The site of perforation is most often in the sigmoid colon or splenic flexure. Perforation occurs usually in patients with toxic megacolon.

(E) Symptoms of toxicity are treated by nasogastric suction, intravenous corticosteroids, antibiotics, and total parenteral nutrition. Potassium and blood transfusion are often needed. If toxic colitis, with or without megacolon, does not improve within 48 hours, emergency abdominal colectomy, with either a Hartmann pouch or mucous fistula, and Brooke ileostomy are performed. Emergency colectomy has a 3 to 6 percent mortality rate if performed within 5 days of admission.

(F) Chronic ulcerative colitis can be intermittent or persistent. When medical therapy such as steroids and nutritional support fails to bring improvement within 6 months, the entire colon is removed. Signs of medical intractability are uncontrolled diarrhea, chronic debilitation, arrested development in children, and fibrosis with stricture.

(G) Extracolonic disease rarely is an indication for colectomy. Ankylosing spondylitis and liver disease do not consistently respond to resection.

(H) The Turnbull blowhole procedure, which consists of one or more colostomies and a diverting loop ileostomy, is rarely necessary but is acceptable treatment when colonic perforation has caused an intraabdominal abscess. When the patient has recovered, elective proctocolectomy is considered.

(I) Patients followed more than 7 years should undergo annual colonoscopy and multiple biopsies to search for epithelial dysplasia. Severe dysplasia on several biopsies is associated with cancer of the colon in half the patients. Patients with severe or moderate dysplasia require colectomy, but mild dysplasia is followed by close surveillance.

(J) The usual elective operation for medically intractable ulcerative colitis is total proctocolectomy. Brooke ileostomy, continent ileostomy, ileorectal anastomosis, or an ileoanal anastomosis after mucosal proctectomy is then performed. Some patients benefit from nutritional repletion before elective operation to help maintain the operative mortality under 3 percent.

REFERENCES

Beart RW Jr, McIlrath DC, Kelly KA, et al. Surgical management of inflammatory bowel disease. Curr Prob Surg 1980; 17:533–584.

Caprilli R, Vernia P, Colaneri O, et al. Risk factors in toxic megacolon. Dig Dis Sci 1980; 25:817–822.

Dozois RR, Goldberg SM, Rothenberger DA, et al. Restorative proctocolectomy with ileal reservoir. Int J Colorec Dis 1986; 1:2–9.

Farmer RG. Clinical features and natural history of inflammatory bowel disease. Med Clin North Am 1980; 64:1103–1115.

Kewenter J, Ahlman H, Hulten L. Cancer risk in extensive ulcerative colitis. Ann Surg 1978; 188:824–828.

Nicholls RJ, Pescatori M, Motson RW, et al. Restorative proctocolectomy with a 3-loop ileal reservoir for ulcerative colitis and familial adenomatous polyposis. Ann Surg 1984; 199:383–388.

Nugent FW, Veidenheimer MC, Zuberi S, et al. Clinical case of ulcerative proctosigmoiditis. Am J Dig Dis 1970; 15:321–326.

Park R, Levy E, Frileus P, et al. Current results: ileorectal anastomosis after total abdominal colectomy for ulcerative colitis. In: Dozois RR, ed. Alternative to conventional ileostomy. Chicago: Year Book Medical Publishers, 1985:81–99.

Singleton JW. Medical therapy of inflammatory bowel disease. Med Clin North Am 1980; 64:1117–1133.

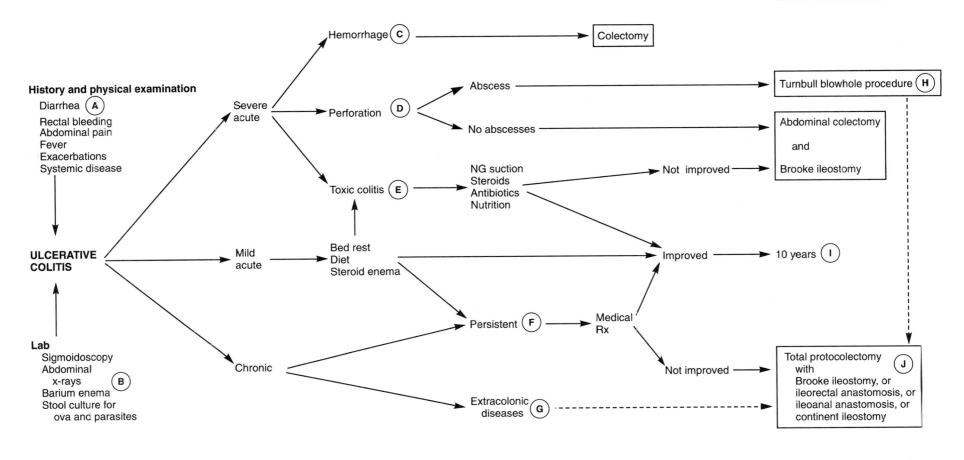

History and physical examination

Diarrhea (A)

Rectal bleeding
Abdominal pain
Fever
Exacerbations
Systemic disease

ULCERATIVE COLITIS

Lab

Sigmoidoscopy
Abdominal
  x-rays   (B)
Barium enema
Stool culture for
  ova and parasites

Severe acute

Mild acute

Chronic

Hemorrhage (C) → Colectomy

Perforation (D)

Abscess → Turnbull blowhole procedure (H)

No abscesses → Abdominal colectomy and Brooke ileostomy

Toxic colitis (E)

NG suction
Steroids
Antibiotics
Nutrition

Not improved

Improved

Bed rest
Diet
Steroid enema

Persistent (F) → Medical Rx

Improved → 10 years (I)

Not improved

Extracolonic diseases (G)

Total protocolectomy with
  Brooke ileostomy, or
  ileorectal anastomosis, or
  ileoanal anastomosis, or
  continent ileostomy (J)

Carcinoma of the Colon

Michael J. Edwards, M.D., and Hiram C. Polk, Jr., M.D.

A The annual incidence of colon carcinoma is greater than 110,000. The average age at presentation is 60 to 65 years. Change in bowel function, the presence of blood in the rectum, and anemia in patients over 40 years old are signs of colon cancer and demand prompt evaluation

B Care for all patients over age 40 should include routine screening for colorectal carcinoma by digital rectal examination and testing for occult blood in the stool. Barium enema, colonoscopy, and tests for fecal occult blood are also important tools for evaluating symptomatic patients and screening high-risk patients with either ulcerative colitis, familial polyposis syndromes, a previous history of colorectal cancer, or a family history of colon or female genital cancer.

C Although carcinoembryonic antigen assay is of limited value in screening for the colorectal carcinoma, it is useful for the detection of recurrent or persistent cancer. A preoperative baseline level is necessary.

D Accurate staging of the extent of the primary lesion and the presence of distant metastasis is imperative for appropriate treatment. Signs and symptoms delineated in a careful history and physical examination may suggest the presence of metastases. The possibility is evaluated by x-ray studies and liver function tests, particularly alkaline phosphatase. The routine use of magnetic resonance imaging, ultrasonography, technetium, and computed tomography scanning is costly and usually not helpful. It subjects patients to possible complications that result from efforts to resolve false-positive findings. This approach is prohibitively expensive at a time when all health care costs are under scrutiny.

Carcinomas of the colon or rectum arising within the pelvis commonly impinge on or invade the adjacent urinary tract. Urinalysis, intravenous py-elography, computed tomography with intravenous contrast, and cystoscopy are valuable tools for staging advanced disease and for planning extended resections.

E Two thirds of patients over age 65 have significant, frequently occult, cardiopulmonary or other systemic illnesses. Preoperative chest radiography and electrocardiography are mandatory. Invasive preoperative monitoring may be required.

F The risk of wound infection (7 to 10 percent) is minimized by mechanical bowel preparation (clear liquid diet and oral cathartics) and safe systemic prophylactic antibiotics of documented efficacy. Some surgeons continue to use preoperative intraluminal antibiotics in addition to the above.

G Perforated cancers have a poor prognosis. The hospital mortality rate is as high as 70 percent. For patients who are unsuitable for primary resection, an end-colostomy, proximal total colonic diversion and drainage, usually avoiding cecostomy, is appropriate. Approximately 30 percent of patients who sustain perforation and undergo resection are long-term survivors.

H Twenty percent of patients have obstruction. Half of them require an emergency operation. Their poor prognosis is due to the innate mortality of intestinal obstruction. Primary resection with end-colostomy is possible in patients of appropriate operative risk. Many patients, however, require relief of obstruction by proximal colostomy followed by resection of the tumor in 10 to 14 days. Primary anastomosis is unjustified (mortality rate, 15 percent). The mortality rate of cecostomy is significantly greater than that of proximal diverting colostomy. Five-year survival for all patients who have obstructive cancers is 25 percent.

I Adjacent contiguous structures involved by cancer should be resected in continuity with the colon. Survival rates after extended extirpation approach those of the colon cancer population as a whole.

J A colonic or paracolonic mass found at laparotomy may be adenocarcinoma, perforative appendicitis, diverticulitis, endometriosis, or tuberculosis. If the diagnosis is questionable, an appropriate cancer operation should be performed.

K Resection and primary anastomosis can be justified for uncontrolled bleeding because intestinal blood acts as a cathartic, accomplishing a mechanical bowel preparation.

L Colorectal cancer metastasizes to the lung in 15 percent of patients. Only 2 percent have solitary metastases. Resection of a solitary lung metastasis carries an operative mortality rate of 2 to 4 percent, a morbidity of 10 to 15 percent, and a 5-year survival rate of 20 percent.

M Patients with hepatic metastases can be cured by resection. Those who should undergo hepatic resection are patients with (1) less than four hepatic metastases localized to one hepatic lobe, (2) tumor-free bowel margins with resection, (3) no evidence of extrahepatic disease, (4) resectable primary colorectal carcinomas, and (5) an appropriate operative risk. Isolated lesions of the left lateral segment may be resected synchronously at the time of primary colorectal resection. Major hepatic lobar resections should be done as a second operation. Selected patients treated by hepatic resection have survival rates of 20 percent at 5 years, and after 5 years have the same risk of death as an age-matched population without cancer.

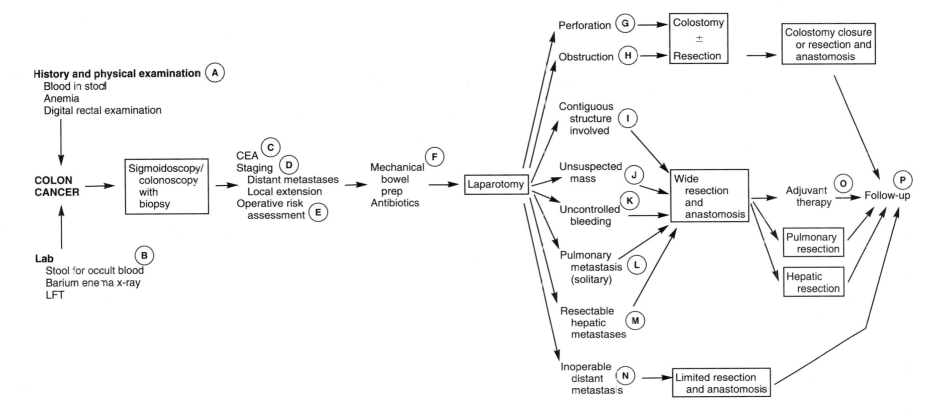

N Patients found to have unresectable metastatic disease at laparotomy should usually undergo resection of the primary lesion for local disease control. Resection of the primary carcinoma prevents obstruction, pain, and bleeding caused by the unimpeded growth of the primary lesion.

O Surgical resection alone results in the cure of nearly half of patients. In the absence of distant metastases, prognosis is determined by the depth of penetration of the carcinoma through the intestinal wall and by the presence of regional lymph node metastases. These two factors are the basis for all current staging systems and delineate subgroups of patients likely to benefit by improved local disease control, adjuvant radiation therapy, or systemic chemotherapy. Patients with rectal wall penetration have increased local disease control with adjuvant postoperative radiotherapy. Patients

with metastatic carcinoma in regional lymph nodes have improved survival with adjuvant systemic levamisole and 5-fluorouracil.

P Evaluation for recurrent disease is important since a few patients can be cured by surgical resection of recurrent disease. Cancer recurs in approximately 40 percent of patients who undergo resection for cure; half are diagnosed within the first 18 months. Curative reexcision of locally recurrent disease is less likely to cure but can result in significant palliation. Radiation therapy for locally extensive disease can also be useful. Chemotherapy is less effective for locally recurrent disease but can be helpful for patients with symptomatic distant metastases. Metachronous cancers occur at a 3 to 5 percent per year rate with a peak incidence at 8.5 years after the initial diagnosis.

REFERENCES

Adson MA, Van Heerden JR, Adson MH, et al. Resection of hepatic metastases from colorectal cancer. Arch Surg 1984; 119:647–651.

Bland KI, Polk HC, Jr. Therapeutic measures applied for the curative and palliative control of colorectal carcinoma. In: Nyhus LM, ed. Surgery annual. New York: Appleton-Century-Crofts, 1983; 123–161.

Goligher JC, Smiddy FG. The treatment of acute obstruction or perforation with carcinoma of the colon and rectum. Br J Surg 1957; 45:270–274.

Polk HC Jr. Extended resection for selected adenocarcinomas of the large bowel. Ann Surg 1972; 175:892–899.

Steele GD Jr, et al. Adjuvant therapy for patients with colon and rectal cancer. JAMA 1990; 264:1444–1450.

Wilkins EW, Head JM, Burke JF. Pulmonary resection for metastatic neoplasm in the lung: experience at the Massachusetts General Hospital. Am J Surg 1978; 135:480–483.

Carcinoma of the Rectum or Anus

J. Milburn Jessup, M.D., and Glenn Steele, Jr., M.D.

(A) History and physical examination yield the diagnosis of rectal or anal carcinoma in over 80 percent of patients. Pain is frequent in anal carcinoma and absent in rectal carcinoma unless the patient has an advanced lesion with tenesmus or perineural involvement causing back pain.

(B) Digital examination of the rectum is important to evaluate the mobility and size of the lesion and to palpate for pararectal nodes. Inguinal regions must also be examined for possible nodal metastases. If inguinal nodes are enlarged, a biopsy (possibly fine-needle aspiration) is done.

(C) Hematest stool examination for occult blood is a cost-effective means of detecting colorectal neoplasms. Cancers detected by occult blood testing usually have a more favorable prognosis than those detected because of symptoms.

(D) Five percent of patients with biopsy-proven carcinoma develop synchronous or metachronous cancer and 30 percent have polyps. Examination of the entire colorectum is mandatory. Barium enema ($48) is cost-effective but has a 5 to 10 percent false-negative rate.

(E) Endorectal ultrasound ($408) accurately identifies the extent of penetration of cancer into the rectal wall in 85 to 93 percent of patients. It does not give information about the status of pararectal lymph nodes. Combined with physical examination by the surgeon, it determines the feasibility of local excision and sphincter preservation.

(F) Computed tomography scan of the pelvis ($1000) is useful because it detects lymph node metastases greater than 1.5 cm. It can define the extent of extramural spread of T3 rectal cancer.

(G) Preoperative serum carcinoembryonic antigen ($38) is an important prognosticator be-cause a level of 5 mg/mL or greater is associated with the subsequent appearance of distant metastasis in 46 to 85 percent of patients. An elevated carcinoembryonic antigen should prompt a thorough evaluation of the liver and lungs, the most common sites of metastasis from rectal carcinoma.

(H) Colonoscopy ($575) has the advantage of permitting a tissue diagnosis. Rigid proctosigmoidoscopy ($50) or flexible sigmoidoscopy ($150) must be done by the surgeon to evaluate resectability of carcinoma or villous adenoma. Biopsy of anal and rectal cancer is the pivotal point in the diagnosis and treatment. Small in situ or noninvasive lesions can be safely excised locally (with negative margins) and given no further therapy. Invasive squamous carcinomas can be cured by chemoradiotherapy and may not need to be excised afterward. Adenocarcinoma of the rectum arises above the dentate line where a biopsy does not cause pain. Regional or general anesthesia is needed for excision, however, because submucosal or deeper dissection is painful.

(I) Carcinoma of the anus that is less than two thirds of the circumference of the anus or invades the anal canal should receive chemoradiotherapy by the Nigro regimen. Patients whose anal carcinoma occupies more than two thirds of the circumference, who are incontinent, or who fail chemoradiotherapy should undergo abdominoperineal resection (APR). Patients with enlarged metastatic inguinal nodes (15 percent) can be palliated by inguinal node dissection but should still receive chemoradiotherapy.

(J) Superficial adenocarcinomas (T1 and T2 lesions that involve but do not penetrate through the muscularis propria) may be locally excised if they are within 10 cm of the dentate line, mobile, and less than 3 cm in diameter. Local excision can be performed transanally or through a trans-sacral approach. Lesions that are greater than 4 cm in diameter and within 5 cm of the anal verge may require APR. Lesions 4 cm in diameter and more than 5 cm from the anal verge usually are removed by anterior resection without permanent colostomy. T1 lesions locally excised with negative margins need no other therapy. The risk of recurrence in T2 lesions (21 percent) warrants the addition of chemotherapy and radiotherapy after surgery. Lesions of between 3 cm and 4 cm in diameter are amenable to local excision depending upon site (e.g., proximity to sphincters).

(K) A deeply penetrating rectal adenocarcinoma (T3 lesion that invades the full thickness of the rectal wall) can be locally excised provided that (1) the margins of resection are free of tumor, (2) the degree of wall invasion is minimal, (3) the lesion is 3 cm or less in diameter, and (4) the patient receives chemotherapy and radiotherapy postoperatively. APR is done for lesions less than 5 cm from the anal verge; anterior resection is reserved for lesions more than 5 cm from the anal verge. All patients should receive adjuvant chemotherapy and radiotherapy, especially if lymph nodes metastases are present. Local recurrence of T3N0 or T3N1 rectal cancer is approximately 25 percent after radical surgery alone and 12 percent after radical surgery and adjuvant chemoradiotherapy. Unfortunately, 20 to 40 percent will develop systemic disease.

(L) Cancer that is fixed to the pelvis, invades pelvic organs, or is more than 5 cm in diameter may benefit from preoperative radiotherapy (with or without chemotherapy) to improve resectability. Patients can then undergo anterior resection or APR. Approximately 60 percent of fixed rectal cancers can be resected after radiotherapy.

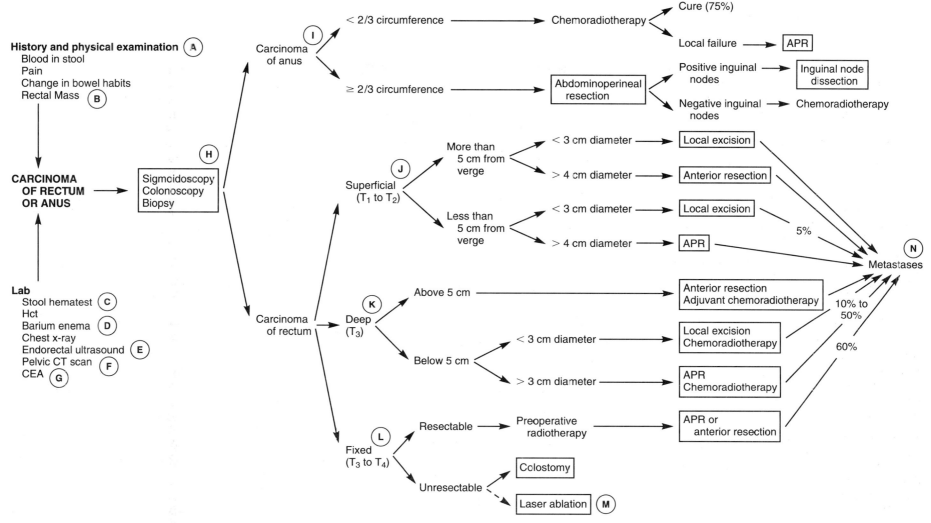

REFERENCES

Jass JR, Atkin WS, Cuzick J, et al. The grading of rectal cancer: historical perspectives and a multivariate analysis. J Cancer Res Clin Oncol 1987; 113:586–592.

Nigro NA, Vaitkevicius VK, Buroker T, et al. Combined therapy for cancer of the anal canal. Dis Colon Rectum 1981; 24:73–75.

Parks JPS, Thompson AG. Per-anal endorectal operative techniques. In: Rob C II, Smith R, Dudley HAF, eds. Operative surgery. London: Butterworth, 1977; 162–163.

Quirke P, Durdey P, Dixon MF, et al. Local recurrence of rectal adenocarcinoma due to inadequate surgical resection. Lancet 1986; 2:1.

York Manson A. Surgical access to the rectum—a transsphincteric exposure. Proc R Soc Med 1970; 64(suppl):92–94.

M Patients whose cancers are unresectable, with obstruction or impending obstruction, need a diverting colostomy. Alternatively, endoscopic laser ablation of the rectal cancer offers good palliation and avoids a diverting colostomy. It may be useful in patients with carcinomas receiving preoperative radiotherapy.

N Systemic metastases are usually multiple and amenable only to systemic therapy. Occasional patients have three or fewer liver or lung metastases. Resection of these lesions with negative margins results in 20 to 42 percent 5-year survival. Resection of four or more lesions does not improve survival. Treatment with 5-fluorouracil and leucovorin can prolong the survival of patients who have metastatic disease and good performance status (out of bed more than 50 percent of the time). An average of approximately 6 months' survival is added in patients who otherwise have a 9-month median survival. This advantage must be balanced against the 1 percent mortality and 15 percent morbidity associated with chemotherapy.

Anorectal Abscess/Fistula

Peter A. Cataldo, M.D., and W. Patrick Mazier, M.D.

(A) Anorectal abscess results from infection of an anal gland in the intermuscular space. Extension may lead to perianal, ischiorectal, intersphincteric, or supralevator abscess. Antibiotic therapy in addition to abscess drainage is appropriate for immunocompromised patients (ie, diabetes, AIDS, leukemia, etc.) Fifty percent of patients with anorectal abscess have an identifiable internal opening at presentation. Therefore, 50 percent of patients treated with external drainage only subsequently develop a fistula-in-ano and require further surgery.

(B) The presence of underlying anorectal pathology (Crohn's disease, ulcerative colitis, pilonidal disease, and hidradenitis suppurativa) as well as systemic disease (AIDS, leukemia, diabetes) must be considered. A history of previous anal surgery, especially prior fistulotomy, should be noted.

(C) Physical examination, either in the office or under anesthesia, should include inspection for areas of fluctuance, bimanual palpation for abscesses as well as fistulous tracts, and anoscopy to identify any internal opening. Pressure on the abscess cavity may accentuate purulent drainage from the internal opening.

(D) Anoscopy and sigmoidoscopy, when tolerated, provide useful information about associated pathology. Sigmoidoscopy can reveal Crohn's disease. Thirty-six percent of patients with Crohn's disease have perianal disease, and 5 to 10 percent initially have perianal complaints. External drainage of abscesses suffices for most patients. Primary fistulotomy may be performed in selected cases, particularly when there is no active Crohn's disease in the anal canal and an internal opening is identified at the dentate line. Setons, used to establish drainage, may be left in place for prolonged periods. Medical management of the underlying disease is essential. Metronidazole is particularly helpful. Colostomy or proctectomy is occasionally necessary.

(E) An intersphincteric (or high intermuscular) abscess can be difficult to diagnose. Patients have dull rectal pain that worsens with defecation. Physical examination can be entirely normal. Careful examination under anesthesia reveals a submucosal mass within the anal canal. Treatment consists of intrarectal drainage.

(F) A supralevator abscess is usually secondary to pelvic infection (inflammatory bowel disease, diverticulitis, pelvic inflammatory disease, previous surgery). It may be of cryptoglandular origin (upward extension of intersphincteric abscess). Differentiation is important. A supralevator abscess secondary to pelvic disease should be drained into the rectum. Those related to cryptoglandular infection should be externally drained with the possible addition of a mucosal flap to close the internal opening.

(G) Fifty percent of patients have an internal opening identified at time of surgery. Those with trans-sphincteric or intersphincteric fistulae should be treated by external drainage and primary fistulotomy. This is an outpatient procedure. Fistulectomy is rarely indicted. Recurrence is from 3 to 6 percent and incontinence is rare if the puborectalis is left intact.

(H) External drainage is performed either as an office procedure or in the hospital with spinal or general anesthesia. The abscess should be drained as close to the anus as possible to shorten the length of the subsequent fistulous tract, should one form. Packing is unnecessary and increases postoperative pain.

(I) Goodsall's rule is used as a guide to identify the internal opening of a fistula. When the external opening lies anterior to the midtransverse plane, the internal opening is located radially. When the external opening lies posterior to the midtransverse plane, the internal opening will be found in the posterior midline. Anterior external openings greater than 3 cm from the anal verge usually have their internal openings located in the posterior midline. The Parks classification should be included in all operative reports when treating abscess or fistula.

(J) Office drainage is relatively inexpensive. This is offset by the cost of a second procedure for the 50 percent who develop a fistula-in-ano. Single-stage fistulotomy and external drainage are the most cost-effective treatment for selected patients.

REFERENCES

Corman M. Colon and rectal surgery. Philadelphia: JB Lippincott, 1989; 125–153.

Goldberg S. Essentials of anorectal surgery. Philadelphia: JB Lippincott, 1980; 100–127.

Levien D, Surrell J, Mazier WP. Surgical treatment of anorectal fistula in patients with Crohn's disease. Surg Gynecol Obstet 1989; 169:133–136.

Parks AG, Gordon PH, Hardcastle JD. A classification of fistula-in-ano. Br J Surg 1976; 63:1–12.

White RA, Eisenstat TE, Rubin RJ, et al. Seton management of complex anorectal fistulas in patients with Crohn's disease. Dis Colon Rectum 1990; 33:587–589.

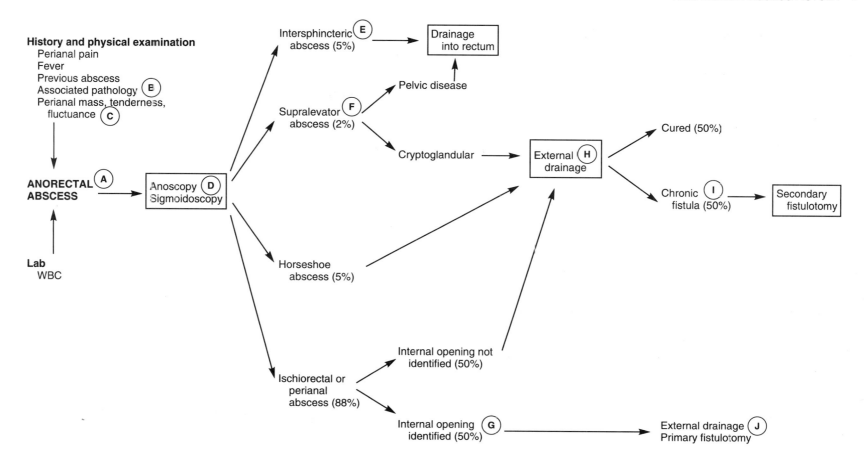

Hemorrhoids

Peter A. Cataldo, M.D., and W. Patrick Mazier, M.D.

(A) Hemorrhoids are prominent cushions that line the anal canal. They consist of submucosa, arteries, veins, smooth muscle, and connective tissue. True hemorrhoids represent a sliding down of these cushions, possibly secondary to chronic straining associated with constipation. They lie in three constant sites: left lateral, right anterior, and right posterior. Five percent of the general population suffer from hemorrhoids.

(B) Hemorrhoids usually cause painless rectal bleeding. Protrusion is also common. Internal hemorrhoids do not cause pain. Pruritus may be associated with prolapsing hemorrhoids, but should not be the sole reason for treatment because cure is unlikely. Constipation is often found in association with hemorrhoids. It may be a causative factor and should be treated before treating hemorrhoids. Rectal bleeding should never be attributed solely to hemorrhoids without careful investigation to rule out colon cancer.

(C) Cirrhotic liver disease, ascites, and chronic lung disease may contribute to the development of hemorrhoids. Hemorrhoids associated with pregnancy usually resolve without treatment.

(D) External hemorrhoids, located below the dentate line, are dilated vessels of the inferior hemorrhoidal plexus. They are covered with sensate squamous epithelium. Asymptomatic external hemorrhoids require no specific treatment.

(E) External skin tags are folds of skin arising outside the anal verge and are the result of previously thrombosed external hemorrhoids. If asymptomatic, they require no specific treatment. Symptomatic skin tags may be excised under local anesthesia.

(F) Internal hemorrhoids, located above the dentate line, are covered with columnar epithelium and, therefore, are insensate. They are classified as first-degree hemorrhoids—painless bleeding; second-degree—bleeding and prolapse with spontaneous reduction; third-degree—prolapse requiring manual reduction; and fourth-degree—irreducible prolapse.

(G) Thrombosed external hemorrhoids present with severe pain and swelling. Excision under local anesthesia is the treatment of choice for acute thrombosis. Simple evacuation of clot is not recommended because recurrence and bleeding are common with this procedure. Minimally symptomatic thrombosis can usually be treated with analgesics and sitz baths.

(H) Bulk agents combined with adequate fluid intake are the mainstay of medical treatment. The goal is to avoid straining with defecation. Eighty to ninety percent of patients with first-degree hemorrhoids can be treated effectively.

(I) Rubber band ligation is the most common form of treatment for first- and second-degree hemorrhoids. A constricting rubber band is placed at the hemorrhoidal apex. This is an office procedure done without anesthesia. Two or three treatments may be required. One percent of patients develop infection or bleeding. Ninety percent of patients are treated successfully.

(J) Sclerotherapy is used to treat first- and second-degree hemorrhoids. From 1 to 3 mL of 5 percent phenol in vegetable oil or sodium morrhuate is injected into the submucosa at the apex of each hemorrhoid. Subsequent scarring causes retraction and fixation of the redundant tissue. Complications include sloughing, infection, and thrombosis. Treatment is 80 percent effective.

(K) Cryosurgery may be used to treat internal and external hemorrhoids. Either local anesthesia or intravenous sedation may be necessary. Unpredictable tissue destruction and prolonged postoperative drainage have limited the utility of this procedure. Seventy percent of patients have resolution.

(L) Anal dilation may be used to treat all stages of hemorrhoids. Incontinence occurs in 5 percent of patients, particularly in the elderly. Eighty percent are improved. Because of fecal incontinence, dilation is no longer commonly used in the treatment of hemorrhoids.

(M) Closed hemorrhoidectomy is recommended for third- and fourth-degree hemorrhoids, and for combined internal and external hemorrhoids. Hospitalization for 1 to 3 days is required. Ninety-nine percent of patients are cured. Complications are rare. They include hemorrhage, infection, and anal stenosis. Office procedures (including sclerotherapy and rubber band ligation) are relatively inexpensive. Patients are able to return to work the following day in most cases. Formal hemorrhoidectomy is more costly; patients are usually able to return to work in 2 or 3 weeks.

REFERENCES

Corman M. Colon and rectal surgery. Philadelphia: JB Lippincott, 1989; 49–73.

Ferguson L. The closed hemorrhoidectomy. J Int Coll Surg 1961; 36:655–662.

Goldberg S. Essentials of anorectal surgery. Philadelphia: JB Lippincott, 1980; 69–83.

MacLeod J. Rational approach to treatment of hemorrhoids based on a theory of etiology. Arch Surg 1983; 118:29–32.

Mazier P. Hemorrhoidectomy—how I do it. Dis Colon Rectum, 1977; 20:202–208.

Muldoon J. The completely closed hemorrhoidectomy. Dis Colon Rectum 1981; 23:211–214.

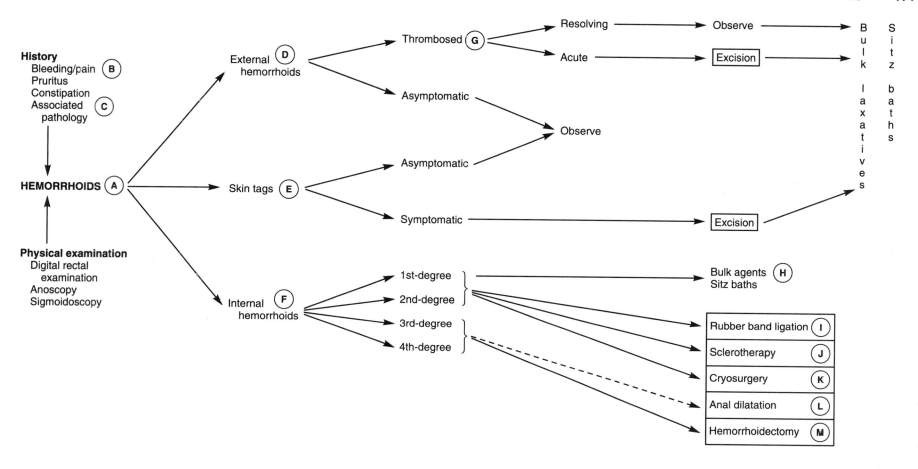

History
Bleeding/pain (B)
Pruritus
Constipation
Associated (C)
pathology

HEMORRHOIDS (A)

Physical examination
Digital rectal
examination
Anoscopy
Sigmoidoscopy

External (D)
hemorrhoids

Skin tags (E)

Internal (F)
hemorrhoids

Thrombosed (G)

Resolving → Observe

Acute → Excision

Asymptomatic

Asymptomatic

→ Observe

Symptomatic → Excision

1st-degree
2nd-degree
3rd-degree
4th-degree

Bulk agents (H)
Sitz baths

Rubber band ligation (I)

Sclerotherapy (J)

Cryosurgery (K)

Anal dilatation (L)

Hemorrhoidectomy (M)

Bulk laxatives

Sitz baths

Pilonidal Disease

Ash Mansour, M.D.

(A) An asymptomatic dimple in the skin of the sacrococcygeal area does not require treatment. In children, attention should be given to differentiate between a sacrococcygeal chordoma or teratoma, which will need further evaluation, and the normal finding of glomus coccygeum.

(B) Debate continues about whether pilonidal cysts are congenital or acquired lesions. The preponderance of pilonidal disease in hirsute people and the presence of a foreign body reaction caused by hairs support an acquired cause.

(C) Poor hygiene or repeated mechanical trauma may precipitate acute inflammation and abscess formation in a chronic cyst or sinus tract.

(D) In the United States, 40,000 patients are hospitalized annually for pilonidal disease. The average hospital stay is 5.2 days.

(E) Incision and drainage on an outpatient basis may be all that is required initially. A high recurrence rate can be expected (40 percent). Recent data suggest that excision of the sinus tract, intravenous antibiotics, and avoidance of flattening of the natal cleft reduce the risk of recurrence. Excision of both acute and chronic sinuses has been achieved using loop diathermy. This method allows for a one-stage operation, usually with satisfactory results.

(F) The wound may be left open to heal by secondary intention with granulation tissue or delayed primary closure may be done in 4 to 8 days. Frequent dressing changes and keeping pressure off the wound allow faster healing but often cause significant absence from work (6 to 12 weeks). Recurrence is relatively infrequent (1 to 20 percent).

(G) Marsupialization is achieved by incision of the cyst wall or tract and suturing the edges of the cyst or tract to the skin. For this to be successful, adequate visualization of the cyst or tract and meticulous suturing to the skin is necessary. Healing time is 20 to 30 days and recurrence is unlikely (0 to 7 percent).

(H) Pilonidal cystotomy is safe and rapid. It can be performed with local anesthesia on an outpatient basis. A significant rate of recurrence (3 to 20 percent) is encountered. Healing is prolonged (2 months).

(I) Phenol injection of the cyst under regional or general anesthesia is usually successful in obliterating a chronic sinus if there is no evidence of infection. Recurrence rates are 17 to 19 percent.

(J) Primary excision should be done meticulously to be certain that all tract or cyst remnants are removed. If primary closure causes tension or loss of the natal cleft, alternatives such as a rotation flap or Z-plasty should be considered. Perioperative intravenous antibiotics, the use of closed suction drains to avoid hematoma, and keeping weight off for at least 5 days have all been shown to enhance healing. Contraindications to primary closure include active infection, significant lateral extension of the sinus, excessive hairiness, or presence of complicating factors such as hidradenitis suppurativa or osteomyelitis of the sacrum. Recurrence rates after primary excision are 2 to 38 percent.

(K) Recurrences are due to incomplete drainage, failure to excise the sinus tract, inadequate postoperative wound care (hematoma, wound dehiscence), and inadequate follow-up.

REFERENCES

Abramson DJ. Excision and delayed closure of pilonidal sinus. Surg Gynecol Obstet 1977; 144:205.

Allen-Mersh TG. Pilonidal sinus: finding the right tract for treatment. Br J Surg 1990; 77:123–132.

Bascom J. Pilonidal disease: origin from follicles of hair and results of follicle removal as treatment. Surgery 1980; 87:567–572.

Fishbein RH, Handelsman JC. A method for primary reconstruction following radical excision of sacrococcygeal pilonidal disease. Ann Surg 1979; 190:231–235.

Shpitz B, Kaufman Z, Kantarovsky A, et al. Definitive management of acute pilonidal abscess by loop diathermy excision. Dis Colon Rectum 1990; 33:441–442.

Solla JA, Rothenberger DA. Chronic pilonidal disease: an assessment of 150 cases. Dis Colon Rectum 1990; 33:758–761.

Williams RS. A simple technique for successful primary closure after excision of pilonidal sinus disease. Ann R Coll Surg Engl 1990; 72:313–315.

History and physical examination
Pain
Mass
Discharge
Previous infection
   or surgery
Dimple
Cyst
Sinus tract

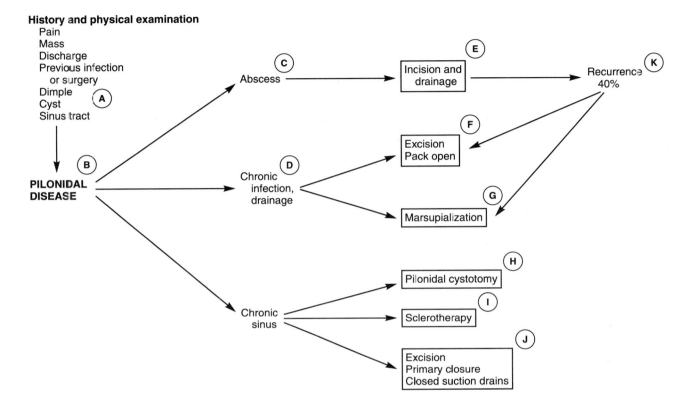

Breast and Soft Tissues

Nipple Discharge

Roger Wotkyns, M.D., and Lawrence W. Norton, M.D.

(A) Nipple discharge is one of six clinical features of benign breast disorders. Others are physiologic cyclic swelling and tenderness, nodularity (cyclic and noncyclic), mastalgia (cyclic and noncyclic), dominant lumps (including gross cysts and fibroadenomas), and infection or inflammation. Secretion from the nipple of any mature woman is common with or without stimulation. The discharge may be clear or cloudy. The color is brown, green, blue, milky, yellow, or a mixture of these.

(B) Factors to be evaluated by history include the nature of the discharge, spontaneity, relation to menses, pregnancy, stimulation, exercise, medications (hormones, central nervous system depressants), and thyroid disorders. Physical examination determines the presence of a breast mass, nipple disease, signs of infection, single or multiple duct discharge, and whether or not pressure at a single site produces fluid.

(C) Mammography is indicated in women over the age of 40 with or without nipple discharge. Onset of discharge should trigger mammography. Ultrasound can be a helpful adjunctive tool. Smearing the discharge for Gram stain or cytologic examination can also be helpful. Guaiac study of nipple discharge is indicated; persistent positivity requires further evaluation.

(D) Nipple disease associated with nipple discharge may be squamous carcinoma (Bowen disease), ductal carcinoma (Paget disease), or duct ectasia. Nipple biopsy should be performed for any nipple lesion that does not resolve promptly when treated.

(E) A palpable breast mass in the presence of nipple discharge is diagnosed by aspiration, fine-needle aspiration cytology, core needle biopsy, or excisional biopsy. Negative cytologic findings imply but do not guarantee benign breast disease. Excision of the mass may control nipple discharge and, at the same time, provide a definitive diagnosis.

(F) Milky nipple discharge from multiple ducts may be the result of increased prolactin secretion from the pituitary gland. Persistent elevation of prolactin requires an endocrine evaluation.

(G) Purulent discharge suggests duct ectasia or abscess. If antibiotic treatment does not control the situation, excision of involved breast tissue is necessary. Recurrent infection after antibiotic therapy alone is not infrequent.

(H) When the drainage emanates from a single duct, it is typically caused by an intraductal papilloma. Drainage may or may not be grossly bloody or guaiac positive. The responsible duct can be identified by pressing at various points around the areola. If discharge occurs as a result of pressure, the underlying ductal tissue can either be excised or explored through microdochectomy.

(I) When nipple discharge is grossly bloody or persistently guaiac positive or when the secretion has a sticky clear character, *further evaluation is indicated*. The most common causes of gross or occult blood in nipple discharge in order of frequency are intraductal papilloma (45 percent), duct ectasia (36 percent), carcinoma (8 percent), infection (8 percent), and other (25 percent). A negative cytology report does not necessarily exclude cancer.

(J) A ductogram can be helpful. Successful visualization of a lesion requires a skilled radiologist.

REFERENCES

Funderburk W, Syphax B. Evaluation of nipple discharge in benign and malignant disease. Cancer 1969; 24:1290–1296.

Harris JR, Hellman S, Henderson IC, Kinne DW. Breast diseases (2nd ed). Philadelphia: JB Lippincott, 1991.

Tabar L, Dean P, Pentek Z. Galactography: the diagnostic procedure of choice for nipple discharge. Radiology 1983; 149:31–38.

Urban JA, Egeli RA. Nonlactational nipple discharge. Cancer 1978; 28:130.

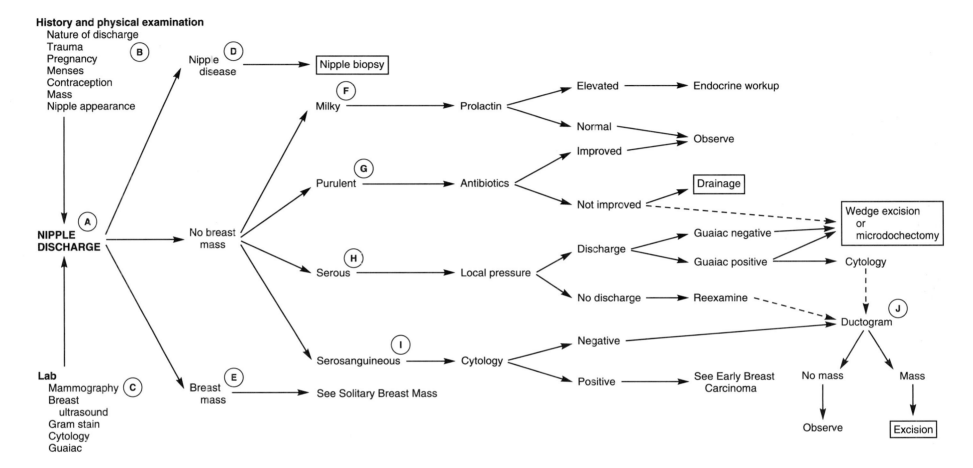

History and physical examination
Nature of discharge
Trauma
Pregnancy
Menses
Contraception
Mass
Nipple appearance

B

D
Nipple disease → Nipple biopsy

F
Milky → Prolactin → Elevated → Endocrine workup
Prolactin → Normal → Observe

G
Purulent → Antibiotics → Improved → Observe
Antibiotics → Not improved → Drainage

A
NIPPLE DISCHARGE → No breast mass

H
Serous → Local pressure → Discharge → Guaiac negative → Wedge excision or microdochectomy
Local pressure → Discharge → Guaiac positive → Cytology
Local pressure → No discharge → Reexamine

I
Serosanguineous → Cytology → Negative → Ductogram
Cytology → Positive → See Early Breast Carcinoma

Lab
Mammography C
Breast ultrasound
Gram stain
Cytology
Guaiac

E
Breast mass → See Solitary Breast Mass

Wedge excision or microdochectomy

J
Ductogram → No mass → Observe
Ductogram → Mass → Excision

Solitary Breast Mass

Lawrence W. Norton, M.D.

(A) It is important to learn the diagnosis of a previously excised breast mass. A history of breast cancer in the family is a significant risk factor. Breast pain and tenderness, common in patients with fibrocystic change, are uncommon (10 percent) in patients with cancer.

(B) A dominant palpable breast mass is distinct from other breast lesions and can be measured. It requires diagnosis by one means or another.

(C) A solitary palpable breast mass is detected by the patient (70 percent), by a physician (20 percent), or by mammography (5 percent). Approximately 80 percent of solitary breast masses are benign.

(D) Mammography is useful to detect breast lesions but cannot establish a diagnosis. Its value in the presence of a palpable breast mass is to exclude occult disease, particularly in the opposite breast. Mammography is not required before biopsy in patients under age 40 unless the patient has a family history of breast cancer occurring at an early age.

(E) Ultrasonography is helpful to establish the nature (cyst vs. solid) of a mammographically detected breast mass. It has little application when a mass is palpable.

(F) Aspiration with a 25- or 22-gauge needle is a logical first step in the diagnosis of a palpable mass. Direct puncture without local anesthesia is usually well tolerated. Care must be exercised to be certain that the needle enters the mass. In a thin patient with a small breast, aspiration can cause pneumothorax.

(G) If clear fluid is obtained by aspiration and the breast mass disappears, the diagnosis of a simple breast cyst is made and no further evaluation is required. The patient should be reexamined within 4 to 6 weeks. If the cyst recurs, it can be reaspirated. Repeated aspirations justify cyst excision.

(H) The presence of blood in aspirated fluid or the persistence of a mass after aspiration raise the small possibility of carcinoma. Bloody fluid should be examined cytologically. If no malignant cells are seen, a follow-up mammogram is advisable. Persistent masses should be excised or diagnosed by fine-needle aspiration (FNA) cytology.

(I) FNA cytology is a rapid, minimally invasive means to diagnose a palpable breast mass. A well-trained cytologist can detect cancer with an accuracy of greater than 95 percent. Breast operations can be performed on the basis of FNA cytologic results.

(J) Excisional biopsy remains the "gold standard" in the diagnosis of breast lumps. Because it is a surgical procedure, it is painful and has the risk of bleeding and infection. Specimens should be kept fresh and cold so that hormone receptors can be measured. The tissue may also be analyzed for DNA ploidy by flow cytometry.

(K) Core needle biopsy is used for larger masses when excisional biopsy would be an extensive procedure. The accuracy of core needle biopsy depends entirely on the operator's skill in obtaining a sample of the palpable mass.

(L) Fibroadenoma very rarely contains carcinoma and probably never becomes cancer. For these reasons, it can remain in the breast if diagnosed by FNA cytology or core needle biopsy.

(M) Other benign masses include intraductal papilloma, duct ectasia, and fat necrosis. After the removal of such masses, the patient can be discharged.

(N) Fibrocystic change encompasses a number of benign breast conditions. Fibrocystic change comprises most breast masses. It presents usually as multiple masses rather than as a solitary lump. Fibrocystic change is frequently associated with pain and tenderness. Despite popular opinion, neither avoiding theophylline (caffeine) nor taking vitamin E consistently relieves symptoms. The only pathologic variant of fibrocystic change that increases the risk of developing breast cancer significantly is atypical ductal hyperplasia. Patients with that diagnosis should be followed by examining the breasts semiannually and obtaining mammograms as often as every year.

REFERENCES

Cusik J, Dotan J, Jaecks R, et al. The role of Tru-Cut needle biopsy in the diagnosis of carcinoma of the breast. Surg Gynecol Obstet 1990; 170:407–410.

deManblanc M, Giraud C, Simondon F, et al. Hormone receptors, fine-needle aspiration and breast cancer. Second International Congress on Neo-Adjuvant Chemotherapy. February 19–21, 1988, Paris, 1988:8.

Ellis L. Techniques for obtaining the diagnosis of malignant breast lesions. Surg Clin North Am 1990; 70:815–830.

Gelabert H, Hsiu J, Mullen J, et al. Prospective evaluation of the role of fine needle aspiration biopsy in the diagnosis and management of patients with palpable solid breast lesions. Am Surg 1990; 56:263–267.

Layfield L, Glasgow B, Cramer H: Fine needle aspiration in management of breast masses. Pathol Ann 1989; 24:23–62.

Leis H. Current methods for biopsy and treatment of potentially curable breast cancers. Int Surg 1990; 75:1–7.

Norton L, Davis J, Wiens J, et al. Accuracy of aspiration cytology in detecting breast cancer. Surgery 1984; 96:806–814.

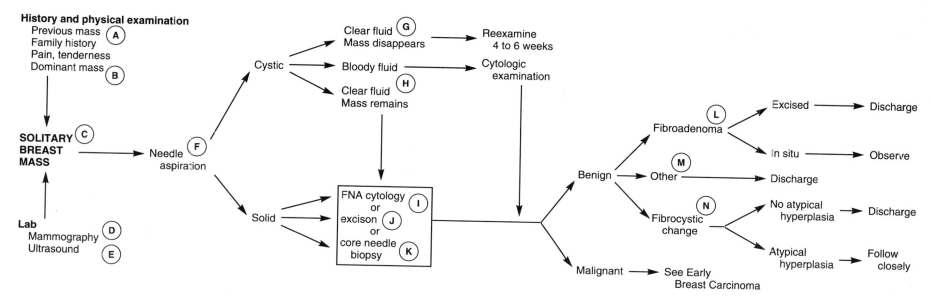

History and physical examination
Previous mass (A)
Family history
Pain, tenderness
Dominant mass (B)

SOLITARY (C)
BREAST
MASS

Lab
Mammography (D)
Ultrasound (E)

Needle (F)
aspiration

Cystic

Clear fluid (G)
Mass disappears → Reexamine
4 to 6 weeks

Bloody fluid (H) → Cytologic examination

Clear fluid
Mass remains

Solid

FNA cytology (I)
or
excison (J)
or
core needle
biopsy (K)

Cytologic examination

Benign

Fibroadenoma (L) → Excised → Discharge
In situ → Observe

Other (M) → Discharge

Fibrocystic change (N)
No atypical hyperplasia → Discharge
Atypical hyperplasia → Follow closely

Malignant → See Early Breast Carcinoma

Early Breast Carcinoma

Lawrence W. Norton, M.D.

A One of nine American women will develop breast cancer. Risk is greatest when a close relative has the disease. Other risk factors are early menarche and late menopause, nulliparity, cancer of the uterus or ovary, and previous breast cancer. Intraductal carcinoma, lobular carcinoma in situ, and atypical ductal hyperplasia increase the risk of invasive cancer. Nipple or skin retraction is an unusual physical finding because most breast cancers are detected before such changes occur.

B Breast carcinoma is second only to lung cancer as a cause of cancer-related death among women. Nearly 45,000 women will die of breast cancer this year. Incidence appears to be increasing. The cause of this increase is unknown.

C Bilateral mammography, if not previously obtained, should be done in all patients with early breast cancer. Mammography can detect multifocal or contralateral cancer. A decision to conserve the breast and to use radiation as primary treatment might be changed if multifocal carcinoma is detected mammographically.

D Chest x-ray and liver function tests are obtained routinely in patients with early breast cancer. Bone scan is positive in fewer than 15 percent of patients with stage I or II disease and is not cost-effective.

E Of tests done on tumor cells, only hormone receptor status, S phase fraction, and possibly cathepsin D levels correlate with outcome. DNA ploidy is not a proven prognostic factor.

F Most breast cancers are invasive. The proportion of noninvasive tumors has increased with the routine use of screening mammography and needle localization biopsy and is reported to be as high as 30 percent.

G Stages I and IIA invasive carcinoma are considered to represent early disease. Stage I (T1, N0, M0) refers to tumors 2 cm or less in diameter that have not metastasized. Stage IIA describes undetectable (T0, N1, M0) or small tumors (T1, N1, M0) with regional metastases and larger primary tumors (T2, N0, M0) without metastases.

H Intraductal carcinoma (ductal carcinoma in situ) is associated with invasive breast cancer, usually ductal, in 30 to 65 percent of patients observed 6 to 10 years. Because of this high risk, patients with intraductal carcinoma must be treated.

I Intralobular carcinoma (lobular carcinoma in situ) is associated with invasive breast cancer, usually ductal, in only 15 to 35 percent of patients observed 20 years. Because of this low risk, patients with intralobular carcinoma can be observed with annual breast examination and mammography.

J Prospective clinical trials confirm that early breast cancer under 4 cm in diameter can be treated by either modified radical mastectomy or a combination of wide local excision of the tumor, axillary dissection, and radiation (breast conservation). Results after either treatment are virtually identical in terms of disease-free interval, overall survival, local recurrence, and distant metastases. Choice of treatment usually depends on patient preference. Contraindications to breast conservation include tumor involvement of the nipple/areolar complex, a small breast (poor cosmesis), and an extensive intraductal component of the cancer (higher recurrence rate after radiation).

K Traditional treatment of intraductal carcinoma is total mastectomy. Breast conservation by wide local excision and radiation is now an option. Local recurrence is greater after conservation (8 to 12 percent) but can be treated by salvage mastectomy without altering chances of survival.

L Node-negative breast cancer less than 1 cm in diameter is associated with 10-year disease-free survival of greater than 90 percent. Survival rates decrease in relation to increasing tumor size (T).

M The presence of positive axillary lymph nodes significantly alters relapse rates. One to three positive nodes are associated with 10-year relapse rates as high as 65 percent. More than three positive nodes are associated with relapse rates approaching 85 percent.

N Chemotherapy or hormone therapy is currently recommended for all node-negative patients with breast cancer. This is based on 10 randomized clinical trials showing that recurrence rates are decreased by one third when adjuvant therapy is given. Mortality is probably reduced as well. No correlation with menopausal or receptor status is reported. The fact remains that some patients with small primary lesions can expect a survival rate of at least 95 percent for 10 years. The advantage of adjuvant chemotherapy in these patients is small.

O Tamoxifen, a hormonal agent with primarily antiestrogen effects, decreases recurrence rates in postmenopausal women with either node-negative or node-positive disease. It is used after chemotherapy in some premenopausal patients. One study suggests that tamoxifen reduces the incidence of contralateral cancer.

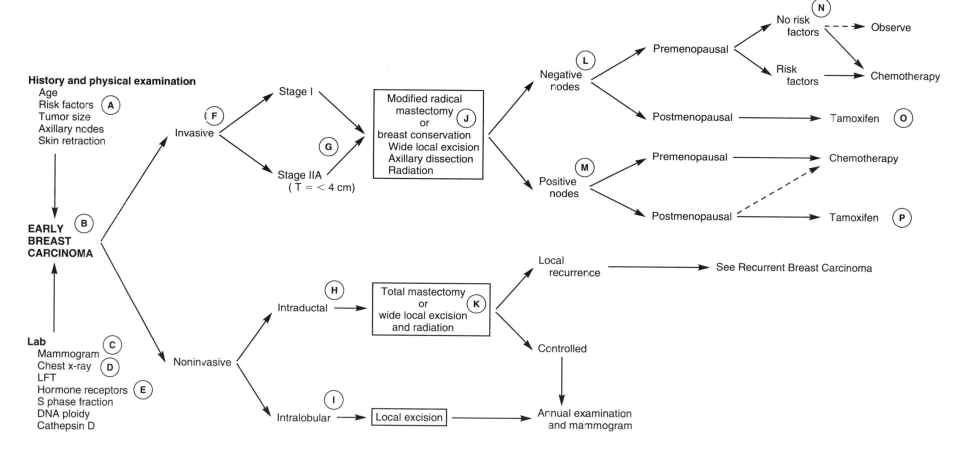

History and physical examination
Age
Risk factors (A)
Tumor size
Axillary nodes
Skin retraction

EARLY BREAST CARCINOMA (B)

Lab
Mammogram (C)
Chest x-ray (D)
LFT
Hormone receptors (E)
S phase fraction
DNA ploidy
Cathepsin D

(P) The benefit of adjuvant chemotherapy in node-positive postmenopausal women is debated.

REFERENCES

Fisher B, Costantino J, Redmond C, et al. A randomized clinical trial evaluating tamoxifen in the treatment of patients with node-negative breast cancer who have estrogen-receptor-positive tumors. N Engl J Med 1989; 320:479–484.

Fisher B, Redmond C, Poisson R, et al. Eight-year results of a randomized clinical trial comparing total mastectomy and lumpectomy with or without irradiation in the treatment of breast cancer. N Engl J Med 1989; 320:822–828.

Holland R, Connolly JL, Gelman R, et al. The presence of an extensive intraductal component following a limited excision correlates with prominent residual disease in the remainder of the breast. J Clin Oncol 1990; 8:113–118.

Mansour EG, Greg R, Shatila AH, et al. Efficacy of adjuvant chemotherapy in high-risk node-negative breast cancer: an intergroup study. N Engl J Med 1989; 320:485–490.

Margolese R, Poisson R, Shibata H. The technique of segmental mastectomy (lumpectomy) and axillary dissection. Surgery 1987; 102:828–834.

Sigurdsson H, Baldetorp B, Borg A, et al. Indicators of prognosis in node-negative breast cancer. N Engl J Med 1990; 322:1045–2053.

Tandon AK, Clark GM, Chamness GC, et al. Cathepsin D and prognosis in breast cancer. N Engl J Med 1990; 322:297–302.

Tejler G, Aspergren K. Complications and hospital stay after surgery for breast cancer: a prospective study of 385 patients. Br J Surg 1985; 72:542–544.

Veronesi U, Salvadori B, Luini A, et al. Conservative treatment of early breast cancer: long term results of 1232 cases treated with quadrantectomy, axillary dissection and radiotherapy. Ann Surg 1990; 211:250–259.

Vinton AL, Traverso LW, Zehring RD. Immediate breast reconstruction following mastectomy is as safe as mastectomy alone. Arch Surg 1990; 125:1303–1308.

Advanced Breast Cancer

David P. Winchester, M.D., and Douglas E. Merkel, M.D.

(A) Clinical staging for patients with bulky or advanced disease should include chest x-ray, bone scan, and, if liver enzymes are elevated, computed tomography scan of the liver. Although routine bone and computed tomography scans are not indicated in the evaluation of asymptomatic patients with early breast cancer, distant metastases are more commonly discovered in association with locally advanced disease.

(B) According to the staging system of the American Joint Committee on Cancer, T0 tumors are in situ, T1 tumors are 2.0 cm or less in greatest dimension, T2 tumors are more than 2.0 cm but not more than 5.0 cm in greatest dimension, T3 tumors are more than 5.0 cm in greatest dimension, and T4 tumors are of any size with direct extension to the skin or chest wall. Stage T4 includes inflammatory carcinoma. N1 represents metastases to moveable ipsilateral axillary nodes, N2 metastases to fixed ipsilateral nodes, and N3 metastases to ipsilateral internal mammary nodes.

(C) The algorithm for stage IV or systemic disease assumes that the breast has been previously treated and controlled.

(D) Incisional or excisional breast biopsies should produce enough tissue for histologic diagnosis, biochemical receptor assays, and flow cytometric ploidy and proliferative fraction determinations. In some settings, immunocytochemical receptor assays are available, permitting the use of a core needle for definitive biopsy. Fine-needle aspiration for cytology may be applicable in some clinical trials. A few laboratories are able to provide a comprehensive prognostic analysis of the tumor based on fine-needle aspiration results.

(E) Fixation to the pectoral fascia is not recorded for staging because its presence or absence

does not influence the stage. Modified radical mastectomy with full axillary lymph node dissection is the preferred procedure for patients without pectoral fascia involvement. If a small area of pectoral fascia is involved, incontinuity resection of an adequate portion of the pectoral muscle is performed. If the muscle is more widely invaded or Rotter nodes are involved, a radical mastectomy may be necessary.

(F) Neoadjuvant chemotherapy before definitive surgical treatment of resectable breast cancer is currently an investigational approach. Cooperative groups in this country are prospectively studying the use of Adriamycin-based chemotherapy before mastectomy.

(G) Neoadjuvant chemotherapy for clinically unresectable breast cancer is given for at least three cycles, or to the point of maximum response. An Adriamycin-based program, such as FAC (fluorouracil, Adriamycin, cyclophosphamide), is recommended.

(H) Systemic adjuvant therapy is given to all patients with advanced breast cancer. This means chemotherapy for all premenopausal women and at least tamoxifen for all postmenopausal, receptor-positive women. Adjuvant chemotherapy in postmenopausal women has not consistently resulted in prolongation of disease-free interval or overall survival. Most positive trials of adjuvant chemotherapy consist of 4 to 6 months of treatment. Adjuvant tamoxifen should be administered for at least 5 years. Chemotherapy and tamoxifen should not be given simultaneously outside of a clinical trial.

(I) Ovarian ablation or suppression with gonadotropin-releasing hormone agonists is first-line therapy in this group of patients. The addition

of chemotherapy is reserved for patients with more rapidly progressive visceral disease.

(J) Tamoxifen is first-line therapy with the addition of chemotherapy for more rapidly progressive disease.

(K) Adjuvant radiotherapy after mastectomy has not been shown to improve survival consistently, but is considered for patients at disproportionate risk for local relapse, that is, with involved surgical margins or 10 or more involved lymph nodes.

(L) Lumpectomy after chemotherapeutic cytoreduction has been reported in European series. After several cycles of chemotherapy, the breast is treated by lumpectomy and adjuvant radiotherapy. The long-term outcome of such an approach is not yet known.

(M) The optimal sequence in which systemic adjuvant therapy and radiotherapy are administered after successful cytoreduction and resection of stage III disease has not been determined. The relative risk for local or distant sites of first relapse should determine the order in which these modalities are administered.

(N) High-dose chemotherapy supported by autologous bone marrow transplantation may be useful in highly selected cases.

(O) Locally directed therapy for metastases in addition to systemic therapy is indicated under special circumstances.

(P) It is unusual for systemic therapy to control pleural effusion. Tube thoracostomy and a sclerosing agent may be required. Recurrent effusion can be treated by repeat sclerosis, thoracen-

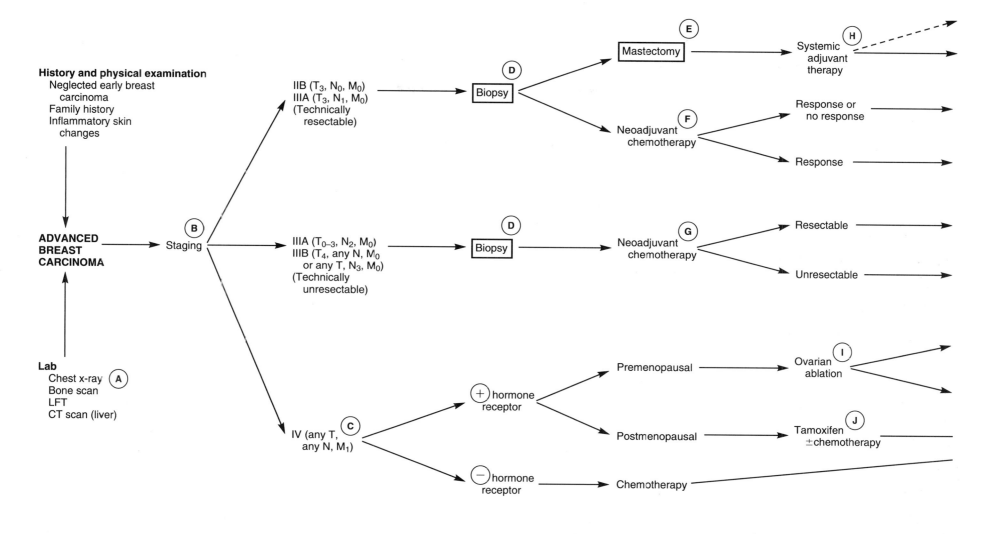

History and physical examination
- Neglected early breast carcinoma
- Family history
- Inflammatory skin changes

ADVANCED BREAST CARCINOMA

Lab
- Chest x-ray (A)
- Bone scan
- LFT
- CT scan (liver)

(B) Staging

IIB (T_3, N_0, M_0)
IIIA (T_3, N_1, M_0)
(Technically resectable)

(D) Biopsy

(E) Mastectomy → Systemic adjuvant therapy (H)

Neoadjuvant chemotherapy (F) → Response or no response

→ Response

IIIA (T_{0-3}, N_2, M_0)
IIIB (T_4, any N, M_0 or any T, N_3, M_0)
(Technically unresectable)

(D) Biopsy → Neoadjuvant chemotherapy (G) → Resectable

→ Unresectable

IV (any T, any N, M_1) (C)

(+) hormone receptor

→ Premenopausal → Ovarian ablation (I)

→ Postmenopausal → Tamoxifen ±chemotherapy (J)

(−) hormone receptor → Chemotherapy

Advanced Breast Cancer (Continued)

tesis, parietal pleurectomy, or pleural–peritoneal shunting.

(Q) Prophylactic stabilization of bony lesions in high-risk weight-bearing areas may be indicated in addition to stabilization of fractures.

REFERENCES

Antman K, Gale RP. Advanced breast cancer: high-dose chemotherapy and bone marrow autotransplants. Ann Intern Med 1988; 108:570–574.

Bonadonna D. Conceptual and practical advances in the management of breast cancer: the Karnofsky memorial lecture. J Clin Oncol 1989; 7:1380–1397.

Bonadonna G, Veronesi U, Brambilla C, et al. Primary chemotherapy to avoid mastectomy in tumors with diameters of three centimeters or more. J Natl Cancer Inst 1990; 82:1539–1545.

DeLena M, Zucali R, Viganotti G, et al. Combined chemotherapy-radiotherapy approach in locally advanced ($T_{3.b}$–T_4) breast cancer. Cancer Chemother Pharm 1978; 1:53–59.

Hery M, Namer M, Moro M, et al. Conservative treatment (chemotherapy/radiotherapy) of locally advanced breast cancer. Cancer 1986; 57:1744–1749.

Ingle JN. Principles of therapy in advanced breast cancer. In: Henderson IC, ed. Hematology/Oncology Clinics of North America, Diagnosis and Therapy of Breast Cancer. Vol 3. December, 1989; 743–764.

Loprinzi CL, Carbone PP, Tormey DC, et al. Aggressive combined modality therapy for advanced local-regional breast cancer. J Clin Oncol 1984; 2:157–163.

Pritchard KI, Sutherland DJA. The use of endocrine therapy. In: Henderson IC, ed. Hematology/Oncology Clinics of North America, Diagnosis and Therapy of Breast Cancer. Vol 3. December, 1989.

Rusch VW, Harper GR. Pleural effusions in patients with malignancy. In: Roth JA, Ruckdeschel JC, Weisenberger TH, eds. Thoracic oncology. Philadelphia: WB Saunders, 1989; 594–605.

Sewa SL. Tamoxifen in the treatment of breast cancer. Ann Intern Med 1988; 109:219–228.

Swain SM, Sorace RA, Bagley CS, et al. Neoadjuvant chemotherapy in the combined modality approach of locally advanced nonmetastatic breast cancer. Cancer Res, 1987; 47:3889–3894.

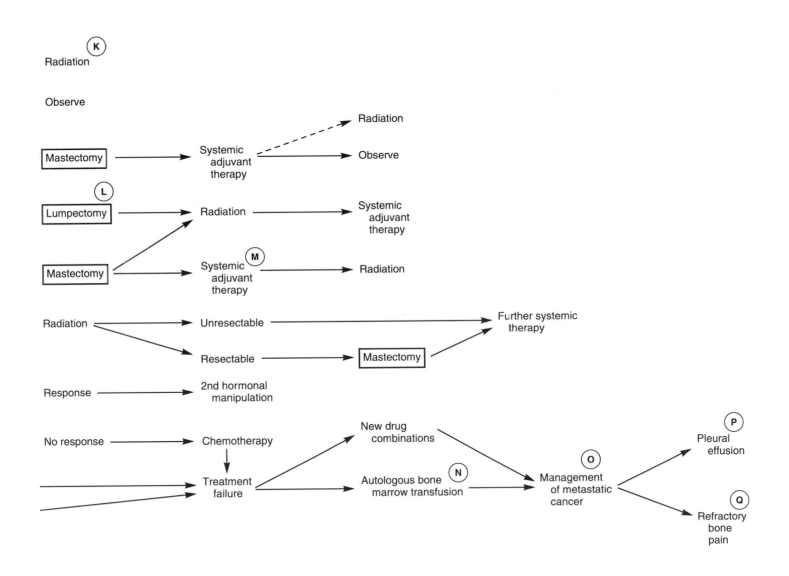

Recurrent Breast Carcinoma

Michael D. Stone, M.D., and Blake Cady, M.D.

(A) The primary determinants of treatment of recurrent breast carcinoma are the nature of the previous treatments and the site and extent of disease recurrence.

(B) Chest computed tomography scan shows additional lesions in up to 50 percent of patients evaluated for local–regional recurrence, including disease in internal mammary nodes, sternal erosion, axillary adenopathy, and rib metastases.

(C) All lesions thought to be breast cancer recurrence should be biopsied, with the exception of suspicious axillary nodes that are amenable to formal axillary dissection. Estrogen and progesterone receptor protein should be measured even if this has been done previously. Estrogen receptor data differ from the primary tumor status in 25 to 35 percent of patients.

(D) Local–regional recurrence after previous mastectomy has a grave prognosis, with 5- and 10-year disease-free survival rates of 30 and 7 percent. Survival patterns vary considerably depending on a number of factors, including size and number of recurrences and disease-free interval. Important palliation may be possible by further treatment. There are occasional patients who experience extended survival. Twenty-five to thirty-three percent of patients with local–regional recurrence of breast cancer have concurrent metastatic disease at the time of local recurrence. Complete staging, consisting of chest x-ray, chest computed tomography scan, bone scan, liver function tests, and liver ultrasonography, should be done.

(E) Local recurrence rate after lumpectomy and radiation therapy is 5 to 10 percent at 5 years. Distant metastatic disease presenting before local recurrence is uncommon, and concurrent distant metastases are found in only 5 to 8 percent of patients. Therefore, complete staging is not appropriate unless the patient is symptomatic or has abnormal alkaline phosphatase, bone scan, liver function tests, or liver ultrasound.

(F) The local recurrence rate after lumpectomy without radiation is reported to be 38 percent at 8 years.

(G) Total field radiation should be used for recurrent breast cancer rather than radiation limited to the specific site of recurrence. Patients previously irradiated require chemotherapy or hormonal treatment. Complete excision of the recurrence should be carried out if at all possible because this treatment, in addition to 4500 cGy, is associated with minimal local recurrence. Doses of 5500 to 6000 cGy are necessary for residual disease. Most patients have complete regression of disease initially, but only 43 percent enjoy local control for 5 years. Most re-recurrences are at the original site of disease in the field of radiation. Treatment should therefore include 4500 cGy boosts to the initial primary site. The previously dissected axilla should not be radiated unless clinically involved or highly suspicious nodes are present.

(H) Patients who develop distant metastatic disease before or concurrent with local regional failure should receive chemotherapy or hormonal therapy initially. Such patients should be watched carefully for evidence of advancing local disease or symptoms that may require therapy. Patients who have a complete response to either chemotherapy or hormonal therapy should be considered for aggressive local therapy including chest wall resection. No clear data are available to indicate that chemotherapy or hormonal therapy for local recurrence increases or lengthens local control or disease-free survival.

(I) Extensive intraductal component (intraductal cancer making up 25 percent or more of the invasive cancer and present in the breast tissue surrounding the invasive component) is associated with local recurrence rates of 22 to 71 percent after gross excision and radiation therapy.

(J) Carefully selected patients can benefit from chest wall resection. Patients with large isolated recurrences, particularly those who have not failed previous radiation therapy, have a 5-year survival as high as 43 percent. Local control can be achieved in most patients with survival of up to 46 months in patients rendered disease-free vs. 21 months in patients with residual disease. The presence of distant metastases is not in itself a contraindication to the procedure, but patients should be expected to survive at least 1 year to justify the procedure.

(K) Standard treatment for recurrence after conservation surgery and radiation therapy is mastectomy. Overall survival rates of 45 to 70 percent at 5 years have been reported. Conservative reexcision may be appropriate for selected patients with small (< 2 cm), mobile lesions without skin or extensive axillary node involvement or for patients with in situ cancer. In carefully selected patients treated by wedge reexcision, 5-year actuarial disease-free survival of 70 percent has been reported. Breast reconstruction is an option for patients after mastectomy. This is best performed with a rectus abdominis myocutaneous flap in patients who have had previous radiation therapy.

(L) The role of adjuvant chemotherapy or hormonal therapy has not been investigated for patients treated for local–regional recurrence. It seems reasonable to treat patients who develop new positive nodes, have positive resection margins after previous radiation therapy, or have skin, blood, or lymphatic vessel invasion. The role of

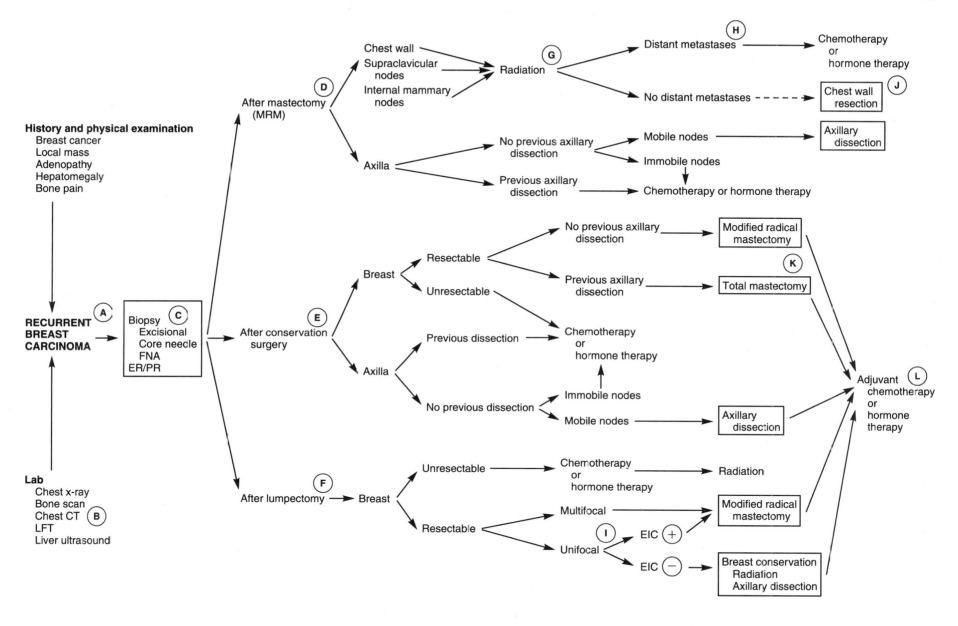

History and physical examination
Breast cancer
Local mass
Adenopathy
Hepatomegaly
Bone pain

RECURRENT BREAST CARCINOMA

Lab
Chest x-ray
Bone scan
Chest CT (B)
LFT
Liver ultrasound

(A) (C) Biopsy
Excisional
Core needle
FNA
ER/PR

(D) After mastectomy (MRM)
Chest wall
Supraclavicular nodes
Internal mammary nodes
→ (G) Radiation → Distant metastases (H) → Chemotherapy or hormone therapy
→ No distant metastases - - -> Chest wall resection (J)

Axilla
→ No previous axillary dissection → Mobile nodes → Axillary dissection
→ Immobile nodes
→ Previous axillary dissection → Chemotherapy or hormone therapy

(E) After conservation surgery
Breast
→ Resectable → No previous axillary dissection → Modified radical mastectomy
→ Previous axillary dissection → Total mastectomy (K)
→ Unresectable → Chemotherapy or hormone therapy

Axilla
→ Previous dissection → Chemotherapy or hormone therapy
→ No previous dissection → Immobile nodes
→ Mobile nodes → Axillary dissection

(F) After lumpectomy → Breast
→ Unresectable → Chemotherapy or hormone therapy → Radiation
→ Resectable → Multifocal → Modified radical mastectomy
→ Unifocal (I) → EIC (+)
→ EIC (−) → Breast conservation Radiation Axillary dissection

Adjuvant chemotherapy or hormone therapy (L)

Recurrent Breast Carcinoma (Continued)

adjuvant systemic treatment for patients who have previously been treated at the time of the primary is not clear.

REFERENCES

Aberizk WJ, Silver B, Henderson IC, et al. The use of radiotherapy for treatment of isolated local regional recurrence of breast cancer after mastectomy. Cancer 1986; 58:1214–1218.

Ames FC, Balch CM. Management of local and regional recurrence after mastectomy or breast conserving treatment. Surg Clin North Am 1990; 70:1115–1124.

Bedwinek JM, Lee J, Fineberg B, et al. Prognostic indicators in patients with isolated local-regional recurrence of breast cancer. Cancer 1981; 47:2232–2235.

Bedwinek JM, Monroe D, Fineberg B. Local regional treatment of patients with simultaneous local regional recurrence and distant metastases following mastectomy. Am J Clin Oncol 1983; 6:295–300.

Fisher B, Redman C, Poisson R, et al. Eight year results of a randomized clinical trial comparing total mastectomy and lumpectomy with or without irradiation in the treatment of breast cancer. N Engl J Med 1989; 320:822–828.

Kurtz JM, Amalric R, Brandone H, et al. Results of salvage surgery for mammary recurrence following breast conserving therapy. Ann Surg 1987; 207:347–351.

Lindfors KK, Meyer JE, Busse PM, et al. CT evaluation of local and regional breast recurrence. AJR 1985; 145:833–837.

Osteen RT, Smith BL. Results of conservative surgery and radiation for breast cancer. Surg Clin North Am 1990; 70:1005–1021.

Recht A, Hayes DF. Specific sites of metastatic disease and emergencies: local recurrence. In: Harris JR, Helman S, Henderson IC, Kinne DW, eds. Breast diseases (2nd ed). Philadelphia: JB Lippincott, 1991:508–524.

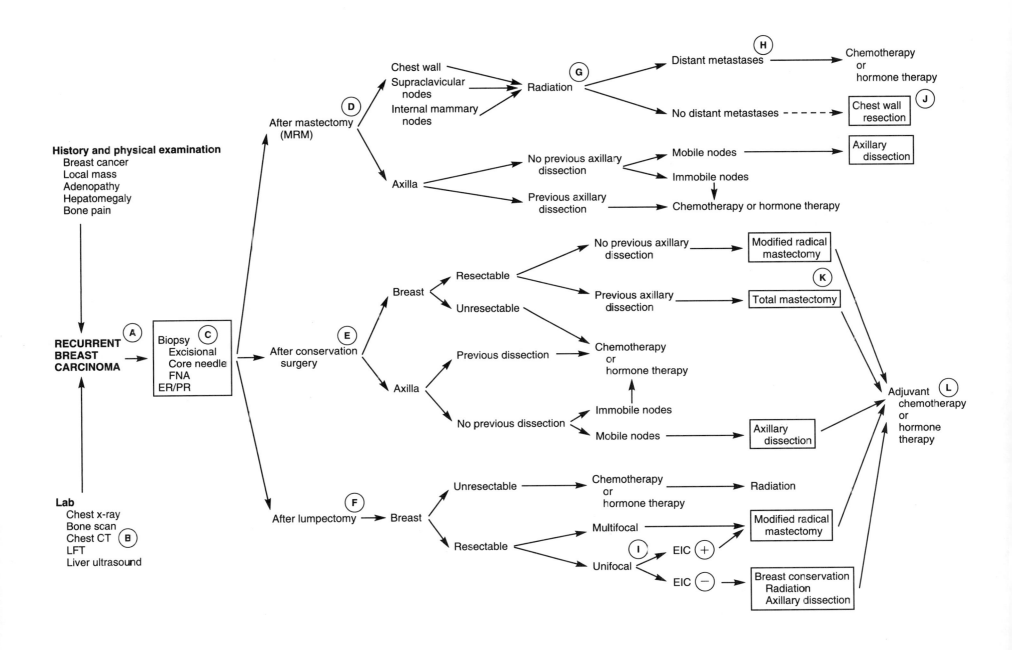

Hodgkin's Disease

Walter D. Holder, Jr., M.D.

(A) The characteristic history of Hodgkin's disease includes progressive adenopathy unresponsive to antibiotics, weight loss, night sweats, and recurrent spiking fever. The usual age of onset is between 15 and 34 years, but Hodgkin's disease may occur after age 50. Males are affected more frequently than females (1.5:1).

(B) In order of frequency, cervical, mediastinal, and retroperitoneal nodes are involved.

(C) Initial laboratory studies include complete blood count (anemia or leukocytosis), liver function tests (liver metastases), and chest x-ray (widened mediastinum and pulmonary infiltrates).

(D) An entire abnormal lymph node should be excised and examined for routine microorganisms, fungi, and acid-fast bacteria. Histologic examination confirms the diagnosis and indicates prognosis. The Lukes-Butler classification from most to least favorable prognosis is lymphocyte predominance (10 to 15 percent), nodular sclerosis (20 to 50 percent), mixed cellularity (20 to 40 percent), and lymphocyte depletion (5 to 15 percent).

(E) An elevated alkaline phosphatase level correlates with a 30 to 40 percent probability of bone marrow involvement. Extensive liver metastases can also increase alkaline phosphatase.

(F) Patients with lymphomas and leukemias frequently have elevated uric acid levels because of rapid nucleic acid turnover in growing cancer cells. The uric acid level must be lowered to prevent gouty nephropathy.

(G) Asymptomatic patients with localized disease almost never have bone marrow involvement, and biopsy may be omitted. The chance of bone marrow involvement is greatest in patients with lymphocytic depletion and mixed cellularity

Hodgkin's disease. The possibility increases progressively in patients with symptoms, widespread adenopathy, liver function abnormalities, elevated alkaline phosphatase levels, and radiographic evidence of skeletal fibrosis.

(H) The diagnostic accuracy of lymphangiography is 80 to 90 percent. Its value is greatest in disease involving iliac and periaortic lymph nodes up to the level of the diaphragm. Contrast remains in the lymph nodes for as long as 2 years, providing a means of measuring response to treatment. Lymphangiography does not visualize celiac, splenic hilar, portal, or mesenteric lymph nodes.

(I) The major advantage of computed tomography scanning is its ability to visualize lymph nodes undetected by lymphangiography. Ultrasound is much less reliable than computed tomography scan and is limited by obesity and bowel gas. Computed tomography scan is limited by cost, radiation exposure, and inability to detect disease in small lymph nodes. It is not helpful in evaluating liver and spleen involvement unless disease is extensive.

(J) Liver or bone scan is obtained if there is clinical or chemical suspicion of involvement (eg, tenderness, jaundice, abnormal liver function). Liver scan is not necessary if abdominal computed tomography shows liver involvement.

(K) Chest computed tomography is useful to define mediastinal adenopathy and pulmonary involvement.

(L) Percutaneous needle biopsy of the liver may be done using computed tomography or ultrasound guidance when a lesion is localized and the bone marrow is negative. A blind biopsy may be done for hepatomegaly and functional abnormalities in the absence of a specific lesion.

(M) Staging laparotomy is used to identify patients who may be treated with radiation therapy alone. Staging laparotomy should not be done unless the outcome of staging will substantially affect treatment. About 10 to 20 percent of patients will have less disease and 20 to 30 percent of patients will have more disease than expected from clinical staging. The procedure is done through a midline laparotomy incision and includes right and left lobe biopsies of the liver (needle and wedge), splenectomy, and lymph node biopsies. Enlarged and lymphangiographically suspicious nodes are sampled, as are bilateral periaortic, splenic hilar, celiac, portal, mesenteric, and bilateral iliac nodes, even if they appear to be normal. Radiopaque clips are placed on the splenic pedicle, sites of node biopsies, and margins of tumor masses to aid the radiation therapist. Oophoropexy (moving the ovaries to the midline behind the uterus) is performed in premenopausal women to protect ovaries from radiation with a midline shield. The incidence of postsplenectomy sepsis with predominantly gram-positive organisms is 3 to 5 percent.

Current recommendations for staging laparotomy in Hodgkin's disease when radiation therapy alone is a treatment option are based on the clinical stage. *Clinical stage I:* IA men and women and anyone with IB should have staging laparotomy. Staging is not indicated in asymptomatic patients with bulky mediastinal disease (requires both radiation and chemotherapy), in women with disease limited to the mediastinum (5 percent risk of disease below diaphragm), and men with lymphocyte-predominant Hodgkin's disease (less than 5 percent risk of disease below diaphragm). *Clinical stage II:* everyone should undergo staging except patients with bulky mediastinal disease (requires both radiation and chemotherapy) and women 27 years of age or younger with minimal disease (9 percent risk of disease below diaphragm). *Clinical*

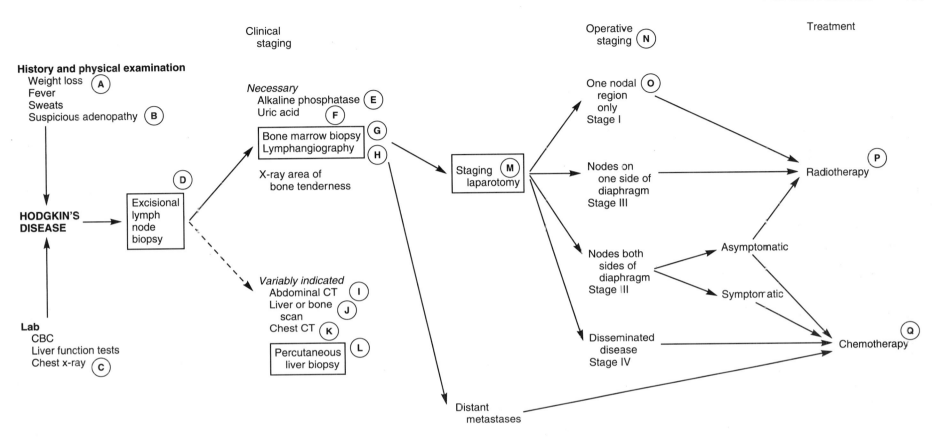

Clinical staging

History and physical examination
Weight loss (A)
Fever
Sweats
Suspicious adenopathy (B)

HODGKIN'S DISEASE

Excisional lymph node biopsy (D)

Necessary
Alkaline phosphatase (E)
Uric acid (F)
Bone marrow biopsy (G)
Lymphangiography (H)
X-ray area of bone tenderness

Variably indicated
Abdominal CT (I)
Liver or bone scan (J)
Chest CT (K)
Percutaneous liver biopsy (L)

Lab
CBC
Liver function tests
Chest x-ray (C)

Staging laparotomy (M)

Operative staging (N)

One nodal region only Stage I (O)

Nodes on one side of diaphragm Stage III

Nodes both sides of diaphragm Stage III

Disseminated disease Stage IV

Asymptomatic

Symptomatic

Distant metastases

Treatment

Radiotherapy (P)

Chemotherapy (Q)

---

stage III: all asymptomatic patients should be staged. Symptomatic patients require treatment with chemotherapy with or without radiation therapy and do not require staging. *Clinical stage IV:* staging is not indicated since all patients require chemotherapy with or without radiation therapy.

(N) After laparotomy, patients are staged according to the Ann Arbor classifications:

Stage I: involvement of a single lymph node region (I) or a single extralymphatic site (IE)
Stage II: involvement of two or more lymph node regions on the same side of the diaphragm (II), which may also include the spleen (IIS), localized extralymphatic involvement (IIE), or both (IISE), if confined to the same side of the diaphragm

Stage III: involvement of lymph node regions on both sides of the diaphragm (III), which may also include the spleen (IIIS), localized extralymphatic involvement (IIIE), or both (IIISE)
Stage IV: diffuse or disseminated involvement of extralymphatic sites (eg, bone marrow, liver, or pulmonary metastases)

Each stage is divided into A (asymptomatic) and B (symptomatic) categories. The latter includes 10 percent or greater unexplained weight loss in 6 months, prolonged fever greater than 38°C, and night sweats. Pruritus alone or short febrile illnesses do not constitute B symptoms.

(O) Surgical excision of lymph nodes in Hodgkin's disease is for diagnosis only and has no therapeutic benefit.

(P) Radiotherapy is usually given as "extended fields" (involved plus adjacent fields) for stages I and II or as "total nodal irradiation" for stage III. Any bulky disease may be treated with combined involved field radiation and chemotherapy. Stages IIIB and IV may be treated with combined radiation and chemotherapy. Complications of radiation therapy include hypothyroidism (20 to 70 percent), pneumonitis and pulmonary fibrosis (up to 90 percent), inhibition of bone growth in children, and possible acceleration of coronary artery disease in patients receiving mantle and mediastinal radiation.

(Q) Effective chemotherapy regimens usually include MOPP: nitrogen mustard (cyclophosphamide), vincristine (Oncovin), procarbazine, and

Hodgkin's Disease (Continued)

prednisone. Other effective combinations are ABVD (Adriamycin [doxorubicin hydrochloride], bleomycin, vinblastine, and dacarbazine) and PAVe (procarbazine, Alkeran [melphalan], and vinblastine). A complete response rate of 70 to 90 percent is usually achieved in patients with disseminated disease. Failure to respond implies mortality rates of 50 percent at 1 year and 90 percent at 2 years. Between 35 and 45 percent of patients have a complete remission relapse within 5 years but may respond to additional chemotherapy. Bone marrow transplantation may be considered in patients with poorly responsive disease. Patients who remain in remission beyond 5 years tend to remain disease-free in over 90 percent of cases. Complications of chemotherapy include sterility (up to 95 percent with MOPP), leukemia, and secondary tumors (10 to 30 percent).

REFERENCES

Cannon WB, Nelson TS. Staging of Hodgkin's disease: a surgical perspective. Am J Surg 1976; 131:224–230.

Carbone PP, Kaplan HS, Musskoff K, et al. Report of the committee on Hodgkin's disease staging classification. Cancer Res 1971; 31:1860.

DeVita VT, Simon RM, Hubbard SM, et al. Curability of advanced Hodgkin's disease with chemotherapy: long-term follow-up of MOPP-treated patients at NCI. Ann Intern Med 1980; 92:587–595.

Holder WD. Current management of lymphomas and Hodgkin's disease. In: Sabiston DC Jr, ed. Textbook of Surgery. 14th ed. Philadelphia: WB Saunders, 1991.

Hoppe R. The contemporary management of Hodgkin's disease. Radiology 1988; 169:297.

Leibenhout M, Hoppe R, Efron B, et al. Prognostic indicators of laparotomy findings in clinical stage I-II supradiaphragmatic Hodgkin's disease. J Clin Oncol 1989; 7:81.

Rosenberg S, Kaplan H. Malignant lymphomas: etiology, immunology, pathology, and treatment. New York: Academic Press, 1982.

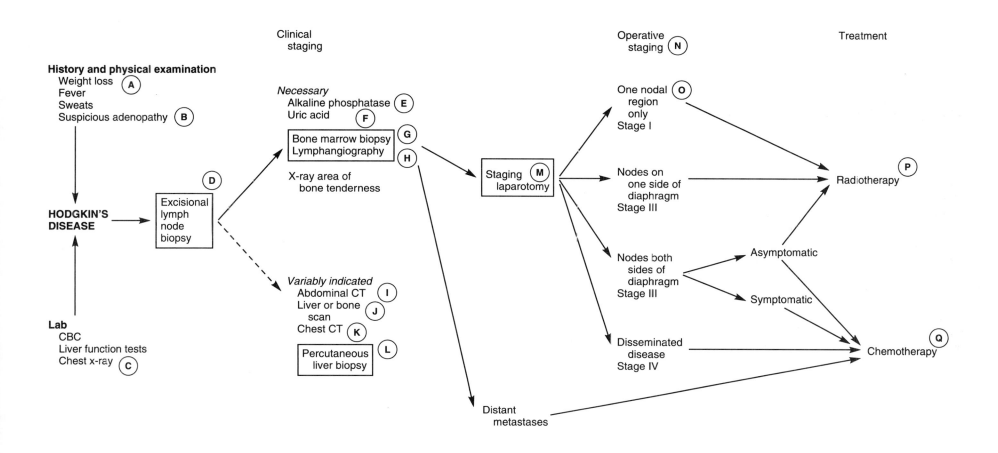

Retroperitoneal Mass

William C. Williard, M.D., and Murray F. Brennan, M.D.

(A) Primary retroperitoneal tumors constitute 0.07 to 0.5 percent of all neoplasms. Most (65 to 85 percent) are malignant. The differential diagnosis includes sarcoma (35 to 45 percent), lymphoma (25 to 35 percent), germ cell tumor (5 percent), retroperitoneal carcinoma (5 percent), undifferentiated malignant tumor, neuroblastoma, metastatic lesion, and malignant tumor of the retroperitoneal organs (pancreas, duodenum, adrenal glands, kidney, ureters, ascending and descending colon). The most common benign lesions are cysts, neurofibromas, paragangliomas, lipomas, leiomyomas, and tumors of the organs of the retroperitoneum.

(B) Complaints include abdominal mass (78 to 87 percent), abdominal or back pain (30 to 69 percent), gastrointestinal symptoms (26 to 49 percent), neurologic symptoms (27 percent), lower extremity pain (15 percent), urinary symptoms (7 to 10 percent), weight loss (7 to 55 percent), anorexia (44 percent), and lower extremity edema (14 percent).

(C) The most sensitive method of diagnosing a retroperitoneal mass is abdominal computed tomography scanning (89 percent). Magnetic resonance imaging may be helpful in determining vascular invasion and differentiating between an adrenal versus a renal mass. It is not as sensitive as computed tomography scanning.

(D) If the computed tomography scan indicates an adrenal mass, one must determine if the mass is functional or nonfunctional, benign or malignant. Tests of 24-hour urinary free cortisol, catecholamines, 17 ketosteroids, and plasma aldosterone will screen for functional tumors. Malignancy is suggested by a size greater than 6 cm, evidence of necrosis, large areas of calcification, enlarged regional lymph nodes, distant metastases, and the presence of virilization or feminization syndromes. T2-weighted images on magnetic resonance imaging can be helpful in differentiating adrenal masses with the signal intensity of the liver used as a standard reference. A high or moderate signal intensity is most consistent with a pheochromocytoma, adrenocortical carcinoma, or metastases; a low signal intensity most commonly represents functional or nonfunctional adenomas. Fine-needle aspiration can confirm malignancy.

(E) Surgery is not primary treatment for patients with lymphoma, retroperitoneal carcinoma, metastatic carcinoma, undifferentiated carcinoma, or germ cell tumors. Fine-needle aspiration should be attempted for diagnosis to prevent exploratory laparotomy in these patients. Fine-needle aspiration, when combined with immunocytochemical stains, is helpful in 66 percent of patients with retroperitoneal lymphoma.

(F) When an adrenal, vascular, lymphatic, or renal retroperitoneal mass is excluded, exploratory laparotomy with frozen-section biopsy of the tumor mass is indicated.

(G) Examination for other areas of lymphadenopathy is crucial for staging the disease and allowing a diagnosis to be made in a less invasive manner. If these diagnostic maneuvers are unsuccessful, exploratory laparotomy with frozen-section biopsy of the tumor is indicated.

(H) Nonfunctioning lesions less than 2.5 cm in diameter are almost always benign and should be followed with serial computed tomography scans at 3 months and yearly. If the mass increases in size, resection should be performed. Nonfunctioning lesions between 2.5 and 5 cm in diameter should be managed individually based on the patient's age and general health.

(I) Treatment of a suspected adrenocortical carcinoma consists of en bloc resection of the adrenal gland with regional lymph nodes and kidney through an anterior approach. Resection of hepatic, omental, and peritoneal metastases should also be performed to relieve endocrine symptoms associated with tumor. Morbidity after resection includes pneumothorax, pancreatitis, prolonged ileus, subphrenic abscess, splenic injury, hemorrhage, and infection. Operative mortality ranges from 0 to 5 percent. Mean overall survival of patients with adrenocortical carcinoma is 3.1 years. Five-year survival is 25 percent.

(J) Benign tumors should be completely resected to prevent recurrence and subsequent development of symptoms, provided the morbidity associated with complete resection is acceptable. If a patient's workup is consistent with paraganglioma, α-adrenergic blockade should be established before exploration.

(K) Every effort should be made to completely resect a retroperitoneal sarcoma. Complete resection is possible in 40 to 75 percent of these patients. Five-year survival for patients with complete resection is 54 to 74 percent and median survival is 60 to 76 months. Five-year survival of patients with incomplete resection is 0 to 33 percent and median survival is only 13 to 24 months, which is no better than results after biopsy alone. The only role for incomplete resection is to palliate or prevent symptoms. Twenty-five to 46 percent of patients with retroperitoneal sarcomas require nephrectomy. A bowel prep should be performed for possible colon resection. En bloc resection of other organs is required in 37 to 83 percent of patients. Major morbidity associated with resection is 6 to 14 percent. Thirty-day operative mortality is 2 to 6 percent. Local recurrence occurs in 40 to 86 percent of patients with complete resection and is a common cause of death. Complete resection of local recurrence (49 percent of local recurrences)

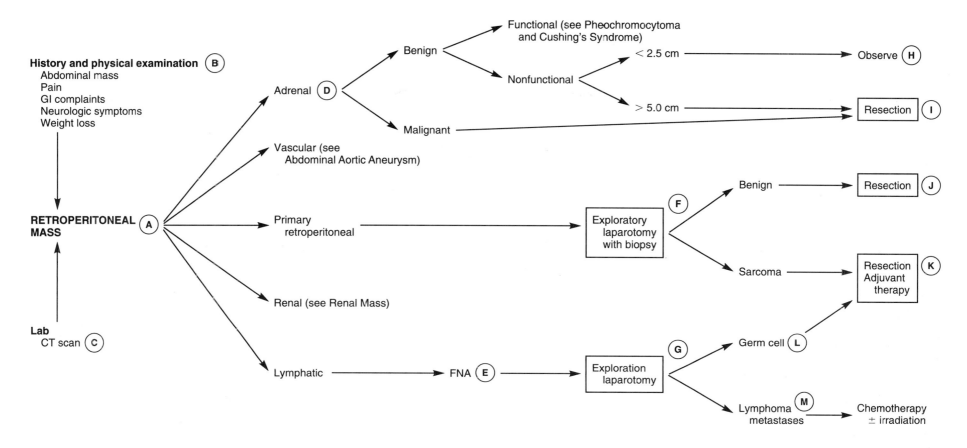

History and physical examination (B)
Abdominal mass
Pain
GI complaints
Neurologic symptoms
Weight loss

RETROPERITONEAL MASS (A)

Lab
CT scan (C)

Adrenal (D)

Benign → Functional (see Pheochromocytoma and Cushing's Syndrome)

Benign → Nonfunctional → < 2.5 cm → Observe (H)

Nonfunctional → > 5.0 cm → Resection (I)

Malignant → Resection (I)

Vascular (see Abdominal Aortic Aneurysm)

Primary retroperitoneal → Exploratory laparotomy with biopsy (F) → Benign → Resection (J)

Exploratory laparotomy with biopsy (F) → Sarcoma → Resection Adjuvant therapy (K)

Renal (see Renal Mass)

Lymphatic → FNA (E) → Exploration laparotomy (G) → Germ cell (L) → Resection Adjuvant therapy (K)

Exploration laparotomy (G) → Lymphoma metastases (M) → Chemotherapy ± irradiation

leads to median survival of 48 months compared with 15 months for patients with unresectable recurrences. Use of adjuvant therapy in retroperitoneal sarcomas is indicated because of the high local recurrence rate. Adjuvant chemotherapy and radiation therapy have not improved disease-free or overall survival or decreased local recurrence rates. Other forms of adjuvant therapy undergoing investigation include brachytherapy, intraoperative radiation therapy, photodynamic therapy, and hyperthermia.

(L) If germ cell tumor is suspected, human chorionic gonadotropin and α-fetoprotein levels should be obtained preoperatively. Testicular ultrasound rules out an occult primary in the testis.

(M) Treatment of patients with lymphoma, retroperitoneal carcinoma, undifferentiated tumors, and germ cell tumors is with chemotherapy and radiation therapy. Five-year survival rates for these tumors are lymphoma, 25 percent; metastatic carcinoma, 6 percent; undifferentiated carcinoma, 5 percent; seminoma, 85 percent; teratoma, 62 percent; choriocarcinoma, 26 percent; and mixed element tumors, 39 percent.

REFERENCES

Bevilacqua RG, Rogatko A, Hajdu S, Brennan MF. Prognostic factors in primary soft tissue sarcomas. Arch Surg 1991; 126:328–334.

Dalton RR, Donohue JH, Mucha P, et al. Management of retroperitoneal sarcomas. Surgery 1989; 106:725–33.

Jacques DP, Coit DG, Hajdu SI, Brennan MF. Management of primary and recurrent soft-tissue sarcoma of the retroperitoneum. Ann Surg 1990; 212:51–59.

Lane RH, Stephens DH, Reiman HM. Primary retroperitoneal neoplasms: CT findings in 90 cases with clinical and pathologic correlation. AJR 1989; 152:83–89.

Pinson CW, ReMine SG, Fletcher WS, Braasch JW. Long-term results with primary retroperitoneal tumors. Arch Surg 1989; 124:1168–1173.

Serio G, Tenchini P, Nifosi F, Iacono C. Surgical strategy in primary retroperitoneal tumors. Br J Surg 1989; 76:385–389.

Zhang G, Chen KC, Manivel C, Fraley EE. Sarcomas of the retroperitoneal and genitourinary tract. J Urol 1989; 141:1107–1110.

Melanoma

William A. Robinson, M.D., Ph.D.

(A) Biopsies should be performed on all suspicious nevi. Such lesions may be irregular in color and shape or be notable by recent growth, nodularity, ulceration, or bleeding.

(B) Patients with disease limited to the primary site (stage I) require complete blood count, liver function tests, and a chest x-ray. Those with regional lymph node metastases (stage II) require liver, brain, and, if indicated, bone scanning.

(C) Excisional biopsy is adequate for accurate microstaging of lesions 2 cm or less in diameter. Shave biopsy does not permit accurate microstaging and should be avoided. Incisional biopsy is used for lesions larger than 2 cm in diameter.

(D) Clark's system classifies primary melanoma histologically according to its microanatomic level of invasion into the dermis. A Clark level I lesion (in situ melanoma) is in the epidermis above an intact basal lamina. It is also known as atypical melanocytic hyperplasia and is regarded as benign. A Clark level II lesion penetrates through the basal lamina into the papillary dermis. A Clark level III lesion extends into the papillary reticular interface. A Clark level IV lesion invades into the reticular dermis, and a Clark level V lesion penetrates subcutaneous fat. The Breslow system quantitates depth of invasion or thickness of the lesion from the basal lamina. Breslow's system is easier to use and more accurate. Clark's levels and depth of invasion correlate with regional lymph node metastases and prognosis.

(E) The width of excision of primary melanoma is more dependent on depth of invasion than on size. For Clark level I and II lesions, 0.5 to 1 cm margins are adequate. For all other lesions, 2 cm margins are now considered reasonable and ensure a low likelihood of local recurrence. When regional nodes are clinically suspicious, regional lymph node dissection is performed. Nodes contain metastatic melanoma in 95 percent of such cases. Elective lymph node dissection in patients with clinically negative nodes is controversial. There may be some benefit in certain patients. Clark level III lesions have a 29 percent incidence of lymph node involvement; level IV lesions, a 42 percent incidence; and level V lesions, a 58 percent incidence. Because microstaging correlates with nodal involvement and nodal involvement correlates with survival, regional lymphadenectomy is the best method for accurate staging, for determining prognosis, and for identifying high-risk patients. Such patients may benefit from postoperative adjuvant therapy, which is of limited therapeutic value in those with clinically negative nodes. Based on currently available data, elective regional node dissection is not recommended in extremity melanomas with clinically negative nodes. For treatment of trunk melanomas, it is recommended only for deep lesions (Clark level IV and V) after lymphosintography.

(F) Melanomas arising on the trunk, particularly near the midline or belt line, and those near the neck can drain to more than one lymphatic area. A technetium (^{99}Tc) sulfur colloid lymphatic scan can determine into which lymph nodes the primary drains. Those nodes are then removed.

(G) Follow-up of stage I patients consists of physical examination, chest x-ray, complete blood count, and liver function tests. The interval for testing is based on the level of invasion of the primary lesion. The number of yearly follow-up visits is roughly equivalent to the Clark level. Patients with node metastases should be seen at least four times per year. New pigmented lesions should be biopsied because multiple primary melanomas occur in up to 5 percent of patients.

(H) Depth of invasion of the primary and the presence or absence of regional lymph node metastases are the two most important prognostic factors.

(I) Patients with regional node metastases have a greater than 50 percent chance of recurrence within the first 5 years after lymphadenectomy. Adjuvant therapy is seldom effective. A number of current studies are underway to evaluate immunotherapy with interferons, interleukin-2, and tumor cell vaccines and should be considered in all patients at high risk for recurrences.

(J) Most patients with local recurrence eventually develop systemic metastatic disease. About 20 percent of patients with local recurrence do not develop systemic disease and are long-term survivors after therapy. Treatment choices include local injection of immunotherapeutic agents, local hyperthermia, and radiation after wide local excision. For multiple skin or subcutaneous recurrences in an extremity, isolated limb perfusion with a number of chemotherapy drugs or hyperthermia has been used.

(K) The most common sites of metastases are lung, liver, brain, and the gastrointestinal tract. Most patients have multiple areas of involvement and die within 6 to 12 months. Surgical excision of brain metastases should be considered since other forms of therapy are of minimum benefit. Solitary lung metastases and bleeding areas of gastrointestinal involvement should also be considered for surgical removal. For bone metastases, radiation therapy can relieve pain. It is of little benefit for other metastases except for multiple brain metastases, where some palliation is possible. Systemic treatment produces responses in 20 to 30 percent, but only rare cures. Current choices are combination chemotherapy (dicarbazine and cis-platinum) with tamoxifen, α-interferon, and,

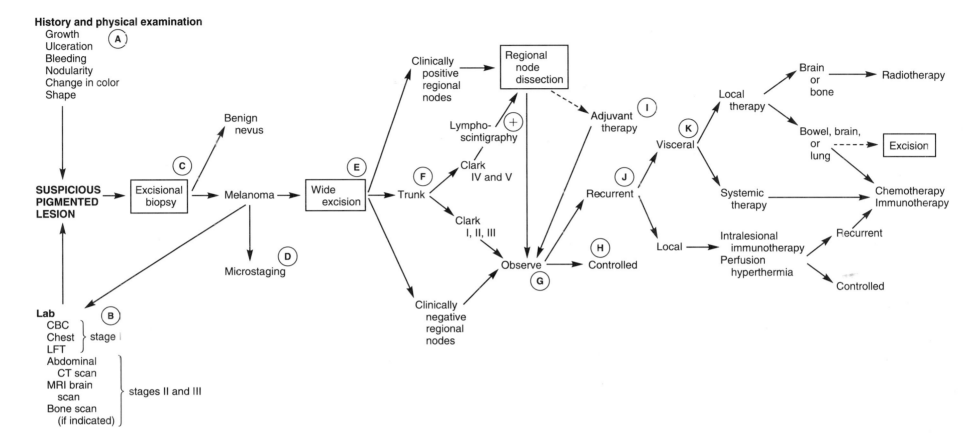

History and physical examination
Growth (A)
Ulceration
Bleeding
Nodularity
Change in color
Shape

experimentally, interleukin-2 in combination with activated immune cells.

REFERENCES

Balch CH. The role of elective lymph node dissection in melanoma: rationale, results, and controversies. J Clin Oncol 1988; 6:163–172.

Brega K, Robinson WA, Winston K, et al. Surgical treatment of brain metastases in malignant melanoma. Cancer 1990; 66:2105–2110

Coit DG, Brennan MF. Extent of lymph node dissection in melanoma of the trunk or lower extremity. Arch Surg 1989; 124:162–166.

Edwards MJ, Soong Seng-Jaw, Boddie AW, et al. Isolated limb perfusion for localized melanoma of the extremity: a matched comparison of wide local excision with isolated limb perfusion and wide local excision alone. Arch Surg 1990; 125:317–321.

Karp NS, Boyd A, Depan HJ, et al. Thoracotomy for metastatic malignant melanoma of the lung. Surgery 1990; 107:256–261.

McClay EF, Mastrangelo MJ, Bellet RE, et al. Combination chemotherapy and hormonal therapy in the treatment of malignant melanoma. Cancer Treat Rep 1987; 71:465–469.

Norman J Jr, Cruse W, Ruas E, et al. The expanding role of lymphoscintography in the management of cutaneous melanoma. Surg 1989; 55:689–694.

Robinson WA, Mughal TI, Thomas MR, et al. Treatment of metastatic malignant melanoma with recombinant interferon Alpha 2. Immunobiology 1986; 172:275–282.

Rosenberg SA, Lotze MT, Muul LM, et al. A progress report on the treatment of 157 patients with advanced cancer using lymphokine-activated killer cells and interleukin-2 or high-dose interleukin-2 alone. N Engl J Med 1987; 316:889–897.

Veronesi U, Cascinelli N, Adamus J, et al. Primary cutaneous melanoma 2 mm less in thickness: results of a randomized study comparing wide with narrow surgical excision—a preliminary report. N Engl J Med 1988; 318:1159.

Veronesi V, Adamus J, Aubert C, et al. A randomized trial of adjuvant chemotherapy and immunotherapy in cutaneous melanoma. N Engl J Med 1982; 307:913–916.

Burns

John F. Hansbrough, M.D.

(A) Depth of burn, partial or full thickness, may be difficult to estimate immediately after injury. In adults, the percentage of body surface area (BSA) burned is estimated by the rule of nines (head, arm, each 9 percent; leg, front, and back of torso, each 18 percent). The extent of full-thickness burn injury determines survival as follows:

BSA Burned (%)	Mortality Rate (%)
<20	<2
20–30	2–5
30–40	10
>50	25 +

The extremes of age and the presence of inhalation injury substantially increase (as much as double or triple) mortality.

Hospitalization time for burn injury approximates 1 day per 1 percent of body surface area of injury. Cost per day in the intensive care unit (ICU) ranges from $3000 to $6000, whereas non-ICU care costs up to $1000 per day of hospitalization.

(B) Airway and pulmonary injuries most often follow burns sustained in closed areas and may require tracheal intubation. Evidence of inhalation injury includes burns about the face, nose, and mouth; singed nasal hairs; glottic edema; hoarseness and stridor; and production of carbonaceous sputum. Bronchoscopy confirms airway and pulmonary injury.

(C) The hematocrit may be high initially as a result of burn edema and resultant hemoconcentration but should fall with fluid replacement. If carboxyhemoglobin content is over 20 percent, 100 percent oxygen is given until levels fall to less than 5 percent or until the sensorium clears, since carbon monoxide accumulates in the brain. Extensive erythrocyte destruction occurs early after major burn injury. The resultant hemoglobinuria is not dangerous. Myoglobinemia and myoglobinuria result from muscle breakdown due to direct muscle

injury or to a compartment syndrome. Vigorous diuresis and bicarbonate therapy are required to prevent renal damage. Since myoglobin is concentrated in urine, serum myoglobin need not be followed.

(D) In an extensively burned patient, blood pressure and arterial blood gases are monitored using an arterial cannula. A catheter is placed to measure urine output every 30 to 60 minutes. A central venous catheter is passed. More invasive (Swan-Ganz) monitoring is helpful with burns in the elderly, with inhalation injury, or with massive burns (>70 percent body surface area).

(E) The volume of Ringer's lactate (mL) given during the first 24 hours is approximated by the formula: percent of total body surface burned × body weight in kilograms × 4. Half this volume is administered intravenously in the first 8 hours after the burn. Colloids are contraindicated until serum proteins fall (albumin < 1.8 g/dL). Blood may be required if erythrocyte destruction is massive. Hypertonic saline can reduce fluid needs and tissue edema but its use requires experience. Infusion rates must be modified according to urine output, vital signs, acid–base balance, and hemodynamic status. Patients with extensive and deep burns and those with inhalation injury usually require substantially more fluid than predicted.

(F) Hypercatabolism, protein wasting, and weight loss are severe after major burns. Enteral nutrition with high protein feedings should be initiated on the first day of injury and advanced as tolerated. Central hyperalimentation often results in catheter and systemic sepsis and should be avoided. With continuous enteral feeding, antacids and H_2 blockers to control stress ulcer bleeding are unnecessary unless the feeding tube traverses the pylorus.

(G) Circumferential, constricting eschars on the extremities lead to deep tissue necrosis. Doppler ultrasonography may detect arterial pulses after tissue blood flow ceases. Direct measurement of compartment pressures with a catheter and transducer accurately diagnoses a compartment syndrome (compartment pressure >30 torr). With massive, deep burns, escharotomy may proceed without evaluation of compartment pressures. Constriction of the chest by eschar can limit respiration. Prompt release is critical.

(H) Silver sulfadiazine and mafenide acetate are the most useful topical antimicrobial agents. Wounds are debrided and topical agents reapplied, usually twice a day. Mafenide acetate penetrates burn eschar better than silver sulfadiazine but causes pain on application and metabolic acidosis. Therapy may be alternated. Systemic antibiotics are not useful in the acute period.

(I) Biologic dressings for superficial partial-thickness wounds include pigskin and Biobrane. They eliminate further dressing changes, reduce pain, promote healing, and may allow earlier discharge from the hospital. Biobrane costs approximately $80 per square foot and pigskin costs approximately $100 per square foot. Cadaver allograft, also effective, is more expensive ($450 to $700 per square foot).

(J) Deep partial-thickness burns that require longer than 3 weeks to heal are candidates for early excision and grafting. Hospitalization time is less and functional outcome may be improved. Hospitalization costs may be increased, however, because of the cost of surgery.

(K) Operative debridement removes a nidus for bacterial growth, allows early graft coverage, improves functional results, and allows earlier hospital discharge. In patients with extensive burns,

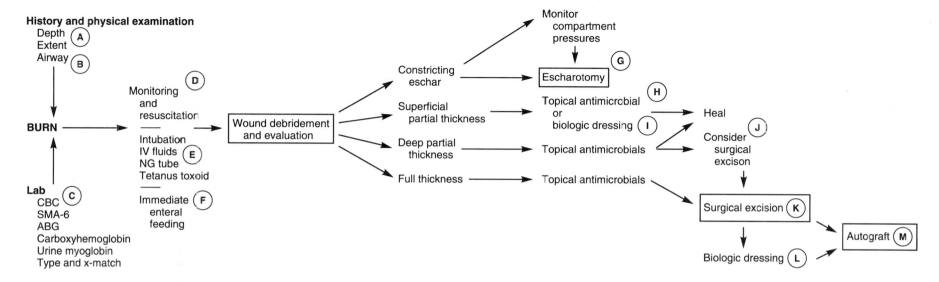

survival is improved compared with allowing gradual eschar separation. Techniques include tangential excision of the wound down to viable tissue with a dermatome or other instruments, or scalpel/electrocautery debridement to fat or fascia. Blood loss with tangential debridement averages as much as 0.5 to 1 unit of blood per percent total body surface area debrided, but graft take is excellent (approaching 100 percent). Blood loss with fascial debridement is much less. The procedure can be disfiguring, but graft take on fascia is excellent (nearly 100 percent). Graft take on fat can be poor (50 to 70 percent). Test grafting of the wound with cadaver allograft is expensive and mandates repeat surgery but it may avoid loss of valuable autograft skin.

L Biologic dressings for excised wounds include fresh or cryopreserved human cadaver allograft skin and Biobrane. Biologic dressings provide temporary coverage until autograft coverage is available. They control bacterial proliferation, reduce fluid loss and pain, and promote vascularization of the wound bed.

M Partial-thickness autografts from unburned areas provide permanent closure of full-thickness wounds. When meshed, they expand the area covered from 1.5 to 9 times. A single donor site may be used every 1 to 2 weeks after healing. Cultured cell sheets and matrices are being used for wound coverage, but graft take is not ideal (30 to 70 percent). The cost of commercial cultured epidermal sheets is high (up to $300,000/patient for extensive grafting).

REFERENCES

Compton C, Gill JM, Bradford DA, et al. Skin regenerated from cultured epithelial autografts on full-thickness wounds from 6 days to 5 years after grafting: a light, electron microscopic and immunohistochemical study. Lab Invest 1989; 60:600.

Dominioni L, Trocki O, Mochizuki H, et al. Prevention of severe postburn hypermetabolism and catabolism by immediate intragastric feeding. J Burn Care Rehab 1984; 5:106–112.

Goodwin CL, Dorethy J, Lam V, et al. Randomized trial of efficacy of crystalloid and colloid resuscitation on hemodynamic response and lung water following thermal injury. Ann Surg 1983; 197:520–531.

Hansbrough JF, Boyce ST, Cooper ML, et al. Burn wound closure with cultured autologous keratinocytes and fibroblasts attached to a collagen-glycosaminoglycan substrate. JAMA 1989; 262:2125–2130.

Hansbrough JF, Field TO, Dominic W, et al. Burns: critical decisions. Prob Crit Care 1987; 1:588–610.

Heimbach D, Luterman A, Burke J, et al. Artificial dermis for major burns: a multicenter randomized clinical trial. Ann Surg 1988; 208:313–320.

Hildreth MA, Herndon DN, Desai MH, et al. Current treatment reduces calories required to maintain weight in pediatric patients with burns. J Burn Care Rehab 1990; 11:405–409.

Saffle JR, Zeluff GR, Warden GD. Intramuscular pressure in the burned arm: measurement and response to escharotomy. Am J Surg 1980; 140:825–831.

Thompson PB, Herndon DN, Traber DL, et al. Effect on mortality of inhalation injury. J Trauma 1989; 26:163–165.

Tompkins RG, Remensnyder JP, Burke JF, et al. Significant reductions in mortality for children with burn injuries through the use of prompt eschar excision. Ann Surg 1988; 208:577–585.

Endocrine

Hyperthyroidism

R. Dale Liechty, M.D.

(A) New, sensitive thyroid stimulating hormone (TSH) assays ($72) have revolutionized thyroid function testing. TSH is always suppressed by elevated tetraiodothyronine (T_4) and triiodothyronine (T_3) levels, with the rare exception of pituitary hypersecretion of TSH. In virtually all other cases, a low TSH coupled with elevation of thyroid hormone levels indicates hyperthyroidism. A normal TSH rules out hyperthyroidism.

(B) In concert with TSH, free thyroxin (FT_4) ($34) and free thyroxin index (FT_4I) ($45) are the most reliable indices of thyroid function. FT_4, measured by direct equilibrium dialysis, is currently the "gold standard" for assessing free thyroxin levels. The FT_4I corrects for thyroid-binding protein abnormalities. The index results from a formula that factors in both T_4 and T_3 resin uptake values.

(C) Radioactive iodine uptake ($400) can clarify some confusing diagnoses. For example, in subacute thyroiditis the injured thyroid cells spill out T_3 and T_4, mimicking hyperthyroidism. The damaged thyroid gland cannot take up iodine as well as the thyrotoxic or normal gland does. The Jod-Basedow effect begins with excessive ingestion of iodine that initiates hyperthyroidism. The iodine flooding blocks the radioactive iodine uptake. Low uptake in the face of clinical toxicity, especially in an older patient with goiters, confirms the Jod-Basedow syndrome.

(D) In the euthyroid "sick" syndrome, acute illnesses (burns, trauma, operation, febrile illnesses, myocardial infarction) and chronic illnesses (renal, hepatic, cancer) inhibit conversion of T_4 to the more active T_3. The result is normal T_4, low T_3, and elevated reverse T_3. A high TSH suggests hypothyroidism. Failure to treat myxedema can be catastrophic in these critically ill patients. In the rare condition T_3 thyrotoxicosis, the patient appears toxic, TSH is suppressed, but FT_4 and FT_4I are normal. An elevated T_3 assay ($96) makes the diagnosis of T_3 toxicosis.

(E) With TSH low, FT_4 high, and radioactive iodine uptake elevated, the diagnosis of thyrotoxicosis is confirmed. The radioactive iodine scintiscan ($400) can differentiate the source of the thyrotoxicosis, for example, diffuse goiter, solitary or multiple toxic nodules.

(F) Medical therapy is used only to control symptoms while awaiting definitive therapy. Toxic nodules require large and often repeated doses of radioactive iodine. Lobectomy and subtotal thyroidectomy are ideal treatments, but often the critical condition of older patients prohibits operative treatment. Although it blocks radioactive iodine uptake, amiodarone, an iodine-containing antiarrhythmic agent, has initiated the Jod-Basedow effect in patients with goiters, necessitating thyroidectomy in some cases.

(G) Thiocarbamides produce remission in about 25 percent of thyrotoxic patients. This is about half as effective as 20 years ago, perhaps because of more iodine in the diet. Dose-related complications such as pruritus and granulocytopenia occur in 4.4 percent of patients. β-blockers control symptoms (cardiac overactivity, sweating, tremulousness, agitation), but serum concentrations of T_3 and T_4 remain elevated. This is the most rapid method of preparing patients for operation, especially useful during pregnancy or when intervening disease (eg, acute cholecystitis) necessitates urgent operation. Available for both oral and parenteral use, β-blockers must be given before, during, and after operative procedures. Contraindications include congestive heart failure and asthma. Atropine is the antidote. β-blockers markedly decrease thyroid vascularity and thus reduce bleeding during thyroidectomy.

(H) Single doses of radioactive iodine ($996) produce remissions in 86 percent of thyrotoxic patients. Myxedema occurs in 15 percent of these patients within 1 year, with an annual increment of 2 to 3 percent. Multiple doses of radioactive iodine increase this risk. Although the incidences of thyroid cancer and leukemia have not increased after ^{131}I treatment, genetic damage is slightly increased. The normal risk is 4.0 percent. After treatment with ^{131}I, it is 4.025 percent.

(I) Subtotal thyroidectomy ($6000) previously produced a 6 to 75 percent incidence of myxedema. Less extensive gland resection, leaving 8 to 16 g intact, is equally effective in curing hyperthyroidism and has a 2 to 9 percent incidence of myxedema. Drug treatment requires excessively large doses of ^{131}I or lifetime administration of antithyroid drugs.

(J) Complications from subtotal thyroidectomy include:

Mortality	0.3%
Hypoparathyroidism	3.7%
Vocal cord paresis	0.6%
Hemorrhage	1.9%

(K) In experienced hands, complications rates after modified subtotal thyroidectomy (also preserving inferior thyroid arteries) are:

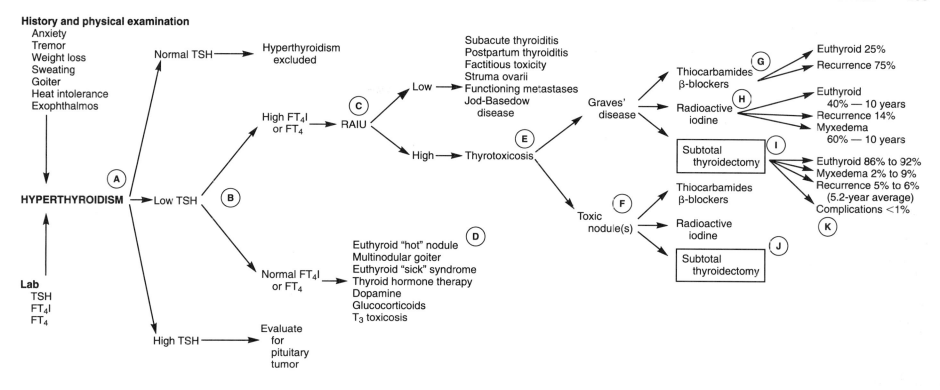

History and physical examination
- Anxiety
- Tremor
- Weight loss
- Sweating
- Goiter
- Heat intolerance
- Exophthalmos

HYPERTHYROIDISM

Lab
- TSH
- FT₄I
- FT₄

A → Normal TSH → Hyperthyroidism excluded

A → Low TSH (B)
- High FT₄I or FT₄ → RAIU (C)
  - Low → Subacute thyroiditis, Postpartum thyroiditis, Factitious toxicity, Struma ovarii, Functioning metastases, Jod-Basedow disease
  - High → Thyrotoxicosis (E)
    - Graves' disease
      - Thiocarbamides β-blockers (G) → Euthyroid 25%, Recurrence 75%
      - Radioactive iodine (H) → Euthyroid 40% — 10 years, Recurrence 14%, Myxedema 60% — 10 years
      - Subtotal thyroidectomy (I)
    - Toxic nodule(s) (F)
      - Thiocarbamides β-blockers
      - Radioactive iodine
      - Subtotal thyroidectomy (J)
  - (I, K) → Euthyroid 86% to 92%, Myxedema 2% to 9%, Recurrence 5% to 6% (5.2-year average), Complications <1%
- Normal FT₄I or FT₄ (D) → Euthyroid "hot" nodule, Multinodular goiter, Euthyroid "sick" syndrome, Thyroid hormone therapy, Dopamine, Glucocorticoids, T₃ toxicosis

A → High TSH → Evaluate for pituitary tumor

Recurrent nerve injury	
Transient bilateral	0%
Transient unilateral	0.6%
Permanent bilateral	0%
Permanent unilateral	0%
Tetany	
Transient	3%
Permanent	0%
Wound	
Infection	1%
Suture reaction	0.5%
Tracheostomy	0%
Deaths	0%

REFERENCES

Bradley EL, Liechty RD. Modified subtotal thyroidectomy for Graves' disease: a two institution study. Surgery 1984; 94:955–960.

Clark OH. Endocrine surgery of the thyroid and parathyroid glands. St. Louis: CV Mosby, 1985:56–90.

DeGroot LJ. The thyroid and its diseases. New York: John Wiley & Sons, 1984.

Edis AJ, Ayala LA, Egdahl RH. Manual of endocrine surgery. New York: Springer-Verlag, 1975:66–79.

Goldsmith RE. Radioisotope therapy for Graves' disease. Mayo Clin Proc 1972; 47:953–963.

Gough AL, Neil RW. Partial thyroidectomy for thyrotoxicosis. Br J Surg 1974; 61:939–943.

Greenfield LJ. Complications in surgery and trauma. Philadelphia: JB Lippincott, 1990.

Greenspan FS. Basic and clinical endocrinology. Norwalk: Lange, 1991:236–244.

Ivy HK, Wahner HW, Gorman CA. Tri-iodothyronine (T₃) toxicosis: its role in Graves' disease. Arch Intern Med 1971; 128:529–533.

Lee TC, Coffey RJ, Mackin J, et al. The use of propranolol in the surgical treatment of thyrotoxic patients. Ann Surg 1973; 177:643–649.

Starling JR, Thomas CG. Experience with the use of propranolol in the surgical management of thyrotoxicosis. World J Surg 1977; 1:251–255.

Wartofsky L. Low remission after therapy for Graves's disease: possible relations of dietary iodine with antithyroid therapy results. JAMA 1973; 225:1083–1090.

Thyroid Nodule

R. Dale Liechty, M.D.

(A) Important factors in a history for thyroid nodule include duration, voice change, age, toxicity, growth rate, and radiation exposure.

(B) Important factors in physical examination include consistency, fixation, regional nodes, and hoarseness.

(C) A normal thyroid stimulating hormone assay (the most precise test) ($72) rules out both hyperthyroidism and hypothyroidism.

(D) Needle aspiration has largely replaced ultrasonography for evaluating nodules. It provides cyst fluid or tissue for gross and cytologic diagnosis. High-resolution (10 MHz) ultrasound images ($220) are helpful in patients with thick necks.

(E) Scintiscans ($280) provide a map of the uptake of technetium by the thyroid gland. Although cancers are "cold," so are all cysts and most adenomas.

(F) Solitary thyroid nodules should be considered malignant (28 percent) until proved benign. Conversely, multinodular glands are benign unless findings suggest malignancy. At least 50 percent of clinically solitary nodules are in fact one dominant nodule in a multinodular gland.

(G) Multinodular goiter is more frequent with increasing age and six to nine times as frequent in women as in men. If it lacks suspicious characteristics, it is treated with a trial of suppression therapy. If nodules continue to grow they are excised.

(H) Fine-needle aspiration cytology ($245) is the single most important diagnostic aid. It detects cysts and yields material for cytologic study. This requires a trained cytologist. The procedure obviates operation in about 80 percent of patients. The false-negative rate is 10 percent. The danger of seeding malignant cells is minimal. Large cutting-needle biopsies ($230) can help in diagnosing equivocal lesions.

(I) Signs that a thyroid nodule may be malignant include firmness, voice change, fixation, local lymphadenopathy and rapid growth. Male gender, occurrence in children, and previous neck radiation also suggest malignancy.

(J) Soft nodules arising during pregnancy warrant a trial of suppression therapy for 3 to 6 months. Most nodules regress postpartum.

(K) Ninety percent of cysts disappear after aspiration. Cysts that persist after two or three aspirations require excision.

(L) Colloid goiter is the most common benign diagnosis (80 percent). Lymphocytic thyroiditis can be confirmed by aspiration of identical material from the opposite lobe. Papillary and medullary cancers are readily recognized. Differentiating follicular cancer from follicular adenomas can become a difficult problem.

(M) Suppression is accomplished with levothyroxine (Synthroid) 100 to 150 µg daily ($60/year).

(N) Selection of patients by fine-needle aspiration cytology has increased the incidence of cancer in surgical specimens from about 28 to 50 percent. The mortality rate of thyroid lobectomy ($5100) for a thyroid nodule is that of the anesthesia. Morbidity includes recurrent nerve injury (permanent <0.1 percent), myxedema (<1 percent), tetany (<0.1 percent), and wound infection (0.1 percent).

(O) The mortality rate with subtotal thyroidectomy is 0.1 percent. Morbidity includes single recurrent nerve injury (0.4 percent), injury to both nerves (0.1 percent), permanent tetany (0.1 percent), myxedema (5 percent), reoperation for bleeding (0.1 percent), and wound infection (0.5 percent). Incidence of malignancy in multinodular glands varies from 4 to 17 percent. Patient selection for operation and the benign course of many malignant thyroid tumors account for the discrepancy between the high incidence of cancer in thyroid nodules and the low death rate from thyroid cancer (6 persons/million/year). Needle biopsy of especially suspicious nodules should precede thyroidectomy.

REFERENCES

Arganini M, Behar R, Wu TC, et al. Hurtle cell tumors: a twenty-five year experience. Surgery 1986; 100:1108–1113.

Brooks JR. The solitary nodule. Am J Surg 1973; 125:477–481.

Colcock BP, King ML. The mortality and morbidity of thyroid surgery. Surg Gynecol Obstet 1962; 144:313–316.

Cole W. The treatment of non-toxic nodular goiter with desiccated thyroid. Surgery 1965; 58:621–627.

Hill LD, Beebe HG, Hipp R, et al. Thyroid suppression. Arch Surg 1974; 108:403–408.

Liechty RD, Graham J, Freemeyer P. Benign solitary thyroid nodules. Surg Gynecol Obstet 1965; 121:511–515.

Lowhagen T, Willem JS, Lundell G. Aspiration biopsy cytology in diagnosis of thyroid cancer. World J Surg 1981; 5:61–73.

Thomas CG Jr, Buckwalter JA, Staab EV, et al. Evaluation of dominant thyroid masses. Ann Surg 1976; 183:463–469.

Thompson NW. The thyroid nodule—surgical management. In: Johnston IDA, Thompson NW, eds. Endocrine surgery. London: Butterworth, 1983; 14–24.

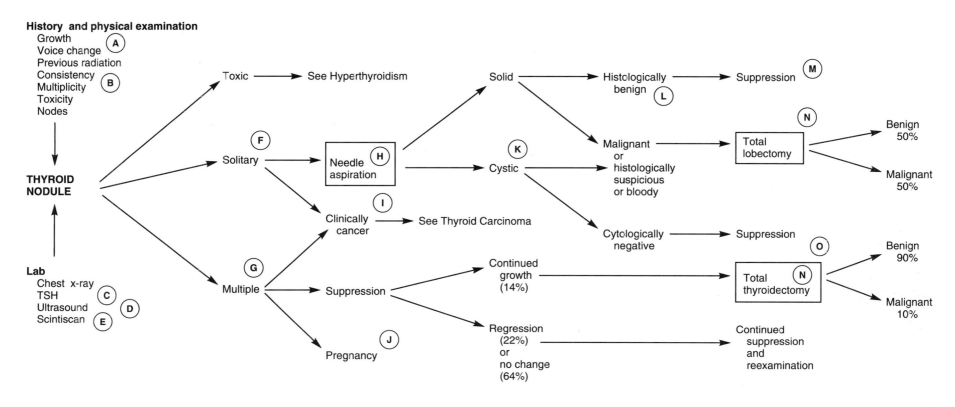

History and physical examination
Growth (A)
Voice change
Previous radiation
Consistency (B)
Multiplicity
Toxicity
Nodes

THYROID NODULE

Lab
Chest x-ray
TSH (C)
Ultrasound (D)
Scintiscan (E)

Toxic → See Hyperthyroidism

Solitary (F) → Needle aspiration (H)

Clinically cancer (I) → See Thyroid Carcinoma

Multiple (G)

Suppression

Pregnancy (J)

Solid → Histologically benign (L) → Suppression (M)

→ Malignant or histologically suspicious or bloody

Cystic (K)

→ Cytologically negative → Suppression

Total lobectomy (N) → Benign 50%
→ Malignant 50%

Continued growth (14%) → Total thyroidectomy (N)(O) → Benign 90%
→ Malignant 10%

Regression (22%) or no change (64%) → Continued suppression and reexamination

Thyroid Carcinoma

Clive S. Grant, M.D.

(A) Four percent of the adult population in the United States has clinical thyroid nodules. Fewer than 5 percent of these nodules are malignant. Previously only 10 to 20 percent of excised thyroid nodules proved malignant and up to 15 percent of proven malignancies may have been incorrectly assessed clinically as benign.

(B) About 25 percent of patients who had neck radiation in childhood will have a palpable thyroid nodule. Of these, about one third (8.5 percent overall) will have thyroid cancer, which may be occult and separate from the nodule. Although some advise total thyroidectomy for all irradiated patients with a nodule, conclusive data to support this advice are lacking.

(C) A hot nodule on scintiscan essentially excludes the chance of malignancy.

(D) Fine-needle aspiration is a safe, reliable, inexpensive, expedient, minimally invasive, and virtually risk-free technique for diagnosing thyroid nodules. It requires experience in thyroid needle aspiration and an expert cytopathologist

(E) With minimal invasion, 10-year and 20-year survival rates approach 100 percent. With extensive invasion, the 10-year survival rate is 40 percent.

(F) Follicular cancers with papillary components behave like papillary cancers and should be so treated. Ten-year and 20-year survival rates are 90 to 95 percent.

(G) Family members of patients with medullary carcinoma should be screened for multiple endocrine neoplasia (MEN-II) syndrome. Up to 10 percent may be index cases for this autosomal dominant disease. If disease is confined to the thyroid, 5-year and 10-year survival rates are 97 percent. With higher stage disease, the 5-year survival rate is 65 percent.

(H) There is no curative treatment for anaplastic thyroid cancer. Preoperative radiotherapy may permit palliative resection. There are few 5-year survivors.

(I) With tumor in the thyroid only, the 5-year survival rate is 86 percent. If the tumor is extrathyroid, the 5-year survival rate is 38 percent.

(J) Near-total thyroidectomy implies total lobectomy on the side of the cancer and contralateral subtotal or near-total lobectomy, leaving only enough thyroid to protect parathyroid vascular supply. Although controversial, this minimizes recurrent laryngeal nerve damage and hypoparathyroidism while excising multicentric lesions, facilitating ^{131}I ablation, and minimizing local recurrence in the thyroid.

(K) Excision may be impossible. Debulking is of questionable value. Tracheostomy may be required.

(L) Preserving the jugular vein, sternocleidomastoid muscle, and spinal accessory nerve during dissection of the posterior triangle and jugular nodes constitutes a modified neck dissection.

(M) ^{131}I thyroid remnant ablation has not proved to either diminish recurrence or prolong survival but its use is reasonably supported in the literature.

Dose ^{131}I
Cervical scan, 1 mCi
Whole-body scan, 3 mCi
Thyroid remnant ablation, 30 mCi
Metastasis therapy, 100 to 200 mCi

(N) Experimental and clinical evidence supports lifelong thyroid hormone suppression postoperatively in patients with papillary and follicular carcinoma.

(O) Thyroid hormone replacement therapy is necessary after total thyroidectomy for medullary carcinoma.

Short term, Cytomel (T_3) 25 μg orally three times a day
Long term, Synthroid (T_4) 0.15 to 0.3 mg orally daily

REFERENCES

Beahrs OH. Irradiation-related thyroid cancer: workshop on late effects of irradiation to the head and neck in infancy and children. Department of Health, Education, and Welfare Publication No (NIH) 77–1120, 1975.

Devine RM, Edis AJ, Banks PM. Primary lymphoma of the thyroid: a review of the Mayo Clinic experience through 1978. World J Surg 1981; 5:33–38.

Grant CS, Hay ID, Gough IR, et al. Local recurrence in papillary thyroid carcinoma: is extent of surgery resection important? Surgery 1988; 104:954–962.

Grant CS, Hay ID, Gough IR, et al. Long-term follow-up of patients with benign thyroid fine needle aspiration cytologic diagnoses. Surgery 1989; 106:980–986.

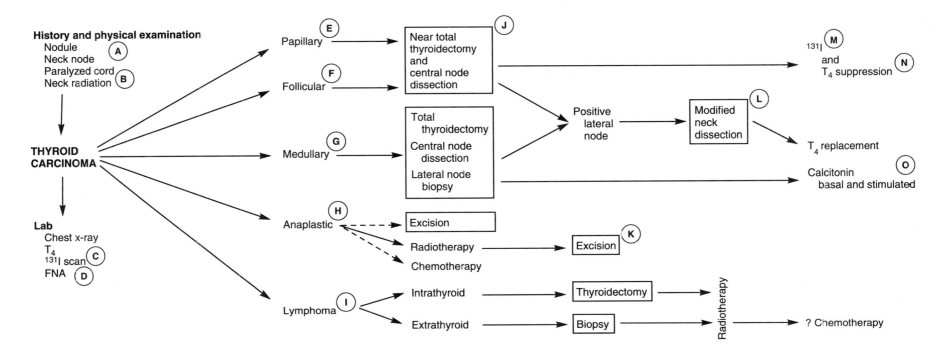

Hamburger JL, Miller JM, Kimi SR. Clinical pathological evaluation of thyroid nodules handbook and atlas. Southfield, MI: Limited edition, private publication, 1979.

Hay ID, Grant CS, Taylor WF, et al. Ipsilateral lobectomy versus bilateral lobar resection in papillary thyroid carcinoma: a retrospective analysis of surgical outcome using a novel prognostic scoring system. Surgery 1987; 102:1088–1095.

Hay ID, Ryan JJ, Grant CS, et al. Prognostic significance of nondiploid DNA determined by flow cytometry in sporacid and familial medullary thyroid carcinoma. Surgery 1990; 108:972–980.

Russell CF, van Heerden JA, Sizemore GW, et al. The surgical management of medullary thyroid carcinoma. Am Surg 1983; 197:42–48.

Snyder J, Gorman C, Scanlan P. Thyroid remnant ablation: questionable pursuit of an ill-defined goal. J Nucl Med 1983; 24:659–665.

Vander J, Gastson EA, Dawher TR. The significance of nontoxic thyroid nodules: final report of a 15-year study of the incidence of thyroid malignancy. Ann Intern Med 1968; 69:537–540.

Hypercalcemia and Hyperparathyroidism

Norman W. Thompson, M.D.

(A) Primary hyperparathyroidism (HPT) occurs in approximately 1 in 1000 people. The cause remains unknown except in those with previous neck radiation or genetic predisposition. Patients with familial HPT have chief cell hyperplasia rather than a single gland adenoma. The disease may be associated with other endocrine gland involvement (multiple endocrine neoplasia [MEN] syndrome, type I and type IIa). HPT is often asymptomatic when first diagnosed. History and physical examination can exclude other causes of hypercalcemia such as malignant disease with or without bone involvement. Two diseases causing hypercalcemia can occur concomitantly.

(B) Elevated serum calcium levels are the basis of diagnosis. Serum phosphorus levels are usually low and chloride is elevated in HPT when renal function is normal. When measured in milligrams per deciliter, the chloride-to-phosphorus ratio is greater than 33 in more than 90 percent of patients. An elevated intact parathyroid hormone (I-PTH) level confirms the diagnosis of HPT in close to 100 percent of patients. Urinary calcium levels are done to rule out benign familial hypocalciuric hypercalcemia, a rare entity that biochemically mimics HPT but requires no treatment. Calcium levels of less than 100 mg in a 24-hour collection suggest this diagnosis.

A chest x-ray is the only roentgenogram needed unless the patient has specific symptoms. Localization studies are neither cost-effective nor necessary in primary cases. A positive study does not rule out multigland disease.

(C) Neck exploration is done after the diagnosis is established. An effort is made to visualize at least four parathyroid glands. Exploration is terminated when an enlarged hyperplastic gland is excised or the surgeon is certain that no enlarged gland remains in the neck or cervically accessible mediastinum. Parathyroid adenoma arising in superior glands can always be excised through a cervical approach. Only 1 percent of inferior gland adenomas or hyperplastic glands require subsequent mediastinal exploration.

(D) Most patients with HPT (80 percent) have single gland enlargement (adenoma). Its excision "cures" the patient. The only reason for biopsy of a normal-sized gland is to be certain that the patient does not have asymmetrical hyperplasia.

(E) Double adenomas occur in about 2 to 4 percent of patients overall and in about 9 to 10 percent of those 65 years of age or older. The remaining normal-sized glands are normal histologically. These patients have neither a family history nor other endocrinopathy. The possibility of double adenomas is the reason for always exploring both sides of the neck.

(F) Normal superior glands can almost always be found just above the junction of the recurrent laryngeal nerve and the inferior thyroid artery. Adenomas are found there also, but in 40 percent they migrate to a retropharyngeal or paraesophageal location. They are rarely, if ever, intrathyroidal but may lie beneath the thyroid sheath. Inferior glands, if not found initially, can often be located in the upper thymus, the lower one third of the thyroid gland, or within the carotid sheath (undescended).

(G) Diffuse chief cell hyperplasia with rough symmetry of all glands occurs in patients with familial or sporadic hyperplasia (7 to 10 percent). Because of the frequency of a fifth or supernumerary gland (10 to 20 percent), cervical thymectomy should be done routinely. All glands are excised except a viable 50 mg remnant of one inferior gland tacked to the trachea with a metal clip. An optional procedure favored by many is total parathyroidectomy and forearm transplant. The MEN I syndrome should be ruled out in all hyperplasia patients.

(H) Hyperplastic parathyroids in MEN I patients are often asymmetrically enlarged. This is a clue to the syndrome. HPT will recur if resection is inadequate. Virtually all patients with MEN I syndrome have HPT.

(I) HPT is seen in only 20 to 30 percent of MEN IIa patients and is usually mild. After conservative surgical treatment by excising only the enlarged gland (1 or 2), recurrence is rare. Near-total or total parathyroidectomy risks needless permanent hypocalcemia and is not indicated. Total thyroidectomy is required in all cases of multicentric medullary carcinoma, however.

(J) Patients with suspected MEN I syndrome should have periodic evaluation for pituitary and pancreatic islet adenomas. The syndrome is an all or none phenomenon, and metachronous expression of disease is common. HPT patients with single adenomas do not need routine studies for other endocrine organ involvement.

(K) MEN IIa patients should have periodic evaluation for possible pheochromocytoma (40 to 50 percent). Hypercalcemia in a patient with suspected pheochromocytoma should be treated after the adrenal disease has been eliminated.

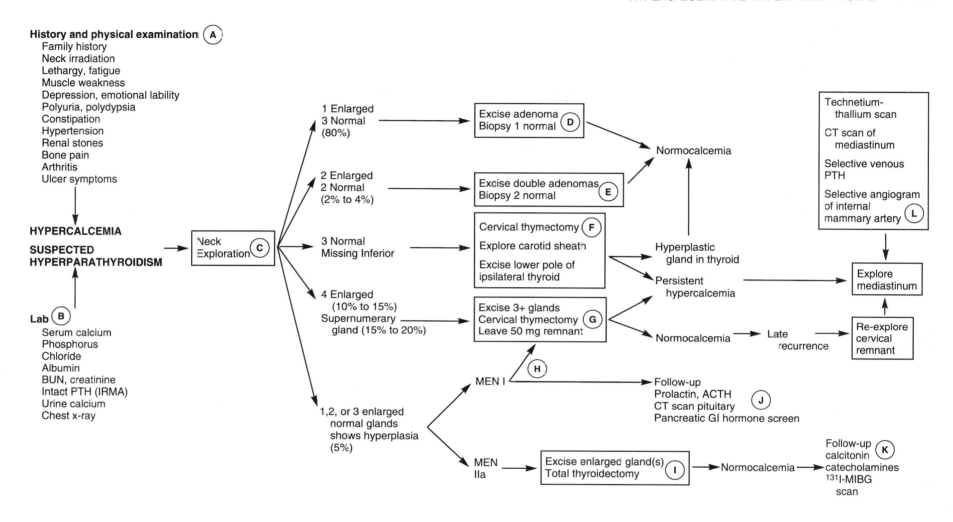

History and physical examination Ⓐ
- Family history
- Neck irradiation
- Lethargy, fatigue
- Muscle weakness
- Depression, emotional lability
- Polyuria, polydypsia
- Constipation
- Hypertension
- Renal stones
- Bone pain
- Arthritis
- Ulcer symptoms

HYPERCALCEMIA

SUSPECTED HYPERPARATHYROIDISM

Lab Ⓑ
- Serum calcium
- Phosphorus
- Chloride
- Albumin
- BUN, creatinine
- Intact PTH (IRMA)
- Urine calcium
- Chest x-ray

Neck Exploration Ⓒ

1 Enlarged
3 Normal
(80%)
→ Excise adenoma Biopsy 1 normal Ⓓ → Normocalcemia

2 Enlarged
2 Normal
(2% to 4%)
→ Excise double adenomas Biopsy 2 normal Ⓔ → Normocalcemia

3 Normal
Missing Inferior
→ Cervical thymectomy Ⓕ / Explore carotid sheath / Excise lower pole of ipsilateral thyroid → Hyperplastic gland in thyroid / Persistent hypercalcemia

4 Enlarged
(10% to 15%)
Supernumerary gland (15% to 20%)
→ Excise 3+ glands Cervical thymectomy Leave 50 mg remnant Ⓖ → Persistent hypercalcemia / Normocalcemia → Late recurrence

1,2, or 3 enlarged normal glands shows hyperplasia (5%)
→ MEN I Ⓗ → Follow-up Prolactin, ACTH CT scan pituitary Pancreatic GI hormone screen Ⓙ
→ MEN IIa → Excise enlarged gland(s) Total thyroidectomy Ⓘ → Normocalcemia → Follow-up Ⓚ calcitonin catecholamines 131I-MIBG scan

Technetium-thallium scan
CT scan of mediastinum
Selective venous PTH
Selective angiogram of internal mammary artery Ⓛ

→ Explore mediastinum

Re-explore cervical remnant

Ⓛ Mediastinal exploration is required in only 1 to 2 percent of all patients with HPT and only after the surgeon is convinced that the diseased gland is not in the neck. Invasive localization studies are justified in this group of patients, but only 60 to 70 percent of adenomas will be identified. Primary mediastinal exploration is done only in patients who have been in hypercalcemic crisis.

REFERENCES

Edis AJ, van Heerdon JA, Scholz DA. Results of subtotal parathyroidectomy for chief cell hyperplasia. Surgery 1979; 86:462–469.

Freeman JB, Sherman BN, Mason EF. Cervical thymectomy. Arch Surg 1979; 112:359–364.

Scholz AA, Purnell DC, Woolner IB, et al. Mediastinal hyperfunctioning parathyroid tumors. Ann Surg 1973; 178:173–178.

Thompson NW, Eckhauser FE, Harness JK. The anatomy of primary hyperparathyroidism. Surgery 1982; 92:814–822.

Thompson NW. The techniques of initial parathyroid exploration and reoperative parathyroidectomy. In: Thompson NW, Vinik AK, eds. Endocrine surgery update. New York: Grune & Stratton, 1983:365–384.

Wang CA. Parathyroid re-exploration, a clinical pathological study of 112 cases. Ann Surg 1977; 186:140–145.

Wells SA, Leight GS, Ross AJ. Primary hyperparathyroidism. Curr Probl Surg 1983: 17:400–483.

Insulinoma

R. Dale Liechty, M.D.

(A) Symptoms of insulinoma are due to cerebral glucopenia and hypoglycemic stimulation of compensatory catecholamines, which tend to correct the "attack." Whipple's diagnostic triad—hypoglycemia (<50 mg/dL) at the time of symptoms, associated low fasting blood glucose, and relief of symptoms by administration of glucose—is usually but not always present during fasting (before breakfast) or after exercise.

(B) An inappropriately high insulin level with synchronous hypoglycemia is the most accurate single sign of hyperinsulinism. Low insulin levels suggest the rare case of mesothelioma. Insulin-to-glucose ratios greater than 0.3 are diagnostic of hyperinsulinism.

(C) If diazoxide controls hypoglycemia preoperatively it should control it postoperatively. In the case of overlooked tumors, this chemical suppression allows time for additional localizing or diagnostic studies.

(D) In equivocal cases, prolonged fasting (by causing hypoglycemia) helps elicit hyperinsulinism.

(E) Arteriography has a diagnostic accuracy of 65 percent, venous insulin sampling has an accuracy of 89 percent, and magnetic resonance imaging has an accuracy of 72 percent. Endoscopic ultrasound, although promising, remains in the trial stage. Venous sampling has the distinct advantage of indicating hyperplasia (with no step-up insulin levels). If arteriography outlines a tumor, many authorities forgo other preoperative tests and proceed with celiotomy.

(F) Surgical palpation is accurate in 76 percent of cases, and intraoperative ultrasound is accurate in 90 percent. Intraoperative ultrasound can rule out multiple adenomas. It has become a reliable asset in localizing pancreatic tumors.

(G) When no tumor is found on exploration, frozen-section biopsy of the tail or the inferior edge of the body of the pancreas may disclose islet hyperplasia or nesidioblastosis. When present, particularly in infants, these lesions requires a total (>85 percent) distal pancreatectomy or diazoxide therapy if insulin release is suppressible.

(H) Most insulinomas (up to 90 percent) are single and benign and can be enucleated. The potential for surgical cure is high. Persistent postexcision hypoglycemia may indicate a second tumor. Hypoglycemia may occur temporarily even in the presence of a second tumor.

(I) When no hyperplasia is found, intraoperative ultrasound should be repeated to search for tumors. Blind distal pancreatectomy should be avoided since the yield (removing a functioning tumor) is less than 50 percent and the risk of diabetes is substantial. Rapid insulin assays (30 minutes) are not widely available.

(J) If an insulin-secreting carcinoma with hepatic metastases is present, palliation may be obtained by excision of the primary lesion (distal pancreatectomy) and intraoperative placement of an intraarterial catheter for hepatic artery chemotherapy with streptozocin. Diazoxide is used if insulin secretion is known to be suppressible.

(K) Prognosis after excision of a single insulinoma is excellent, but long-term follow-up shows that 25 percent of patients develop other endocrinopathies. If a patient has proven multiple endocrine neoplasia (MEN-I) syndrome, some authorities recommend subtotal pancreatectomy with enucleation of any tumors in the pancreatic head. This tactic recognizes the multiple nature of the tumor.

REFERENCES

Doherty GM, Doppman JL, Shawker TH. Results of a prospective strategy to diagnose, localize and resect insulinoma. Surgery 1991; 110:989–997.

Friesen SR. Tumors of the endocrine pancreas. N Engl J Med 1982; 306:580–593.

Galbut DL, Markowitz AM. Diagnosis, surgical management and long-term follow-up: review of 41 cases. Am J Surg 1980; 139:682–689.

Grant CS, van Heerden J, Charboneau JW. Insulinoma, the value of intra-operative ultrasound. Arch Surg 1988; 123:843–848.

Harrison TS. The hypoglycemic syndrome: endogenous hyperinsulinism. In: Friesen SR, ed. Surgical endocrinology: clinical syndromes. Philadelphia: JB Lippincott, 1978:150–167.

Sigel B, Durate B, Coelho JC, et al. Localization of insulinomas of the pancreas at operation by real-time ultrasound scanning. Surg Gynecol Obstet 1983; 156:145–151.

Vinik A, Delbridge L, Moattari R, et al. Transhepatic portal vein catheterization for localization of insulinomas: a ten-year experience. Surgery 1991; 100:1–11.

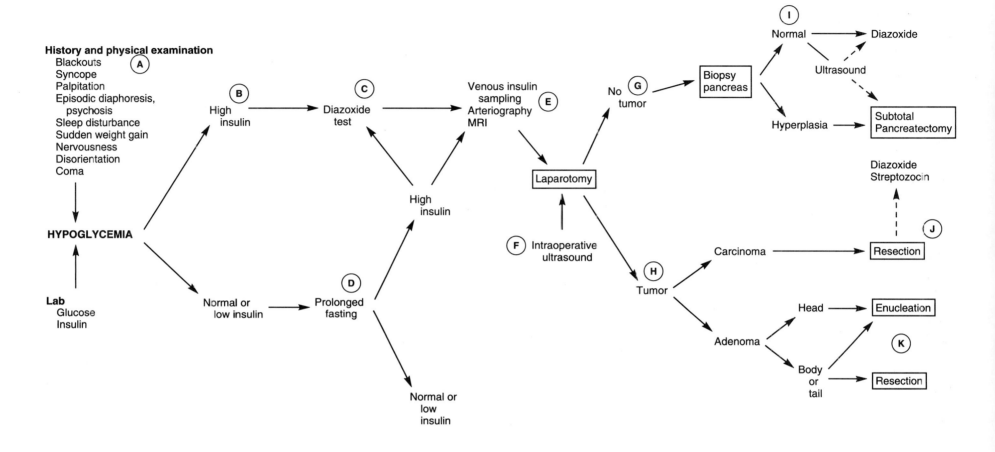

History and physical examination
(A)
Blackouts
Syncope
Palpitation
Episodic diaphoresis,
  psychosis
Sleep disturbance
Sudden weight gain
Nervousness
Disorientation
Coma

HYPOGLYCEMIA

Lab
Glucose
Insulin

(B) High insulin

(C) Diazoxide test

High insulin

(D) Prolonged fasting

Normal or low insulin

Normal or low insulin

Venous insulin sampling
Arteriography
MRI
(E)

Laparotomy

(F) Intraoperative ultrasound

No tumor (G)

Tumor (H)

Biopsy pancreas

Normal (I)

Hyperplasia

Diazoxide

Ultrasound

Subtotal Pancreatectomy

Carcinoma

Resection (J)

Diazoxide Streptozocin

Adenoma

Head → Enucleation

Body or tail

Enucleation

Resection (K)

Zollinger-Ellison Syndrome (Gastrinoma)

E. Christopher Ellison, M.D.

(A) Zollinger-Ellison syndrome (ZES) is caused by a gastrin-producing tumor (gastrinoma) that may arise primarily in the pancreas (65 percent), duodenum (20 percent), stomach (5 percent), or ectopic locations (10 percent).

(B) ZES should be suspected in cases of severe refractory ulcer disease, recurrence after medical or surgical treatment, and peptic ulcer disease in the very young or elderly. About 20 to 25 percent of patients have multiple endocrine neoplasia (MEN), usually MEN I.

(C) Fasting gastrin is measured in high-risk patients. An elevated gastrin is diagnostic of ZES only when acid hypersecretion is demonstrated (basal acid output [BAO] > 10 to 15 mEq/hr, BAO/maximal acid output [MAO] > 0.6). Normal or low acid secretion may be observed in a postoperative stomach in ZES. The most common cause of elevated gastrin is pernicious anemia. Gastric analysis identifies this group and eliminates unnecessary secretin provocation ($600). A test meal will cause gastrin to rise (usually twofold) in G cell hyperplasia. Secretin causes gastrin to rise in ZES (usually two- to three-fold). Elevations of 200 pg/mL over baseline are diagnostic.

(D) It is important to screen all patients for MEN I by analyzing calcium, parathormone, prolactin, and cortisol levels. A few patients may have MEN II (pheochromocytoma, medullary carcinoma of thyroid, hyperparathyroidism) or variations of these syndromes.

(E) Medical treatment is initiated with H_2 blockers (cimetidine, ranitidine, famotidine). Treatment should begin with twice the standard dose

and be titrated to maintain a BAO of less than 10 mEq/hr 1 hour before the next dose. H_2 blockers should be stopped 48 hours before the initial diagnostic gastric analysis. H_2 blockers may be continued during secretin provocation and a test meal, since they do not alter the response. H_2 blockers should be continued if good acid control and symptomatic relief are observed. Omeprazole, a hydrogen-potassium inhibitor, is the most effective method of acid control in ZES but also the most expensive. The starting dose of omeprazole (20 mg PO BID) is increased as needed. Because the effect of omeprazole on fasting gastrin and secretin provocation in ZES is not known, it should be discontinued before these tests.

(F) The initial goal of tumor location is to identify patients with hepatic metastases. Magnetic resonance imaging is 100 percent accurate. Computed tomography accuracy in identifying the primary tumor is 25 to 70 percent. Adding angiography to computed tomography doubles the accuracy. Upper endoscopy can identify duodenal primaries preoperatively. Portal venous sampling, a risky, costly ($1000), and work-intensive procedure, does not improve primary tumor localization and should not be done routinely. The negative predictive value of all localization procedures is only 40 percent. These tests cannot be used to predict a negative laparotomy.

(G) If elevated parathyroid hormone is identified, parathyroidectomy (3.5 glands) is warranted to allow better acid control. Aggressive resection of gastrinoma in this group is controversial. There are usually no cures (ie, normal gastrin) with aggressive

tumor resection in MEN patients and no prolongation or improvement in quality of life.

(H) Laparotomy is indicated in sporadic ZES without liver metastases even in the face of negative preoperative localization. Primary tumors amenable to resection are usually found in the gastrinoma triangle. An adequate exploration includes complete pancreatic mobilization and bimanual and visual inspection of the duodenum, necessitating pyloroplasty or duodenotomy. Intraoperative ultrasound may be helpful but is operator and instrument dependent and not reproducible. Laparotomy is not indicated in MEN because it does not alter outcome.

(I) Chemotherapy is indicated for liver metastases in selected situations. Fluorouracil and streptozotocin give a 60 percent response rate. It is not known whether chemotherapy prolongs survival. It does improve quality of life if used for symptoms related to the mass of tumor. Without chemotherapy, 5-year survival with liver metastases is 40 percent. Lymph node metastases are not an indication for chemotherapy. New agents such as chlorozotocin can improve response. Somatostatin analogues rarely cause tumor regression and are impractical for controlling acid hypersecretion.

(J) In 10 to 15 percent of patients no tumor is found. These patients have an excellent long prognosis (90 percent 10-year survival). Few develop liver or lymph node metastases and none die of the disease.

(K) Gastrinoma excision for isolated or multiple tumors in sporadic ZES results in cure in 20 to 30 percent of cases. Gastrin levels return to normal within 24 to 48 hours. Acid hypersecretion

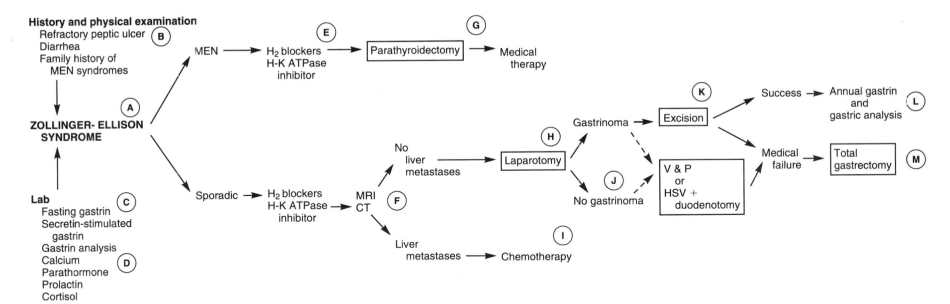

persists 3 months until regression of increased parietal cell mass. It is necessary to remeasure BAO after treatment before discontinuing medical therapy. Survival in this group exceeds 5 to 10 years. Recurrence rates are not known and yearly gastrin determinations are indicated. Controversy exists about the merits of highly selective vagotomy and duodenotomy vs. truncal vagotomy and pyloroplasty to further reduce acid secretion. Liver metastases preclude cure. Debulking may be indicated on a selective basis for tumor pain.

Ⓛ Long-term observation with yearly gastrin measurement is indicated in all patients. A rising gastrin level should prompt a search for late liver metastases. Magnetic resonance imaging is most efficient for this purpose.

Ⓜ Total gastrectomy is indicated only for medical failure or when complications such as gastrojejunocolic fistula occur after previous surgery.

REFERENCES

Andersen DK. Current diagnosis and management of Zollinger-Ellison syndrome. Ann Surg 1989; 210:685–703.

Cherner JA, Doppman JL, Norton JA, et al. Selective venous sampling for gastrin to localize gastrinomas. Ann Intern Med 1986; 105:841–847.

Ellison EC, Carey LC, Sparks J, et al. Early surgical treatment of gastrinoma. Am J Med 1987; 82:17–24.

Kvols LK, Buck M. Chemotherapy of metastatic carcinoid and islet cell tumors: a review. Am J Med 1987; 82(suppl 5B):77–83.

Maton PN, Miller DL, Doppman JL, et al. Role selective

angiography in the management of patients with Zollinger-Ellison syndrome. Gastroenterology 1987; 92:913–918.

Maton PN, Vinayek R, Frucht H, et al. Long-term efficacy and safety of omeprazole in patients with the Zollinger-Ellison syndrome: a prospective study. Gastroenterology 1989; 97:827–836.

Norton JA, Doppman JL, Gardner JD, et al. Aggressive resection of metastatic disease in selected patients with malignant gastrinoma. Ann Surg 1986; 203:352–359.

Sawicki MP, Howard TJ, Dalton M, et al. The dichotomous distribution of gastrinomas. Arch Surg 1990; 125:1584–1587.

Stabile BE, Morrow DJ, Passaro E. The gastrinoma triangle: operative implications. Am J Surg 1984; 147:25–31.

Wank SA, Doppman JL, Miller DI, et al. Prospective study of the ability of computed axial tomography to localize gastrinomas in patients with Zollinger-Ellison syndrome. Gastroenterology 1987; 92:905–912.

Wise SR, Johnson J, Ellison EC, et al. Gastrinoma: the predictive value of preoperative localization. Surgery 1989; 106:1087–1093.

Pheochromocytoma

Glenn W. Geelhoed, M.D., M.P.H.

(A) Screening all hypertensive patients for pheochromocytoma is not cost effective. The expected yield is less than 1 percent. Screening is reserved for those with features such as diabetes, arrhythmia, paroxysms, or panic attacks. The yield in such patients is 10 percent.

(B) Screening measures vanillylmandelic acid ($75), metanephrine ($90), and catecholamine ($85) in a 24-hour urine sample. Diagnosis is made by radioimmunoassay of plasma catecholamines ($230). High levels are found in 10 percent of atypical hypertensives who screen positively.

(C) Localization of pheochromocytoma is best accomplished by computed tomography scanning, although iodine-131 meta-iodobenzylguanidine (MIBG) scanning is an alternative. Computed tomography scan ($1070) sensitivity exceeds 95 percent. It should not be done with enteric contrast and glucagon to avoid catecholamine release. Ultrasonography ($360) can demonstrate large tumors but has a sensitivity of only 60 percent. Localization by arteriography is obsolete. Caval sampling by laminar flow techniques can lateralize tumors (75 percent) when catecholamine-to-steroid ratios are compared.

(D) Perioperative management consists of blood volume expansion, arrhythmia control, antihypertensive support, and crisis prevention. Hemoconcentration is a problem when the pheochromocytoma secretes predominantly norepinephrine. α-adrenergic blockade with phenoxybenzamine is used for significant hypertension and contracted blood volume (hematocrit > 50 percent). β-adrenergic blockade (propranolol) is useful for arrhythmia or tachycardia, particularly ectopic foci of ventricular origin, but β blockade alone without previous and concomitant α-adrenergic blockade risks pulmonary edema.

(E) Combined α and β blockade (labetalol) is useful for intraoperative instability, especially when preoperative preparation is rapid or contracted. Nitroprusside has replaced phentolamine as a short-acting agent for intraoperative hypertensive crisis. It is also useful if invasive localization studies are needed.

(F) Pheochromocytoma patients can be managed using calcium channel blockers alone. Avoiding antiadrenergic drugs reduces the time and cost of monitoring gradual vasodilation.

(G) An anterior transabdominal approach allows exploration of both adrenal glands and the entire chromaffin chain below the diaphragm. Because 10 percent of foci of multicentric pheochromocytoma are missed by preoperative localization, intraoperative ^{125}I MIBG scintiscanning can be used in the operating room. The keystone of adrenalectomy is early occlusion of the central adrenal vein. Only then is provocative testing for disease in the chromaffin chain or elsewhere appropriate. Operation is not concluded until the likelihood of intraabdominal second loci of chromaffin neoplasm is excluded.

(H) Adrenalectomy cures adrenal pheochromocytoma. Bilateral or ectopic tumors suggest the presence of multiple endocrine adenopathy. The multiple endocrine adenopathy patient should be screened for hyperparathyroidism and medullary thyroid cancer. The patient's family should be screened for multiple endocrine adenopathy.

(I) In some familial kindreds, the rate of multicentricity at the time of presentation is as high as 20 percent and the rate of malignancy is as high as 30 percent. Multiple agents are available to manage unresectable pheochromocytoma or recurrent disease until reoperation can reduce or remove tumor. Patients with slow-growing malignancies are unlikely to benefit from chemotherapy and irradiation. Prognosis is generally good after tumor debulking, and patients with metastatic pheochromocytoma can survive many years.

REFERENCES

Bravo EL, Tarazi RC, Gifford RW, et al. Circulating and urinary catecholamine in pheochromocytoma. N Engl J Med 1979; 301:682–686.

Geelhoed GW. CAT scans and catecholamines. Surgery 1980; 87:719–720.

Geelhoed GW. Pheochromocytoma. In: Problem management in endocrine surgery. Chicago: Yearbook Medical Publishers, 1983.

Gough IR, Thompson NW, Shapiro B, et al. Limitations of ^{123}-MIBG scintigraphy in locating pheochromocytomas. Surgery 1985; 98:115–119.

Harrison TS, Seaton JF, Cerny JC. Localization of pheochromocytoma by caval catheterization. Arch Surg 1967; 95:339.

Harrison TS, Gann DS, Edis AJ, et al. Surgical disorders of the adrenal gland. New York: Grune & Stratton, 1975.

Lipson A, Hsu IH, Sherwin B, et al. Nitroprusside in the management of a patient with pheochromocytoma. JAMA 1978; 239:427–428.

Manger WM, Tifford RW Jr. Pheochromocytoma. New York: Springer-Verlag, 1977.

Scott HW Jr. The panic syndrome: pheochromocytoma. In: Friesen SR. Surgical endocrinology, ed. 2. Philadelphia: JB Lippincott, 1991:163–181.

Sisson JC, Frager MS, Valk TW, et al. Scintigraphic localization of pheochromocytoma. N Engl J Med 1981; 305:12–17.

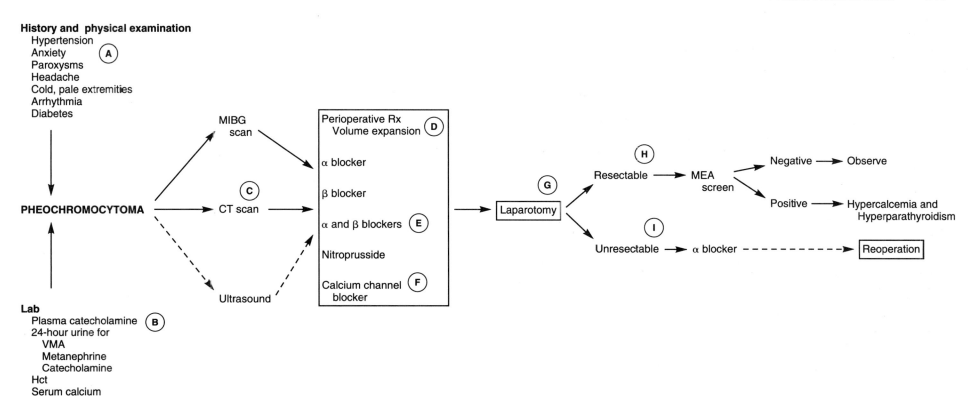

History and physical examination
- Hypertension
- Anxiety (A)
- Paroxysms
- Headache
- Cold, pale extremities
- Arrhythmia
- Diabetes

PHEOCHROMOCYTOMA

MIBG scan

CT scan (C)

Ultrasound

Lab
- Plasma catecholamine (B)
- 24-hour urine for
  - VMA
  - Metanephrine
  - Catecholamine
- Hct
- Serum calcium
- Serum calcitonin

Perioperative Rx
Volume expansion (D)

α blocker

β blocker

α and β blockers (E)

Nitroprusside

Calcium channel (F)
blocker

Laparotomy (G)

Resectable → MEA screen (H)

Negative → Observe

Positive → Hypercalcemia and Hyperparathyroidism

Unresectable (I) → α blocker ----→ Reoperation

Cushing Syndrome

Donald S. Gann, M.D.

(A) The earliest consistent feature of Cushing syndrome is loss of the normal negative feedback response in which adrenocorticotropic hormone (ACTH), and thus cortisol secretion, is suppressed by elevation of cortisol or an analogous steroid. This is demonstrated by administration of 1 mg of dexamethasone orally at 11 PM. In normal subjects, the cortisol level measured at 8 AM should be less than 50 percent of that measured before the test, and less than 10 g/dL. Although urinary free cortisol may be used as an alternative, the dexamethasone suppression test is now taken as the operational definition of Cushing syndrome.

(B) The high-dose dexamethasone suppression test (8 mg at 11 PM) differentiates adrenal tumor from ACTH causes of Cushing syndrome. Immunoradiometric assay for ACTH is precise and sensitive. ACTH is low and cortisol is not suppressed in the presence of adrenal tumor. ACTH is normal or high in ectopic ACTH syndrome or in pituitary tumor. Cortisol is suppressed in the latter case.

(C) Computed tomography scan is an excellent indicator of malignancy, as demonstrated by irregularity of the tumor or by loss of margins between the adrenal and the cava, liver, kidney, or pancreas. Venous sampling (with aldosterone as a control for catheter placement) can be used to lateralize a benign tumor. Venography can demonstrate invasion of the vena cava. Androgens may be elevated in the case of malignancy.

(D) A pituitary tumor (usually a chromophobe microadenoma) is the cause of Cushing disease if it results in ACTH overproduction and hypercortisolemia. Treatment is transsphenoidal hypophysectomy. If tumor has been lateralized by selective venous catheterization, partial anterior hypophysectomy might be possible. Replacement of adrenal steroids is necessary after this operation or after adrenalectomy for Cushing syndrome of adrenal origin. Patients usually require supraphysiologic doses of cortisol or its equivalent for an extended period of time.

(E) In contrast to benign tumors, malignant adrenal tumors must be approached by an anterior or flank approach to permit wide excision and possible vascular reconstruction, as well as to allow search for metastases. Radical nephrectomy has supplanted simple adrenalectomy and appears to yield somewhat better results. If there is evidence of distant disease, debulking of the tumor appears to be valuable.

(F) Ectopic ACTH syndrome generally results from overproduction of ACTH by small-cell carcinoma of the lung. Big ACTH may also be produced and is detected by most ACTH assays. The response of the tumor to chemotherapy may be assessed by assessing changes in ACTH. Aminoglutethimide is used to limit cortisol secretion; adrenalectomy is not indicated.

(G) Benign adrenal tumors should be explored through the posterior approach, unless they are very large. This approach yields low perioperative morbidity and a short hospital stay. There is no postoperative ileus, and pulmonary complications are minimal.

(H) Metastatic disease is usually signaled by persistence or recurrence of Cushing syndrome. Multiple agents can limit or prevent production of cortisol but only mitotane (o,p'-DDD) is cytotoxic to adrenal cortical cells and prevents steroid secretion. Patients who respond to this drug uniformly develop adrenal insufficiency. Replacement of both cortisol and aldosterone is required.

REFERENCES

Gann DS, DeMaria EJ, Campbell RW. Adrenal gland. In: Davis JH, Drucker WR, Foster RS Jr, et al, eds. Clinical surgery. St. Louis: CV Mosby, 1987:2616–2710.
Gann DS, DeMaria ED. Adrenals. In: Schwartz SI, Shires GT, Spencer FG, et al, eds. Principles of surgery, 5th ed. New York: McGraw-Hill, 1989:1557–1612.

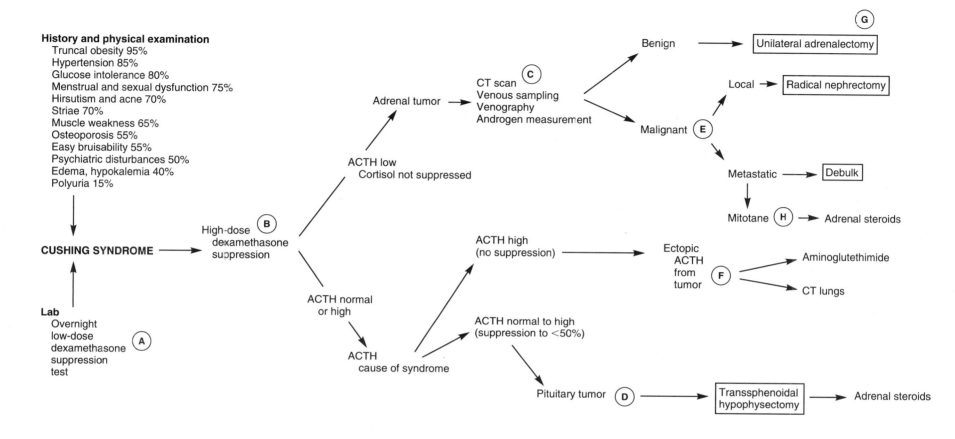

History and physical examination
Truncal obesity 95%
Hypertension 85%
Glucose intolerance 80%
Menstrual and sexual dysfunction 75%
Hirsutism and acne 70%
Striae 70%
Muscle weakness 65%
Osteoporosis 55%
Easy bruisability 55%
Psychiatric disturbances 50%
Edema, hypokalemia 40%
Polyuria 15%

CUSHING SYNDROME

Lab
Overnight low-dose dexamethasone (A) suppression test

High-dose dexamethasone suppression (B)

Adrenal tumor

ACTH low
Cortisol not suppressed

ACTH normal or high

ACTH cause of syndrome

CT scan (C)
Venous sampling
Venography
Androgen measurement

Benign → Unilateral adrenalectomy (G)

Malignant (E)
Local → Radical nephrectomy
Metastatic → Debulk
Mitotane (H) → Adrenal steroids

ACTH high
(no suppression) → Ectopic ACTH from tumor (F)
→ Aminoglutethimide
→ CT lungs

ACTH normal to high
(suppression to <50%)

Pituitary tumor (D) → Transsphenoidal hypophysectomy → Adrenal steroids

Vascular

Thoracic Outlet Syndrome

David B. Roos, M.D.

(A) Neurologic symptoms of thoracic outlet syndrome include fatigue, pain, and paresthesias of the arm, especially with use or elevation. Signs include tenderness of the brachial plexus; weakness of grip and of the interosseous and triceps muscles with diminished sensation in C8 and T1 dermatomes of the inner forearm, ring, and small fingers; and reproduction of the usual symptoms with repeated hand opening and closing for 3 minutes with arm elevation in the "surrender" position. When the upper nerves of the plexus (C5, C6, and C7) are affected by anomalous scalene muscles, pain is felt from the clavicle to the ear and into the upper back, upper chest, top of shoulder, and outer arm. The upper trunk of the plexus is tender to palpation and percussion and is painful when the neck is turned or tilted.

(B) Venous insufficiency is manifested by swelling, fatigability, and cyanosis of the limb with use or, paradoxically, with arm elevation. Arterial insufficiency is manifested by coldness, pallor, fatigability, weak pulse, subclavian bruit with the arm down, and asymmetrical blood pressure difference over 15 mmHg. Emboli from a plaque or aneurysm may cause finger pallor or cyanosis, pain, and gangrene.

(C) Chest and cervical roentgenograms are required to exclude pulmonary disease, sulcus tumor, scoliosis, spondylosis, fractures, and bone anomalies. They may demonstrate a cervical rib or long C7 transverse process, but they are not conclusive because radiolucent congenital bands may compress the nerves or vessels to the arm. Cervical myelograms are occasionally indicated to exclude cervical root or spinal cord disease. Computed tomography and magnetic resonance scans, electromyography, nerve conduction studies, and somatosensory-evoked potentials are seldom helpful, usually are inconclusive, and in most patients are not worth the great expense and pain.

(D) Indications for operation are intolerable pain, progressive weakness, loss of hand function, and muscle atrophy.

(E) Sudden swelling, cyanosis, and upper extremity heaviness characterize acute subclavian vein thrombosis. Urgent venograms confirm the diagnosis. Treatment is with urokinase with follow-up venogram and heparin. Early first rib resection may relieve congestion, enhance collaterals, and avoid the postphlebitic syndrome seen in 85 percent of cases treated with anticoagulants and elevation alone.

(F) Nonoperative management includes avoidance of aggravating arm positions and activities; shoulder exercises and trials of medication, heat, massage, and stretch exercises for muscle spasm; and symptomatic relief.

(G) Surgical sympathectomy is rarely indicated. Symptoms may be associated with collagen vascular disease, which responds poorly to sympathectomy. Medical management involves avoidance of tobacco, protection of the hands from cold and trauma, and oral use of sympatholytic drugs such as phenoxybenzamine (Dibenzyline), guanethidine (Ismelin), or prazosin (Minipress). Anti-platelet drugs (aspirin, sulfinpyrazone [Anturane], dipyridamole [Persantine]) can prevent small vessel thrombosis. Calcium channel blockers (nifedipine) can also be helpful.

(H) Selective arteriograms are indicated to determine the source of emboli, to evaluate a bruit at rest, to investigate a significant upper extremity pulse or blood pressure deficit, or to exclude aneurysm.

(I) The transaxillary approach for removal of the first rib and anomalous fibromuscular bands is used for lower plexus (C8, T1) involvement and decompression of the subclavian vessels. Favorable results are expected in 90 percent of cases depending on careful patient selection and meticulous removal of the first rib and cervical rib, if present, along with all abnormal fibromuscular bands.

(J) Complete excision of the anterior scalene muscle relieves compression of the upper nerves of the brachial plexus. Indications for scalenectomy alone are severe pain in the C5, C6, and C7 distribution, affecting the anterior aspect of the neck from the clavicle to the ear, and the scapular and trapezius areas, with pain radiating down the outer aspect of the arm in the radial nerve distribution. If the lower plexus nerves C8 and T1 are also involved, causing ulnar nerve symptoms through the inner arm and hand, transaxillary first rib resection should be performed along with supraclavicular total anterior scalenectomy. Good to excellent relief of thoracic outlet symptoms is reported in 85 to 90 percent of patients after 2 years. Scar tissue recurrence is

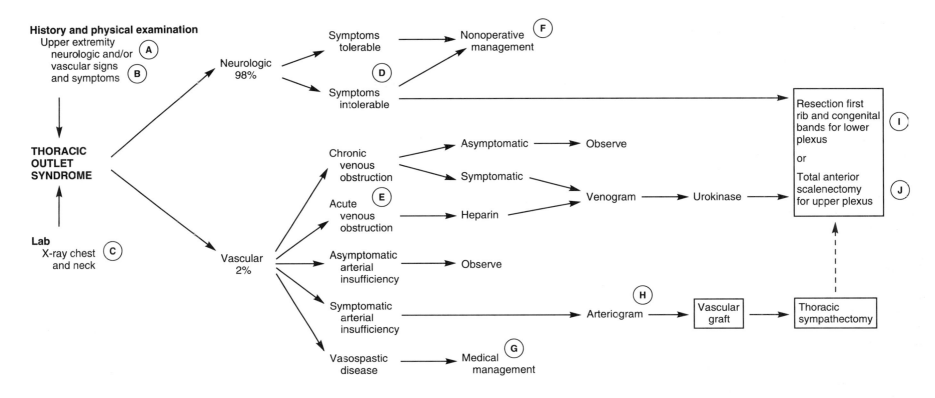

more frequent after scalenectomy (20 to 50 percent) than after transaxillary first rib resection alone (5 to 25 percent).

REFERENCES

Abu Rhama AF, Sadler D, Stuart P, et al. Conventional versus thrombolytic therapy in spontaneous (effort) axillary-subclavian vein thrombosis. Am J Surg 1991; 161:459–465.

Aziz S, Straehley CJ, Whelan TJ. Effort-related axillosubclavian vein thrombosis: a new theory of pathogenesis and a plea for direct surgical intervention. Am J Surg 1986; 152:57–60.

Blunt RJ, Porter JM. Raynaud syndrome. Semin Arthritis Rheum 1981; 10:282–308.

Qvarfordt PG, Ehrenfeld WK, Stoney RJ. Supraclavicular radical scalenectomy and transaxillary first rib resection for the thoracic outlet syndrome: a combined approach. Am J Surg 1984; 148:111–114.

Roos DB. Congenital anomalies associated with thoracic outlet syndrome—anatomy, symptoms, diagnosis and treatment. Am J Surg 1976; 132:771–778.

Roos DB. The place for scalenectomy and first rib resection in thoracic outlet syndrome. Surgery 1982; 92:1077–1085.

Roos DB. Subclavian-axillary vein occlusion. In: Rutherford RB. Vascular surgery, 2nd ed. Philadelphia: WB Saunders, 1984:1385–1393.

Roos DB. Thoracic outlet syndrome: update 1987—the Edgar J. Poth Lecture. Am J Surg 1987; 154:568–573.

Sanders RJ, Monsour JW, Gerber WF, et al. Scalenectomy versus first rib resection for treatment of the thoracic outlet syndrome. Surgery 1979; 85:109–121.

Leg Claudication

Richard F. Kempczinski, M.D., and Richard J. Fowl, M.D.

(A) Claudication is the most common manifestation of chronic peripheral arterial insufficiency and is characterized by cramping pain or fatigue that develops after walking a predictable distance. It is relieved promptly by rest in the standing position and recurs after walking a similar distance. When extremity pain is present at rest, it is not claudication. Instep claudication can occur in the arch of the foot and indicates obstruction of the crural arteries or plantar arch. Calf claudication occurs when a lesion exists at or proximal to the sural artery, which arises from the midpopliteal artery. Thigh claudication implies obstruction at or proximal to the profunda femoris artery, and buttock pain is usually seen with lesions that impair hypogastric artery perfusion. History may reveal previous stroke, myocardial infarction, angina pectoris, or hypertension. Common risk factors include diabetes mellitus, hyperlipidemia, regular use of tobacco, or a strong family history of atherosclerosis.

(B) Findings on physical examination may include absence or diminution of peripheral pulses, the presence of arterial bruits, pallor on elevation of the affected extremity with rubor on dependency, and decreased skin temperature with atrophy of skin appendages. Occasionally with aortoiliac arterial occlusive disease, pulses may be normal at rest. If a patient has exercised until symptoms occur and pedal pulses remain easily palpable, claudication is unlikely. Appropriate neurologic examination includes motor, sensory, and reflex testing of both lower extremities. The lumbar spine is examined for point tenderness, paraspinal muscle spasm, and pain on hyperextension or straight leg raising.

(C) The vascular diagnostic laboratory can document the level of arterial occlusion, its hemodynamic significance, its relevance to the patient's symptoms, and the presence of occult proximal or contralateral disease. Vascular diagnostic laboratory findings can exclude nonarterial causes of leg pain such as herniated intervertebral disk, compression of the cauda equina, arthritis, McArdle syndrome, venous claudication, and muscle cramps.

(D) Symptoms of less than 3 months' duration are consistent with recent onset of claudication.

(E) Cessation of smoking and graded, active exercise can significantly improve maximum walking time. Some patients with moderately severe claudication experience significant improvement in walking distance after the use of pentoxyphylline (Trental). This drug must be given for a minimum of 6 to 8 weeks before its effectiveness can be judged. Weight loss in obese patients reduces demand on the circulation and can result in increased walking distance. The result of nonoperative treatment can be a virtually asymptomatic patient.

(F) The definition of disability is relative. Some patients with a significant hemodynamic lesion will be more limited by chronic obstructive pulmonary disease or coronary artery disease. Younger, more active patients with less significant occlusive disease may be limited economically and emotionally by claudication. In selecting patients for arteriography, it is important to weigh potential benefits of surgical correction against hazards.

(G) Most patients with intermittent claudication have an absolute ankle/brachial pressure between 70 and 200 mmHg and an ankle/brachial index of 0.5 to 0.8.

(H) Eighty percent of patients with intermittent claudication improve or remain stable without surgical revascularization. Only 10 percent come to amputation within 10 years.

(I) Occlusion of distal vessels makes bypass impossible. A patient with popliteal artery occlusion should not be considered for bypass unless claudication is severely disabling or rapidly progressive. Some patients with claudication, especially diabetics, have such heavy calcification or diffuse atherosclerotic involvement that bypass surgery is impossible despite patent vessels.

(J) The choice of a revascularization procedure depends on the location of lesions seen on arteriography. The most proximal of a series of hemodynamically significant occlusions must be corrected first. Restoring systemic pressure to the profunda femoris artery often obviates the need for distal reconstruction. Prosthetic grafts should be carried below the knee only for limb salvage. Unilateral aortoiliac or aortofemoral reconstruction is rarely indicated. In high-risk patients with significant proximal disease, revascularization by a variety of extraanatomic bypasses or percutaneous transluminal angioplasty is safe. The expected 5-year patency after aortoiliac or aortofemoral grafting is 85 to 90 percent. Femorofemoral grafts have an 80 percent 5-year patency and axillofemoral grafts have a 5-year patency rate varying from 35 to 76 percent. The 4-year patency rate is 60 to 70 percent for above-the-knee femoropopliteal grafts. For below-the-knee femoropopliteal grafts, the patency rates range from 40 to 77 percent with vein grafts having significantly better patency than prosthetic grafts. The 4-year patency rate for femorotibial grafts ranges from 21 to 68 percent, with vein grafts having greatly superior patency rates. The operative mortality for direct aortic reconstructive procedures is less than 5 percent. The operative mortality for extraanatomic grafts(femorofemoral, axillofemoral) ranges from 2 to 15 percent. This is related to the severity of underlying illness. The mortality rate for infrainguinal procedures is less

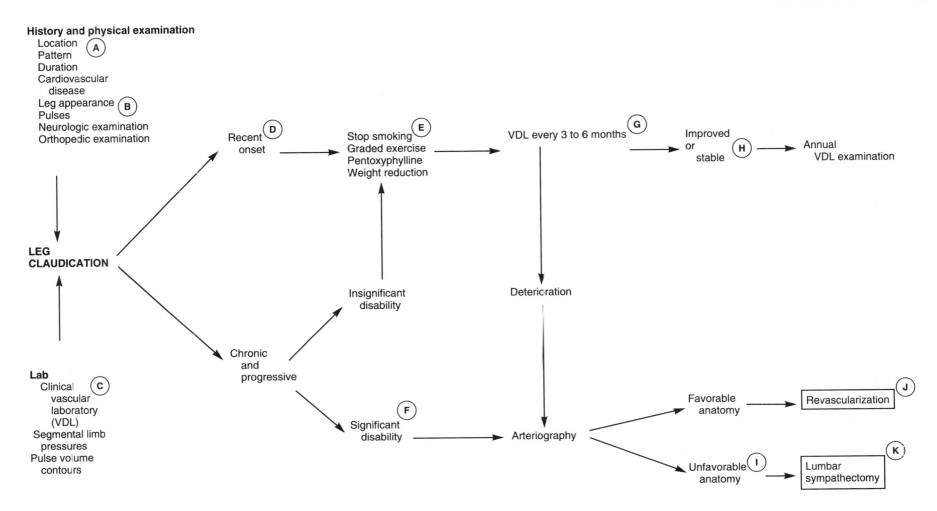

History and physical examination
Location (A)
Pattern
Duration
Cardiovascular
    disease
Leg appearance (B)
Pulses
Neurologic examination
Orthopedic examination

**LEG
CLAUDICATION**

Lab
Clinical (C)
    vascular
    laboratory
    (VDL)
Segmental limb
    pressures
Pulse volume
    contours

Recent (D)
onset

Stop smoking (E)
Graded exercise
Pentoxyphylline
Weight reduction

VDL every 3 to 6 months (G)

Improved
or (H)
stable

Annual
    VDL examination

Insignificant
disability

Deterioration

Chronic
and
progressive

Significant (F)
disability

Arteriography

Favorable
anatomy

Revascularization (J)

Unfavorable (I)
anatomy

Lumbar
sympathectomy (K)

than 3 percent. The most common acute complications after all types of reconstructive procedures include hemorrhage (<3 percent), graft thrombosis (2 to 20 percent), and graft infection (2 to 6 percent).

(K) Lumbar sympathectomy is never indicated in the treatment of intermittent claudication. It is reserved for patients with nonreconstructable, limb-threatening vascular occlusions who suffer rest pain or superficial gangrene. About 50 percent of such patients will obtain objective benefit from the procedure.

REFERENCES

AbuRahma AF, Woodruf BA. Effects and limitations of pentoxifylline therapy in various stages of peripheral vascular disease of the lower extremity. Am J Surg 1990; 160:266–270.

Ascer E, Veith FJ. Extra-anatomic bypasses. In: Haimovici H, ed. Vascular surgery: principles and techniques. Norfolk: Appleton & Lange, 1989:526–538.

Dalman RL, Taylor LM. Basic data related to infrainguinal revascularization procedures. Ann Vasc Surg 1990, 4:309.

Imparato AM, Kim GE, Davidson T, et al. Intermittent claudication: its natural course. Surgery 1975; 78:795–799.

Johnson WC, LoGerfo FW, Vollman RW, et al. Is axillo-bilateral femoral graft an effective substitute for aortic-bilateral iliac/femoral graft? Ann Surg 1977; 186:123–129.

Kempczinski RF. The role of noninvasive testing in the evaluation of extremity arterial insufficiency. In: Kempczinski RF, Yao JST, eds. Practical noninvasive vascular diagnosis. Chicago: Year Book Medical Publishers, 1987:229–259.

Szilagyi DE, Smith RF, Scerpella JR, et al. Lumbar sympathectomy: current role in the treatment of arteriosclerotic occlusive disease. Arch Surg 1967, 95:753–761.

Szilagyi DE, Elliott JP, Smith RF, et al. A thirty-year survey of the reconstructive surgical treatment of aortoiliac occlusive disease. J Vasc Surg 1986; 3:421–436.

Peripheral Arterial Embolism

F. William Blaisdell, M.D., and Richard E. Ward, M.D.

(A) Characteristic features of an arterial embolus that differentiate it from arterial thrombosis include a previous episode; a cardiac source as suggested by arrhythmia (atrial fibrillation), recent myocardial infarct, valve disease, or cardiac surgery (valve replacement); an abdominal aneurysm; normal arteries; and a sudden onset. Characteristic features of arterial thrombosis include underlying atherosclerosis; previous trauma or vascular surgery; ergot ingestion; clotting defects such as polycythemia, leukemia, or coagulopathy; and relatively slow onset.

(B) Physical examination should include evaluation of pulses, skin color and temperature, motor function, and sensory function. Iliac emboli produce midthigh demarcation, femoral bifurcation emboli produce midcalf demarcation, and popliteal emboli result in ankle demarcation.

(C) Noninvasive vascular laboratory studies can only supplement a good physical examination in making the diagnosis. Vascular testing is used to follow trends as assessed by Doppler ultrasonographic pressure measurements.

(D) Arteriography may document the extent of coexisting atherosclerosis and collateral supply. It is useful when the diagnosis of embolism versus thrombosis is in question.

(E) A nonviable limb is blue or mottled with severe pain, anesthesia, and no motor function. Muscles are firm or hard.

(F) A viable limb is pale or cool with minimal or no pain and normal sensation and motor function. A marginally viable limb is waxy, white, and cold with moderate to severe pain; sensation is decreased or absent, and motor function may be present or absent. Muscles are soft.

(G) If ischemia is severe and less than 6 to 8 hours old, the risk of surgery is acceptable and thrombectomy is indicated.

(H) When ischemia exceeds 6 to 8 hours and motor and sensory deficits are present, the limb will contain considerable nonviable tissue. Reperfusion of a nonviable limb results in a high mortality rate. Attempts to revascularize are usually unsuccessful. In these circumstances, nonoperative management is indicated.

(I) Anticoagulation is indicated for ischemia of 8 to 24 hours' duration or more than 24 hours' duration.

(J) For the nonviable or potentially nonviable limb, high-dose heparin therapy is indicated. This consists of heparin 300 U/kg as an initial bolus and at least 50 to 70 U/kg/hour by continuous intravenous infusion over the following 24 to 48 hours. On this regimen, pain should decrease markedly and collateral perfusion should improve within 24 hours. To monitor a patient receiving heparin, a hematocrit is obtained two to four times daily and platelets are counted once daily. Platelet consumption is marked by a precipitous fall in platelet count. Clotting tests such as the activated clotting time or the activated partial thromboplastin time are done daily to verify heparin effect but not to determine the dose, since there is little correlation between the anticoagulant effect of heparin as measured in an antecubital vein and that in the ischemic limb.

(K) If the limb is clearly nonviable initially or does not respond to 24 hours of anticoagulant therapy, amputation is indicated.

(L) For viable limbs, heparin can be administered in more conventional doses while awaiting an effect from simultaneously administered warfarin. The latter is needed for prophylaxis against recurrent embolism.

(M) The source of the embolus should be looked for and treated if possible. In patients who have recurrent emboli and have unidentifiable or surgically untreatable sources, permanent warfin (Coumadin) therapy or low-dose subcutaneous heparin is indicated. If disability is mild or minimal, an operation to remove the emboli may not be necessary. For moderate to severe disability, several weeks of anticoagulant therapy precede revascularization.

(N) At the point of noticeable improvement, oral warfarin is initiated at 10 mg/day and the heparin is decreased by 10 to 15 U/kg/hour daily as long as benefit is maintained. The therapeutic level for warfarin is reached when the prothrombin time rises to twice normal. This requires approximately 3 days. After this, heparin can be discontinued gradually provided that therapeutic benefit is maintained.

(O) Arteriography, if not previously obtained, is performed, and reconstructive surgery, if possible, is carried out.

REFERENCES

Cabin HS, Clubb KS, Hall C, et al. Risk for systemic embolization of atrial fibrillation without mitral stenosis. Am J Cardiol 1990; 65:1112–1116.

Takolander R, Lannerstad O, Bergquist D. Peripheral arterial embolectomy: risks and results. Acta Chir Scand 1988; 154:567–572.

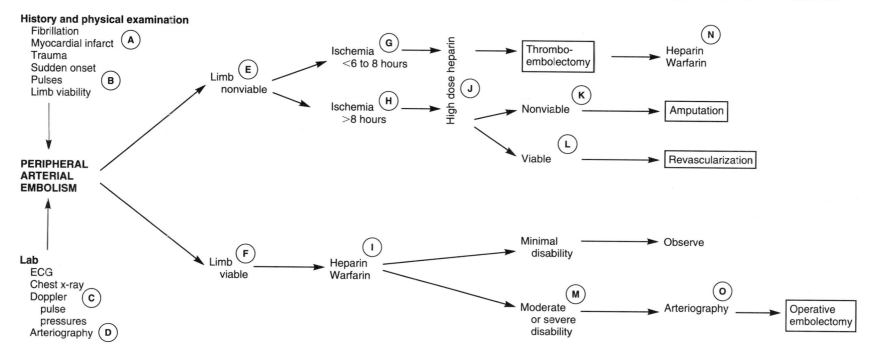

History and physical examination
Fibrillation
Myocardial infarct (A)
Trauma
Sudden onset
Pulses (B)
Limb viability

**PERIPHERAL
ARTERIAL
EMBOLISM**

Lab
ECG
Chest x-ray
Doppler (C)
  pulse
  pressures
Arteriography (D)

Limb (E)
nonviable

Ischemia (G)
<6 to 8 hours

Ischemia (H)
>8 hours

High dose heparin (J)

Thrombo-
embolectomy

Heparin (N)
Warfarin

Nonviable (K) → Amputation

Viable (L) → Revascularization

Limb (F)
viable

Heparin (I)
Warfarin

Minimal
disability → Observe

Moderate (M)
or severe
disability → Arteriography (O) → Operative
embolectomy

Abdominal Aortic Aneurysm

Ronald Stoney, M.D., and Joseph H. Rapp, M.D.

(A) Seventy percent of abdominal aortic aneurysms are diagnosed by palpation.

(B) Back, flank, or abdominal pain in a patient with a palpable aneurysm must be treated as evidence of impending rupture and demands urgent operation.

(C) Coexisting disease is common; coronary atherosclerosis, hypertension, and obstructive pulmonary disease exist in at least 50 percent of those with abdominal aortic aneurysm. Peripheral arterial occlusive disease, other aneurysms, and cerebrovascular disease are found in at least 5 to 15 percent. This, together with advanced age (>80 years), accounts for most of the hospital deaths after elective graft replacement.

(D) Abdominal x-ray studies outline the aneurysm when it is calcified (70 percent). Chest x-ray may suggest thoracic aortic enlargement. True thoracic aortic enlargement is rare (2 percent).

(E) Ultrasonography and computed tomography scan quantitate the diameter and extent of the aneurysm with equal accuracy. The latter also indicates the size of the aortic lumen.

(F) Aortography is not required in every case. It defines proximal aortic dimension, visceral and renal artery branches, vascular anomalies, and peripheral atherosclerosis. Carotid or coronary arteriography is used only if symptomatically indicated.

(G) Rate of growth and probability of rupture vary directly with external diameter. The cutoff between "large" and "small" aneurysms is a diameter of ±5 cm.

Transverse Diameter (cm)	Approximate Rupture Rate (%/year)
<4	5
4–5	8
5–6	12
6–7	17
>7	25

(H) Characteristically there is a symptomatic period of 4 to 12 hours between the onset of pain and free intraperitoneal rupture.

(I) Those with small aneurysms should be examined (plus ultrasonography) every 6 months to exclude enlargement. Even small aneurysms of less than 4 cm in diameter have a 15 percent probability of rupture within 3 years.

(J) A patient with a rupturing aneurysm is resuscitated en route to the operating room, where bleeding is controlled and graft replacement is undertaken. About half the patients with a ruptured abdominal aortic aneurysm reach definitive care, and of these only half survive. With free intraperitoneal rupture the mortality rate is 80 percent.

(K) Immediate preoperative preparation includes pulmonary and cardiac evaluation, prophylactic antibiotics, two intravenous lines, central venous pressure or Swan-Ganz catheter monitoring, clotting profile, indwelling urinary catheter, and four units of cross-matched blood.

(L) A prosthetic bifurcation graft is required when significant iliac aneurysmal disease coexists. Tubular grafts are used for abdominal aortic aneurysms whenever possible to save operating time, especially in cases of rupture. Woven prostheses reduce blood loss in these cases.

(M) Postoperative complications include pulmonary dysfunction (20 to 40 percent), heart failure (20 to 37 percent), myocardial infarct (2 to 15 percent), renal failure (4 to 7 percent), and rarely, colon ischemia and limb amputation.

(N) Hospital mortality rates are 40 to 50 percent for a ruptured abdominal aortic aneurysm and 2 to 10 percent for elective abdominal aortic aneurysm repair, depending on the degree of associated disease.

(O) Life expectancy of 2 years after graft replacement is 75 percent; of 5 years, 50 percent. Death is usually due to associated atherosclerosis, principally myocardial infarction or rupture of another aneurysm (often thoracic aortic).

REFERENCES

Diehl JT, Cali RF, Hertzer NR, et al. Complications of abdominal aortic reconstruction: an analysis of peri-operative risk factors in 557 patients. Ann Surg 1983; 197:49–56.

Johnston KW, Scobie TK. Multicenter prospective study of nonruptured abdominal aortic aneurysms: I. Populations and operative management. J Vasc Surg 1988; 7:69–81.

Rvewster DC, Franklin DP, Cambria RP, et al. Intestinal ischemia complicating abdominal aortic surgery. Surgery 1991; 109:447–454.

Wakefield TW, Whitehouse WM, Wu SC, et al. Abdominal aortic aneurysm rupture: statistical analysis of factors affecting outcome of surgical treatment. Surgery 1982; 91:586–596.

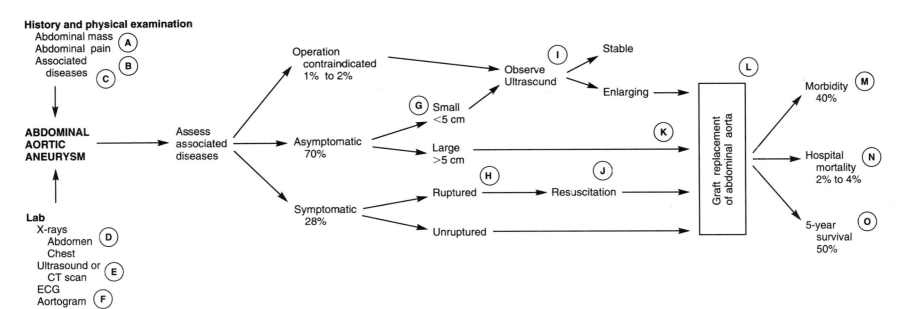

History and physical examination
Abdominal mass (A)
Abdominal pain (B)
Associated
  diseases (C)

**ABDOMINAL
AORTIC
ANEURYSM**

Lab
X-rays
  Abdomen (D)
  Chest
Ultrasound or (E)
  CT scan
ECG (F)
Aortogram

Assess
associated
diseases

Operation
contraindicated
1% to 2%

Asymptomatic
70%

Symptomatic
28%

(G) Small
    <5 cm

Large
>5 cm

(H) Ruptured

Unruptured

Observe
Ultrasound (I)

Stable

Enlarging

(K)

(J) Resuscitation

Graft replacement
of abdominal aorta (L)

Morbidity
40% (M)

Hospital
mortality
2% to 4% (N)

5-year
survival
50% (O)

Cerebrovascular Insufficiency

Robert G. Scribner, M.D.

(A) The term cerebrovascular insufficiency includes the entire neurologic spectrum of focal neurologic deficits.

(B) Important factors in history include known previous attacks or signs and symptoms suggesting previous disease. Associated diseases that can mimic cerebral insufficiency are brain tumor, heart disease, migraine, and hypoglycemia. Transient ischemic attacks last less than 24 hours. A reversible ischemic neurologic deficit lasts more than 24 hours. Factors of importance in physical examination include a neurologic deficit, evidence of cholesterol embolism, fundoscopy, and cervical bruit (90 percent) associated with carotid disease.

(C) Laboratory studies should exclude heart disease (electrocardiogram, chest x-ray, echocardiography). Computed tomography scan can exclude other intracranial disease and may demonstrate new or old cerebral infarction.

(D) About 75 percent of all transient ischemic attacks are caused by extracranial atherosclerosis. Untreated, 30 percent of such patients will have strokes. Another 30 percent will be dead in 5 years.

(E) Carotid bruit can indicate any degree of internal or external carotid stenosis. The bruit often disappears with a stenosis greater than 85 percent. Only 37 percent of arteries with a bruit have a significant obstruction. The risk of stroke in patients with an asymptomatic stenosis greater than 75 percent has been found to be 20 percent at 2 years. Stroke often occurs without a preceding transient ischemic attack.

(F) Patients with crescendo transient ischemic attacks should undergo immediate vascular laboratory studies and computed tomography scanning, anticipating a possible emergency operation. Management of an evolving stroke is controversial. The options are observation (preferred) or emergency operation after laboratory study.

(G) Patients with a completed stroke are at risk of having a second stroke. They should have noninvasive vascular laboratory studies to determine the presence of carotid plaque, its degree of stenosis, and its morphology (ulcerated or unstable).

(H) Carotid duplex scanning with spectral analysis or color flow Doppler should be done on all patients. Diagnostic accuracy is 82 to 98 percent. In patients with asymptomatic carotid stenosis greater than 75 percent and in patients with focal symptoms, carotid endarterectomy can be done without preoperative angiography.

(I) Conventional arteriography ($1500) studies all vessels from the aortic arch to the intracranial arteries in at least two planes.

(J) Digital subtraction arteriography allows a small intraarterial injection of contrast to be used and gives excellent detail of the cervical carotid vessels.

(K) Vertebral artery stenosis seldom requires vascular reconstruction. Operative indications for symptomatic patients include contralateral vertebral artery occlusion or hypoplasia and an unreconstructible carotid artery.

(L) Tortuous or kinked carotid arteries, unless clearly correlated with symptoms, do not require correction.

(M) Significant stenosis begins with 40 to 50 percent reduction of the diameter of the internal carotid. This represents 75 percent reduction in cross-sectional luminal area. Near-occlusive lesions (over 75 percent) carry a high risk of stroke (20 percent at 2 years) and require endarterectomy. Any degree of stenosis can be significant if associated with ulceration or necrotic, hemorrhagic, unstable plaques.

(N) Completely occluded internal carotid arteries cannot be reopened. Rarely, external carotid artery endarterectomy is beneficial.

(O) Dilation of the internal carotid involves minimal risk. Subsequent transient ischemic attacks are almost completely prevented in women (90 percent).

(P) Technical considerations in carotid endarterectomy include use of general or local anesthesia, internal shunt, and patch closure. The hospital mortality rate is 1 to 2 percent, and a neurologic deficit occurs in 1 to 4 percent of patients. The 5-year mortality rate of 35 to 65 percent is primarily due to coronary artery disease. Freedom from subsequent transient ischemic attacks is 95 percent.

REFERENCES

Caracci BF, Zukowski AF, Hurley JJ, et al. Asymptomatic severe carotid stenosis. J Vasc Surg 1989; 9:361–366.

Geuder JW, Lamparello PJ, Riles TS, et al. Is duplex scanning sufficient valuation before carotid endarterectomy? J Vasc Surg 1989; 9:193–201.

Langsfeld M, Gray-Weale AC, Lusby RJ. The role of plaque morphology and diameter reduction in the development of new symptoms in asymptomatic carotid arteries. J Vasc Surg 1989; 9:548–557.

Mackey WC, O'Donnell TF, Callow AD. Cardiac risk in patients undergoing carotid endarterectomy: impact on peri-operative and long-term mortality. J Vasc Surg 1990; 11:226–234.

Piotrowski JJ, Bernard VM, Rubin JR, et al. Timing of carotid endarterectomy after acute stroke. J Vasc Surg 1990; 11:45–52.

Towne JB, Weiss DG, Hobson RW II. First phase report of cooperative Veterans Administration asymptomatic carotid stenosis study—operative morbidity and mortality. J Vasc Surg 1990; 11:252–259.

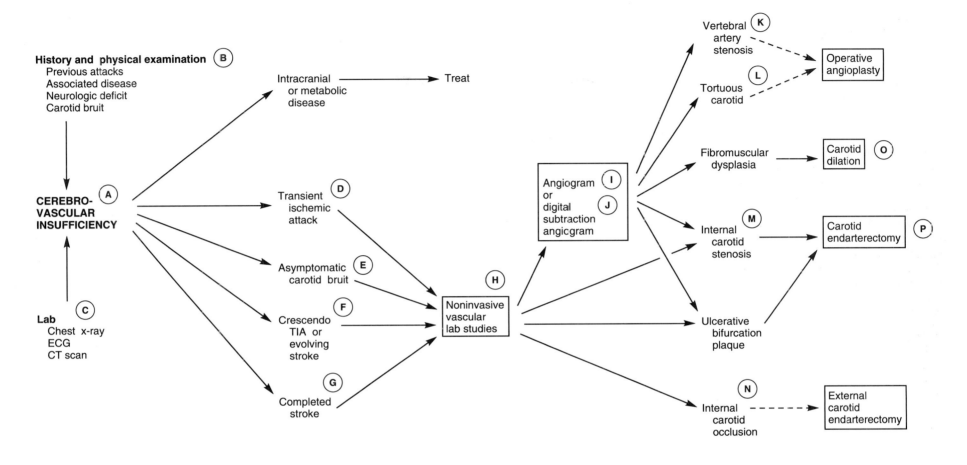

Renovascular Hypertension

Gary Alan Tannenbaum, M.D., and Frank W. LoGerfo, M.D.

(A) The diagnosis of renovascular hypertension requires demonstration of both anatomic and functional abnormalities related to renal artery pathology. The diagnosis is established only after demonstrating improvement of hypertension after surgery or percutaneous transluminal angioplasty.

(B) No combination of clinical findings can reliably distinguish renovascular hypertension from essential hypertension. Severe hypertension (diastolic > 105 mmHg) at the extremes of life carries the greatest probability of being renovascular in origin. Atherosclerotic disease accounts for 60 percent of renovascular hypertension; it usually occurs in older people with evidence of other arterial disease. Fibromuscular dysplasia more often affects young women.

(C) Noninvasive modalities that may prove valuable in screening are renal artery duplex ultrasonography and captopril-enhanced renal scintigraphy.

(D) Determination of plasma renin activity before and after a single dose of captopril, an angiotensin converting enzyme inhibitor, appears to separate patients with renovascular hypertension from those with essential hypertension accurately.

(E) Renal vein renin levels are useful to confirm the diagnosis of renovascular hypertension when a renal artery stenosis is visualized. Renal vein renin and inferior vena cava renin samples can be obtained during angiography. The incremental increase between renal vein renin and inferior vena cava renin is more predictive of renovascular hypertension than is a simple ratio. If renal vein renin − inferior vena cava renin/inferior vena cava renin ≥ 48 percent, more than 90 percent of lateralizing lesions will improve after intervention.

(F) Once renovascular hypertension is confirmed, determination of a pathologic lesion is indicated. Conventional angiography allows the best definition of renal artery pathology and may be augmented with selective injections to delineate branch lesions. Intravenous digital subtraction angiography is less reliable.

(G) Hypertension that is difficult to control medically or diminished renal function after angiotensin converting enzyme inhibitors raises the possibility of renovascular hypertension. Medical management of renovascular hypertension does not prevent progression of renal dysfunction.

(H) Favorable lesions include fibromuscular dysplasia and a nonorificial atherosclerotic lesion.

(I) Percutaneous transluminal angioplasty is technically feasible in up to 95 percent of cases. Blood pressure is lowered in 80 to 90 percent with persistence for over 2 years in many. A 5 to 10 percent complication rate is reported. A prospective randomized study comparing surgery with percutaneous transluminal angioplasty has not been reported.

(J) Surgery is indicated for osteal lesions, for recurrent renovascular hypertension after percutaneous transluminal angioplasty or unsuccessful percutaneous transluminal angioplasty, and when concomitant aortic disease requires operation. Recent series report improvement of blood pressure in 75 to 95 percent of patients, with less than 5 percent mortality.

(K) Autogenous saphenous vein is preferred in the treatment of atherosclerotic renal artery stenosis. Autogenous hypogastric artery is used in young patients with fibromuscular dysplasia. When an autologous conduit is unavailable, a prosthetic may be substituted.

(L) When the aorta is severely diseased, the splenic or hepatic artery may be used for bypass, with or without an intervening conduit of vein or prosthetic.

(M) With distal renal artery fibromuscular dysplasia, ex vivo reconstruction and autotransplantation can be used.

(N) Nephrectomy is reserved for the severely impaired kidney with little hope of functional recovery.

REFERENCES

Maxwell MH, Waks AU. Application of diagnostic procedures in patient management. In: van Schilfgaarde R, Stanley JC, Brummelen P, Overbosh EH, eds. Clinical aspects of renovascular hypertension. Boston: Martinus Nijhoff Publishers, 1983:74–79.

Meier GH, Sumpio B, Black HR, et al. Captopril renal scintigraphy—an advance in the detection and treatment of renovascular hypertension. J Vasc Surg 1990; 11:770–777.

Muller FB, Sealey JE, Case DB, et al. The captopril test for identifying renovascular disease in hypertensive patients. Am J Med 1986; 80:633–644.

Ram CVS. Renovascular hypertension. Cardiol Clin 1988; 6:483–508.

Stanley JC, Messina LM. Renal artery fibrodysplasia and renovascular hypertension. In: Rutherford RB, ed. Vascular surgery, 3rd ed. Philadelphia: WB Saunders, 1989:1218–1230.

Strandness DE Jr. Duplex scanning in diagnosis of renovascular hypertension. Surg Clin North Am 1990; 70:109–117.

Thibonnier M, Joseph A, Sassano P, et al. Improved diagnosis of unilateral renal artery lesions after captopril administration. JAMA 1984; 251:56–60.

van Bockel JH, van Schilfgaarde R, van Brummelen P, et al. Renovascular hypertension. Surg Gynecol Obstet 1989; 169:467–478.

Vaughan ED Jr. Pathophysiology of renovascular hypertension. In: Rutherford RB, ed. Vascular surgery, 3rd ed. Philadelphia: WB Saunders, 1989:1218–1230.

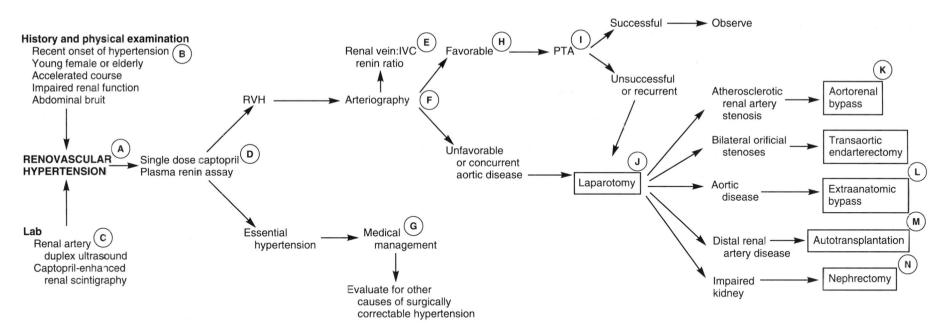

Varicose Veins

Robert B. Rutherford, M.D., and Glenn Kelly, M.D.

(A) Inherent defects, particularly a missing or weak femoral sentinel valve, often predispose to "primary" varicose veins.

(B) Cosmetic reasons are a valid indication for operation in early varicosities still amenable to simple surgery.

(C) A history of deep venous thrombosis suggests probable subsequent deep vein insufficiency and incompetence of the perforating veins connecting the deep and superficial systems. This is the major cause of secondary varicose veins.

(D) Tourniquet tests identify incompetence of the saphenofemoral/popliteal valves and the presence of incompetent perforator valves. Although they are part of the physical examination, they have been largely replaced by noninvasive testing.

(E) Photoplethysmography identifies inefficiency in the venomotor pump and venous reflux. It measures the rate of subcutaneous venous emptying with a photoelectric cell. If an upper thigh tourniquet corrects reflux and produces normal venous return, this indicates saphenofemoral incompetence. Correction by tourniquets applied at lower levels suggests either saphenopopliteal or perforator vein incompetence. Failure to correct suggests deep venous incompetence.

(F) Doppler ultrasound tests are performed by listening over the saphenous, femoral, popliteal, and posterior tibial veins with a directional velocity detector and by performing compressive maneuvers. These tests can localize incompetent valves in the greater and lesser saphenous systems, incompetent perforators or valves in the deep venous system, and sites of deep venous obstruction.

(G) Incompetent saphenofemoral (frequent) and saphenopopliteal (infrequent) valves account for 85 percent of varicosities. Perforator valves may become incompetent as well because of back pressure and increased retrograde flow. Most patients with primary varicosities have legitimate indications for operative treatment.

(H) Venographic visualization of valvular incompetence is rarely (5 percent) required for diagnosis. Color Duplex scanning is better for this purpose. Duplex scanning can also show if the main saphenous trunks are merely dilated, not varicose, so they may be preserved in early cases.

(I) Secondary varices are primarily caused by defects in the deep veins or multiple incompetent perforators. Patients with this problem do not benefit from operation or injection. Their condition can be made worse if venous flow is primarily through the superficial system.

(J) Injection of sodium tetradecyl sulfate is made into the empty varicose vein with the patient supine (injection sites are marked with the patient erect) and at perforator sites (points of control). It is safer to perform small injections at multiple sites than to give a large bolus or an infusion. Firm compression with cotton balls and elastic bandages is maintained for at least 1 week following major sclerotherapy. Sclerotherapy followed by compression is used for patients whose proximal saphenous valves are competent. This technique is also useful for residual or recurrent varices after surgery. It does not produce lasting results in the face of continued saphenofemoral/popliteal incompetence. Therefore, in selected (early) cases, it is combined with high ligation under local anesthesia.

(K) Good risk patients deserve intervention (surgery, sclerotherapy, or a combination) if there is an expectation that all underlying defects (eg, saphenofemoral or perforator incompetence) and the varicosities can be obliterated effectively. Discomfort and evidence of progressive deterioration are obvious indications for treatment. Cosmetic reasons alone are acceptable in early cases. Treatment at an early stage is simpler and more effective.

(L) Firm, custom-fitted elastic stockings are required in conjunction with compulsive intermittent elevation. Stocking length depends on the degree of proximal venous distention. Usually knee-length support is sufficient.

(M) Operative management consists of high ligation of the saphenous vein and division of its three to seven proximal tributaries. This is followed by stripping the saphenous vein proximally to distally. Incompetent perforator veins are ligated and divided. This can be done subfascially through one or two strategically placed incisions. Small to moderate tributary varicosities can be cosmetically controlled with sclerotherapy. Large clusters of varicosities are excised.

(N) The principle of the Linton and Cockett operations is subfascial ligation of all incompetent perforating veins so deep vein hypertension cannot be transmitted to the superficial venous system. Varicosities may be removed at the same time. The numerous incisions once used are unnecessary. Incompetent perforators are localized by color duplex scanning and marked. Through a few strategically placed incisions, using a lighted retractor, these perforators can be clipped readily at a distance.

(O) Valve transplantation or valvuloplasty is indicated rarely for secondary varicose veins. Even in chronic deep venous insufficiency, the

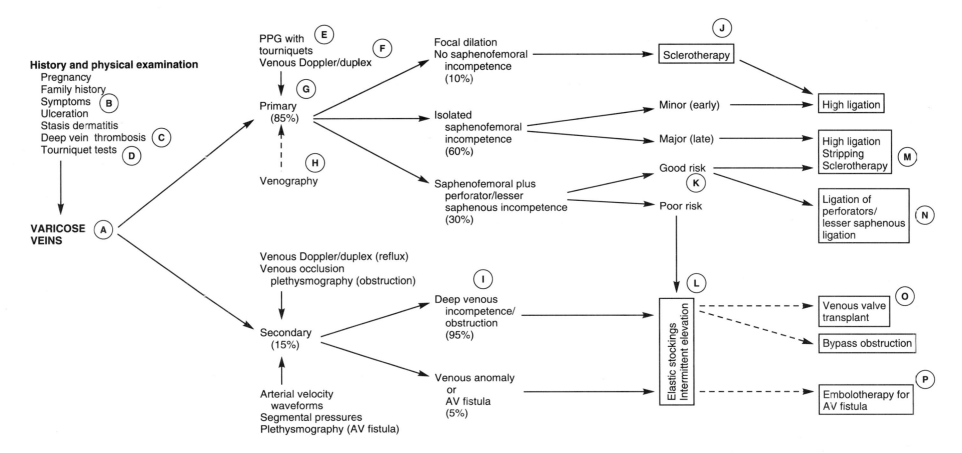

value of these procedures is improved. Femoro-femoral (cross pubic) venous bypass is useful when iliac obstruction (rather than distal reflux) is the primary problem.

(P) Congenital arteriovenous fistulas are a rare cause of varicose veins but an important one to recognize. Surgery is rarely curative. Embolo-therapy is safer although usually palliative and is reserved for complications (eg, ischemic ulcer, bleeding lesion, chronic disseminated intravascular coagulation, unrelenting pain, forward heart fail-ure). In some, venous hypertension is controlled by elastic support and intermittent elevation.

REFERENCES

Bishop CCR, Fronek HS, Fronek A, et al. Real-time color duplex scanning after sclerotherapy of the greater saphenous vein. J Vasc Surg 1991; 14:505–510.

Hobbs JT. A random trial of the treatment of varicose veins by surgery and sclerotherapy. In: Hobbs JT, ed. The treatment of venous disorders. Lancaster: MTP Press Ltd, 1977; 195–207.

Kistner RL, Ferris III EB, Randhawa G, et al. The evolving management of varicose veins: Straub Clinic experience. Postgrad Med J 1986; 80:51–59.

O'Donnell TF Jr. Surgical treatment of incompetent communicating veins. In: Bergan JJ, Kistner RL, eds. Atlas of venous surgery. Philadelphia: WB Saunders, 1992; 111–124.

O'Donnell TF Jr, Burnand KG, Clemenson G, et al. Doppler examination vs clinical and phlebographic detection of the location of incompetent perforator veins: Prospective study. Arch Surg 1977; 112:31–35.

Rollins DL, Semrow CM, Friedell ML, et al. Use of ultrasonic venography in the evaluation of venous valve function. Am J Surg 1987; 154:189–191.

Rutherford RB, Anderson BO. The evaluation of congenital vascular malformations of the extremities by non-angiographic methods. In: Ernst CB, Stanley JC, eds. Current therapy in vascular surgery, ed 2. Philadelphia: BC Decker, 1991; 902–906.

Semrow CM, Laborde A, Buchbinder D, et al. Preoperative mapping of varicosities and perforating veins. J Vasc Tech 1990; 14:72–74.

Sladen JG. Flush ligation and compression sclerotherapy for the control of venous disease. Am J Surg 1986; 152:535–538.

Venous Stasis Ulcers

Roy E. Carlson, M.D.

(A) Most lower extremity ulcers (90 percent) are due to chronic venous insufficiency. Clinically apparent deep venous thrombophlebitis precedes 40 to 50 percent of venous ulcerations. It is important to prevent perioperative deep venous thrombophlebitis. The risk can be minimized by low-dose subcutaneous heparin, compression boots, subtherapeutic Coumadin (sodium warfarin), low molecular weight dextran, and early ambulation. Advanced age; obesity; malignancy; myocardial infarction; cerebrovascular accident; congestive heart failure; and deficiencies of antithrombin III, protein S, and protein C increase the risk of deep venous thrombophlebitis. Fibrinolytic agents in low-risk patients increase clot lysis and decrease long-term sequelae.

(B) Arterial insufficiency occasionally (4 to 5 percent) coexists with venous insufficiency.

(C) Venous ulceration occurs characteristically in a gaiter location (area above medial malleolus) near the ankle. It is surrounded by pigmented dermatitis and thickened tissue (liposclerosis). Ulcers due to arterial insufficiency are usually located distal to the ankle. They are deeper and more painful than venous stasis ulcers. Pulses are weak or absent. The status of pulses can be evaluated by laboratory studies including pulse volume recordings, segmental pressures, and, if necessary, arteriography. Other causes of ulceration are bacterial infection, mycotic infection, hematologic disease such as sickle cell disease, and collagen vascular disease.

(D) A coagulation profile should include prothrombin time, partial thromboplastin time, platelet count, fibrinogen level, bleeding time, AT-3 level, protein S, and protein C.

(E) Noninvasive testing confirms the presence or absence of obstruction or reflux in both the superficial and deep venous systems with an accuracy of greater than 90 percent. Photoplethysmography with tourniquets differentiates superficial from deep venous incompetence (95 percent accuracy). Doppler ultrasonography (90 percent accuracy) and color duplex scanning (96 percent accuracy) outline the anatomy and define the location and severity of reflux.

(F) Superficial venous insufficiency is rarely (<1 percent) the sole cause of ulceration. When it is, ulcers can be healed with compression bandages (Unna paste boot), vein stripping and ligation (100 percent), or sclerotherapy (90 to 95 percent).

(G) Large or infected ulcerations (<10 percent of cases) are treated initially with hospitalization, elevation of the leg above the heart level, wet-to-dry dressings with normal saline, and, if cellulitis exists, systemic antibiotics. Topical antibiotics and enzymes are of little help. Subcutaneous heparin (5000 U subcutaneously every 8 to 12 hours) decreases risk of clot formation while the patient is on bedrest.

(H) Outpatients with venous stasis ulcer can be treated by applying an Unna paste boot (gauze impregnated with zinc oxide, calamine, and gelatin). The boot is changed weekly. Most ulcers heal in 3 to 4 weeks. Superficial varicosities and large perforators in the area of the ulcer can be obliterated using sclerotherapy (sodium tetradecyl sulfate, 1 percent).

(I) Ascending and descending venography with or without duplex scanning is used in patients with recalcitrant ulcers (15 percent) being considered for surgery. Ambulatory venous pressure measurements may be helpful in this group of patients.

(J) After healing, recurrence is minimized by wearing a custom-fitted, graded compression, below-the-knee stocking (30 to 40 mmHg for severe edema). Stockings are of little help in patients on bedrest and are contraindicated if severe arterial insufficiency coexists.

(K) Iliac and common femoral venous occlusions can cause disability due to severe edema of the entire leg, venous claudication, or ulceration. Cross-femoral venous bypass offers a 75 percent patency rate and gives excellent clinical results in 63 percent of selected patients.

(L) Incompetent perforating veins can be obliterated with sclerotherapy. In severe cases, subfascial ligation of perforating veins followed by elastic stockings reduces recurrence rates to less than 15 percent (17 percent wound complication rate). Superficial vein stripping is performed if major varicosities coexist.

(M) Restoration of valvular competence by valvuloplasty (60 to 70 percent good results), venous segment transfer (75 percent success), or vein valve transplantation (40 percent success at 2 years) can be accomplished in selected patients.

(N) Meshed split-thickness skin grafting increases speed of healing of large ulcers.

REFERENCES

Bergan JJ, Yao J. Surgery of the veins. Orlando: Grune and Stratton, 1985.

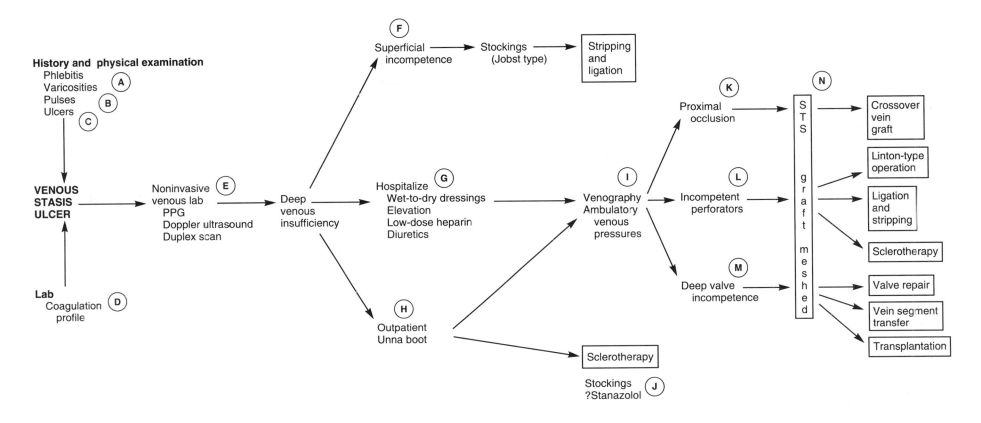

History and physical examination
Phlebitis (A)
Varicosities
Pulses (B)
Ulcers (C)

VENOUS STASIS ULCER

Lab
Coagulation (D)
profile

Noninvasive (E)
venous lab
PPG
Doppler ultrasound
Duplex scan

Deep
venous
insufficiency

Superficial (F)
incompetence

Hospitalize (G)
Wet-to-dry dressings
Elevation
Low-dose heparin
Diuretics

Outpatient (H)
Unna boot

Stockings
(Jobst type)

Stripping
and
ligation

Venography (I)
Ambulatory
venous
pressures

Sclerotherapy

Stockings (J)
?Stanazolol

Proximal (K)
occlusion

Incompetent (L)
perforators

Deep valve (M)
incompetence

S
T
S
g
r
a
f
t
m
e
s
h
e
d (N)

Crossover
vein
graft

Linton-type
operation

Ligation
and
stripping

Sclerotherapy

Valve repair

Vein segment
transfer

Transplantation

Comerota AJ. An overview of thrombolytic therapy for venous thromboembolism. In: Comerota AJ, ed. Thrombolytic therapy. Orlando: Grune and Stratton, 1988:65.

Dale WA. Peripheral venous reconstruction. In: Dale WA, ed. Management of vascular surgical problems. New York: McGraw-Hill, 1985:493.

Ferris EB, Kistner RL. Femoral vein reconstruction in the management of chronic venous insufficiency. Arch Surg 1982; 117:1571–1579.

Flinn WR, O'Mara CS, Peterson LK, et al. The use of photophlethysmography in the assessment of chronic venous insufficiency. In: Kempczinski RF, Yao J, eds. Practical non-invasive vascular diagnosis. Chicago: Year Book Medical Publishers, 1982.

Haeger K. Leg ulcers. In: Hobbs JT, ed. The treatment of venous disorders. Philadelphia: JB Lippincott, 1977:272–292.

Hobbs JT. A random trial of treatment of varicose veins by surgery and sclerotherapy. In: Hobbs JT, ed. The treatment of venous disorders. Philadelphia: JB Lippincott, 1977:195–210.

Karl R, Garlick I, Zarins C, et al. Surgical implications of antithrombin III deficiency. Surgery 1981; 89:429–433.

Rajir S. Venous insufficiency of the lower limb and stasis ulceration: changing concepts and management. Ann Surg 1983; 197:688–696.

Silver D, Cikrit D. Operative management of perforator vein incompetence. In: Rutherford RB, ed. Vascular surgery. Philadelphia: WB Saunders, 1989:1068.

Szendro G, Nicolaides AN, Zukowski AJ, et al. Duplex scanning in the assessment of deep venous incompetence. J Vasc Surg 1986; 4:237–242.

Pediatrics

Tracheoesophageal Fistula

Roberta J. Hall, M.D., Frederick M. Karrer, M.D.,
and John R. Lilly, M.D.

(A) Twenty-five to 40 percent of neonates with the tracheoesophageal fistula (TEF) malformation are premature or have low birth weight.

(B) Fifty percent of patients with TEF have associated congenital defects. The most common are cardiac malformations (30 to 40 percent) and gastrointestinal malformations (20 percent). The acronym VACTERL (vertebra defects, anorectal malformations, cardiovascular anomalies, tracheoesophageal fistula, renal anomalies, limb defects) summarizes possible defects. The limb defects (7 percent) suggest that a teratogen may influence the developing fetus at a critical time.

(C) The most characteristic signs are choking, coughing, and regurgitation with the first feeding. There is often gastric distention secondary to air expired through the TEF.

(D) Current classification is by description of the anatomic defect, not by complex categorization with numbers and letters (see illustration).

(E) X-rays of chest and abdomen should be studied for evidence of pneumonitis, air in the gastrointestinal tract (which rules out esophageal atresia without TEF), and associated anomalies, such as duodenal atresia, vertebral and other skeletal anomalies, and sacral malformations.

(F) A soft radiopaque catheter, size 6 to 10 French, passed through the mouth or nose into the esophagus as far as it will go, with lateral x-ray confirmation, determines the level of the proximal esophageal remnant. If esophageal atresia with proximal TEF is suspected, barium sulfate (1 to 2 mL) should be instilled in the nasogastric tube for diagnosis.

(G) An H-type fistula represents about 5 percent of TEF malformations. Most occur in the cervical esophagus, and diagnosis is made in later infancy or early childhood because of repeated episodes of pneumonia. Bronchoscopy makes the diagnosis.

(H) Esophageal atresia without fistula occurs in approximately 10 percent of infants with the TEF malformation. Diagnosis is suspected because of the absence of intestinal air on abdominal x-ray examination and confirmed by contrast studies through subsequent gastrostomy. The short distal esophagus makes primary repair impossible. After several weeks, there is often impressive elongation of the esophageal pouch that may permit end-to-end anastomosis. Livaditis's method of lengthening the upper pouch by circular myotomy helps bridge the gap.

(I) This is the most common type of malformation (85 percent). Diagnosis is made by the inability of nasogastric tube passage into the stomach and visualization of intestinal air on abdominal x-ray.

(J) Esophageal atresia with proximal TEF is rare. Because the esophageal sump catheter often cannot prevent tracheal aspiration, immediate primary repair is mandated.

(K) Occasionally in infants with severe compromised pulmonary status in which the presence of the TEF prevents adequate oxygenation, the fistula is divided as a temporizing measure.

(L) In patients with severe pneumonitis or life-threatening malformations, a gastrostomy is done, the patient is placed on sump aspiration of the upper esophageal segment, and total parenteral nutrition is given until clinical status is optimized.

(M) In patients diagnosed in less than 24 hours, without pneumonitis and without life-threatening associated malformations, primary anastomosis is done.

(N) Most H-type fistulas may be divided by a transcervical operation. Thoracotomy is indicated for unusual fistulas located in the thorax. Mortality of repair is less than 3 percent, and morbidity is minor.

(O) In patients in whom the gap remains too long for anastomosis, a cervical esophagostomy is done, gastrostomy feedings are continued, and esophageal replacement with colon or gastric tube is performed at 1 year.

(P) Morbidity and mortality from immediate primary repair and from staged repair are not substantially different. In general, mortality follows Waterson's patient risk classification. Complications consist of abnormal motility (100 percent), esophageal stricture (10 to 25 percent), gastroesophageal reflux (10 to 25 percent), anastomotic leak (8 to 12 percent), and recurrent fistula and clinical tracheomalacia (both 3 to 5 percent). Anastomotic leaks usually seal spontaneously but contribute to stricture. In most cases, strictures are successfully managed by dilation during the first postoperative year. Recurrent fistula requires reoperation. Clinical tracheomalacia requires aortopexy in 3 to 5 percent of infants with TEF.

REFERENCES

Livaditis A. Esophageal atresia: a method of overbridging large segmental gaps. Z Kinderchir 1973; 13:298.

Randolph JG, Altman P, Anderson KD. Selective surgical management based upon clinical status in infants with esophageal atresia. J Thorac Cardiovasc Surg 1977; 74:335–342.

Waterston DJ, Carter RT, Aberdeen E. Tracheoesophageal fistula: a study of survival in 218 infants. Lancet 1962; 1:819–826.

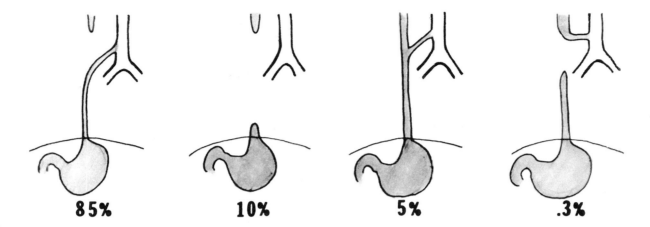

85%   10%   5%   .3%

History and physical examination

Prematurity Ⓐ
Congenital defects Ⓑ
Respiratory and gastrointestinal Ⓒ
   signs

TRACHEOESOPHAGEAL FISTULA Ⓓ → Nasogastric tube passage Ⓕ

Lab
Chest and abdominal Ⓔ
   x-rays

→ Esophageal atresia without TEF Ⓗ

→ Esophageal atresia with distal TEF Ⓘ

→ Esophageal atresia with proximal TEF Ⓙ

→ TEF without esophageal atresia Ⓖ → Bronchoscopy → Fistula division Ⓝ

Gastrostomy Sump aspiration of esophagus → Cervical esophagostomy Ⓞ → Esophageal replacement

Fistula division G tube Ⓚ

Gastrostomy Sump aspiration of esophagus TPN Ⓛ → Delayed (staged) repair Ⓟ

Primary repair Ⓜ

Infantile Pyloric Stenosis

Jeffrey A. Lowell, M.D.

(A) Progressively more frequent, nonbilious projectile vomiting is the most common presenting symptom in infantile pyloric stenosis. Symptoms typically begin in the third week of life. Signs of dehydration (sunken fontanelles, dry mucous membranes, decreased skin turgor) are usually present to some degree. Visible gastric peristaltic waves may be present. An olive-shaped tumor palpable in the upper abdomen is pathognomonic of pyloric stenosis. Boys are affected four times more frequently than girls. Pyloric stenosis is more common in first-born children and in children of affected parents.

(B) A palpable pylorus is present in nearly 90 percent of infants with pyloric stenosis. It is best felt from the left side, with the stomach decompressed and the infant relaxed.

(C) Pyloric stenosis is the most common cause of gastric outlet obstruction in the newborn. There is both hypertrophy and hyperplasia of the circular layer pyloric myocytes. This may be due to a decrease either in the number or function of ganglion cells. Pyloric obstruction can lead to gastritis and subsequent hematemesis.

(D) Ultrasound is specific but has a false-negative rate of 10 percent.

(E) Barium upper gastrointestinal series that typically show a string sign are both sensitive and specific for pyloris stenosis.

(F) Hypochloremic, hypokalemic alkalosis is the most common metabolic derangement. Varying degrees of dehydration are nearly always present. Surgical repair of pyloric stenosis is not an emergency procedure and should be performed only after correction of fluid and electrolyte abnormalities. Indirect hyperbilirubinuria may be present in a small percentage of infants due to decreased activity of hepatic glucuronyl transferase, which resolves 5 to 10 days after surgical repair.

(G) Pyloric atresia, antral webs, duplications of the pylorus, or aberrant pancreatic rests are much rarer causes of gastric outlet obstruction in newborns. These abnormalities, in addition to gastroesophageal reflux, a more common cause of newborn vomiting, are identifiable by barium upper gastrointestinal studies.

(H) Ramstedt performed the first successful pyloromyotomy in 1912, and the procedure is performed today essentially as was initially described. The hypertrophied pylorus muscle is divided along its anterior surface from pyloric vein to antrum. Oral feedings can begin shortly after repair. Perforation of the duodenal mucosa must be recognized and repaired immediately to avoid potential postoperative catastrophe.

(I) Prolonged postoperative vomiting due to incomplete myotomy is uncommon and can be detected by barium upper gastrointestinal examination.

REFERENCES

Benson CD. Infantile hypertrophic pyloric stenosis. In: Welch KJ, Randolph JG, Ravitch MM, et al, eds. Pediatric surgery, 4th ed. Chicago: Year Book Medical Publishers, 1986:811–815.

Conran AG, Behrendt DM, Weintraub WH, et al. Pyloric stenosis and spontaneous gastric perforation. In: Conran AG, Behrendt DM, Weintraub WH, et al, eds. Surgery of the neonate. Boston: Little, Brown & Co, 1978:135–143.

Raffensperger JG. Pyloric stenosis. In: Raffensperger JG, ed. Swenson's pediatric surgery, 4th ed. New York: Appleton-Century-Crofts, 1980:181–189.

Stevenson RJ. Non-neonatal intestinal obstruction in children. Surg Clin North Am 1986; 65:1217–1226.

History and physical examination

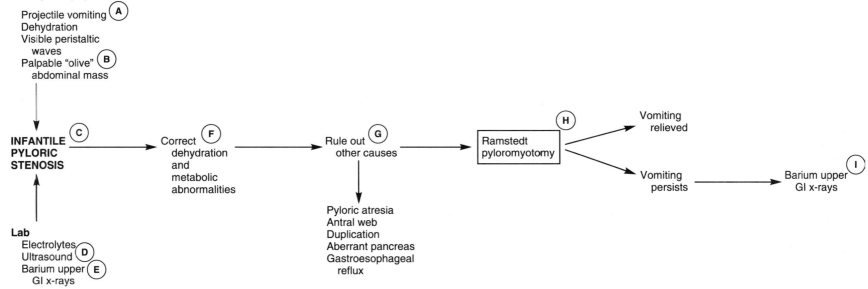

Projectile vomiting (A)
Dehydration
Visible peristaltic
    waves
Palpable "olive" (B)
    abdominal mass

INFANTILE (C)
PYLORIC
STENOSIS

Lab
Electrolytes
Ultrasound (D)
Barium upper (E)
    GI x-rays

Correct (F)
    dehydration
    and
    metabolic
    abnormalities

Rule out (G)
    other causes

Pyloric atresia
Antral web
Duplication
Aberrant pancreas
Gastroesophageal
    reflux

Ramstedt (H)
pyloromyotomy

Vomiting
    relieved

Vomiting
    persists

Barium upper (I)
    GI x-rays

Neonatal Bowel Obstruction

Frederick M. Karrer, M.D., and John R. Lilly, M.D.

(A) Bowel obstruction in the newborn is suggested by a maternal history of polyhydramnios (high obstruction due to reduced intestinal absorption of swallowed amniotic fluid) or diabetes (small left colon syndrome). Cardiac, genitourinary, and skeletal defects occur most commonly with duodenal atresia and imperforate anus. One quarter of infants with duodenal atresia have Down syndrome. Prematurity, especially if associated with hypoxia or hypotension, predisposes to necrotizing enterocolitis. Bowel obstruction presents with bilious emesis and a variable degree of abdominal distention. The more distal the obstruction, the greater the distention and the later the presentation. Failure to pass meconium in the first 24 hours of life suggests a more distal obstruction, eg, ileal or colonic atresia, meconium ileus, meconium plug, small left colon syndrome, imperforate anus, and especially Hirschsprung disease.

(B) Volume and electrolyte derangements are unusual unless the diagnosis is delayed and vomiting is protracted. Abdominal radiographs are helpful for diagnosis. Intestinal atresias have air–fluid levels in the distended proximal bowel but no intestinal air distal to the obstruction. The number and size of bowel loops correlate with the site of atresia, eg, the classic "double bubble" sign of duodenal obstruction and multiple bowel loops seen in ileal atresia. Webs or stenoses have small amounts of air distal to the obstruction. Pneumatosis intestinalis is almost pathognomic of necrotizing enterocolitis, and portal venous gas (an ominous sign) is sometimes present. In meconium ileus, the thick secretions prevent air–fluid levels; instead small trapped air bubbles produce a radiographic "ground glass" appearance. Calcification, a sign of intrauterine bowel perforation, signifies meconium peritonitis. Upper gastrointestinal barium studies (never done with complete obstruction) help differentiate duodenal obstruction due to malrotation and volvulus from duodenal stenoses or webs. Barium enema shows a "microcolon" in distal intestinal atresia and meconium ileus.

(C) Intravenous fluid therapy should precede an operation. Nasogastric suction adequately decompresses high but not low intestinal obstruction. Broad-spectrum antibiotics are started preoperatively. Total parenteral nutrition should be anticipated in situations in which return of gastrointestinal function is delayed.

(D) Almost always associated with cystic fibrosis, meconium ileus results from pancreatic enzyme deficiency and abnormally tenacious meconium. Contrast enema examination shows a microcolon that also demonstrates unusual intraluminal pelletlike concretions. Hypertonic contrast enema may relieve the obstruction by drawing fluid into the bowel lumen and loosening the thick meconium. If unsuccessful, or for complicated meconium ileus (ie, atresia, volvulus, meconium peritonitis), operative intervention by (1) enterotomy and irrigation to relieve obstruction, (2) resection with Bishop-Koop enterostomy, or (3) resection and reanastomosis is indicated. The major morbidity is pulmonary. Survival exceeds 85 percent, even in complicated meconium ileus.

(E) Unlike meconium ileus, meconium plug syndrome is not a sequela of cystic fibrosis. Microcolon, seen on barium enema, extends to the descending or transverse colon. The colon becomes dilated proximally with thick intraluminal meconium. Gastrografin enema can expel inspissated plugs and relieve obstruction. A number of these infants have Hirschsprung disease. A rectal biopsy should always be done. In infants of diabetic mothers, dysmotility of the narrow left colon may produce the small left colon syndrome. Obstruction is permanently relieved by contrast enema.

(F) Duodenal atresia or stenosis, usually located in the second portion, is corrected by duodenoduodenostomy (preferred) or duodenojejunostomy. Duodenal dilation can cause a prolonged functional obstruction, and proximal duodenal tapering or plication is often done to prevent this. Annular pancreas requires identical treatment since there is almost always an intrinsic duodenal obstruction. (Division of the pancreas fails to relieve the obstruction.) Survival is 90 percent except when major anomalies are associated.

(G) If the diagnosis is delayed, malrotation with volvulus infarcts the midgut. Viability must be assessed and a decision made whether to close the abdomen and accept a fatal outcome or to attempt resection with proximal intestinal exteriorization. The latter is usually followed by short gut syndrome, long-term hyperalimentation, and cholestatic liver disease resulting from total parenteral nutrition. If the gut is viable after detorsion by counterclockwise rotation, then Ladd's procedure is performed. The peritoneal bands across the duodenum are divided, the narrow mesenteric root is separated and splayed open, and the duodenum and jejunum are placed on the right side of the abdomen and the colon on the left side. Inversion appendectomy is recommended because of the resultant ectopic location of the appendix.

(H) Mucosal webs in the duodenum can be above, below, or at the same level as the ampulla of Vater. The location is determined by passage of an intraluminal tube until the indentation at the level of the web is seen. Duodenotomy

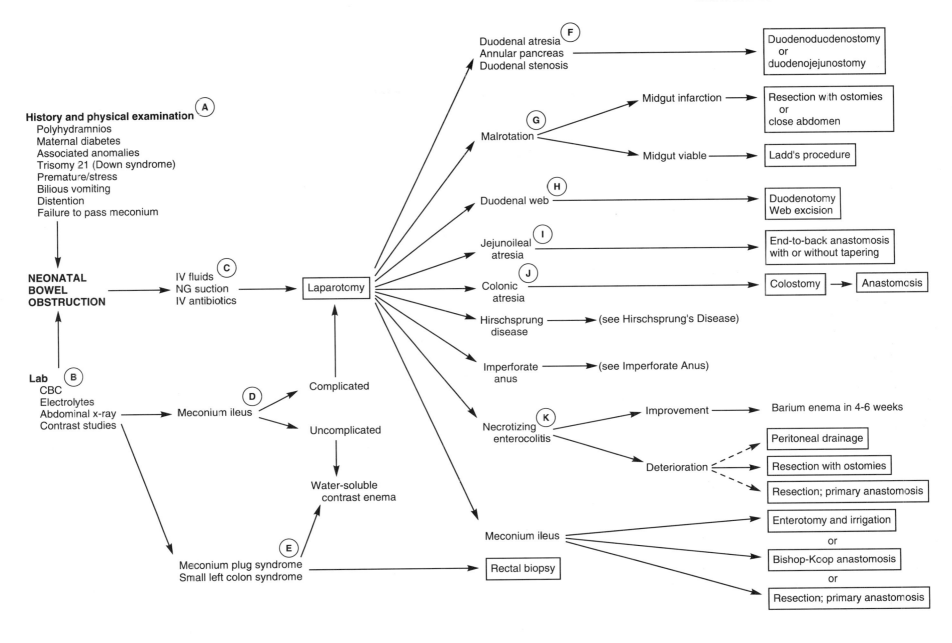

History and physical examination (A)
- Polyhydramnios
- Maternal diabetes
- Associated anomalies
- Trisomy 21 (Down syndrome)
- Premature/stress
- Bilious vomiting
- Distention
- Failure to pass meconium

NEONATAL BOWEL OBSTRUCTION

Lab (B)
- CBC
- Electrolytes
- Abdominal x-ray
- Contrast studies

(C)
IV fluids
NG suction
IV antibiotics

Laparotomy

Meconium ileus (D)
- Complicated
- Uncomplicated

Water-soluble contrast enema

Meconium plug syndrome (E)
Small left colon syndrome

Rectal biopsy

Duodenal atresia (F)
Annular pancreas
Duodenal stenosis
→ Duodenoduodenostomy or duodenojejunostomy

Malrotation (G)
→ Midgut infarction → Resection with ostomies or close abdomen
→ Midgut viable → Ladd's procedure

Duodenal web (H)
→ Duodenotomy Web excision

Jejunoileal atresia (I)
→ End-to-back anastomosis with or without tapering

Colonic atresia (J)
→ Colostomy → Anastomosis

Hirschsprung disease → (see Hirschsprung's Disease)

Imperforate anus → (see Imperforate Anus)

Necrotizing enterocolitis (K)
→ Improvement → Barium enema in 4-6 weeks
→ Deterioration
  - Peritoneal drainage
  - Resection with ostomies
  - Resection; primary anastomosis

Meconium ileus
→ Enterotomy and irrigation
or
→ Bishop-Koop anastomosis
or
→ Resection; primary anastomosis

Neonatal Bowel Obstruction (Continued)

at this level permits careful excision, leaving the medial portion of the web intact to avoid injury to the pancreaticobiliary ducts.

(I) In jejunal and ileal atresia there is a 10 percent incidence of multiple atresias. Confirmation of distal patency by injection of fluid must be done. The distended proximal segment is usually atonic and should be resected up to the more normal-sized bowel. The distal bowel is opened obliquely, the proximal bowel at right angles, and a single layer end-to-back anastomosis is performed. When the proximal segment is too short for excision, it should be tapered along the antimesenteric border. In all midgut atresias, survival exceeds 90 percent. Mortality results primarily from sepsis and cholestasis due to total parenteral nutrition.

(J) Contrast enema determines the level of obstruction in low intestinal obstruction. Contrast enema may be therapeutic as well in cases of meconium ileus, meconium plug, or small left colon syndrome. Atresia of the colon usually presents with massive proximal distention and is best treated by colostomy and delayed anastomosis.

(K) Indications for operation in necrotizing enterocolitis are pneumoperitoneum, abdominal wall cellulitis/edema, abdominal mass, a radiographic fixed loop of dilated bowel, and clinical deterioration as evidenced by thrombocytopenia, leukocytosis, acidosis, and shock. Treatment is usually by resection of necrotic bowel with proximal and distal exteriorization. Placement of peritoneal drains in premature infants (<1000 g) and resection with primary anastomosis in low-risk patients are accepted alternatives. Fifty to eighty percent of infants recover after operation. Barium enema should be done at 4 to 6 weeks to identify the 10 to 20 percent with colonic stricture, usually left-sided.

REFERENCES

Bishop HC, Koop CE. Management of meconium ileus: resection, Roux-en-Y anastomosis and ileostomy irrigation with pancreatic enzymes. Ann Surg 1957; 145:410–414.

Ein SH, Shandling B, Wesson D, et al. A 13-year experience with peritoneal drainage under local anesthesia for necrotizing enterocolitis perforation. J Pediatr Surg 1990; 25:1034–1037.

Harberg FJ, McGill CW, Saleem MM, et al. Resection with primary anastomosis for necrotizing enterocolitis. J Pediatr Surg 1983; 18:743–746.

Kimura K, Tsujawa C et al. Diamond-shaped anastomosis for congenital duodenal atresia. Arch Surg 1977; 112:1262–1263.

Noblett HR. Treatment of uncomplicated meconium ileus by Gastrografin enema: a preliminary report. J Pediatr Surg 1990; 4:190–197.

Rescorla FJ, Grosfeld JL. Intestinal atresia and stenosis: analysis of survival in 120 cases. Surgery 1985; 98:668–676.

Rescorla FJ, Grosfeld JL, West KJ, et al. Changing patterns of treatment and survival in neonates with meconium ileus. Arch Surg 1989; 124:837–840.

Ross MN, Wayne ER, Janik JS, et al. A standard of comparison for acute surgical necrotizing enterocolitis. J Pediatr Surg 1989; 24:998–1002.

Smith EI. Malrotation of the intestine. In: Welch KJ, Randolph JG, Ravitch MM, et al, eds. Pediatric surgery, 4th ed. Chicago: Year Book Medical Publishers, 1986:882–895.

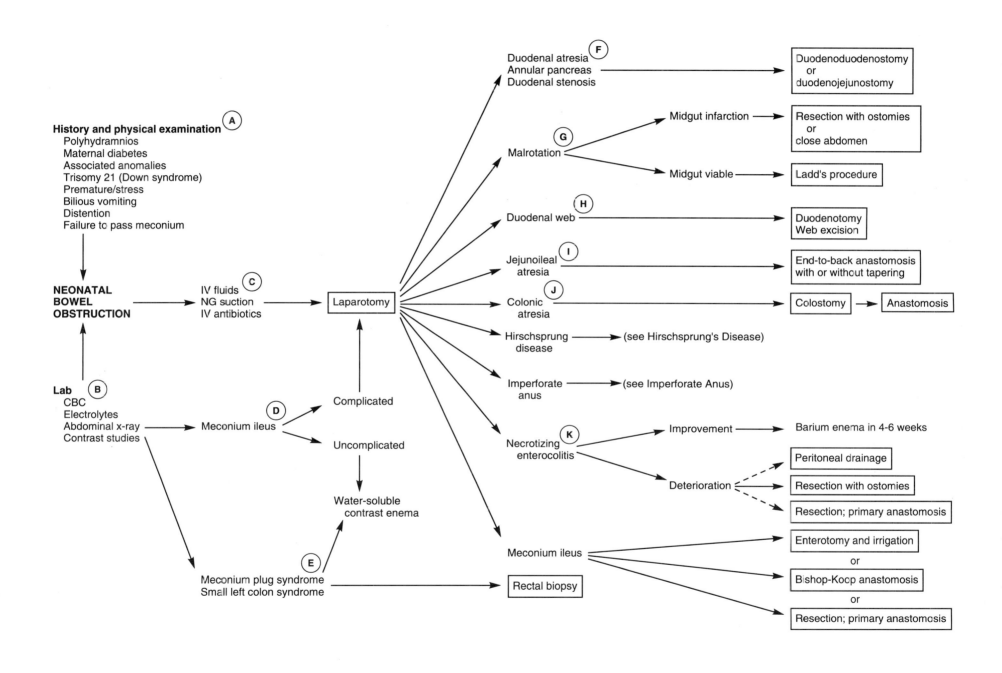

History and physical examination (A)
  Polyhydramnios
  Maternal diabetes
  Associated anomalies
  Trisomy 21 (Down syndrome)
  Premature/stress
  Bilious vomiting
  Distention
  Failure to pass meconium

NEONATAL BOWEL OBSTRUCTION

IV fluids (C)
NG suction
IV antibiotics

Lab (B)
  CBC
  Electrolytes
  Abdominal x-ray
  Contrast studies

Meconium ileus (D)
  Complicated
  Uncomplicated
  Water-soluble contrast enema

Meconium plug syndrome (E)
Small left colon syndrome

Laparotomy

Duodenal atresia (F)
Annular pancreas
Duodenal stenosis
→ Duodenoduodenostomy or duodenojejunostomy

Malrotation (G)
  → Midgut infarction → Resection with ostomies or close abdomen
  → Midgut viable → Ladd's procedure

Duodenal web (H) → Duodenotomy Web excision

Jejunoileal atresia (I) → End-to-back anastomosis with or without tapering

Colonic atresia (J) → Colostomy → Anastomosis

Hirschsprung disease → (see Hirschsprung's Disease)

Imperforate anus → (see Imperforate Anus)

Necrotizing enterocolitis (K)
  → Improvement → Barium enema in 4-6 weeks
  → Deterioration ⇢ Peritoneal drainage
                  ⇢ Resection with ostomies
                  ⇢ Resection; primary anastomosis

Rectal biopsy

Meconium ileus
  → Enterotomy and irrigation
  or
  → Bishop-Koop anastomosis
  or
  → Resection; primary anastomosis

Hirschsprung Disease

Walton Shim, M.D.

(A) Hirschsprung disease, or congenital megacolon, occurs about once in every 500 births, ranking third (16 percent) among the causes of neonatal intestinal obstruction after intestinal atresia and meconium ileus.

(B) Delayed passage of the first meconium stool beyond 24 hours after birth is present in 94 percent of infants with Hirschsprung disease and should alert the clinician to the possibility of the diagnosis. Other signs include abdominal distention, vomiting, and poor feeding. Digital rectal examination is not diagnostic. Constipation alternating with diarrhea due to enterocolitis occurs in 35 percent of infants with megacolon and may cause lethal dehydration. Immediate supportive therapy should include rectal irrigations, anal dilation, and intravenous fluids. Older children may have abdominal distention, vomiting, and a history of constipation dating from infancy. Fecal masses frequently are palpable through the abdominal wall. Rectal examination usually reveals an empty ampulla.

(C) An aganglionic infant who has not passed meconium during the first day of life may show diffuse gaseous distention of the intestine with a large sentinel colonic loop and no rectal air. Barium enema is then necessary.

(D) Barium is injected into unprepared colon by hand to prevent overfilling, which might obscure the transition zone between normal and abnormal bowel. A balloon catheter should not be placed in the rectum because this may dilate the narrow segment.

(E) In children over 1 year of age, barium enema usually discloses a transition zone. This study is less accurate in younger children and is falsely negative in 23 percent of neonates. If a transition zone is not seen, rectal biopsy is justified before

proceeding with an operation. If a transition zone is obvious, colostomy is done under frozen section guidance for proper placement in a ganglionated area.

(F) Barium retention for more than 24 hours is strongly suggestive of Hirschsprung disease. Confirmation is obtained by rectal mucosal biopsy.

(G) If the barium enema shows an irregular or "sawtooth" mucosa indicating enterocolitis, and no transition zone is evident, rectal mucosal biopsy is performed.

(H) If a microcolon is discovered, ileal atresia and meconium ileus must be excluded as well as total colonic aganglionosis. This may require rectal mucosal biopsy and diagnostic exploratory laparotomy.

(I) Hirschsprung disease is not excluded because an infant begins to pass stools regularly. Rectal examination may induce defecation. Failure to sustain a normal pattern of stooling should prompt barium enema followed by biopsy if the enema is not diagnostic.

(J) Although barium enema is frequently diagnostic, rectal mucosal biopsy may be necessary to confirm aganglionosis. This biopsy is taken proximal to the area of hypoganglionosis extending about 2 cm cephalad to the pectinate line of the infant. Immature ganglion cells or neural units in the newborn are not easily recognized. An inexperienced pathologist may render a false diagnosis of aganglionosis. Rectal mucosal suction biopsy requires no anesthesia and is performed with a Rubin or Crosby suction capsule through which 15 to 20 mmHg of negative pressure is transmitted to elevate tissue deep to the muscularis mucosa, where ganglion cells of Meissner's plexus are located. Cells here are less populous than in the deeper Auerbach's plexus between the circular and

longitudinal muscles. Auerbach's plexus is sampled by a full-thickness rectal wall biopsy under general anesthesia. Both mucosal and full-thickness rectal wall biopsies are taken 2.5 to 3.5 cm from the anal verge. A suction specimen is obtained from each side, whereas the single full-thickness specimen is taken from the posterior wall. Full-thickness biopsies require anesthesia and jeopardize the dissection at the definitive surgical procedure. Less dependable means of identifying congenital megacolon are abnormal rectal manometry, atypical histochemical distribution of neurotransmitters such as acetylcholinesterase, and measurement of acetylcholine levels. In cases of ultrashort-segment aganglionosis both histochemical and manometric studies may be helpful since the terminal 2 cm of rectum contains few ganglion cells.

(K) Colostomy is performed under frozen-section guidance, locating the stoma in a normally ganglionated area immediately proximal to the transition zone.

(L) The timing of resection balances the need for early correction with operative safety. The balance is best when the patient weighs 15 to 20 lb. Three techniques—abdominoperineal resection with everted anastomosis (Swenson), posterior spur-crushing rectal anastomosis (Duhamel), and endorectal pull-through anastomosis (Soave)—are used currently. Any of the three can yield good results, but none avoids significant morbidity. The author finds that the Swenson procedure yields excellent results. Most resections are performed months after colostomy. The internal sphincter and smooth muscles of the rectum atrophy and make the everted (Swenson) anastomosis more difficult. Preoperative anorectal dilation twice daily for a month by insertion and repetitive flexion of the gloved thumb by a parent results in a thicker muscle coat around the rectal stump, to which the

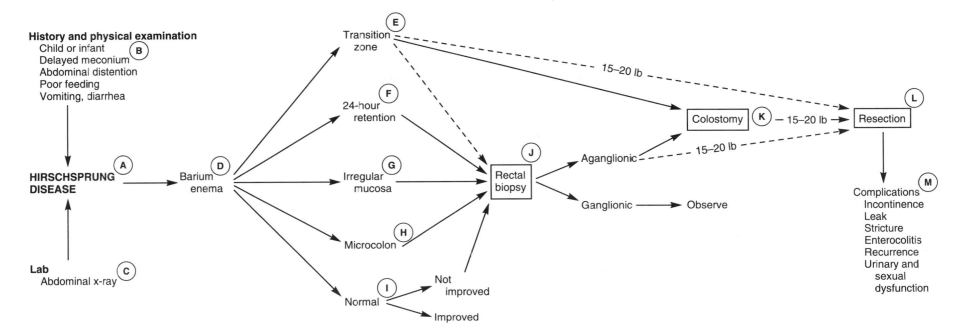

History and physical examination (B)
Child or infant
Delayed meconium
Abdominal distention
Poor feeding
Vomiting, diarrhea

HIRSCHSPRUNG DISEASE (A) → Barium enema (D)

Lab (C)
Abdominal x-ray

Transition zone (E)

24-hour retention (F)

Irregular mucosa (G)

Microcolon (H)

Normal (I) → Not improved
          → Improved

Rectal biopsy (J) → Aganglionic
                  → Ganglionic → Observe

Colostomy (K) — 15–20 lb → Resection (L)

15–20 lb

Complications (M)
Incontinence
Leak
Stricture
Enterocolitis
Recurrence
Urinary and sexual dysfunction

normally ganglionated proximal segment can be more easily sutured. This maneuver, together with preoperative mechanical and antibiotic bowel preparation, tension-free anastomosis, and operative systemic antibiotic coverage, virtually obviates anastomotic leaks. Infants who can be decompressed by rectal irrigations and colonic stimulation performed by the parents may undergo a primary Swenson procedure without prior colostomy.

(M) The mortality rate of each operation is 3 to 6 percent. It is higher in infants under 4 months of age. Normal continence is obtained in 80 to 90 percent of infants. Incontinence may improve with time. Some children require 10 or more years to become continent. Anastomotic leak occurs in 5 to 9 percent. If immediately treated by diverting colostomy, a leak will seal spontaneously and the colostomy can be closed after 6 to 8 weeks. Leak occurs more often in patients with Down syndrome,

previous colonic shortening operations, and short-segment disease. Strictures occur in 6 to 12 percent. Few of these require operative treatment. Postoperative enterocolitis occurs episodically in about 25 percent and may require intravenous support, rectal irrigations, and anal dilation for dehydration and diarrhea. Inadequate resection of the residual rectum in the Swenson procedure, improper preparation of the anterior rectal pouch in the Duhamel operation, and cuff abscesses and retraction of the pulled-through colon in the Soave procedure can occur. The reoperation rate is about 2 to 3 percent. Urinary and sexual dysfunctions occur rarely.

REFERENCES

Aldridge RT, Campbell PE. Ganglion cell distribution in the normal rectum and anal canal: a basis for the diagnosis of Hirschsprung's disease by anorectal biopsy. J Pediatr Surg 1968; 3:475–490.

Carcassonne M, Guys JM, Morrison-Lacombe G, et al. Management of Hirschsprung's disease: corrective surgery before three months of age. J Pediatr Surg 1989; 24:1032–1034.

Larsson LT, Sandler F. Neuronal markers in Hirschsprung's disease with special reference to neuropeptides. ACTC Histochem Suppl 1990; 38:115–125.

Puri P, Nixon HH. Long-term results of Swenson's operations for Hirschsprung's disease. Progr Pediatr Surg 1977; 10:87–102.

Santulli TV, Amoury RA. Congenital anomalies of the G.I. tract. Pediatr Clin North Am 1967; 14:21–45.

Shim WKT, Swenson O. Treatment of congenital megacolon in 50 infants. Pediatrics 1966; 38:185–193.

Soave F. Megacolon: long-term results of surgical treatment. Prog Pediatr Surg 1977; 10:141–149.

Swenson O, Sherman J, Fisher J. Diagnosis of congenital megacolon: an analysis of 501 patients. J Pediatr Surg 1973; 8:587–594.

Swenson D, Sherman JO, Fisher JH, et al. The treatment and postoperative complications of congenital megacolon. Ann Surg 1975; 182:266–273.

Imperforate Anus

J. Laurance Hill, M.D.

(A) Imperforate anus is life-threatening because of sepsis, bowel obstruction, or associated congenital anomalies. The latter two are recognized readily. Sepsis is less obvious and occurs as a result of contamination of the urinary tract through a colourinary fistula or translocation of organisms secondary to stasis in a rectal pouch with no outlet or with a tiny fistula providing inadequate decompression.

(B) Although mortality for imperforate anus should be rare, associated anomalies can cause death (70 percent). Genitourinary anomalies are responsible for 30 percent of mortality. Cardiac, central nervous system, and gastrointestinal (eg, esophageal atresia) defects each cause 10 percent of deaths.

(C) Ultrasonography has become the procedure of choice to differentiate high vs. low lesions in the absence of a perineal fistula and meconium staining. The Rice-Wangensteen inversion "babygram" can be performed in infants over 18 hours of age to determine the level of obstruction. A lateral x-ray is obtained with the infant's knees flexed and an opaque marker at the anal "wink" or dimple.

(D) Sepsis is diagnosed by thermal instability, lethargy, falling platelet counts, and positive blood cultures. Treatment is systemic antibiotics followed by relief of obstruction.

(E) A urinary fistula is assumed for all high pouches until proved otherwise. It can be diagnosed by the presence of meconium in urine (gross or microscopic), by the escape into the urine of carmine red instilled into the gut, or by cystoscopy, voiding cystourethrogram, or vaginogram.

Urinary fistula demands total fecal diversion by colostomy with separated stomas.

(F) The pubococcygeal line indicates the level of the levator ani sphincter. Gas in the rectal pouch 2 cm or more above the pubococcygeal line (supralevator) excludes the possibility of primary anoplasty. "Two centimeters is too far." Meconium in the rectal pouch can cause error on the "high pouch" side.

(G) Gas in the rectal pouch caudal to the pubococcygeal line (infralevator) defines a low pouch and permits anoplasty.

(H) A perineal fistula is associated with a low pouch in 90 percent of girls and 66 percent of boys.

(I) Supralevator obstruction requires a primary separated double-barrel colostomy. A transverse colostomy better ensures adequate length and blood supply for later colon pull-through than does a sigmoid colostomy. A sigmoid colostomy avoids the problems of bacterial overgrowth and hyperchloremic acidosis in the long segment distal to a transverse colostomy, however.

(J) Septicemia can be avoided by irrigation of the rectal pouch with 0.1 percent neomycin in Ringer's lactate solution through the distal limb of the colostomy and by administration of systemic antibiotics.

(K) Contraindications to anoplasty are prematurity and poor condition of the infant due to delayed diagnosis, sepsis, or associated anomalies.

(L) After the infant is 6 to 12 months of age or 10 kg in weight, a second-stage repair can be done with relative safety and ease. Some surgeons advocate earlier reconstruction. The anterior perineal approach of Mollard and the posterior (sagittal anorectoplasty) procedures of Stephens and Smith or deVries and Pena have anatomic and physiologic advantages over the earlier abdominoperineal pull-through techniques.

(M) Programmed neorectoanal dilations for 6 to 12 months are an essential part of care after repair of imperforate anus.

(N) Colostomy closure follows 6 to 12 weeks after the neoanus is constructed.

(O) Functional assessments at least 5 years after treatment (with more objective data by manometry, electromyograph, and newer imaging techniques instead of clinical criteria) demonstrate that continence depends on anatomic level and sacral integrity rather than on the technical differences of the perineal operations. Sixty-five to eighty-five percent of children with low pouches managed by perineal operations or simple anoplasty have good to excellent continence. At best, high pouches have good results in about one third of children. Another third with bad results may have the equivalent of a perineal colostomy.

(P) Cost varies proportionally to the severity of the anomaly. Least cost occurs after discharge to trustworthy parents 3 days after a simple anoplasty with the expectation of complete continence by 3 years of age. Greatest cost is associated with at least three major operations, an initial 3 to 5 weeks of hospitalization, numerous complications from infection or associated anomalies, and incontinent constant soiling with the attendant psycho-

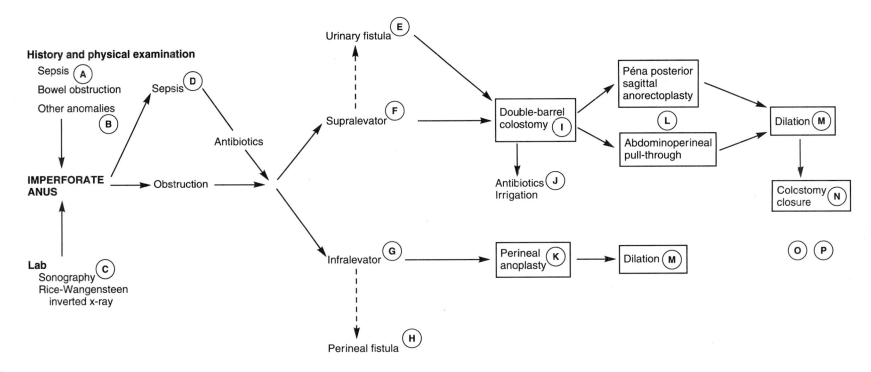

social maldevelopments in the child and the parents.

REFERENCES

Kiesewette WB, Chang JHT. Imperforate anus: a five to thirty year follow-up perspective. Prog Pediatr Surg 1977; 10:111–120.

Mollard P, Marechal JM, deBeaujeu MJ, et al. Anterior perineal approach. J Pediatr Surg 1978; 13:499–504.

Pena A, deVries PA. Posterior sagittal anorectoplasty. J Pediatr Surg 1982; 17:796–811.

Rehbein F. Imperforate anus: experience with abdomino-perineal and abdomino-sacroperineal pull-through procedures. J Pediatr Surg 1967; 2:99–105.

Santulli TV, Schullinger JN, Kiesewetter WB, et al. Imperforate anus: a survey from the members of the Surgical Section of the American Academy of Pediatrics. J Pediatr Surg 1971; 6:484–487.

Stephen FD, Smith ED. Ano-rectal malformations in children: update 1988. New York; Alan R. Liss. 1988.

Wangensteen OH, Rice CO. Imperforate anus. Ann Surg 1930; 92:77–81.

Surgical Jaundice in Infancy

Gianna Stellin, M.D., and John R. Lilly, M.D.

A Jaundice in an infant with "butterfly" vertebrae and pulmonary peripheral stenosis is consistent with Alagille syndrome, a familial disease also called intrahepatic biliary atresia or arteriohepatic dysplasia. Jaundice is due to paucity of the intrahepatic ducts. About 10 percent of infants with extrahepatic biliary atresia have associated malformations such as polysplenia, situs inversus, and intestinal malrotation.

B Impaired excretion of bile is manifested by steatorrhea and acholic stools. Infant stools are never completely acholic even in the absence of bile.

C Splenic enlargement occurs in Rh incompatibility, sepsis, and hemolysis. After 6 months, splenomegaly indicates portal hypertension secondary to neonatal hepatitis, biliary atresia, α_1-antitrypsin deficiency, Alagille syndrome, or cystic fibrosis.

D Ascites in the newborn suggests spontaneous perforation of bile ducts. It is due to bile peritonitis and is usually sterile.

E Leukocytosis suggests infection. A neonate normally has 50 to 70 percent lymphocytosis and a white blood cell count of 14,000 to 20,000/mm^3.

F Conjugated bilirubin is increased in infants with obstructive jaundice but rarely exceeds 15 mg/100 mL. Fluctuations are common. An elevated indirect serum bilirubin level excludes mechanical jaundice and suggests hemolysis due to Rh incompatibility, sepsis, or red blood cell defects. An elevated alkaline phosphatase level suggests mechanical biliary obstruction. Serum glutamic oxaloacetic transaminase and serum glutamic

pyruvic transaminase elevations suggest neonatal hepatitis.

G A coagulation profile includes prothrombin time, partial thromboplastin time, and bleeding time.

H α_1-Antitrypsin deficiency causes cholestatic jaundice in 5 to 10 percent of infants. Some with micronodular cirrhosis die within months. Jaundice remits in others but alterations of liver function tests may persist. The mechanism of hepatocyte damage is unknown. Treatment is supportive. Liver transplantation may correct the enzymatic defect.

I Iminodiacetic acid compound scan is the best diagnostic tool for obstructive jaundice in infants. The combined values for hepatocellular uptake and excretion give the correct diagnosis in over 70 percent of patients. In early obstructive jaundice, eg, biliary atresia, there is uptake but no excretion. In parenchymal disease, eg, neonatal hepatitis, cellular function is as poor as excretion. α_1-Antitrypsin deficiency closely simulates an obstructive process and a serum level of the protein must be obtained before operation.

J Ultrasound evaluates the size of the gallbladder and the intrahepatic ducts. It can visualize choledochal cysts.

K In these conditions there may be indirect hyperbilirubinemia as in Rh and ABO incompatibility, hemolysis due to spherocytosis, and Crigler-Najjar disease, or direct hyperbilirubinemia as in sepsis, leptospirosis, and hepatitis B.

L Choledochal cysts are excised and not drained because of potential malignancy and

a propensity for stricture if the cyst is anastomosed to the intestine.

M Spontaneous perforation usually occurs at the junction of the cystic duct with the common bile duct. Treatment is drainage. A cholecystostomy catheter is left in place for postoperative cholangiography.

N Extrahepatic biliary atresia is the most common and life-threatening cause of cholestatic jaundice in infancy. Diagnosis within 3 months of age is the key to survival. In total extrahepatic biliary atresia, the entire extrahepatic biliary tree is a fibrous cord and the gallbladder either has no lumen or is tiny and filled with white bile. In proximal extrahepatic biliary atresia, the fibrous cord extends from the liver hilus to the cystic duct. The gallbladder, cystic duct, and common bile duct have small lumens. Distal extrahepatic biliary atresia ("correctable" biliary atresia) is characterized by a visible lumen in the hepatic duct and complete atresia of the distal duct.

O A small right subcostal incision is made for liver biopsy and for placement of a cholangiography catheter in the gallbladder.

P If the cholangiogram shows a patent but tiny biliary tree, the incision is closed. Biliary hypoplasia is caused by neonatal hepatitis, Rotor syndrome, Dubin-Johnson syndrome, cystic fibrosis, galactosemia, α_1-antitrypsin deficiency, and Alagille syndrome. Because the primary defect is intrahepatic, operation has little to offer.

Q Massive hemolysis due to ABO and Rh incompatibility can cause the inspissated bile syndrome. It is rare today because of prompt exchange transfusion.

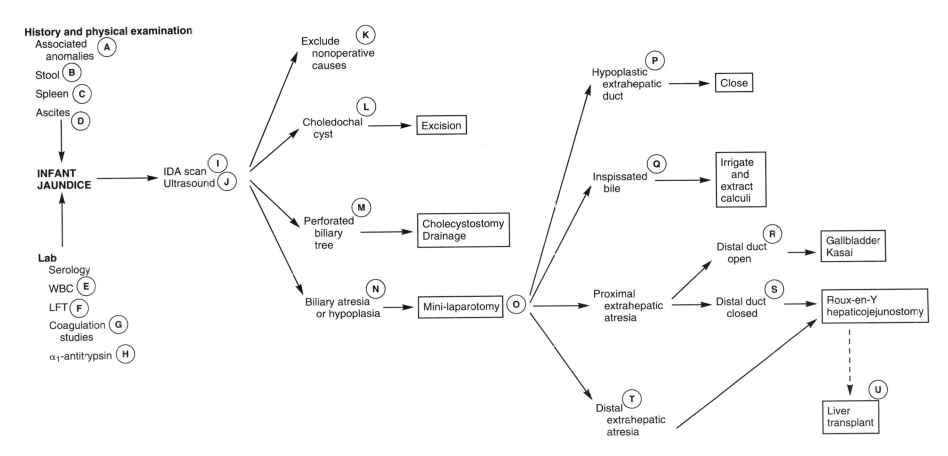

R In proximal extrahepatic biliary atresia with a patent distal duct (10 percent), the gallbladder can be anastomosed to the transected common hepatic duct at the liver hilus. An autoanastomosis occurs between the gallbladder and the microscopic intrahepatic bile ducts.

S A Roux-en-Y limb of jejunum is sutured to the transected common hepatic duct at the liver hilus. Even without visible hepatic ducts, biliary drainage will develop in about two thirds of patients if the procedure is performed before 3 months of age.

T If a cyst can be seen at the porta hepatis and the hepatic ducts are visible, a procedure similar to that described in **S** must be performed. A Roux-en-Y jejunostomy is anastomosed to the patent common hepatic duct at the liver hilus.

U Homograft liver replacement has been performed in patients who had an ''unsuccessful'' Kasai operation with a 1-year survival rate of 65 percent.

REFERENCES

Alagille D, Odievre M, Gautier M, et al. Hepatic ductular hypoplasia associated with characteristic facies, vertebral malformations, retarded physical, mental and sexual development and cardiac murmur. J Pediatr 1975; 86:63–71.

Esquivel CO, Koneru B, Karrer F, et al. Liver transplantation in infants younger than 1 year of age. J Pediatr 1987; 110:545–548.

Lilly J, Karrer FM, Hall RJ, et al. The surgery of biliary atresia. Ann Surg 1989; 210:289–296.

Lilly J, Stellin GP, Karrer FM. Forme fruste choledochal cyst. J Pediatr Surg 1985; 20:449–451.

Lilly JR, Weintraub WH, Altman RP. Spontaneous perforation of the extrahepatic bile ducts and bile peritonitis in infancy. Surgery 1974; 75:664–673.

Ohi JR, Hanamatsu M, Mochizuki I, et al. Progress in the treatment of biliary atresia. World J Surg 1985; 2:285–293.

Retroperitoneal Mass in Infancy

Ann M. Kosloske, M.D.

(A) Most abdominal masses in the infant (birth to 2 years of age) are retroperitoneal. Because many are malignant and rapidly growing, the workup must be expeditious and should be completed within 36 to 48 hours. Differentiation of retroperitoneal from intraperitoneal and pelvic masses begins with physical examination but depends primarily on diagnostic studies and, ultimately, exploration. A cystic mass within the peritoneal cavity may be an intestinal duplication, mesenteric cyst, or choledochal cyst. A solid intraperitoneal mass usually arises from the liver (eg, hepatoblastoma, hemangioendothelioma). Lymphoma can be either intraperitoneal or retroperitoneal. Pelvic masses include hydrometrocolpos, ovarian cyst, ovarian teratoma, malignant ovarian tumor (eg, teratocarcinoma, entodermal sinus tumor), pelvic kidney, and rhabdomyosarcoma.

(B) A retroperitoneal mass in infancy is typically asymptomatic and is frequently discovered by the person bathing the infant or by a practitioner performing routine physical examination. Malignant masses may be unaccompanied by pain, fever, or weight loss.

(C) Abdominal x-rays reveal calcifications in 50 percent of patients with neuroblastoma. Wilms tumor and adrenal hemorrhage calcify less commonly.

(D) Abdominal ultrasonography is the best way to distinguish cystic from solid masses. In children, cystic tumors are generally benign; solid tumors are generally malignant. Some masses such as adrenal hemorrhage have mixed echodensity. Sonography should include the renal veins and inferior vena cava, since Wilms tumor sometimes has tumor thrombi floating in these vessels. They can extend as far as the right atrium. Intravenous pyelogram has been supplanted by computed tomography and ultrasound. Sonography is limited by excessive bowel gas often found in infants. Computed tomography is more expensive, uses ionizing radiation, and usually requires sedation of the child to eliminate motion artifacts.

(E) Computed tomography scan with both intravenous and gastrointestinal contrast is performed on every infant with a solid retroperitoneal mass. It distinguishes a renal mass from one of extrarenal origin and determines the extent of the mass as well as its relationship to adjacent structures. Delineation of organs by computed tomography is limited by a child's relative paucity of perivisceral and retroperitoneal fat. A limited intravenous pyelogram may be obtained after injection of contrast material for computed tomography. The intravenous pyelogram remains useful in determining renal size and position, particularly if postoperative radiotherapy is needed. Renal opacification on intravenous pyelogram reflects the kidney's ability to concentrate and gives a rough estimate of renal function.

(F) Children with extrarenal solid tumors should have a bone scan or a bone survey for metastases. Bone marrow aspiration is done in all suspected cases of neuroblastoma or lymphoma because marrow involvement establishes a tissue diagnosis and negates the need for surgical exploration and biopsy. Analysis of urine and serum for tumor markers, such as catecholamine products in neuroblastoma, is helpful for follow-up, but operation should not be delayed until these results are obtained.

(G) A cystic extrarenal mass may be a retroperitoneal lymphangioma or a pancreatic pseudocyst. Lymphangiomas are benign tumors identical histologically to mesenteric cysts and cystic hygromas. They should be excised as completely as possible without sacrificing vital structures. Pancreatic pseudocyst in children occurs most often after trauma. It usually resolves spontaneously. If the pseudocyst persists or becomes symptomatic, internal drainage into the gastrointestinal tract is recommended.

(H) Mesoblastic nephroma is a benign renal tumor that occurs primarily in infants under 6 months of age. It generally is large and rapidly growing and can be distinguished from Wilms tumor only histologically. Treatment is by excision without chemotherapy or radiation.

(I) The most common abdominal mass palpable at birth is a multicystic dysplastic kidney. Other cystic masses include hydronephrosis and duplication. Evaluation of cystic masses of the kidney include a voiding cystourethrogram to assess urethral patency and the presence or absence of reflux and an intravenous pyelogram or renal scan to assess renal function. Nonfunctioning congenital cystic kidneys should be removed to prevent subsequent infection, trauma, or hypertension and to rule out a cystic renal tumor. The operation is not urgent. Reconstruction may be possible for anomalies in which functioning renal parenchyma remains, eg, duplications.

(J) Adrenal hemorrhage in neonates follows birth stress or trauma. The usual presentation is jaundice and a right suprarenal mass that develops rim calcification and gradually regresses. Adrenal hemorrhage may be observed without operation.

(K) Excision of a Wilms tumor is by radical nephrectomy with low division of the ureter. The essential steps of the staging operation are

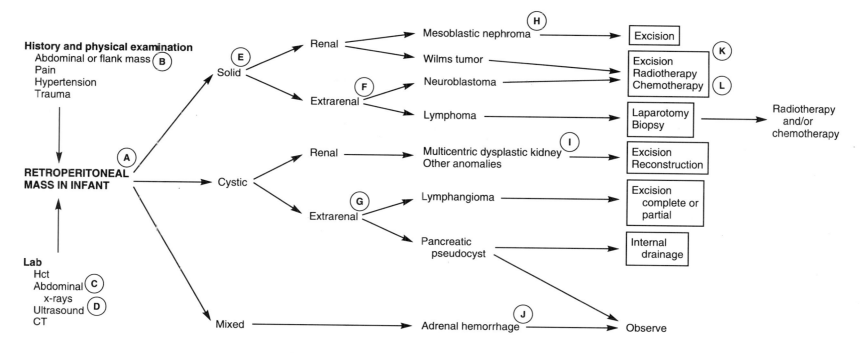

periaortic node sampling, direct exploration of the opposite kidney (which includes opening of Gerota's fascia, inspection and palpation of both anterior and posterior surfaces), and marking the tumor bed for the radiotherapist. The clips used for marking should be of a material that does not interfere with subsequent scanning procedures. The prognosis of Wilms tumor is good, depending on the stage.

(L) The prognosis of abdominal neuroblastoma is generally poor. Complete excision is rarely possible because of extensive local invasion. Tumor may extend through the intervertebral foramina to compress the spinal cord. Radiation and chemotherapy add little to survival. The prognosis is best in infants under the age of 1 year.

REFERENCES

Brasch RC, Abols IB, Gooding CA, et al. Abdominal disease in children: a comparison of computed tomography and ultrasound. Am J Radiol 1980; 134:153–158.

Cooney DR, Grosfeld JL. Operative management of pancreatic pseudocysts in infants and children: a review of 75 cases. Ann Surg 1975; 182:590–596.

Eaton DR, Cohen H. Pediatric abdominal calcifications. In: Baker SR, Elkin M, eds. Plain film approach to abdominal calcifications. Philadelphia: WB Saunders, 1982: 188.

Fletcher BD, Pratt CB. Evaluation of the child with a suspected malignant solid tumor. Pediatr Clin North Am 1991; 38:223–248.

Longino LA, Martin LW. Abdominal masses in the newborn infant. Pediatrics 1958; 21:596–604.

Otherson HB Jr. Wilms' tumor (nephroblastoma). In: Welch KJ, Randolph JG, Ravitch MM, et al, eds. Pediatric surgery, 4th ed. Chicago: Year Book Medical Publishers, 1986.

Smith EI, Castleberry RP. Neuroblastoma. Curr Probl Surg 1990; 27:575–620.

Swischuk LE, Hayden CK. Abdominal masses in children. Pediatr Clin North Am 1985; 32:1282–1298.

Transplantation

Kidney Transplantation

Roberta J. Hall, M.D., and Igal Kam, M.D.

(A) No longer are kidney transplant recipients limited to those over 12 months or under 50 years of age. Infants less than 12 months of age have a 60 to 70 percent 5-year graft survival rate for living related donors and 40 percent for cadaveric donors. Many centers restrict pediatric kidney transplantation to children over the age of 2 years.

(B) Common indications in adults are chronic glomerulonephritis, chronic pyelonephritis, or diabetic nephropathy. In children, congenital or hereditary diseases account for most renal failure treatable by transplantation.

(C) Indications for the occasional bilateral nephrectomy include (1) uncontrollable renin-dependent hypertension; (2) persistent upper urinary tract infection; (3) polycystic kidney disease complicated by significant pain, infection, bleeding, or excessive size; and (4) massive proteinuria.

(D) Previous transplantation complicates repeat transplantation for both technical and immunologic reasons. If the previous graft was lost by acute rejection, prognosis was reduced 15 to 20 percent in the pre-cyclosporine era.

(E) Pretransplant transfusion can improve graft survival but risks sensitization in approximately 20 percent. Because improved immunosuppression (cyclosporine) has nearly obliterated any advantage of pretransplant transfusion, at least half of all centers have now abandoned the practice.

(F) Pretransplant immunologic studies include ABO blood group determination; human lymphocyte antigen (HLA) typing of the A, B, C, and DR loci; panel-reactive antibody screen (PRA), and donor–recipient cross-match.

(G) Absolute immunologic requirements are ABO compatibility and negative cross-match. PRA screening measures the degree of cytotoxic antibodies in the recipient's serum against a panel of T and B lymphocytes. The more highly sensitized the recipient, the longer the waiting time will be to find a cross-match negative donor. Approximately 20 percent of patients awaiting kidney transplant are so highly sensitized that they are unlikely ever to find a graft.

(H) In 1988 and 1989, annual renal transplants numbered 9000 in the United States. Most recipients were dialysis dependent. Average cost of transplantation is approximately $40,000 for the first year and $4,000 per year thereafter. Hemodialysis costs exceed $20,000 per year for life. When risk factors are controlled (age, primary disease, associated illness) patient survival curves are identical for cadaveric transplantation and dialysis.

(I) HLA identical living donor kidney transplantation consistently provides the best chance for long-term graft survival (95 percent) with less immunosuppression and fewer complications. In recipients where donors are one or two haplotype mismatched, the 2-year survival is 85 percent. A living donor must be in good physical health and between the ages of 19 and 65 years. The donor should have a normal creatinine clearance and intravenous pyelogram and be free of coercion.

(J) Seventy-five percent of transplanted kidneys are from cadavers. A cadaveric donor must be under 65 years of age, have a normal blood urea nitrogen and creatinine (preterminal creatinine up to 3 mg/dL), and be free of sepsis, malignancy, significant hypertension, and AIDS.

(K) Kidneys flushed with cold saline are viable for 6 to 12 hours. Use of preservation fluids such as Euro-Collins or University of Wisconsin solutions extends preservation up to 72 hours.

(L) Cyclosporine, azathioprine, and corticosteroids (prednisone) are the mainstay of current immunosuppression. Cyclosporine, used since 1983, has revolutionized clinical transplantation. It inhibits the induction phase of immune response by blocking transcription of interleukin-2 and interferon-gamma. FK-506 acts similarly but is 100 times more potent. Antilymphocyte globulin, a polyclonal antiserum produced by repeated inoculation of human lymphocytes into animals, and OKT_3, a monoclonal anti-T cell antibody preparation made in mice, are powerful biologic immunosuppressive agents used to abort rejection crises.

(M) One- to two-year graft survival using both living related and cadaveric donor grafts is 74 to 95 percent. A graft that survives 2 years has a 64 percent probability of functioning 21 years.

(N) With cyclosporine, 1-year patient survival rates are 90 to 98 percent. Diabetic patients have a lower 5-year life expectancy (63 percent) compared with patients with glomerulonephritis (83 percent). Infection and cardiovascular events are major causes of death.

(O) In spite of the steroid-sparing effects of cyclosporine, infection continues to be a major source of morbidity and mortality. Infections in the first month are usually bacterial. Opportunistic infections with herpes viruses such as cytomegalovirus, Epstein-Barr virus, herpes simplex, and varicella-zoster usually occur after the first 2 to 4 weeks after steroid or OKT_3 treatment of acute rejection.

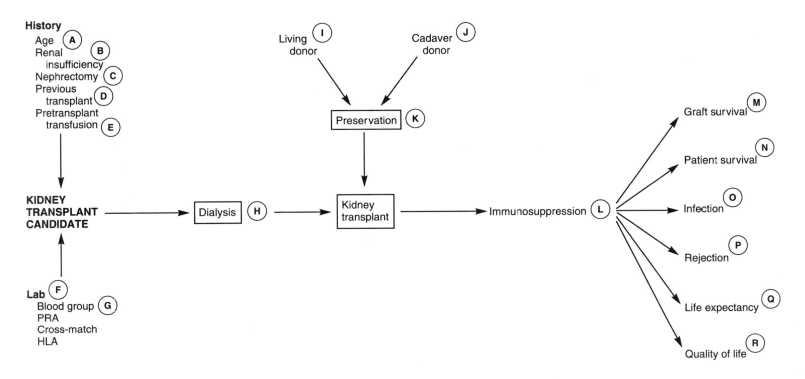

P Acute rejection causes most graft loss in the first year but less than 10 percent thereafter. Chronic rejection accounts for 80 percent of late graft failure. It is heralded by proteinuria, hypertension, and slow deterioration in renal function, is unresponsive to pulse steroid treatment, and progresses inexorably to chronic renal failure over a period of 6 months to 5 years.

Q Many patients have survived 10 to 20 years after kidney transplantation. After 5 years, patient survival and graft survival become similar.

R Quality of life significantly favors transplantation over hemodialysis. Seventy-two percent of transplantation patients and only 30 percent of dialysis patients are actively working.

REFERENCES

Blagg CR. Dialysis or transplantation? JAMA 1983; 250:1072–1073.

Carpenter CB. Immunosuppression in organ transplantation. N Engl J Med 1990; 322:1224–1226.

Gaudier FL, Santiago-Delpin E, Rivera J, et al. Pregnancy after renal transplantation. Surg Gynecol Obstet 1988; 167:533–543.

Hickey DP, Lutins JA, Lopatin WB. Lack of effect of DR matching on five-year renal allograft and patient survival with cyclosporine. Transplantation 1989; 3:83–86.

Najarian JS, Frey D, Matas A, et al. Renal transplantation in infants. Ann Surg 1990; 212:353–365.

Nylander WA, Sutherland DER, Bentley FR, et al. Fifteen to twenty year follow-up of renal transplant performed in the 1960s. Trans Proc 1985; 17:104–105.

Rubin RH, Wolfson JS, Losini AS, et al. Infection in the renal transplant recipient. Am J Med 1981; 70:405–411.

Terasaki PI, Toyotome A, Mickey MR, et al. Patient, graft and functional survival rates: an overview. In: Terasaki PI, ed. Clinical Kidney Transplants 1985. Los Angeles: UCLA Tissue Typing Lab, 1985:1.

Pancreas Transplantation

Roberta J. Hall, M.D., and Everett E. Spees, M.D., Ph.D.

(A) Pancreas transplantation is performed in diabetic patients (types I or II) in three settings: (1) pancreas transplant alone in a preuremic patient (PTA); (2) pancreas transplant after successful kidney transplant (PAK); and (3) simultaneous kidney and pancreas transplant (SPK). Because graft survival in the latter group is superior to that in either the PTA or PAK groups (approximately 75 percent 1-year graft survival compared with 55 percent 1-year graft survival, respectively), many centers restrict transplantation to patients who need both kidney and pancreas replacement.

(B) There are no strict age restrictions. Half of all pancreas transplants are performed in patients between the ages of 30 and 40 years. Few are performed in patients less than age 20 years or in those over age 50 years. Most patients have had diabetes for 10 to 20 years but one third have had diabetes for less than 10 years.

(C) Pretransplant laboratory evaluation is identical to that for kidney transplantation and includes ABO blood group and human lymphocyte antigen (HLA) typing. Absolute prerequisites are ABO compatibility and a negative cross-match. Close HLA matching for A, B, and DR loci is preferred. A significantly higher 1-year graft survival is expected when the degree of mismatch is less than three loci (68%) than when the mismatch is four or greater (59%).

(D) Recipient evaluation includes a thorough physical examination with special emphasis on neurologic, ophthalmologic, and cardiac function. Transplantation should be performed before the patient develops severe secondary complications such as disabling neuropathy, extensive vascular disease, and advanced retinopathy. Contraindications are presence of malignancy, active infection, advanced cardiovascular disease, major amputations, or blindness.

(E) A potential cadaver donor should be age 10 to 55 years with no family history of diabetes, pancreatitis, or significant hypertension. The donor should be hemodynamically stable on minimal vasopressors with no pancreatic trauma or peritoneal contamination. Serum amylase may be elevated but lipase should be normal.

(F) The ureters, abdominal vena cava, aorta, and major vascular branches are surgically dissected. Then the liver and heart are removed. Finally, the pancreas and duodenum are harvested. Care is taken to identify vascular anomalies, particularly a right hepatic artery arising from the superior mesenteric artery, and to ensure that both pancreas and liver allografts have adequate blood supply. A portal cannula may be inserted into the inferior mesenteric vein for liver precooling. The duodenum is irrigated with antibiotics through the nasogastric tube. It is then divided proximally and distally with a stapler knife. Heparin is administered. The abdominal organs are perfused and refrigerated by aortic cannula flush while the thoracic allografts are removed. After adequate cooling, the abdominal allografts are removed en bloc.

(G) The abdominal (but not the thoracic) allograft viscera are usually perfused with University of Wisconsin solution (Viaspan), using 2 to 3 L for the average adult. External cooling is employed using a sterile saline slush solution. After removal of the pancreas and liver, verapamil is added to the renal allograft perfusate to reduce vasospasm. The abdominal viscera can be placed in sterile containers and maintained at 4°C for 24 hours or longer before transplantation.

(H) The abdomen is opened through a midline incision. Vascular anastomoses are made between the donor splenic vein and recipient common iliac vein and between the donor splenic artery (to which the donor superior mesenteric artery has already been attached) and the recipient common iliac artery. By tradition, when simultaneous kidney and pancreas transplantation is performed, the pancreas is placed on the right and the kidney on the left. Both are drained via the bladder, ie, the pancreas by anastomosis of a donor duodenal patch containing the pancreatic duct to the bladder, the kidney by ureterocystostomy.

(I) Adequate pancreatic endocrine function can be provided by segmental transplantation of the body and tail. Transplanting the entire pancreas is more commonly done because it provides more islet cells and allows monitoring of exocrine excretion in the urine after pancreaticocystostomy.

(J) Whole pancreas drainage into the bladder through the attached duodenal allograft is commonly used. It provides less danger of leakage and has fewer complications than drainage into a Roux-en-Y ileal loop. Bladder drainage also allows monitoring of urine amylase. Levels of amylase parallel the degree of function of the pancreas allograft.

(K) The highest graft survival rates follow combined pancreas and kidney transplant. High HLA-DR matched pancreas transplants, alone or subsequent to a previous successful kidney transplant, also have good survival rates.

(L) Pancreas transplants tend to be rejected frequently and strongly. Histocompatibility matching, especially for the HLA-DR antigens, reduces this risk. Immune induction with horse, goat, or mouse antiserum is usually used in combination with prednisone and Imuran. Cyclosporine is started after 1 to 2 weeks of antiserum.

(M) With simultaneous kidney transplant and bladder drainage, a fall in urine amylase usually accompanies allograft rejection. Elevation of the serum creatinine and blood urea nitrogen

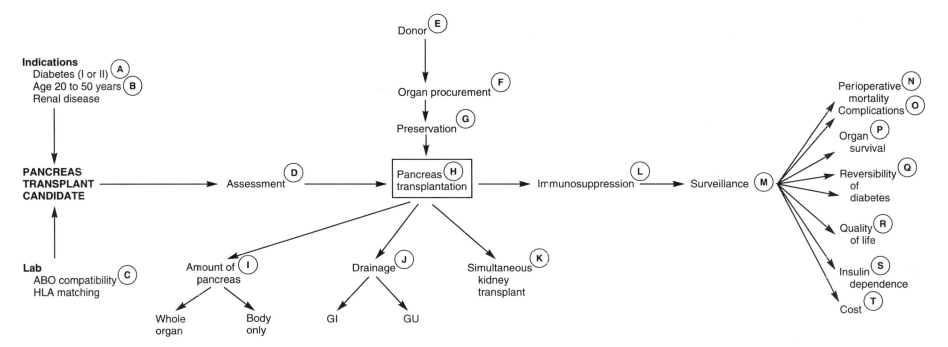

frequently accompany this fall. Renal and pancreas ultrasound examination and renal needle biopsy help confirm rejection.

(N) Perioperative mortality is 1 percent or less. Occasionally, cardiovascular catastrophe or reaction to mouse monoclonals cause death.

(O) Complications include accelerated rejection, primary graft nonfunction, early pancreatic venous thrombosis, infections (especially cytomegalovirus), hematuria, pancreatitis, and pancreatic fistula.

(P) One-year pancreas graft survival is 60 to 75 percent and kidney graft survival is 75 to 85 percent.

(Q) After successful transplant, recipients may stabilize their vision and improve or stabilize

their neuropathy. The pancreas transplant may protect kidney allografts from diabetic nephropathic changes.

(R) Quality of life is greatly improved, especially in those who had unstable diabetes before transplantation and in those who have functioning eyes, limbs, and hearts.

(S) Successful recipients are insulin independent within hours to days and have normal glucose tolerance test results and glycosylated hemoglobin levels. Unstable diabetics are free of the danger of insulin reactions as well as hyperglycemia. Hyperglycemia can occur transiently with rejections and infections or permanently if the allograft is rejected.

(T) The cost is about $60,000. This does not include postdischarge care or medications.

The cost of pancreas transplant accompanying kidney transplantation is about $20,000, since much of the overhead is included in the kidney transplant cost.

REFERENCES

Frohnert PP, Velosa JA, Munn SR, et al. Morbidity during the first year after pancreas transplantation. Transplant Proc 1990; 22:577–578.

Groth CG, ed. Pancreatic transplantation. Philadelphia: WB Saunders, 1988.

Johnson JL, Schellberg J, Munn SR, et al. Does pancreas transplantation really improve the patient' quality of life? Transplant Proc 1990; 22:575–576.

Sutherland DER. International pancreas transplantation registry analysis. Transplant Proc 1990; 22:571–574.

Liver Transplantation

Luis G. Podesta, M.D., Linda S. Sher, M.D., Todd K. Howard, M.D., and Leonard Makowka, M.D., Ph.D.

(A) In adults, the most frequent indications for liver transplantation are postnecrotic cirrhosis, sclerosing cholangitis, and primary biliary cirrhosis. In children, primary indications are biliary atresia, inborn errors of metabolism, and cirrhosis.

(B) Infection imposes an obvious added risk in the immunodepressed recipient.

(C) Pretransplant evaluation includes liver enzymes, coagulation profile, hematologic profile, nutritional evaluation, infectious disease evaluation, electrocardiogram, and tumor markers.

(D) ABO blood group and donor–recipient crossmatch are the only absolute requirements for transplant but human leukocyte antigen (HLA) typing of the A,B,C, and DR loci and panel-reactive antibody screening evaluate the degree of cytoxic antibodies in the recipient's serum.

(E) Imaging evaluations include computed tomography scan of the abdomen to determine liver volume and evidence of metastases.

(F) Metastatic workup is needed where liver tumor is involved.

(G) Doppler ultrasound evaluates patency of the extrahepatic vasculature and the bile ducts. Arteriography, cholangiography, or magnetic resonance imaging may be indicated.

(H) A multispecialty evaluation committee determines a patient's relative priority for transplantation compared with other recipients. Absolute contraindications include AIDS, severe infection outside the hepatobiliary tract, extrahepatic malignancy, multiple organ failure not reversible by liver transplant, irreversible brain damage, technical impossibility, and inability of the patient to comply with postoperative requirements.

(I) The potential donor must be pronounced brain dead by standards established in the local community. The donor must have normal liver function studies and no history of liver disease.

(J) Successful procurement includes adequate oxygenation and circulation to the liver and satisfactory liver function as shown by coagulation profile, enzymes, and bilirubin. Multiple organ procurement (kidney, heart, pancreas, etc.) has become increasingly common.

(K) Hepatic allografts can be preserved up to 24 hours using the University of Wisconsin solution.

(L) Although whole orthotopic allografts are usual, variants include segmental portions of donor livers for children, splitting the liver for use in two recipients, living related donation of a liver segment, piggy-back liver implantation, hepatic arterial and portal venous grafting, and grafting with other abdominal or thoracic organs.

(M) Immunosuppression involves administration of cyclosporine, azathioprine, steroids, monoclonal antibodies, polyclonal antibodies, or FK-506.

(N) Rejection is suggested by jaundice, elevated liver enzymes, fever, feeling of illness, decrease in quantity of bile, ascites, or pleural effusion. Proof is by liver biopsy.

(O) Technical complications include hepatic artery thrombosis, biliary stricture, biliary leak, and postoperative hemorrhage. Hepatic artery thrombosis is manifested by fulminant hepatic failure. In most cases retransplantation is necessary.

(P) In the immediate posttransplantation period most infections are bacterial in origin. After a month most are viral, usually cytomegalovirus.

Fungal infections usually occur in severely debilitated patients.

(Q) Indications for retransplantation include primary graft nonfunction, unremitting rejection, hepatic artery thrombosis, portal vein thrombosis, multiple intrahepatic strictures, and recurrence of primary disease (eg, hepatitis B or Budd-Chiari syndrome).

(R) Five-year survival rates are 65 to 75 percent. Variation primarily depends on case selection. For hepatocellular carcinoma, one-year survival is about 40 percent. With the fibrolamellar variant, 1- and five-year survival rates are 75 percent and 30 percent, respectively.

(S) Side effects of immunosuppressive drugs include hypertension, hyperkalemia, hirsutism, central nervous system toxicity, renal and hepatotoxicity, increased fat deposition, poor wound healing, and fluid retention.

(T) After successful transplantation, over 85 percent of patients return to near-normal lifestyles, including employment, school, and family responsibilities.

REFERENCES

Iwatsuki S, Starzl TE, Todo S, et al. Experience in 1000 liver transplants under cyclosporine-steroid therapy: a survival report. Transplant Proc 1988; 20(Suppl 1):498–504.

Maddrey WC, ed. Transplantation of the liver. New York: Elsevier Science Publishers, 1988.

Makowka LM, Van Thiel DH. Liver transplantation. Gastroenterol Clin North Am 1988; 1:1–233.

Starzl TE, Demetris AJ, Van Thiel DH. Liver transplantation (first of two parts). N Engl J Med 1989; 321:1014–1022.

Starzl TE, Demetris AJ, Van Thiel DH. Liver transplantation (second of two parts). N Engl J Med 1989; 321:1092–1099.

Starzl TE. Liver transplantation. Chicago: Mosby Year Book Medical Publishers, 1990.

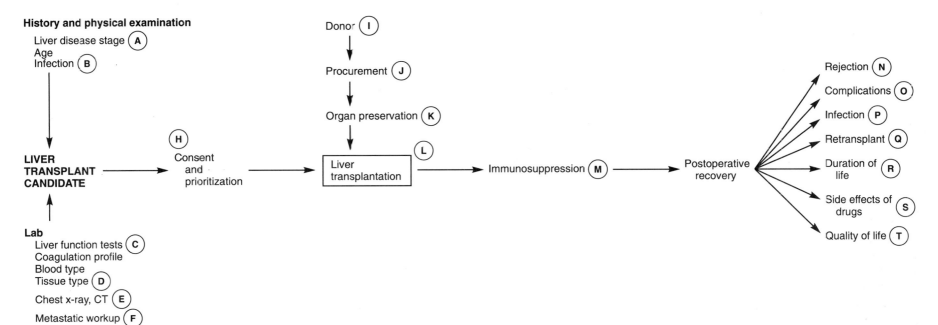

History and physical examination

Liver disease stage (A)
Age
Infection (B)

Donor (I)

↓

Procurement (J)

↓

Organ preservation (K)

↓

(H)

LIVER TRANSPLANT CANDIDATE → Consent and prioritization → Liver transplantation (L) → Immunosuppression (M) → Postoperative recovery

Rejection (N)
Complications (O)
Infection (P)
Retransplant (Q)
Duration of life (R)
Side effects of drugs (S)
Quality of life (T)

Lab
Liver function tests (C)
Coagulation profile
Blood type
Tissue type (D)
Chest x-ray, CT (E)
Metastatic workup (F)
Ultrasound (G)

Heart Transplantation

Robert L. Kormos, M.D., and Henry T. Bahnson, M.D.

(A) Myocardial failure refractory to all alternative therapy is the essential indication for heart transplantation. By definition, all patients have class III or IV heart failure with restricted physical activity and fluid intake and are receiving maximal pharmacologic treatment. Idiopathic cardiomyopathy was once the most common preoperative diagnosis. Because of improved techniques and results, ischemic heart disease has now become the most common diagnosis. The average age of recipients has increased; 60 percent of patients are over age 45 years.

(B) Right heart catheterization determines reactivity of the pulmonary vasculature. Pulmonary vascular resistance greater than 5 Wood units or a transpulmonary gradient greater that 17 torr, unresponsive to prostaglandin E_1 or nitroglycerin, is an indication for heterotopic cardiac transplantation or, in some cases, heart–lung transplantation.

(C) Significant primary disease in other vital organs is a contraindication for transplantation. Obstructive or restrictive lung disease, which requires bronchodilator therapy, is a contraindication. The psychosocial resources of patient and family are important in selecting candidates because of the lifelong need for medication and surveillance for rejection or infection. Other contraindications are conditions worsened by immunosuppression, specifically infection, malignancy, and recent pulmonary embolism.

(D) A panel-reactive antibody level measures potential reactivity to donor human leukocyte (HLA) antigens. Patients with reactivity greater than 25 percent have an actuarial 1-year freedom from death due to rejection of only 58 percent compared with 95 percent for patients with reactivity less than 10 percent.

(E) Screening for reactivity to Epstein-Barr nuclear antigen, cytomegalovirus, and toxoplasmosis helps guide postoperative therapy.

(F) Hemodynamic deterioration while waiting for a donor heart may require a pharmacologic or mechanical bridge to transplantation. This involves use of intravenous dopamine, dobutamine, and amrinone, and then possibly insertion of an intraaortic balloon pump or assist devices for the left or both ventricles. Ventricular arrhythmias may require implantation of an automatic defibrillator.

(G) A donor who is brain dead with a beating heart must have a compatible blood type. A matching blood type is desired. Restraints of time and logistics usually preclude a preoperative crossmatch for HLA. The donor should be under age 45 years with no known heart disease, systemic infection, trauma to the heart, prolonged hypotension or arrest, or great need for cardiotonic or vasopressor drugs. Echocardiography provides a reliable assessment of ventricular function. For donors over the age of 45 years and for those with a family history of coronary artery disease, coronary angiography should be considered. A consent for donation must be obtained from next of kin.

(H) Procurement of multiple organs by different teams from the same donor is common. Kidneys, liver, heart, and lungs are obtained in that order of frequency. Viability of other organs depends on preservation of cardiac function until the final swift isolation and removal of the heart. Preservation of the heart is with cold blood cardioplegia containing potassium 40 mEq/L. Heart size of donor and recipient should match within 10 percent.

(I) Operation is standardized with little change from earlier techniques. After the ischemia of implantation, the heart usually needs unloaded perfusion for some minutes and then pharmacologic support for 1 to 3 days by cardiotonic drugs (dobutamine, dopamine), vasodilators (nitroglycerin or nitroprusside), and vasopressors.

(J) Heterotopic implantation is indicated for high pulmonary vascular resistance or when a small heart or one with questionable function is used. It is less desirable because of the threat of pulmonary emboli from the hypofunctioning recipient heart. Angina may persist and the two hearts, by compressing each other, can jeopardize function. Heart–lung transplantation is used for severe pulmonary hypertension or disease of both heart and lungs. Donors are fewer. About half of recipients survive 1 year.

(K) Immunosuppression consists of azathioprine, cyclosporine, low-dose steroids, and sometimes antithymocytic globulin. Rabbit antithymocytic globulin, OKT3, or equine antilymphocytic globulin is often used prophylactically during the first weeks to selectively reduce the T lymphocyte count.

(L) Endomyocardial biopsy is performed weekly and then at increasing intervals during the first year. Drug dosages are adjusted to combat renal toxicity and the reciprocal problems of infection and rejection. Annual reevaluations look for lymphoproliferative disease as well as fungal, viral, and parasitic infections and nephrotoxicity of immunosuppressive agents. Cardiac catheterization is used to monitor atherosclerosis of the coronary arteries, which develops in 5 percent of patients at

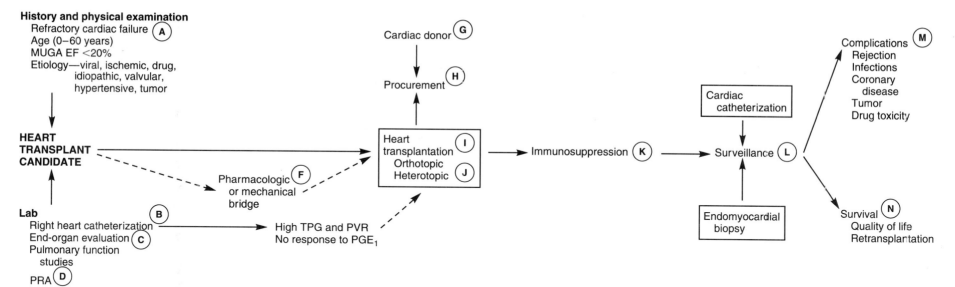

History and physical examination
Refractory cardiac failure (A)
Age (0–60 years)
MUGA EF <20%
Etiology—viral, ischemic, drug,
    idiopathic, valvular,
    hypertensive, tumor

HEART TRANSPLANT CANDIDATE

Pharmacologic or mechanical bridge (F)

Lab
Right heart catheterization (B)
End-organ evaluation (C)
Pulmonary function studies
PRA (D)
Blood group
Absence of infection (E)

High TPG and PVR
No response to PGE$_1$

Cardiac donor (G)

Procurement (H)

Heart transplantation (I)
Orthotopic
Heterotopic (J)

Immunosuppression (K)

Cardiac catheterization

Surveillance (L)

Endomyocardial biopsy

Complications (M)
Rejection
Infections
Coronary disease
Tumor
Drug toxicity

Survival (N)
Quality of life
Retransplantation

---

1 year and subsequently in 10 percent per year to an incidence of 60 percent at 5 years.

(M) Rejection occurs with inadequate immunosuppression. It is inversely related to infection, which results from over immunosuppression. Hypertension in 95 percent of patients is a nephrotoxic side effect of cyclosporine. It can be treated by diuretics, acetylcholinesterase inhibitors, or calcium channel blockers. Diabetes mellitus and osteoporosis occur with the overuse of corticosteroids. Lymphoproliferative tumors and malignant neo-

plasms occur in 4 percent of patients as a result of immunosuppression and infection with the Epstein-Barr virus.

(N) Perioperative mortality is 5 to 7 percent. It is higher in children, in the elderly, in women, and in those who are transplanted urgently. Primary graft failure occurs in approximately 7 percent of patients, one third of whom have hyperacute rejection. Perioperative mortality for patients with pulmonary hypertension and a transpulmonary

gradient less than 15 torr is approximately 10 percent; for a gradient over 15 torr it is 20 percent.

REFERENCES

Levett JM, Karp RB. Heart transplantation. Surg Clin North Am 1985; 65:613–631.
Miller LW. Long-term complications of cardiac transplantation. Prog Cardiovasc Dis 1991; 33:229–282.
Reichenspurner H, Odell JA, Cooper DX, et al. Twenty years of heart transplantation at Groote Shuur Hospital. J Heart Transplant 1987; 6:317–323.

Urologic

Traumatic Hematuria

Norman E. Peterson, M.D.

(A) Gross or microscopic (>5 red blood cells per high power field) hematuria after trauma warrants investigation. Survivable trauma rarely involves both the upper and lower urinary tract. Diagnostic priority is given to the site of maximum apparent injury (abdomen vs. pelvis). Complicating factors such as pelvic fracture, arterial hemorrhage, and rectal injury must be considered. Urgent laparotomy may preclude preoperative urologic evaluation. If unsuspected retroperitoneal hematoma is encountered, its significance often correlates with the pattern of hematuria. Intraoperative urography (or arteriography, $1030) can be obtained or the kidney can be explored.

(B) Retrograde urethrography ($142) defines urethral integrity: total, partial, or avulsion. Bladder opacification accompanying urethral extravasation connotes subtotal avulsion and warrants cystostomy diversion ($1100). Total avulsion can be managed initially by cystostomy diversion but requires delayed urethroplasty ($1800) or bridging catheterization at laparotomy ($284).

(C) Excretory urography ($235) defines the presence and functional status of the kidneys and the presence of renal extravasation.

(D) Computerized tomography ($650) is favored by some as a screening examination for renal trauma. It may obviate urography. When computerized tomography scanning is done to survey the total abdomen, intravenous pyelogram may be unnecessary.

(E) Extraperitoneal bladder injury commonly responds to 5 to 7 days of urethral catheterization. Intraperitoneal bladder injury requires operative repair ($1100) and evaluation for other injury (bowel, mesentery).

(F) Renal extravasation is usually transitory. If repeat urography (48 to 72 hour) shows improvement, recovery is likely to be complete. Otherwise, repair ($1100) will be necessary.

(G) Renal parenchymal laceration is amenable to spontaneous recovery. Gross hematuria that diminishes noticeably within several hours of injury reflects injury that usually can be managed nonoperatively.

(H) Urographic nonfunction is an indication for either ultrasonic scanning ($234) or computed tomography scanning to verify renal presence, and for isotope flow scanning ($340) to evaluate pedicle integrity. Arterial thrombosis or avulsion causes surprisingly little bleeding and can be managed conservatively. Renal fragmentation bleeds extensively and requires nephrectomy ($1513).

(I) Undiminishing gross hematuria warrants consideration of therapeutic selective embolization ($1021) or operative intervention (repair vs. nephrectomy, $1100). Delayed hematuria often responds to temporary bed rest.

REFERENCES

Brosman SA, Paul JG. Trauma of the bladder. Surg Gynecol Obstet 1976; 143:605–608.

Peterson NE. Traumatic posterior urethral avulsion. Monogr Urol 1986; 7:61–82.

Peterson NE. Current management of urethral injuries. In: Rous SN, ed. 1988 urology annual. East Norwalk, CT: Appleton-Century-Crofts, 1988: 143–179.

Peterson NE. Complications of renal trauma. Urol Clin North Am 1989; 16:221–236.

Peterson NE. Blunt trauma to the kidney. In: Callaham MC, Barrou CW, Schumaker HM, eds: Decision making in emergency medicine. Philadelphia: BC Decker, 1990: 151–179.

Peterson NE. Current management of acute renal trauma. In: Rous SN, ed. 1991 urology annual. New York: Appleton and Lange, 1991.

Peterson NE, Pitts JC III. Penetrating injuries of the ureter. J Urol 1981; 126:587–590.

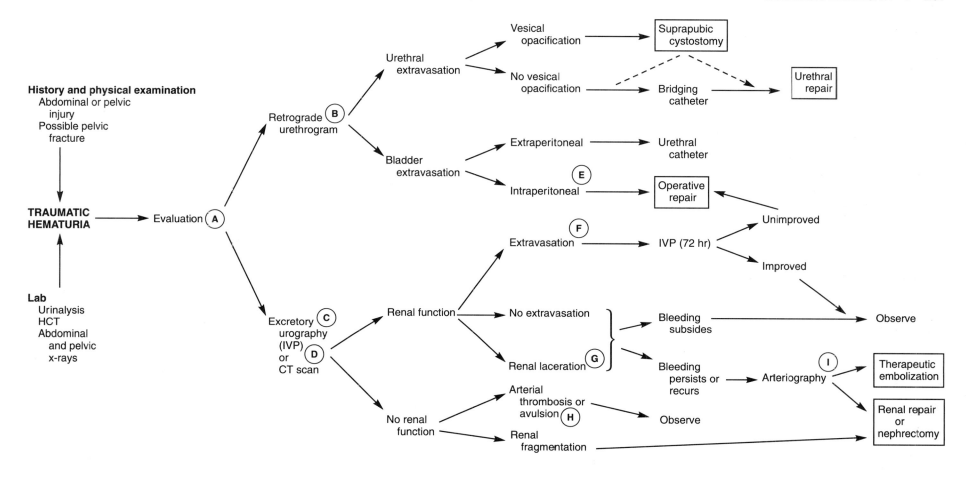

History and physical examination
 Abdominal or pelvic
  injury
 Possible pelvic
  fracture

**TRAUMATIC
HEMATURIA**

Lab
 Urinalysis
 HCT
 Abdominal
  and pelvic
  x-rays

Evaluation Ⓐ

Retrograde Ⓑ
urethrogram

Excretory Ⓒ
urography
(IVP) Ⓓ
or
CT scan

Urethral
extravasation

Bladder
extravasation

Vesical
opacification → Suprapubic
cystostomy

No vesical
opacification → Bridging
catheter

Urethral
repair

Extraperitoneal → Urethral
catheter

Intraperitoneal Ⓔ → Operative
repair

Renal function

No renal
function

Extravasation Ⓕ → IVP (72 hr)

No extravasation

Renal laceration Ⓖ

Arterial
thrombosis or
avulsion Ⓗ

Renal
fragmentation

Unimproved

Improved

Bleeding
subsides

Bleeding
persists or
recurs → Arteriography Ⓘ

Observe

Observe

Therapeutic
embolization

Renal repair
or
nephrectomy

Adult Urinary Tract Infection

Richard Heppe, M.D.

(A) Clinically significant bacteriuria is generally more than 100,000 colonies per milliliter of the same organism in a midstream clean-catch urine specimen. Lower titers are occasionally pathogenic. Pyuria is significant when there are more than 5 white blood cells per high power field.

(B) Pyelonephritis is marked by fever, flank pain, pyuria, bacteriuria, and leukocytosis. Etiologic factors include vesicoureteral reflux, ureteral obstruction, and hematogenous spread.

(C) Lower urinary tract infections are associated with frequency, urgency, dysuria, suprapubic pain, hematuria (hemorrhagic cystitis), pyuria, and bacteriuria. Most commonly, these infections arise from organisms ascending through the urethra. Hematogenous spread and extension from adjacent organs (eg, from diverticulitis) are rarely responsible.

(D) When the patient presents with upper tract findings the kidneys must be evaluated. Intravenous pyelography can be performed safely when serum creatinine is less than 1.5 mg/dL. Ultrasound should be considered in patients with renal insufficiency, diabetes, or dehydration. A contrast-enhanced computed tomography scan is useful for renal imaging, especially if other intraabdominal pathology is suspected. Cystoscopy is always necessary to complete the urinary tract workup in pyelonephritis.

(E) Four specimens are collected as follows. After cleansing the glans, the first voided 10 mL are collected (VB 1); a midstream specimen is then obtained (VB 2); a prostatic massage is carried out and if there are any expressed prostatic secretions these are sent for culture; finally, the patient is again asked to void and the first 10 mL are collected and analyzed (VB 3). No growth in VB 1 or VB 2 with growth in expressed prostatic secretions or VB 3 indicates a bacterial prostatitis.

(F) The renal pelvis and ureter can be obstructed by calculi, intrinsic tumors, sloughed papillae secondary to sickle cell anemia or phenacetin abuse, blood clots, and mycelial bezoars (fungus balls).

(G) Symptomatic or asymptomatic bacteriuria during pregnancy should always be treated with the appropriate antibiotic. Individual episodes can be treated with a short course. Persistent bacteriuria, however, should be managed with chemoprophylaxis until term.

(H) Asymptomatic bacteriuria in a nonpregnant, unobstructed woman requires no therapy.

(I) If all cultures of the three-glass urine are negative, a nonbacterial prostatitis is most likely. Antibiotics are of no value in this situation. Therapy should be directed toward palliation of local symptoms.

REFERENCES

Schoenbeck J, Anderson L, Lingarch G, et al. Ureteric obstruction caused by yeast like fungi. Scand J Urol Nephrol 1970; 4:171–174.

Stamey TA, Sexton CC. The role of vaginal colonization with enterobacteriaceae in recurrent urinary infections. J Urol 1975; 113:214–217.

Stamey TA. Protogenesis and treatment of urinary infections. Baltimore: Williams & Wilkins, 1980.

Stamm WE, Counts GW, Running KR, et al. Diagnosis of coliform infection in acutely dysuric women. New Engl J Med 1982; 307:463–468.

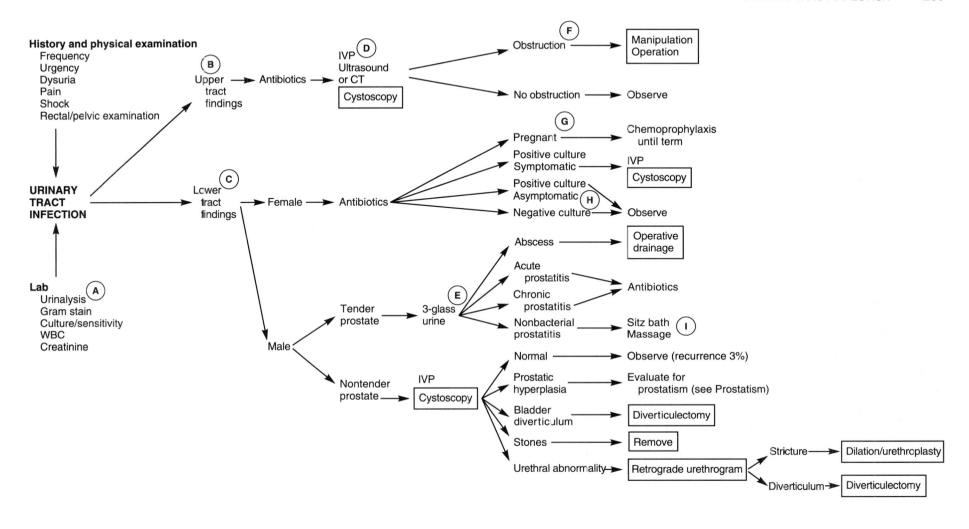

History and physical examination
- Frequency
- Urgency
- Dysuria
- Pain
- Shock
- Rectal/pelvic examination

URINARY TRACT INFECTION

Lab (A)
- Urinalysis
- Gram stain
- Culture/sensitivity
- WBC
- Creatinine

(B) Upper tract findings → Antibiotics → (D) IVP Ultrasound or CT / Cystoscopy

Obstruction (F) → Manipulation Operation

No obstruction → Observe

(C) Lower tract findings → Female → Antibiotics

- Pregnant (G) → Chemoprophylaxis until term
- Positive culture Symptomatic → IVP / Cystoscopy
- Positive culture Asymptomatic (H) → Observe
- Negative culture → Observe

Male → Tender prostate → (E) 3-glass urine

- Abscess → Operative drainage
- Acute prostatitis → Antibiotics
- Chronic prostatitis → Antibiotics
- Nonbacterial prostatitis → Sitz bath Massage (I)

Male → Nontender prostate → IVP / Cystoscopy

- Normal → Observe (recurrence 3%)
- Prostatic hyperplasia → Evaluate for prostatism (see Prostatism)
- Bladder diverticulum → Diverticulectomy
- Stones → Remove
- Urethral abnormality → Retrograde urethrogram → Stricture → Dilation/urethroplasty
- Retrograde urethrogram → Diverticulum → Diverticulectomy

Renal or Ureteral Calculus

George W. Drach, M.D.

(A) Renal colic is intermittent flank or abdominal pain caused by impaction of a calculus somewhere in the upper urinary system. It is severe and crescendos in intensity. The patient often writhes and can find no position of comfort. Pain is often referred to the ipsilateral testicle or labium majorum. Tenderness on deep palpation or percussion of the abdomen or flank, especially the costovertebral angle, is common. A personal or family history of renal calculus is common.

(B) Urinalysis reveals microscopic or gross hematuria in 90 percent of patients. Since over 90 percent of calculi in Americans are radiodense, a plain abdominal x-ray (KUB) should be obtained. If a stone is not obvious on KUB, intravenous urography (IVP) confirms the intraurinary system position of a stone or visualizes a radiolucent stone. Follow-up of patients proved by IVP to have a stone is possible with interval KUB films, radioisotopic studies, or ultrasound scans.

(C) Radiolucent stones composed primarily of uric acid respond to treatment with oral or parenteral alkali such as sodium bicarbonate. They either dissolve rapidly and completely or decrease in size and pass spontaneously. Radiolucent cystine stones respond in the same way but require more

intense alkalization. Those that do not dissolve should be treated as in **D**.

(D) Radiopaque calculi consist of either calcium oxalate, calcium phosphate, or struvite. Treatment of struvite stones that result from urinary infection is with antibiotics.

(E) Calculi less than 4 mm in diameter have a 90 percent chance of passing.

(F) Stones measuring 4 to 6 mm in diameter have only a 60 percent chance of passing.

(G) Stones over 6 mm in diameter have only a 20 percent chance of passing and usually require procedural intervention such as shock-wave lithotripsy.

(H) Ninety-five percent of stones in the upper urinary tract that previously required operation can now be handled by some manipulative technique. Success rates for complete elimination approach 80 percent.

(I) Persistent calculi in the kidney or ureter are seldom removed operatively. They are treated instead by percutaneous or extracorporeal stone destruction. Endoscopic antegrade or retrograde renal or ureteral stone destruction is per-

formed with or without electrohydraulic or ultrasonic techniques. The fragments are extracted by baskets or pass spontaneously. Extracorporeal shock-wave lithotripsy can destroy stones without surgical invasion and has become the management of choice for renal and ureteral calculi.

(J) Calculi retained in the middle or lower third of the ureter can be removed by transurethral stone manipulation or shock-wave lithotripsy. A few require open surgical procedures.

REFERENCES

Drach GW. Urinary lithiasis. In: Walsh PC, Gittes RF, Perlmutter AD, Stamey TA, eds. Campbell's urology. Philadelphia: WB Saunders, 1986:1093–1190.

Drach GW. Stone manipulation: modern usage and occasional mishaps. Urology 1978; 12:286–289.

Furlow WL, Bucchiere JJ. The surgical fate of ureteral calculi: review of Mayo Clinic experience. J Urol 1976; 116:559–561.

Lutzeyer W, Herin FJ, Vander H, et al. Ureteral calculus: experience with 521 stone extractions. Trans Am Assoc Genitourin Surg 1979; 70:19–21.

O'Flynn JD. The treatment of ureteric stones: report on 1120 patients. Br J Urol 1980; 52:436–438.

Wickham JEA, Kellet MJ. Percutaneous nephrolithotomy. Br J Urol 1981; 53:297–299.

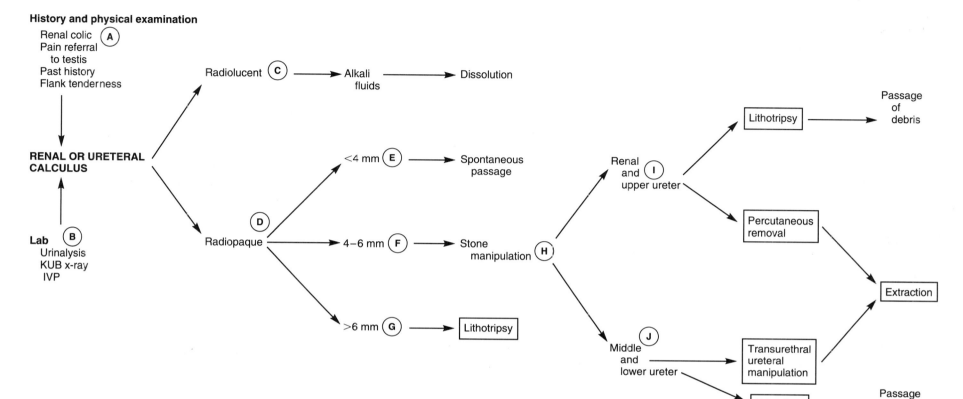

History and physical examination
Renal colic (A)
Pain referral
to testis
Past history
Flank tenderness

RENAL OR URETERAL
CALCULUS

Lab (B)
Urinalysis
KUB x-ray
IVP

Radiolucent (C) → Alkali fluids → Dissolution

Radiopaque (D)

<4 mm (E) → Spontaneous passage

4–6 mm (F) → Stone manipulation (H)

>6 mm (G) → Lithotripsy

Renal and upper ureter (I)
→ Lithotripsy → Passage of debris
→ Percutaneous removal → Extraction

Middle and lower ureter (J)
→ Transurethral ureteral manipulation → Extraction
→ Lithotripsy → Passage of debris

Renal Mass

Robert E. Donohue, M.D.

(A) The most common renal mass is a simple renal cyst. A cyst can achieve great size, produce symptoms at times, and be difficult to distinguish from renal tumor. Other benign lesions occur less frequently but can also be confused with renal tumor. They are renal adenoma, renal angiomyelolipoma, multiloculated cyst, parapelvic cyst, renal abscess, hypertrophied column of Bertin, lobar nephronia, and xanthogranulomatous pyelonephritis.

(B) Renal cell carcinoma is the most common symptomatic renal malignancy. A history of flank pain or hematuria is suggestive of renal cell carcinoma. The presence of an upper abdominal mass increases the suspicion of renal tumor. Other factors in the history or physical examination that increase suspicion of malignancy include a family history of renal cell cancer, tuberous sclerosis, sudden appearance of a varicocele, erythrocytosis, hypercalcemia, or a renal mass with punctate calcification within it. Metastases from lung and breast cancer are more common renal masses than renal cell carcinoma but are often asymptomatic. Hematologic malignancies, such as leukemia and lymphoma, frequently involve the kidney and must be considered in the differential diagnosis of a renal mass. Transitional cell carcinoma of the renal pelvis and calyces also occurs.

(C) Excretion urography (IVP), transabdominal ultrasonography (US), and computed tomography scanning are the imaging studies that can most commonly detect a renal mass. IVP is useful for evaluation of hematuria, urinary tract infection, ureteral and renal colic, flank pain, and the presence of a flank mass. It costs $175 for the procedure and $55 for interpretation. It is an invasive study, and up to 5 percent of patients have unto-

ward reactions ranging from nausea and vomiting to renal failure and death. Ultrasonography is performed during pregnancy, in patients with right upper quadrant pain or an abdominal mass, in jaundiced patients, and for the staging of many malignancies. It costs $185 for the procedure and $70 for interpretation. Ultrasonography is noninvasive and has no side effects. Computed tomography scanning is the first study employed by many clinicians in the above conditions. It costs $730 for the procedure and $115 for interpretation. With the administration of intravenous contrast, the incidence and nature of the side effects are the same as for IVP.

(D) The first study that should be performed after the detection of a renal mass is ultrasonography. The lesion may be cystic, indeterminate, or solid. A simple cyst has sharply defined borders, no internal echoes, and increased through-transmission of sound. If these signs are present no further evaluation of the simple cyst is required. If any suspicion persists after ultrasonography, cyst puncture with aspiration of the fluid for color, enzyme studies, and cytology can usually resolve the question. The cost is $970. Computed tomography scanning or angiography can also be used before exploration is considered. An indeterminate mass and a solid mass require further evaluation. Ultrasonography detects and defines hydronephrosis clearly but it is insensitive in the diagnosis of transitional cell carcinoma.

(E) Computed tomography scanning is more sensitive than ultrasonography in detecting a cystic mass. Ultrasonography is more specific in confirming that the mass is a simple cyst. Ultrasonography is superior for detecting focal mass, adenoma, renal cell carcinoma, or metastatic tumor.

Angiomyelolipoma, lobar nephronia (focal pyelonephritis), renal abscess and perinephric abscess, lymphoma, and leukemia are more accurately defined by computed tomography scanning than by ultrasonography. Computed tomography scanning is also useful to evaluate the status of the renal vein and the inferior vena cava when tumor extension is suspected.

(F) Renal angiography, formerly a mainstay in evaluating solid renal masses, is reserved for indeterminate lesions, for demonstration of renal arterial distribution when surgical difficulty is expected, and for preoperative embolization. It costs $700 for the procedure and $100 for interpretation. It is invasive and has the aforementioned side effects. Such effects are more frequent after the intravenous administration of contrast. The role of magnetic resonance imaging is being defined at present. Studies are underway as to its value in distinguishing cystic versus solid masses and renal vein thrombosis and in staging renal cell carcinoma.

(G) If an infiltrative or inflammatory process is considered, renal biopsy under computed tomography control can establish the diagnosis and allow in situ therapy. The cost is $638. It is invasive. Bleeding and fistula formation are risks. For renal cell carcinoma, radical nephrectomy is the best treatment. Radical partial nephrectomy for polar lesions and for lesions in the solitary kidney is an option that is currently under study.

REFERENCES

Balfe DM, McClennan BL, Stanley RJ, et al. Evaluation of renal masses considered indeterminate on computed tomography. Radiology 1982; 142:421–428.

Bosniak M. The current radiological approach to renal cysts. Radiology 1986; 158:1–10.

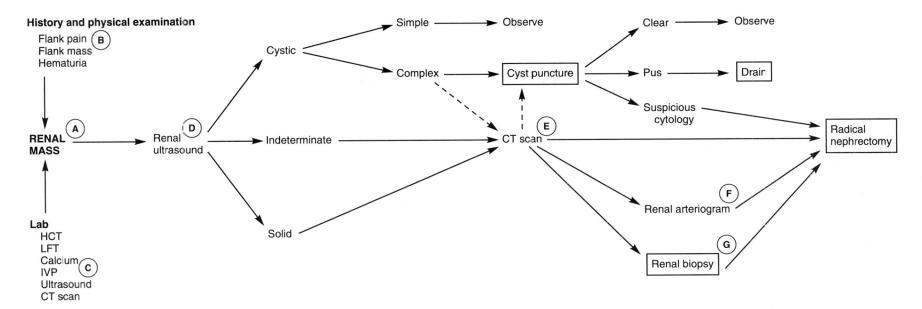

History and physical examination
Flank pain (B)
Flank mass
Hematuria

RENAL MASS (A)

Lab
HCT
LFT
Calcium (C)
IVP
Ultrasound
CT scan

Renal ultrasound (D)

Cystic

Simple → Observe

Complex → Cyst puncture

Indeterminate → CT scan (E)

Solid

Cyst puncture

Clear → Observe

Pus → Drain

Suspicious cytology → Radical nephrectomy

CT scan

Renal arteriogram (F)

Renal biopsy (G)

Radical nephrectomy

Bladder Tumor

Thomas H. Stanisic, M.D.

(A) For practical purposes, all bladder tumors are malignant. About 95 percent are transitional cell carcinomas. The remainder are adenocarcinomas, squamous cell carcinoma, or mixed tumors.

(B) Patients with bladder tumors usually have intermittent gross painless hematuria, microscopic hematuria, irritative bladder symptoms, or a combination of each. Tumors are sometimes detected incidentally by intravenous pyelography (IVP).

(C) IVP, urinary cytologic examination, urinary flow cytometry, and cystoscopy are the best means of evaluating a patient with suspected bladder tumor. IVP will miss 40 percent of tumors, especially small ones. Urinary cytologic study has limited accuracy (60 to 70 percent) in detecting low-grade tumors. Further experience is needed with flow cytometry, a relatively new modality, in this setting. Cystoscopy is essential to complete evaluation.

(D) When tumors are detected cystoscopically they are transurethrally resected (TURBT) as completely as possible. The lamina propria and muscle of the tumor base are examined for evidence of tumor invasion. Random biopsy of grossly normal-appearing areas of the bladder is performed to rule out occult carcinoma in situ. Bimanual examination is performed under anesthesia to delineate possible extravesical tumor extension. A workup for metastases including chest x-ray, liver function tests, IVP, abdominal computed tomography scan, and bone scan is indicated when invasive tumor is found.

(E) Treatment depends on tumor stage. Stages are:

Carcinoma in situ, histologically high-grade flat or velvety lesions, no invasion below the basement membrane, usually diffuse

Stage O, no invasion, usually histologically low grade and papillary in configuration

Stage A, invasion into lamina propria

Stage B, invasion into muscle

Stage C, penetration through bladder muscle into perivesical fat

Stage D_1, regional (pelvic) lymph node metastases

Stage D_2, distant metastases

(F) Papillary low-stage lesions (O, A) are treated by complete transurethral resection (TUR), by segmental resection, or by intravesical chemotherapy. TUR is the most frequently used and generally applicable treatment for superficial tumors. Recurrence is common (75 to 80 percent over 15 years). Most recurrent tumors are superficial. Invasive high-stage recurrence is found in 10 to 15 percent of patients. The risk for invasive recurrence is highest when carcinoma in situ is found on random biopsy in association with a superficial tumor. When the tumor is not amenable to TUR because of size or location, segmental resection of a portion of bladder containing a localized tumor is used. The remainder of the bladder must be free of both carcinoma in situ and gross tumor. This combination of circumstances occurs in less than 10 percent of cases.

Intravesical chemotherapy with thiotepa, doxo-

rubicin, or mitomycin or intravesical immunotherapy with bacille Calmette-Guérin (BCG) is useful in treating superficial tumors (both papillary and carcinoma in situ) and as prophylaxis against recurrence after resection. Thiotepa is effective in about one third of patients. It is inexpensive (less than $100/treatment) and is generally used as first-line treatment for prophylaxis of papillary disease. Adriamycin and mitomycin are two to four times more expensive but are often effective when thiotepa fails. BCG is also effective in this role and is relatively inexpensive. BCG produces a sustained complete response (>70 percent) when used to treat carcinoma in situ. Most urologists consider it to be the agent of choice when treating this disease. Chemotherapeutic agents are less effective (30 to 50 percent) in treating carcinoma in situ.

(G) After a superficial tumor is resected, the patient is followed with cystoscopy every 3 months for 1 to 2 years, every 6 months for another 2 to 5 years, and then annually for life. If recurrence is noted on cystoscopy, the cycle begins again. Annual or biannual intravenous pyelography is advisable to search the upper tracts for transitional cell lesions. Urinary cytologic examination is performed at each cystoscopy to screen for carcinoma in situ. Flow cytometry is useful in detecting urothelial populations with aneuploid clones that may serve as an indicator of high recurrence risk status, which warrants especially close surveillance.

(H) Standard therapy for muscle invasive disease (B,C) consists of radical cystectomy and some form of urinary diversion. This involves 10 to 14

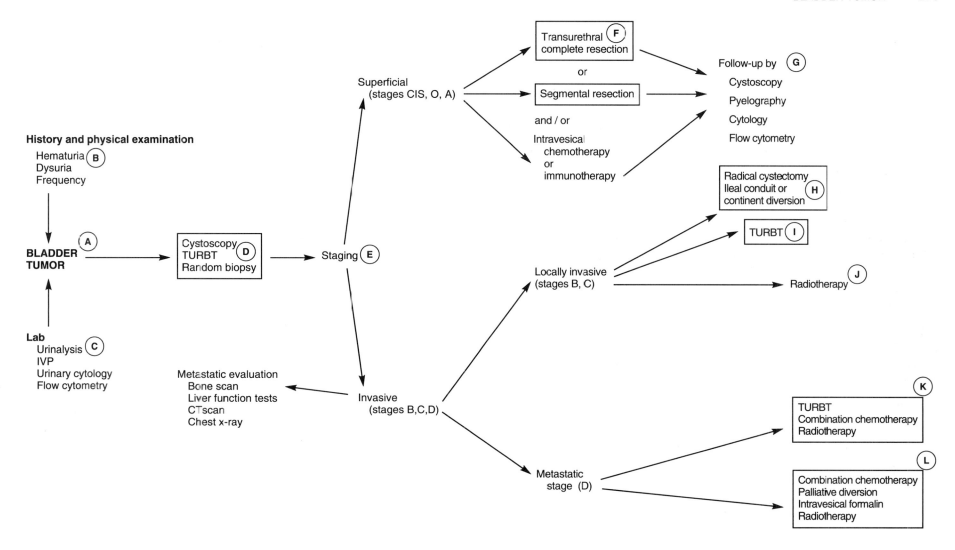

History and physical examination

Hematuria (B)
Dysuria
Frequency

Lab
Urinalysis (C)
IVP
Urinary cytology
Flow cytometry

BLADDER TUMOR (A)

Cystoscopy
TURBT (D)
Random biopsy

Staging (E)

Superficial
(stages CIS, O, A)

Transurethral (F)
complete resection

or

Segmental resection

and / or

Intravesical
chemotherapy
or
immunotherapy

Follow-up by (G)

Cystoscopy
Pyelography
Cytology
Flow cytometry

Radical cystectomy
Ileal conduit or (H)
continent diversion

TURBT (I)

Locally invasive
(stages B, C)

Radiotherapy (J)

Invasive
(stages B,C,D)

Metastatic evaluation
Bone scan
Liver function tests
CTscan
Chest x-ray

Metastatic
stage (D)

TURBT (K)
Combination chemotherapy
Radiotherapy

Combination chemotherapy (L)
Palliative diversion
Intravesical formalin
Radiotherapy

---

days of hospitalization. Five-year survival approximates 50 percent. In addition to the standard ileal conduit, cystectomy patients who are interested and capable of pursing an intermittent catheterization program should be offered the option of continent urinary diversion (Koch pouch, Indiana reservoir, Le Bag, etc.). A urethral stoma can be built when tumor does not involve the prostatic

urethra. Involvement requires urethrectomy to protect the patient from recurrence. In cystectomy series, 7 to 15 percent of patients undergo simultaneous or delayed urethrectomy for prostatic carcinoma in situ, urethral carcinoma in situ, or frank urethral tumor. When the urethra is spared, the remnant must be regularly examined cytologically or endoscopically.

(I) A small number of patients with invasive disease may benefit from thorough transurethral section alone. This approach involves a brief operation and short hospital stay.

(J) Radiotherapy (6000 to 7000 rad over 6 to 8 weeks) offers nonsurgical control in 15 to 35 percent of patients. If invasive recurrence is noted,

Bladder Tumor (Continued)

salvage cystectomy is possible in 20 percent but the complication rate is high.

(K) A bladder-sparing approach can be used in selected patients, in which transurethral resection is followed by systemic chemotherapy using cisplatin in combination with other drugs (cisplatin, methotrexate, vinblastine; methotrexate-vinblastine, Adriamycin [doxorubicin hydrochloride], cisplatin) and subsequent radiotherapy (4000 to 6000 rad). At median follow-up of 2 to 3 years, 50 to 72 percent of patients so treated are alive and 30 to 43 percent have maintained their bladders in situ without recurrent tumor. Cystectomy is possible in local failures.

(L) Cisplatin-based combination chemotherapy produces response rates of 60 to 70 percent in patients with metastatic disease. Complete response is seen in approximately 20 percent and is sustained long term in about 10 percent. Urinary diversion, palliative transurethral resection, intravesical formalin instillation, and irradiation are useful in dealing with hematuria when the tumor-bearing bladder remains in situ. Irradiation can also palliate painful metastases.

REFERENCES

Greene LF, Hanash A, Farrow GM. The benign papilloma or papillary carcinoma of the bladder. J Urol 1973; 110:205–207.

Herr HW. Conservative management of muscle-infiltrating bladder cancer: prospective experience. J Urol 1987; 138:1162–1163.

Rowland R, Mitchell M. Alternative techniques for a continent urinary reservoir. Urol Clin North Am 1987; 14:797–804.

Soloway MS. Intravesical therapy for bladder cancer. Urol Clin North Am 1988; 15:661–669.

Wajsman Z, Marino R, Parsons J, et al. Bladder sparing approach in the treatment of invasive bladder cancer. Semin Urol 1990; 8:210–215.

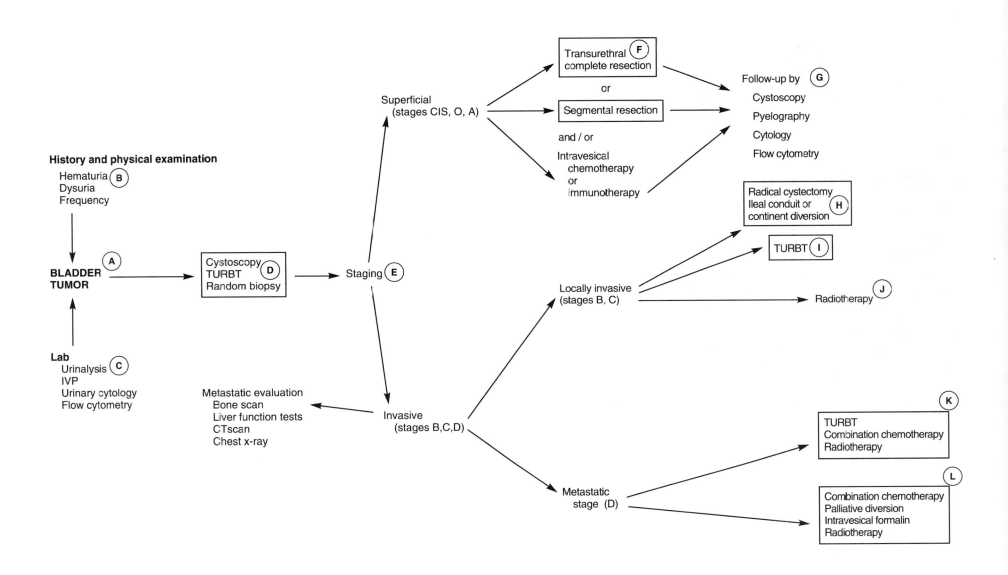

Transurethral complete resection (F)

or

Segmental resection

and / or

Intravesical chemotherapy or immunotherapy

Superficial (stages CIS, O, A)

Follow-up by (G)
Cystoscopy
Pyelography
Cytology
Flow cytometry

History and physical examination
Hematuria (B)
Dysuria
Frequency

Radical cystectomy
Ileal conduit or (H)
continent diversion

TURBT (I)

Radiotherapy (J)

BLADDER TUMOR (A)

Cystoscopy (D)
TURBT
Random biopsy

Staging (E)

Locally invasive (stages B, C)

Lab
Urinalysis (C)
IVP
Urinary cytology
Flow cytometry

Metastatic evaluation
Bone scan
Liver function tests
CTscan
Chest x-ray

Invasive (stages B,C,D)

TURBT (K)
Combination chemotherapy
Radiotherapy

Metastatic stage (D)

Combination chemotherapy (L)
Palliative diversion
Intravesical formalin
Radiotherapy

Prostatism

John Wettlaufer, M.D., and J. Brantley Thrasher, M.D.

(A) Prostatism is a urinary symptom complex secondary to lower urinary tract obstruction or bladder dysfunction and characterized by urinary frequency, nocturia, and diminished urinary stream. Urinary retention, azotemia, and infection may be complications.

(B) A prostate nodule or area of induration is highly suspicious of cancer in all men over the age of 40 years, and biopsy should be performed.

(C) Symptoms of prostatism and congestive obstruction revealed by endoscopy are often related to prostatitis (bacterial or nonbacterial).

(D) Needle biopsy of the prostate is usually performed by the transperineal or transrectal route. The use of transrectal ultrasonography to aid in localization of prostate carcinoma is helpful. Lesions often appear hypoechoic with transrectal ultrasonography. Infection, bleeding, and urinary retention can follow both perineal and transrectal needle biopsy procedures. The incidence of infection after transrectal needle biopsy is 5 percent. After transperineal biopsy, it is less than 3 percent. Prophylactic antibiotics appear to decrease the risk of infection. Repeat needle biopsy is justified when the initial specimen is negative for cancer. Transurethral resectional biopsy is used for obvious diffuse obstructive tumor.

(E) Median bar hypertrophy is a fibromuscular inflammatory obstruction at the posterior vesical outlet. It generally causes symptoms of prostatism earlier (ages 25 to 40 years) than benign hypertrophy. Recurrent cystoprostatitis or hydronephrosis may require transurethral incision of the bladder neck or transurethral resection of the prostate. Both procedures relieve outlet obstruction with similar efficacy and complications. The incidence of retrograde ejaculation is much higher with

transurethral resection of the prostate (40 to 50 percent) than with transurethral incision of the bladder neck (15 to 20 percent). It is prudent to attempt transurethral incision of the bladder neck first, especially in younger patients. Treatment with α-blockers such as phenoxybenzamine (Dibenzyline) or prazosin (Minipres) can improve symptoms and delay surgery.

(F) Periodic massage, frequent ejaculation, warm sitz baths, and tetracycline (for chlamydia) are conventional treatments for congestive prostatitis. Associated bacterial cystitis or chronic gram-negative bacterial prostatitis identified by culture of ejaculate, expressed prostatic secretions, or final voided urine is treated with specific antimicrobials.

(G) Urethral stricture often exists although the digital rectal examination is normal, especially in men under age 50 years.

(H) Several new therapeutic options can now be considered in the management of benign prostatic hypertrophy. α-Blockers cause direct relaxation of the bladder neck and prostatic capsule smooth muscle, decreasing bladder outlet resistance. They are a useful adjuvant for short term partial relief of obstruction. Antiandrogens (luteinizing hormone-releasing hormone agonists) and 5-alpha reductase inhibitors can decrease prostatic volume by as much as 30 percent after 3 to 6 months. Impotence is the primary drawback of luteinizing hormone-releasing hormone agonists. Transurethral incision of the prostate is as effective as transurethral resection of the prostate in treating the small obstructing prostate (<30 g) with similar complications and cost. Posttransurethral resection of the prostate bladder neck contracture occurs in 3 percent and retrograde ejaculation is more common after transurethral resection (40 to 50 percent) than after transurethral incision of the prostate (5 to 10 percent). Transurethral incision is not suitable

for large prostates. Stainless steel stents can be placed in the prostatic urethra of surgically unfit patients with benign prostatic hypertrophy. Disadvantages of prostatic stents are the expense and the tendency for intravesical migration. Transurethral balloon dilation of the prostate is an investigative treatment option for symptomatic benign prostate hypertrophy. The virtues of transurethral balloon dilation are simplicity, safety, speed, cost saving, and reduced convalescence. Its effectiveness is unpredictable and duration of benefits is uncertain. It is contraindicated in the presence of large elongated prostates (>75 g), median lobe hypertrophy, and urinary retention.

(I) Evaluation for metastases includes serum prostatic acid phosphatase assay and measurement of prostate-specific antigen, radioisotope bone scan, skeletal x-rays, chest x-ray, and intravenous pyelogram. Computed tomography scanning, magnetic resonance imaging and transrectal ultrasonography can be used to define extraprostatic soft tissue or nodal spread of cancer.

(J) Prolonged, recurrent, or resistant symptomatic bacterial prostatitis may respond to transurethral resection.

(K) Urodynamic evaluation includes residual urine measurement, cystometry, electromyography, and uroflowmetry.

(L) Uncomplicated, short urethral strictures usually respond to endoscopic direct-vision cold knife urethrotomy. Complex or recurrent strictures in high-risk patients with refractory strictures often require open urethroplasty or intraurethral stents. Stents are made of stainless steel woven into a self-expanding tubular mesh. When placed in the urethra, they expand to become a flexible but stable cylinder. Urothelium grows through the pores by 3 months to cover the stent. Stents are best suited

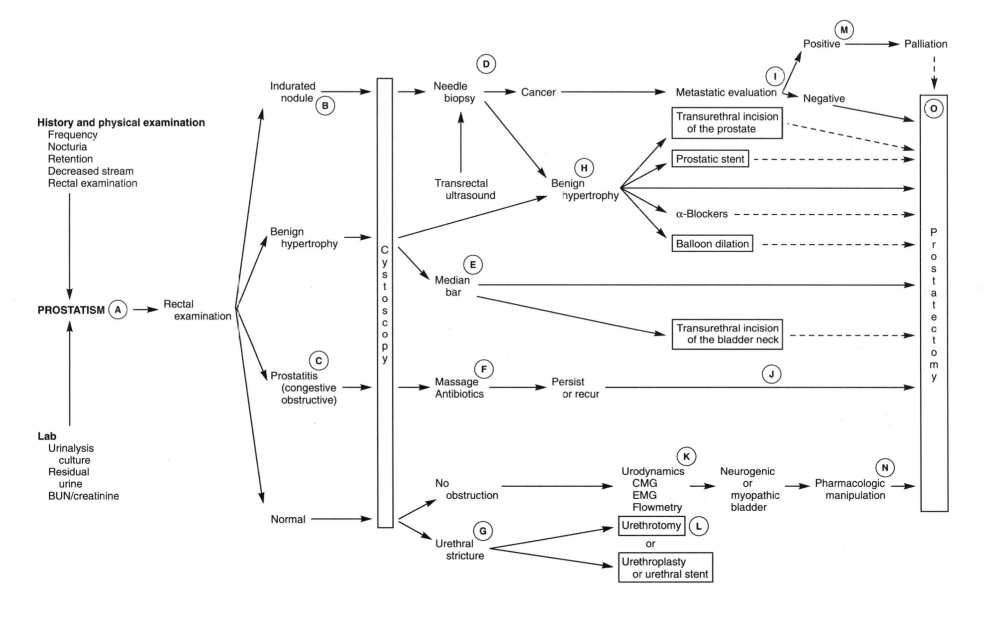

History and physical examination
 Frequency
 Nocturia
 Retention
 Decreased stream
 Rectal examination

PROSTATISM (A)

Lab
 Urinalysis
  culture
 Residual
  urine
 BUN/creatinine

Prostatism (Continued)

for bulbar urethral strictures. They are expensive and their use in young, healthy patients is controversial due to limited long-term experience.

(M) Therapy of metastatic cancer is palliative and reserved for progressive or symptomatic disease. Palliation includes hormonal manipulation (castration, estrogens, antiandrogens) or local radiotherapy. Local obstruction is managed by hormonal therapy or transurethral resection of the prostate. The latter risks urinary incontinence. A subset of patients have recurrent growth of the carcinoma after hormonal manipulation or do not respond at all, mandating the use of transurethral resection for relief of obstruction.

(N) Pharmacologic measures include decreasing resistance at the vesical outlet (phenoxybenzamine or prazosin) or at the external sphincter (baclofen [Lioresal] or diazepam). For high-pressure or uninhibited bladders propantheline (Pro-banthine), oxybutynin (Ditropan), or imipramine may be used. For significant residual urine unresponsive to drugs, clean, intermittent self-catheterization is often effective. Empirically, transurethral resection of the bladder neck, the prostate, or both, or sphincterotomy may result in satisfactory bladder emptying when conservative measures fail.

(O) Choice of technique of prostatectomy depends on the size of the gland. Transurethral resection of the prostate is the most commonly used surgical treatment for benign prostatic hypertrophy. Open procedures are reserved for large glands and coexisting intravesical disease (stones and symptomatic diverticula). Unsuspected prostatic cancer found incidentally in the surgical specimen (if undifferentiated or more than focal) is managed according to its clinical and pathologic stage. Persistent focal well-differentiated cancer found by repeat transurethral resection is best managed expectantly.

REFERENCES

Carlton EC, Scardino PT. Urologic examination: initial evaluation. In: Walsh PC, Gittes RF, Perlmutter AD, Stamey TA, eds. Campbell's urology, 5th ed, vol 1. Philadelphia, WB Saunders, 1986; 276–310.

Chapple CR, Milroy EJ, Rickards D. Permanently implanted urethral stent for prostatic obstruction in the unfit patient. Preliminary report. Br J Urol 1990; 66:58–65.

Gittes RF. Carcinoma of the prostate: review. N Engl J Med 1991; 324(4):236–245.

Lepor H. Nonoperative management of benign prostatic hyperplasia. J Urol 1989; 141:1283–1289.

Mobb GE, Moisey CU. Long-term follow-up of unilateral bladder neck incision. Br J Urol 1988; 62:160–162.

Orandi A. Transurethral resection versus transurethral incision of the prostate. Urol Clin North Am 1990; 17:601–612.

Thrasher JB, Kreder KJ. Balloon dilatation of the prostate. In: Chapple CR, ed. Recent advances in the treatment of benign prostatic hyperplasia. London, Springer-Verlag (in press).

Wein AJ. Drug treatment of voiding dysfunction. Part 1: Evaluation of drugs; treatment of emptying failure. Part II: Drug treatment of storage failure. AUA Update Series, Lessons 14 and 15, Vol VII:106–119, 1988.

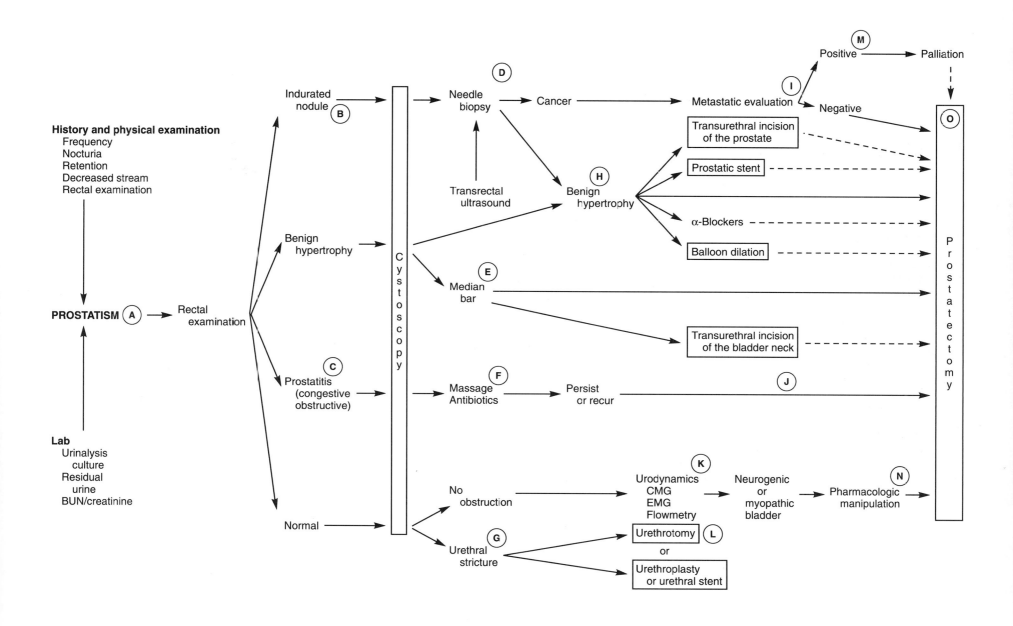

History and physical examination
 Frequency
 Nocturia
 Retention
 Decreased stream
 Rectal examination

PROSTATISM (A) → Rectal examination

Lab
 Urinalysis
  culture
 Residual
  urine
 BUN/creatinine

Indurated nodule (B)

Benign hypertrophy

Prostatitis (C) (congestive obstructive)

Normal

Cystoscopy

Needle biopsy (D) → Cancer → Metastatic evaluation (I)

Transrectal ultrasound

Benign hypertrophy (H)

Median bar (E)

Massage Antibiotics (F) → Persist or recur (J)

No obstruction → Urodynamics CMG EMG Flowmetry (K) → Neurogenic or myopathic bladder → Pharmacologic manipulation (N)

Urethral stricture (G) → Urethrotomy (L) or Urethroplasty or urethral stent

Positive (M) → Palliation

Negative

Transurethral incision of the prostate

Prostatic stent

α-Blockers

Balloon dilation

Transurethral incision of the bladder neck

Prostatectomy (O)

Carcinoma of the Prostate

Jerome P. Richie, M.D.

(A) Diagnosis of prostate carcinoma often follows the discovery of a firm or hard nodule on routine rectal examination. Approximately 10 percent of patients who have transurethral resection of the prostate for obstructive symptoms have prostate cancer within the resected specimen.

(B) Prostate-specific antigen has not been advocated as a screening test. Values between 4 and 10 may indicate benign prostatic hypertrophy or carcinoma of the prostate. Values greater than 100 generally indicate metastatic disease. Enzymatic acid phosphatase, when elevated, implies extension outside of the prostate capsule either to seminal vesicles, regional lymph nodes, or elsewhere locally. Approximately one third of prostate cancers are hypoechoic, and in this instance, ultrasound can be used to direct needle biopsy.

(C) Prostate cancers are divided into well-differentiated, moderately differentiated, and poorly differentiated tumors. The Gleason pattern of glandular appearance gives a primary (1 to 5) and a secondary (1 to 5) score, the sum of which has prognostic implication.

(D) In addition to enzymatic acid phosphatase, two standard tests include bone scan and pelvic computed tomography scan. Pelvic lymphadenectomy, a surgical staging procedure, is often used to further define the accuracy of clinical stage.

(E) Incidentally discovered cancer (following transurethral resection or open prostatectomy) with less than three foci of well-differentiated (Gleason 2, 3, or 4) prostate cancer is stage A_1.

(F) Incidentally discovered prostate cancer that is more diffuse in nature or less than well-differentiated is stage A_2.

(G) A palpable nodule less than 2 cm in diameter confined to one lobe of the prostate is stage B_1.

(H) A palpable nodule involving more than 2 cm of one lobe of the prostate or evidence of bilateral involvement is stage B_2.

(I) Extension to the seminal vesicle or beyond the confines of the prostatic capsule is stage C.

(J) Regional nodal involvement is stage D_1.

(K) Metastases above the true pelvis, usually to bone, define stage D_2.

(L) Patients with minimal A_1 disease have a limited likelihood of progression. Follow-up should include transrectal ultrasound to be certain that there are no other foci of tumor and prostate-specific antigen. In younger patients (less than 60 years old) radical prostatectomy through a nerve-sparing technique can be considered.

(M) Radical prostatectomy, with unilateral or bilateral nerve sparing, offers the best chance for long-term survival and, hopefully, cure. For patients with organ-confined disease, 100 percent age-adjusted survival can be expected after radical prostatectomy. The rate of incontinence persisting beyond 6 months should be less than 1 percent. Nerve-sparing techniques allow return of potency in approximately 70 percent of men, generally within 1 year. Prostate-specific antigen is a specific test to follow patients after radical prostatectomy because levels should be unmeasurable (<0.3 ng/IU) in the absence of cancer.

(N) Radiation therapy of approximately 6500 cGy results in local control for most patients.

In clinically staged series, radiation therapy has not resulted in long-term survival equal to that in pathologically staged radical prostatectomy series. Of concern is elevation of prostate-specific antigen or positive biopsies more than 1 year after completion of radiation therapy. Radiation therapy is generally the treatment of choice in patients older than 70 years or in patients with significant comorbid disease.

(O) Deprivation of testosterone stimulation provides excellent palliation for patients with symptomatic prostate cancer. Controversy exists as to how much this affects overall survival rates. Many authorities advocate delayed hormonal therapy when the patient is symptomatic. Alternative methods of hormonal therapy include orchiectomy, luteinizing hormone-releasing hormone agonists (injected on a monthly basis), or diethylstilbestrol. Because of the increased risk of cardiovascular or thromboembolic phenomena, diethylstilbestrol is used sparingly, if at all. Total androgen ablation by the addition of antiandrogens offers modest benefit in some patients.

REFERENCES

Bagshaw MA, Cox RS, Ray GR. Status of radiation treatment of prostate cancer at Stanford University. NCI Monograph 1988; 7:47–52.

Paulsen DR. Randomized series of treatment with surgery versus radiation for prostate adenocarcinoma. J Urol 1979; 7:127–129.

Stamey TA. Cancer of the prostate. Monog Urol 1983; 4:67–74.

Walsh PC, Epstein JI, Lowe FC. Potency following radical prostatectomy with wide unilateral excision of the neurovascular bundle. J Urol 1987; 138:823–827.

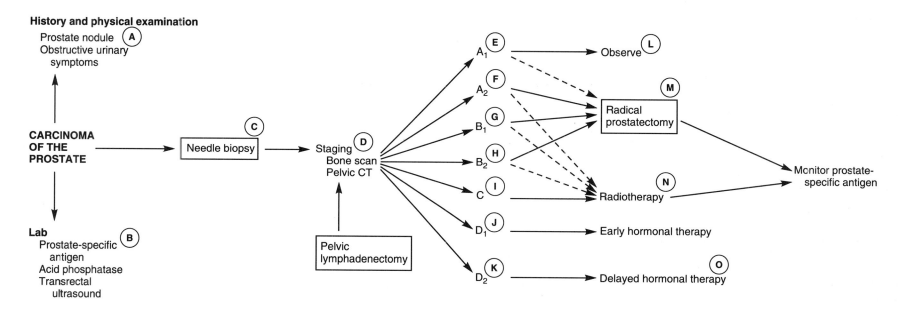

History and physical examination
Prostate nodule (A)
Obstructive urinary
symptoms

CARCINOMA OF THE PROSTATE

Lab (B)
Prostate-specific
antigen
Acid phosphatase
Transrectal
ultrasound

Needle biopsy (C)

Staging (D)
Bone scan
Pelvic CT

Pelvic lymphadenectomy

A₁ (E) → Observe (L)
A₂ (F)
B₁ (G)
B₂ (H)
C (I)
D₁ (J) → Early hormonal therapy
D₂ (K) → Delayed hormonal therapy (O)

Radical prostatectomy (M)
Radiotherapy (N)

Monitor prostate-specific antigen

Scrotal Mass

Norman E. Peterson, M.D.

(A) A scrotal mass may be evaluated by ultrasonic ($234), Doppler ($107), or isotope scanning ($340). These studies should be subjugated to clinical impression.

(B) Posttraumatic testicular enlargement may call attention to an existing mass (tumor) but is more commonly due to intratesticular bleeding (hematocele). Severe pain, collapse, and vomiting may occur. Surgical repair ($1,100) will abbreviate convalescence.

(C) Severe testis pain of abrupt onset, often accompanied by vomiting and scrotal enlargement, reflects spermatic cord torsion. This must be treated as a surgical emergency. Hemorrhage into a tumor presents similarly but is rarely encountered. Serum tumor markers should be obtained before inguinal orchiectomy is performed. Torsion of testis appendages creates similar but less intense symptoms. Management is unchanged.

(D) A newborn or childhood hydrocele (10 percent) of static dimensions usually recedes spontaneously (75 percent); if it waxes or wanes in size, reflecting a patent processus vaginalis, it requires operative repair ($1,100). Persistent static hydrocele may remain decompressed after aspiration ($289). Adult hydroceles may be managed by aspiration and injection of sclerotics ($289), surgically corrected ($500), or merely observed for complication (unusual).

(E) A spermatocele can be painful when small or painless when larger. Complete excision ($686), when symptoms dictate, is curative.

(F) Suspicion of testis tumor requires that preoperative serum tumor markers be obtained (α-fetoprotein, $53; human chorionic gonadotropin, $43; alkaline phosphatase, $7; chest x-ray, $67).

(G) Varicocele in a young adult or adolescent (15 percent) can cause discomfort or, because of poor semen quality, infertility. Either spermatic vein ligation ($688) or radiographic embolization ($1,021) is corrective. Varicocele commonly regresses spontaneously before midlife. A varicocele in preadolescents or older patients or right-sided involvement (2 percent) requires evaluation of the retroperitoneum by computed tomography scanning ($650) or vena cavagram ($275) for the presence of an obstructing mass.

(H) Other scrotal masses occasionally encountered include testicular inclusion cyst, epididymal adenomatoid tumor, testicular nongerminal tumor, paratesticular sarcoma, and spermatic cord lipoma.

(I) Incarcerated indirect inguinal hernia produces a groin or scrotal mass distinct from the testis. Auscultation and x-ray ($55) for gas may assist diagnosis. Emergency surgical reduction is necessary ($1,100).

(J) Acute epididymitis produces gradually increasing testicular pain and swelling. Spermatic cord block (5 mL procaine) permits examination and provides relief. Antibiotics and rest are therapeutic. Worsening symptoms and fever indicate abscess (<5 percent) for which drainage or orchiectomy ($1,100) is required. Chronic epididymitis (local pain, mass) may be managed by maintenance antibiotics or epididymectomy ($600), vasectomy ($450), or orchiectomy ($1,100). If epididymitis recurs, a voiding cystourethrogram ($140) may identify complicating factors such as urethral stricture or vasal reflux.

REFERENCES

Berger RE, Alexander ER, Hamisch JP, et al. Etiology, manifestations and therapy in acute epididymitis. J Urol 1979; 121:750–754.

Donohue JP, Einhorn LH, Williams DS. Is adjuvant chemotherapy following retroperitoneal lymph node dissection for nonseminomatous testis cancer necessary? Urol Clin North Am 1980; 7:747–756.

Javadpour N. Germ cell tumor of the testis. CA 1980; 30:242–245.

Javadpour N. Management of seminoma based on tumor markers. Urol Clin North Am 1980; 7:773–781.

Lange PH, Fraley EE. Serum alpha-fetoprotein and human chorionic gonadotropin in the treatment of patients with testicular tumors. Urol Clin North Am 1977; 4:393–406.

Peterson NE. Physical examination and differential diagnosis of scrotal masses. Emerg Med Rep 1986; 7:1–7.

Ransler CE III, Allen TD. Torsion of the spermatic cord. Urol Clin North Am 1982; 9:245–250.

Skinner DB. Non-seminomatous testis tumors: a plan of management. J Urol 1976; 115:65–69.

Wettlaufer JN. State III germinal testis tumors: aggressive approach. J Urol 1979; 116:593–597.

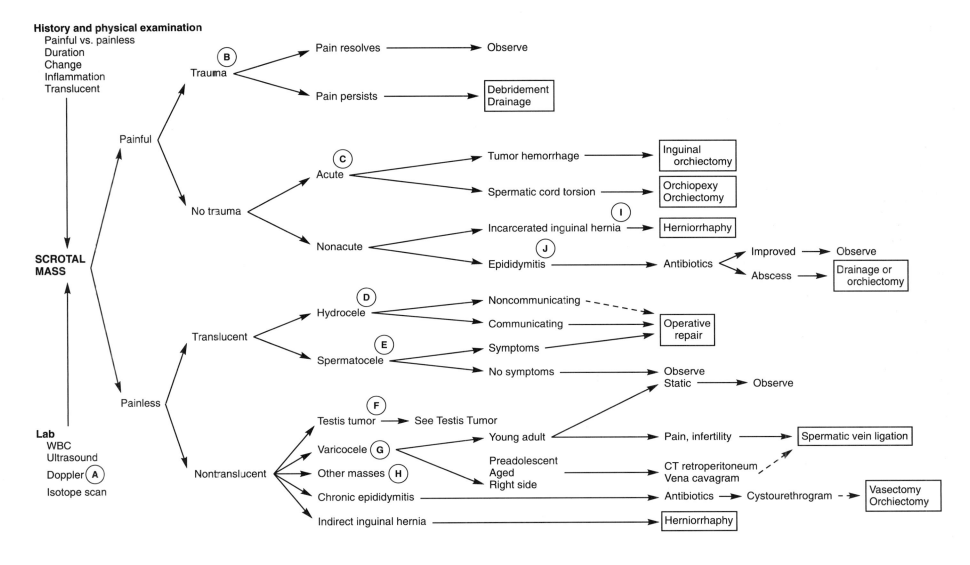

History and physical examination
Painful vs. painless
Duration
Change
Inflammation
Translucent

SCROTAL MASS

Lab
WBC
Ultrasound
Doppler (A)
Isotope scan

Painful

Trauma (B)
- Pain resolves → Observe
- Pain persists → Debridement / Drainage

No trauma

Acute (C)
- Tumor hemorrhage → Inguinal orchiectomy
- Spermatic cord torsion → Orchiopexy / Orchiectomy

Nonacute
- Incarcerated inguinal hernia (I) → Herniorrhaphy
- Epididymitis (J) → Antibiotics
  - Improved → Observe
  - Abscess → Drainage or orchiectomy

Painless

Translucent

Hydrocele (D)
- Noncommunicating ⇢ Operative repair
- Communicating → Operative repair

Spermatocele (E)
- Symptoms → Operative repair
- No symptoms → Observe

Nontranslucent

Testis tumor (F) → See Testis Tumor

Varicocele (G)
- Young adult
  - Static → Observe
  - Pain, infertility → Spermatic vein ligation
- Preadolescent / Aged / Right side → CT retroperitoneum / Vena cavagram ⇢ Spermatic vein ligation

Other masses (H)

Chronic epididymitis → Antibiotics → Cystourethrogram ⇢ Vasectomy / Orchiectomy

Indirect inguinal hernia → Herniorrhaphy

Testis Tumor

Michael J. Schutz, M.D., and E. David Crawford, M.D.

(A) Testis cancer is a disease of young men. The peak incidence is between the ages of 20 to 40 years. It is more common among whites and hispanics than blacks. About 6300 new cases of testis cancer were diagnosed in 1992. The incidence is increasing. Associated risk factors include cryptorchidism and exogenous estrogen exposure in utero. Few testis tumors (2 to 3 percent) are bilateral. Seminoma is the most common histologic type.

(B) Patients usually have painless testicular enlargement, a mass, or a feeling of heaviness in the scrotum. In 10 percent of patients, the presenting signs and symptoms are related to metastatic disease and include supraclavicular adenopathy, abdominal mass or pain, cough, dyspnea, central nervous system disturbances, and bone or back pain. Gynecomastia is seen in 5 percent of patients and is related to hormonal products from the tumor. Scrotal ultrasound can reveal a mass that is equivocal on physical examination.

(C) If testis tumor is suspected, serum α-fetoprotein, β-subunit of human chorionic gonadotropin, lactic dehydrogenase, and a chest x-ray should be obtained preoperatively. Levels of α-fetoprotein or β-human chorionic gonadotropin, if elevated preoperatively, should be measured postoperatively according to their half lives (α-fetoprotein, 5 days; β-human chorionic gonadotropin, 24 hours) to help assess residual disease. Levels should be determined every month thereafter, along with repeat chest x-rays, to monitor for recurrence. Luteinizing hormone cross-reacts with β-human chorionic gonadotropin and can cause false elevation of β-human chorionic gonadotropin.

(D) Any suspicion of testis cancer requires exploration. Early control of the spermatic cord is important. This minimizes the possibility of local recurrence and tumor spread.

(E) These tumors rarely metastasize. Inguinal orchiectomy is the only treatment necessary.

(F) Yolk sac tumors comprise two thirds of childhood testis tumors. Most children have local disease. Inguinal orchiectomy is usually adequate treatment. Only 10 to 15 percent of patients develop metastatic disease. Surveillance with chest x-ray, abdominal computed tomography scanning, and serum markers is necessary to recognize early metastatic disease. Combination chemotherapy with or without surgery and irradiation can salvage two thirds of relapsing patients.

(G) Seminoma presents as localized disease in 75 percent of patients. Of clinical stage I patients, 10 to 20 percent have occult metastases. About 10 percent have minimal retroperitoneal disease. Seminoma is very radiosensitive. At least 95 percent of clinical stage I and 80 percent of clinical stage II patients with minimal disease are cured by radiotherapy to the retroperitoneal lymph node areas. Close follow-up is necessary. Relapse occurs most commonly in the lungs and can be treated with combination chemotherapy, after which cure rates of 99 percent are expected.

(H) Germ cell tumors with bulky retroperitoneal disease or distant metastatic disease (ie, lung, viscera, bone, central nervous system) require platinum-based chemotherapy. Nonseminomatous tumors usually have elevated serum markers but the markers can be normal in up to 25 percent of patients. Bulky seminomas commonly have elevated lactic dehydrogenase. This will fall with response to therapy. Platinum-based chemotherapy gives complete response in 80 to 90 percent of patients. Residual disease can be treated with surgery or salvage chemotherapy. Relapse rates are 10 percent. Relapse can be treated with salvage chemotherapy with good results.

(I) Patients with clinical stage I nonseminomatous germ cell tumor or minimal or moderate stage II disease should be treated with retroperitoneal lymph node dissection. Current nerve-sparing techniques in low-stage disease reduce the incidence of loss of ejaculation to 10 percent. Surveillance is best accomplished in protocol situations where patients are closely observed. With adjuvant chemotherapy for stage II tumors, survival rates of 99 percent for stage I tumors and 97 percent for stage II tumors are achieved.

REFERENCES

Boring CC, Squires TS, Tong J. Cancer statistics 1992. CA 1992; 42:19–38.

Donohue JP. Options in management of low stage testicular cancer. AUA Update Series 1987; 6:27.

Einhorn LH. Chemotherapy of disseminated testicular cancer. In: Skinner DG, Lieskovsky G, eds. Diagnosis and management of genitourinary cancer. Philadelphia: WB Saunders, 1988:526–531.

Kaplan GW. Testicular tumors in children. AUA Update Series 1983; 2:12.

Kaplan GW, Cromie WC, Kelalis PP, et al. Prepubertal yolk sac testicular tumors—report of the Testicular Tumor Registry. J Urol 1988; 140:1109–1112.

Lightner DJ, Lange PH. Tumor markers in the management of urologic neoplasms. AUA Update Series 1987; 6:36.

Loehrer PJ, Williams SD, Einhorn LH. Status of chemotherapy for testis cancer. Urol Clin North Am 1987; 14:713–720.

Richie JP. Diagnosis and staging of testicular tumors. In: Skinner DG, Lieskovsky G, eds. Diagnosis and management of genitourinary cancer. Philadelphia: WB Saunders, 1988: 498–507.

Wettlaufer JN. The management of advanced seminoma. AUA Update Series 1990; 9:11.

History and physical examination
Painless scrotal mass (B)

TESTIS TUMOR (A)

Inguinal orchiectomy (D)

Lab
Serum markers (C)
Chest x-ray
Scrotal ultrasound

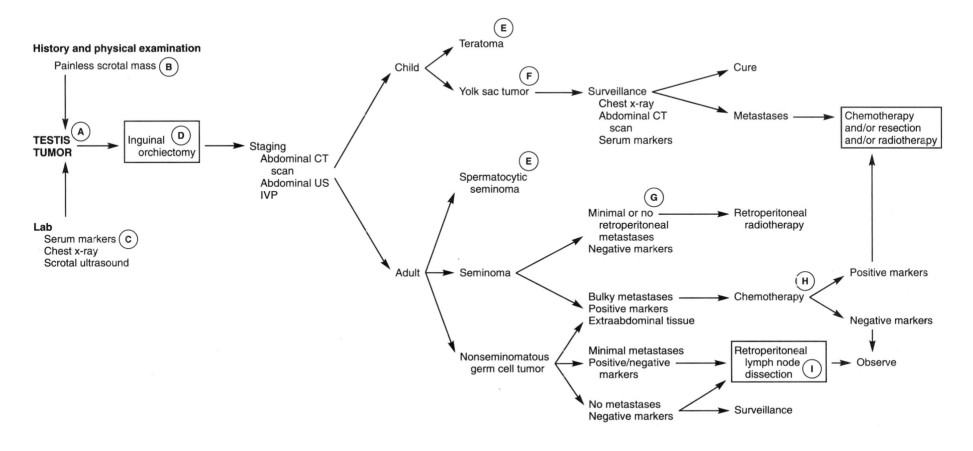

Staging
Abdominal CT scan
Abdominal US
IVP

Child
- Teratoma (E)
- Yolk sac tumor (F) → Surveillance
  Chest x-ray
  Abdominal CT scan
  Serum markers
  → Cure
  → Metastases → Chemotherapy and/or resection and/or radiotherapy

Adult
- Spermatocytic seminoma (E)
- Seminoma
  - Minimal or no retroperitoneal metastases Negative markers (G) → Retroperitoneal radiotherapy
  - Bulky metastases Positive markers Extraabdominal tissue → Chemotherapy (H) → Positive markers → Chemotherapy and/or resection and/or radiotherapy
    → Negative markers → Observe
- Nonseminomatous germ cell tumor
  - Minimal metastases Positive/negative markers → Retroperitoneal lymph node dissection (I) → Observe
  - No metastases Negative markers → Surveillance

Gynecologic

Vaginal Bleeding in Reproductive Years

Marilyn Milkman, M.D., and Paul Wexler, M.D.

(A) Important factors in menstrual history include duration, amount of flow, and interval between menses; use of an intrauterine device, removal of which may stop bleeding; endometriosis, which may require danazol, gonadotropin-releasing hormone (Gn-RH) agonist/antagonist, oral contraceptives, or a surgical procedure; and a history of pelvic infection.

(B) Important factors in pelvic examination include uterine size and consistency, adnexal masses, tenderness, appearance and consistency of cervix, and vaginitis.

(C) In women over age 30 years whose childbearing is over, hysterectomy or yittrium aluminum garnet (YAG) laser vaporization of the endometrium may be preferred.

(D) Dysfunctional (anovulatory) uterine bleeding is treated with conjugated estrogens (Premarin), oral contraceptives, antiprostaglandins, antifibrinolytics, or danazol. Persistent or recurrent bleeding in those over age 30 years may require hysterectomy. Two or more dilation and curettage (D & C) procedures may be tried before surgery. YAG laser vaporization of the endometrium to reduce or eliminate bleeding can be used.

(E) Endometrial biopsy or sampling can be performed by fractional dilation and curettage, Vabra curettage, endometrial biopsy with curette, or use of small aspiration catheters.

(F) With a positive pregnancy test and an adnexal mass, some surgeons forego ultrasound and perform culdocentesis or laparoscopy and then proceed to laparotomy when indicated. With intra-uterine pregnancy, serum human chorionic gonadotropin doubles every 48 to 72 hours. Values with ectopic pregnancy tend to be lower and rise more slowly. Unruptured ectopic pregnancy in a stable patient with an adnexal mass <3 cm in diameter can be treated with methotrexate.

(G) Benign hyperplasia, if estrogen induced, can be premalignant (atypical adenomatous hyperplasia). Exogenous estrogens (Premarin) should be withdrawn. If bleeding continues cancer is suspected. Progesterone is an estrogen antagonist and can be used to treat benign hyperplasia. When adenomatous hyperplasia is managed with progesterone, a 3- to 4-month follow-up sampling of the endometrium should be performed.

(H) Bleeding can be due to an endocervical or endometrial polyp or to a submucus myoma. Local excision can be performed by hysteroscopy or, if childbearing is not completed, YAG laser vaporization. Hysterectomy is indicated in those with recurrent or excessive bleeding. Bilateral salpingo-oophorectomy is indicated for patients over age 50 years. Preoperative use of Gn-RH agonist/antagonist can decrease operative blood loss and time.

(I) D & C is both diagnostic and therapeutic for miscarriage.

(J) Suction D & C is the preferred treatment of molar pregnancies. Follow-up includes measurement of human chorionic gonadotropin titers. Metastasis is excluded by chest x-ray and liver function tests. Elevation of human chorionic gonadotropin may represent invasive mole, which requires chemotherapy.

(K) Decidua without products of conception can occur with corpus luteum cyst. An Arias-Stellar reaction in cells may imply ectopic pregnancy. Decidua can also be found with complete abortion (miscarriages).

(L) A double sac image in the uterus suggests pregnancy and decidua, which helps to confirm intrauterine pregnancy. A single sac image is seen rarely with ectopic pregnancy. Bleeding and an intrauterine gestational sac may represent threatened miscarriage or placenta previa, depending on the gestational age. Patients with these findings should be under close observation with bed rest and pelvic rest.

(M) A large-bore (18- to 20-gauge) spinal needle is inserted into the posterior vaginal cul-de-sac between the uterosacral ligaments. Uterine retroversion is a relative contraindication to culdocentesis. A few drops of serous fluid is considered a negative tap; 5 to 10 mL of blood-tinged serous fluid suggest a ruptured functional cyst that is resolving. If frank blood is returned, the hematocrit (Hct) of the fluid should be compared with the venous Hct to exclude a traumatic tap. An Hct of the culdocentesis fluid higher than the peripheral venous Hct probably indicates blood that has been present for some time. Nonclotting blood is most consistent with hemoperitoneum from a ruptured ectopic pregnancy. Pus may occasionally be aspirated (unusual in the presence of a positive pregnancy test). It represents pelvic inflammatory disease (PID) with possible pelvic abscess or tuboovarian abscess. Gram stain and culture of the aspirate should be performed and the patient treated with parenteral antibiotics covering both

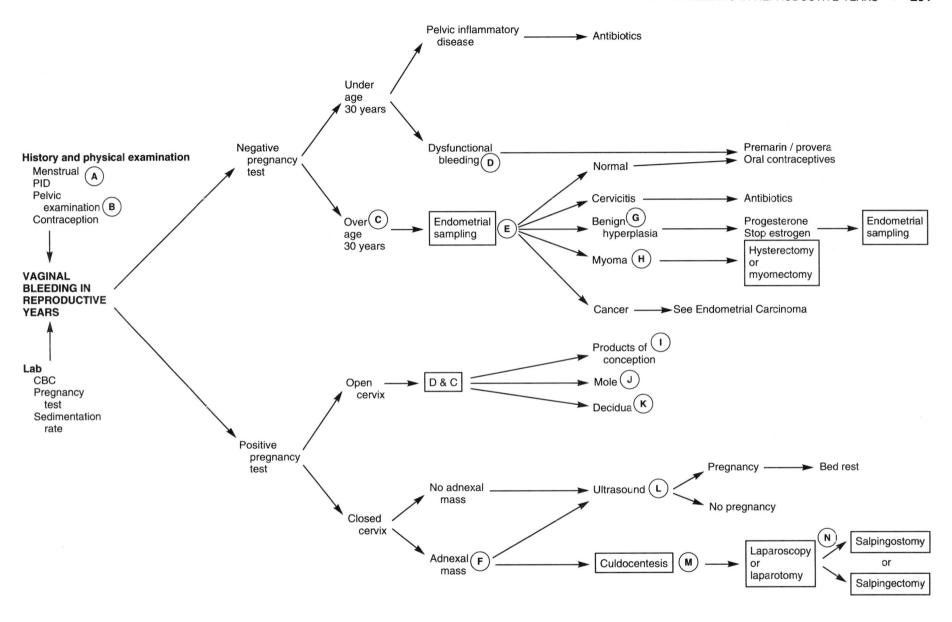

History and physical examination

Menstrual (A)
PID
Pelvic
examination (B)
Contraception

↓

VAGINAL BLEEDING IN REPRODUCTIVE YEARS

↑

Lab

CBC
Pregnancy test
Sedimentation rate

Negative pregnancy test

Under age 30 years → Pelvic inflammatory disease → Antibiotics

Dysfunctional bleeding (D) → Premarin / provera / Oral contraceptives

Over (C) age 30 years → Endometrial sampling (E)

Normal → Premarin / provera / Oral contraceptives

Cervicitis → Antibiotics

Benign (G) hyperplasia → Progesterone Stop estrogen → Endometrial sampling

Myoma (H) → Hysterectomy or myomectomy

Cancer → See Endometrial Carcinoma

Positive pregnancy test

Open cervix → D & C

Products of conception (I)

Mole (J)

Decidua (K)

Closed cervix

No adnexal mass → Ultrasound (L)

Pregnancy → Bed rest

No pregnancy

Adnexal mass (F) → Culdocentesis (M) → Laparoscopy or laparotomy (N)

Salpingostomy

or

Salpingectomy

Vaginal Bleeding in Reproductive Years (Continued)

aerobic and anaerobic organisms. A dry tap (no fluid obtained) is nondiagnostic.

Ⓝ Treatment of an ectopic pregnancy depends on the site in and condition of the tube and the patient's desire for future fertility. Options include linear salpingostomy, with removal of the products of conception either by laparoscopy and at laparotomy, and salpingectomy. Recent experimental methods to avoid operative intervention include systemic methotrexate and citrovorum or tubal instillation of methotrexate and prostaglandins.

REFERENCES

Cope E. The treatment of unexplained menorrhagia. Ir J Med Sci 1983; 152(Suppl 2):29–32.

DeVore GR, Owen O, Kase N. Use of intravenous Premarin in the treatment of dysfunctional uterine bleeding—a double-blind randomized control study. Obstet Gynecol 1982; 59:285–290.

DiSala PJ, Coeassman WT. Clinical gynecologic oncology. St. Louis: CV Mosby, 1981.

Dysfunctional uterine bleeding. ACOG Technical Bulletin No. 66, September 1982.

Greydanus DE, McAnavney ER. Menstruation and its disorders in adolescence. Curr Probl Pediatr 1982; vol 10.

Schaffer RM, Stein K, Shih YH, et al. The echoic pseudogestational sac of ectopic pregnancy simulating early intrauterine pregnancy. J Ultrasound Med 1983; 2:215–218.

Speroff L, Glass RH, Kase NG. Clinical gynecologic endocrinology and infertility, 3rd ed. Baltimore: Williams & Wilkins, 1983.

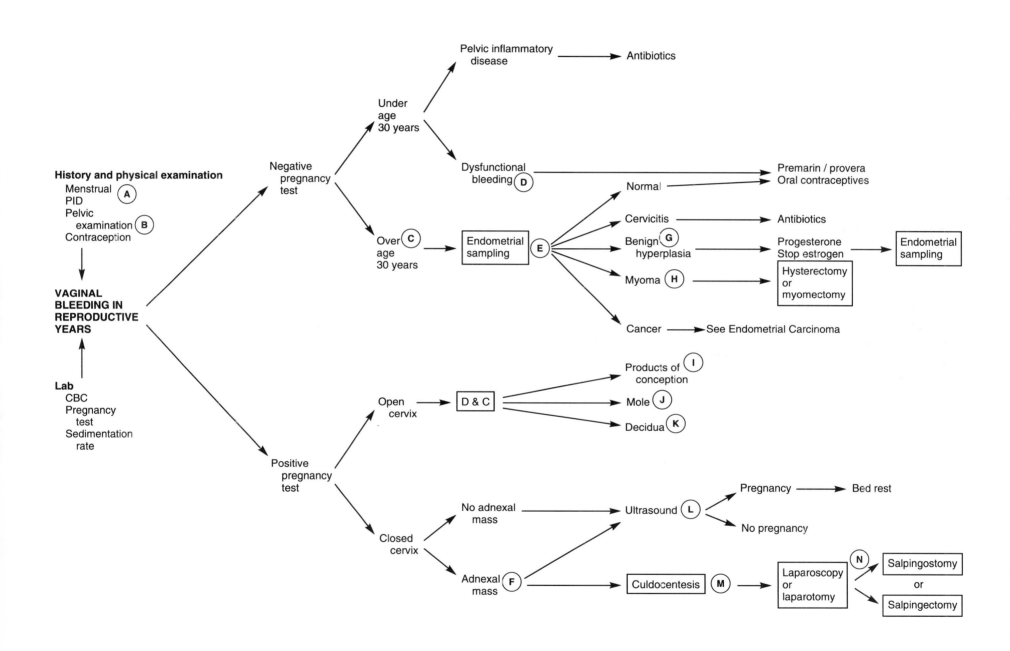

Vaginal Bleeding in Nonreproductive Years

Marilyn Milkman, M.D., and Paul Wexler, M.D.

(A) The risk of developing clear cell adenocarcinoma of the vagina or cervix (or both) through age 24 years in patients with a history of in utero exposure to diethylstilbestrol is 0.14 to 0.4/1000. The mean age of presentation is 19.5 years. The 5-year survival rate is about 75 percent.

(B) Drugs that can be associated with vaginal bleeding are anticoagulants (heparin, Coumadin, and aspirin) and digitalis.

(C) Accepted methods for endometrial sampling include Vabra curettage, endometrial biopsy with curette, fractional dilation and curretage (D&C) or small catheter aspiration.

(D) Infection can cause vaginal bleeding in prepubertal females. Examples are:

1. Vulvar moniliasis. This most commonly presents with intense vulvar pain, itching, and burning. The vulva is often erythematous and sometimes excoriated. Treatment is with local antifungal creams (clotrimazole, nystatin, terconazole).
2. Trichomoniasis. This is rare in virgins. It often presents as a frothy vaginal discharge and pruritus. The cervix can be friable. The treatment of choice is metronidazole.
3. Gardnerella vaginitis (nonspecific). The preferred treatment for this is metronidazole. Op-

tional drugs include ampicillin or triple sulfa cream.
4. Necrotic vulvovaginal condylomata acuminata. There are various treatments for venereal warts, including podophyllin for external lesions, cryotherapy, laser therapy, trichloroacetic acid, or 5-fluorouracil.

(E) Endometrial cancer must be the prime suspect in any postmenopausal woman with vaginal bleeding. Rarely, bleeding is the first manifestation of lymphoma, leukemia, or even metastatic cancer.

(F) Vaginitis in postmenopausal women is due to either infection or, more likely, atrophic vaginitis. Either local estrogen cream or systemic estrogen is effective in restoring the integrity of the vaginal epithelium.

(G) If bleeding persists or recurs and the diagnosis of recurrent dysfunctional uterine bleeding is made, hysterectomy is recommended. Often two or more D & Cs are performed before proceeding to hysterectomy. Some women request yittrium aluminum garnet (YAG) laser vaporization of the endometrium to avoid hysterectomy.

(H) Fractional D & C samples the cervix and the uterus separately. It determines the extent of

uterine involvement and provides for predicting outcome.

(I) Workup for these neoplasms should include liver function tests, excretory pyelogram (IVP), chest x-ray, ultrasonography, directed biopsies, and, occasionally, barium enema. The usual treatment is total abdominal hysterectomy and bilateral salpingo-oophorectomy followed by radiotherapy or chemotherapy. For clear cell adenocarcinoma and sarcoma botryoides, vaginectomy may also be required. In unilateral malignant ovarian disease, unilateral oophorectomy alone may be performed. Chemotherapy or limited radiotherapy may also be required.

(J) Benign hyperplasia, if estrogen induced, may be premalignant (atypical adenomatous hyperplasia). Exogenous estrogens (Premarin) should be withdrawn. If bleeding persists, cancer is suspected. Progesterone, as an estrogen antagonist, can be used to treat benign hyperplasia. If adenomatous hyperplasia is present and progesterone is used, follow-up endometrial sampling should be done in 3 to 4 months.

REFERENCE

Huffman JW, Dewhurst CJ Sr, Caprano VJ. The gynecology of childhood and adolescence. Philadelphia: WB Saunders, 1981.

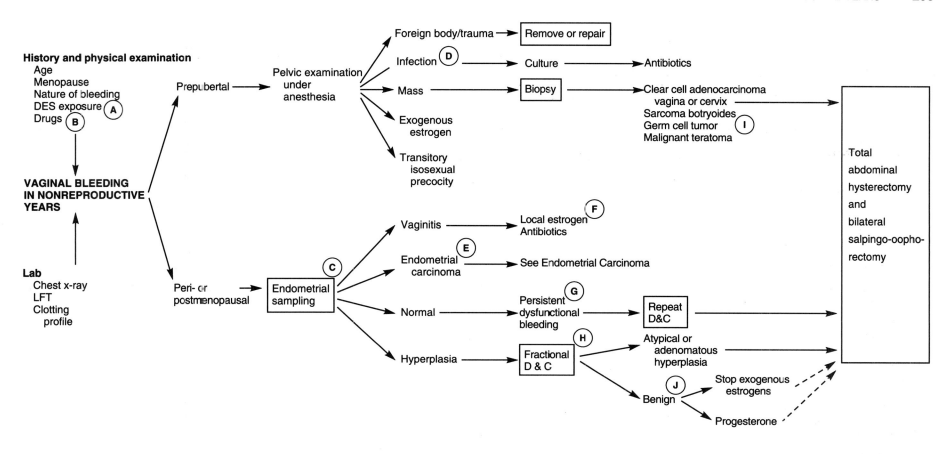

Pelvic Inflammatory Disease

R. Phillip Heine, M.D., and William Droegemueller, M.D.

(A) Pelvic inflammatory disease (PID) is a major health concern in the United States. In 1989 the Centers for Disease Control (CDC) reported approximately 750,000 new cases. In 1990 the estimated medical cost of PID and its sequelae was $3.5 billion.

(B) Variables that increase the incidence of PID include teenage years, multiple sexual partners, previous PID, intrauterine device (2 months after insertion only), and uterine instrumentation. The use of mechanical or oral contraceptives decreases the incidence of upper tract pelvic infections.

(C) The clinical diagnosis of acute PID is often imprecise. Laparoscopic evaluation shows that one third of patients hospitalized for the disease do not have it. Pain (99 percent) and pelvic tenderness (95 percent) are common. Only one third of patients have a temperature greater than 38°C. A pelvic mass or swelling is palpable in 48 percent of patients. Vaginal discharge is found in 80 percent. It is prudent to treat suspected disease because tubal obstruction follows an initial episode of PID in approximately 11 percent of cases.

(D) Laboratory testing sometimes aids in diagnosis. Less than 50 percent of patients have a white cell count above 10,000. Only 30 percent and 25 percent, respectively, have positive chlamydia or gonorrhea cultures. Because PID is a polymicrobial infection involving endogenous aerobes and anaerobes as well as sexually transmitted pathogens, endocervical cultures have limited value in selecting antibiotic therapy. They

should be obtained, nevertheless, because of an increasing incidence of multiple antibiotic-resistant gonorrhea. If cultures are positive, the patient's sexual partner should also be treated. A wet prep to rule out *Trichomonas vaginalis* and a syphilis serology should also be obtained because of the frequent associations of these infections with other sexually transmitted diseases. HIV screening test should be performed if risk factors are present.

(E) If results of pelvic examination are inconclusive, ultrasonography is helpful to establish the presence or absence of a pelvic abscess.

(F) An important therapeutic decision is the choice between outpatient treatment and hospitalization. If outpatient treatment is used, it is important to reexamine the patient after 48 to 72 hours. If response is suboptimal, the patient needs to be hospitalized and intravenous antibiotics initiated.

(G) Indications for hospitalization include the presence of a tuboovarian complex or abscess, uncertain diagnosis, significant gastrointestinal symptoms, nulliparity, and pregnancy.

(H) CDC recommendations for outpatient therapy of PID include (1) cefoxitin 2 g IM and probenecid 1 g PO concurrently, or (2) ceftriaxone 250 mg IM and doxycycline 100 mg PO 2 times a day for 10 to 14 days, or (3) tetracycline 500 mg PO 4 times a day for 10 to 14 days. As an alternative for patients who do not tolerated tetracyclines, erythromycin 500 mg PO 4 times a day for 10 to 14 days may be substituted.

(I) CDC recommendations for hospitalized patients with PID include: For patients without a mass, intrauterine device or recent history of uterine instrumentations, administer cefoxitin 2 g IV every 6 hours or cefotetan 2 g IV every 12 hours (other cephalosporins that provide adequate gonococcal and other facultative gram-negative anaerobic coverage may be used in appropriate doses) and doxycycline 100 mg every 12 hours PO or IV. The above regimen is continued for at least 48 hours after the patient clinically improves. After discharge the patient receives doxycycline 100 mg PO 2 times a day for a total of 10 to 14 days.

For patients with a mass, intrauterine device or history of recent uterine instrumentation, administer clindamycin 900 mg IV every 8 hours and gentamicin 2 mg/kg IV, followed by gentamicin 1.5 mg/kg IV 3 times per day. This regimen is continued for at least 48 hours after the patient improves. After discharge the patient receives doxycycline 100 mg PO 2 times a day for a total of 10 to 14 days. If a patient cannot tolerate doxycycline, clindamycin, 450 mg PO 4 times a day for 10 to 14 days, may be substituted.

(J) Laparoscopy is indicated when the diagnosis of PID is in doubt or when the patient is not responding to medical therapy.

(K) Other complications of PID include ectopic pregnancy (rate six to ten times normal), infertility (rate increase proportional to the number of episodes of acute PID: one episode, 11 percent; two episodes, 23 percent; three episodes, 54 per-

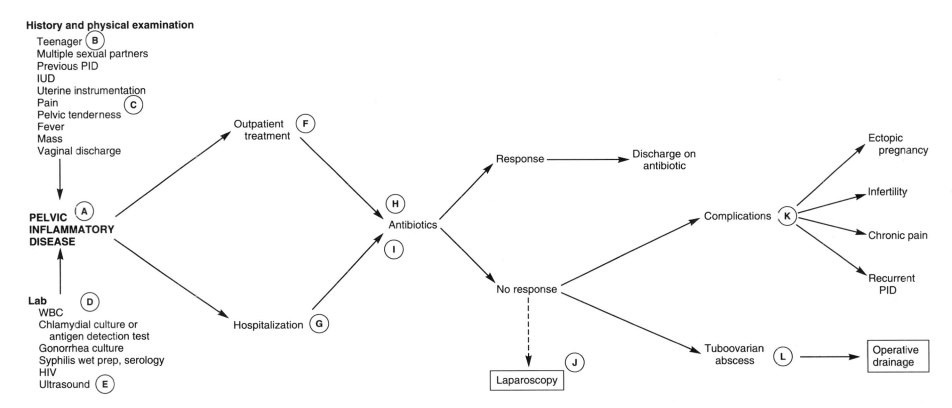

History and physical examination
Teenager (B)
Multiple sexual partners
Previous PID
IUD
Uterine instrumentation
Pain (C)
Pelvic tenderness
Fever
Mass
Vaginal discharge

Lab (D)
WBC
Chlamydial culture or
  antigen detection test
Gonorrhea culture
Syphilis wet prep, serology
HIV
Ultrasound (E)

cent), chronic pelvic pain (approximately 20 percent), and recurrent pelvic inflammatory disease (approximately 25 percent).

(L) Approximately 10 percent of patients with the diagnosis of PID have a documented tuboovarian abscess. With appropriate antibiotics most abscesses regress and do not require operative drainage. If surgery becomes necessary, conservatism is appropriate to protect childbearing potential and continued hormonal function.

REFERENCES

Centers for Disease Control: 1989 Sexually transmitted disease treatment guidelines. MMWR 1989; 38(No. S-8).

Centers for Disease Control: Surveillance Section, 1989.

Droegemueller W, Herbst AL, Mishell DR Jr, et al. Comprehensive Gynecology. St. Louis: CV Mosby, 1987.

Eschenbach DA. Epidemiology and diagnosis of acute pelvic inflammatory disease. Obstet Gynecol 1980; 55:142S–152S.

Westrom L. Incidence, prevalence, and trends of acute pelvic inflammatory disease and its consequences in industrialized countries. Am J Obstet Gynecol 1980; 138:880–892.

Endometriosis

Bradley S. Hurst, M.D.

(A) Endometriosis is a common disease in women of reproductive age. Presenting symptoms may include pelvic pain, dysmenorrhea, dyspareunia, infertility, or a combination of these. Endometriosis is identified in approximately 50 percent of women with dysmenorrhea, 20 percent of women with chronic pelvic pain and dyspareunia, and 40 percent of women with infertility. The extent of endometriosis has no correlation with severity of pain. Even small endometriosis lesions distant from the adnexae can be associated with infertility.

(B) Uterosacral nodularity and tenderness, generalized pelvic or uterine tenderness, fixation of the pelvic organs, retroversion of the uterus, and adnexal masses are identified in some but not all patients with endometriosis.

(C) Evaluation includes a careful search for other causes of pain. Pelvic inflammatory disease, urinary tract infection, and gastrointestinal disorders are common sources of chronic pelvic pain. A trial of nonsteroidal antiinflammatory drugs is warranted before surgery. An infertile couple deserves a complete evaluation before surgery, including semen analysis, a postcoital test, a hysterosalpingogram, and an endometrial biopsy. Nonsteroidal antiinflammatory drugs can be given for relief of symptoms.

(D) Endometriosis is diagnosed by direct visualization of the endometriosis implants. Laparoscopy is the diagnostic procedure of choice, although laparotomy is indicated for the patient with a persistent large adnexal mass. The average cost for laparoscopy is $1,000. Complications include perforation of the bowel, bladder, or pelvic vessels.

(E) The appearance of endometriosis may be quite varied. Typically, one sees brown "powder burn" lesions on peritoneal surfaces or the ovary. This represents an old endometriosis implant. Fresh endometriosis implants are typically red and contain glands and stroma. Endometriosis also can appear as blue nodules, white plaques, small petechial areas, or stellate areas of peritoneal scarring. A directed biopsy may be obtained if the diagnosis is questioned. Care should be taken to avoid rupture of an endometrioma.

(F) Expectant management is recommended when infertility is the major complaint and minimal or mild endometriosis is present. Fifty to sixty percent of these patients conceive. Patients who fail to conceive after a period of observation may elect superovulation with intrauterine insemination, gamete intrafallopian transfer, or in vitro fertilization to maximize fertility. Surgery and medical therapy are often advocated, but pregnancy rates are no higher with these therapies.

(G) Medical therapy is the treatment of choice for patients who have moderate to severe pain and wish to preserve fertility. It is not appropriate when large endometriomas are present. Therapy generally requires 6 months. Gonadotropin-releasing hormone (GnRH) analogues, danazol, and progestins are frequently used medications. GnRH analogues create a hypoestrogenic state and cause atrophy of endometriosis implants by down-regulation of pituitary GnRH receptors. Side effects include hot flashes, headaches, insomnia, and vaginal dryness. Depression is possible. Osteoporosis may occur but does not appear to be severe with a 6-month regimen. Treatment cost is $1,100 to $1,800. Danazol, an androgen derivative, directly

reduces ovarian estrogen production. It binds to estrogen and progesterone receptors in endometriosis implants. Side effects include weight gain, muscle cramps, reduced breast size, nausea, headaches, oily skin, and acne. Irreversible hirsutism and a deepening of the voice may occur. Treatment cost is $1,000 to $1,500. Medroxyprogesterone causes decidualization and atrophy of endometriosis. Side effects include breakthrough bleeding, weight gain, fluid retention, and nausea. Significant depression has been reported. Treatment cost is $150 to $270. Pregnancy rates (50 percent) are not improved after medical treatment. Improvement of pain is comparable with all of these agents (75 to 90 percent) although relief may be greater with GnRH analogues and danazol than with progestins.

(H) Laparoscopic surgery is advised for patients with moderate to severe endometriosis, infertility, or pain. Endometriomas smaller than 5 cm may be removed with laparoscopic surgery. Some advocate uterosacral ablation for pain relief, but there are no controlled prospective studies to indicate a benefit. Pain relief is less than that expected with medical therapy. Approximately 60 to 80 percent of patients report some improvement in pain relief, however. Pregnancy results are 50 percent for patients with moderate to severe endometriosis.

(I) Abdominal conservative surgery is recommended for endometriosis with severe anatomic distortion associated with infertility or pain. A presacral neurectomy may be performed to relieve severe midline dysmenorrhea. The goal of conservation surgery is the removal of all visible endometriosis implants and preservation of normal

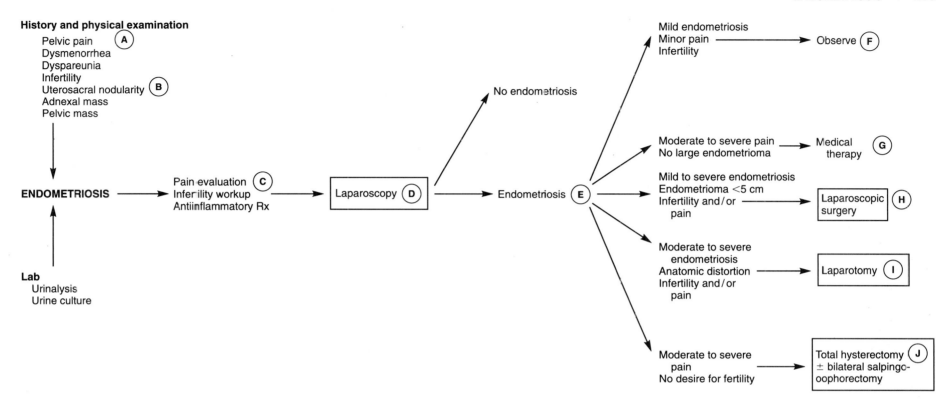

History and physical examination

Pelvic pain (A)
Dysmenorrhea
Dyspareunia
Infertility
Uterosacral nodularity (B)
Adnexal mass
Pelvic mass

ENDOMETRIOSIS → Pain evaluation (C)
Infertility workup
Antiinflammatory Rx

Lab
Urinalysis
Urine culture

→ Laparoscopy (D)

No endometriosis

Endometriosis (E)

Mild endometriosis
Minor pain → Observe (F)
Infertility

Moderate to severe pain → Medical (G)
No large endometrioma   therapy

Mild to severe endometriosis
Endometrioma <5 cm
Infertility and/or → Laparoscopic (H)
pain   surgery

Moderate to severe
endometriosis
Anatomic distortion → Laparotomy (I)
Infertility and/or
pain

Moderate to severe
pain → Total hysterectomy (J)
No desire for fertility   ± bilateral salpingo-
oophorectomy

pelvic structures. Seventy-five to ninety percent of patients experience excellent pain relief after conservative surgery. Fifty to sixty percent of infertile patients conceive after conservative surgery.

(J) Total abdominal hysterectomy with or without bilateral salpingo-oophorectomy is recommended for moderate to severe pain when fertility is no longer desired. Ovarian conservation may be attempted for patients remote from menopause, but recurrence rates are high when bilateral oophorectomy is not performed. Eighty to ninety

percent of patients can expect relief after total abdominal hysterectomy with bilateral salpingo-oophorectomy ($1,800). Estrogen replacement therapy may be safely started 6 weeks after surgery.

REFERENCES

The American Fertility Society. Revised American Fertility Society classification of endometriosis: 1985. Fertil Steril 1985; 43:351–352.

Buttram VC. Conservative surgery for endometriosis in the infertile female: a study of 206 cases with implications for both medical and surgical therapy. Fertil Steril 1979; 36:117–123.

Hammond CB, Rock JA, Parker RT. Conservative treatment of endometriosis: the effects of limited surgery and hormonal pseudopregnancy. Fertil Steril 1976; 27:756–766.

Hurst BS, Rock JA. Endometriosis: pathophysiology, diagnosis and treatment. Obstet Gynecol Surv 1989; 44:297–304.

Olive DL, Stohs GF, Metzger DA. Expectant management and hydrotubations in the treatment of endometriosis associated with infertility. Fertil Steril 1985; 44:35–41.

Schenken RS, ed. Endometriosis: Contemporary concepts in clinical management. Philadelphia; JB Lippincott, 1989.

Carcinoma of the Cervix

Theodore C. Barton, M.D.

(A) All sexually active women are at risk for carcinoma of the cervix.

(B) Cervical intraepithelial neoplasia on PAP smear requires tissue biopsy to confirm the diagnosis. Colposcopy-directed biopsies, serial punch biopsies, and endocervical curettage are required. Cone biopsy of the cervix may be necessary. Cervical staining techniques (Schiller test) may aid in identifying abnormal areas of the cervix for biopsy.

(C) Staging for carcinoma of the cervix is done with the patient under anesthesia. Cystoscopy, sigmoidoscopy, and intravenous pyelogram are part of the staging process. Magnetic resonance imaging and computed tomography scans may facilitate staging.

(D) Stage I carcinoma is strictly confined to the cervix. Stage IA is microinvasive, less than 3 mm (5-year survival, 90 percent); stage IB is frank invasion (5-year survival, 78 percent).

(E) In stage II, the carcinoma extends beyond the cervix but not to the pelvic side walls. Tumor may involve the upper two thirds of the vagina but not the lower one third (5-year survival, 57 percent).

(F) In stage III, the carcinoma extends to the pelvic side walls or involves the lower one third of the vagina (5-year survival, 31 percent).

(G) In stage IV, the carcinoma extends beyond the true pelvis and involves the bladder or rectum (5-year survival, 8 percent).

(H) The operation of radical hysterectomy and pelvic lymphadenectomy is applicable as primary treatment only for stage I and stage IIA lesions. In these cases, surgery and radiation give comparable results. Surgery is usually selected for younger patients who are good operative risks in whom sexual function will be maintained. The ovaries can be preserved.

(I) Radical radiation therapy consists of external beam plus intracavitary radium or cesium. It is used for advanced disease or in patients with marginal operative risk. Points to evaluate in comparing operation with radiation are the immediate complications of radical surgery and the long-term complications of radiation to the bladder and rectum.

(J) Interstitial brachytherapy is used for bulky pelvic disease.

(K) Radiation therapy is used for local palliation of extrapelvic disease. Chemotherapy can be used as a radiation sensitizer. At the present time, systemic chemotherapy for carcinoma of the cervix is of limited use.

(L) Bulky cervical disease is synonymous with "barrel-shaped" cervix.

REFERENCES

Beahrs O, et al. Manual for the staging of cancer. Philadelphia: JB Lippincott, 1988; 151–156.

Downey GO, Potish RA, Adcock LL, et al. Pretreatment surgical staging in cervical carcinoma. Am J Obstet Gynecol 1989; 160:1055–1061.

Kim SI, Choi BI, Lee HP, et al. Uterine cervical carcinoma: comparison of CT and MR findings. Radiology 1990; 175:45–51.

Larson DM. Diagnosis of recurrent carcinoma of the cervix after radical hysterectomy. Obstet Gynecol 1988; 71:6–9.

Richart RM. Causes and management of cervical intraepithelial neoplasia. Cancer 1987; 60:1951–1959.

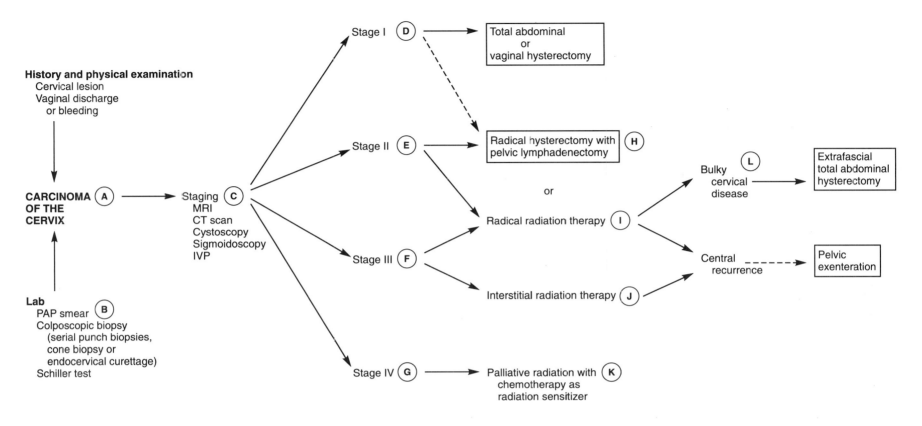

History and physical examination
Cervical lesion
Vaginal discharge
or bleeding

CARCINOMA (A)
OF THE
CERVIX

Staging (C)
MRI
CT scan
Cystoscopy
Sigmoidoscopy
IVP

Lab
PAP smear (B)
Colposcopic biopsy
(serial punch biopsies,
cone biopsy or
endocervical curettage)
Schiller test

Stage I (D) → Total abdominal
or
vaginal hysterectomy

Stage II (E) → Radical hysterectomy with (H)
pelvic lymphadenectomy

or

Radical radiation therapy (I)

Stage III (F)

Interstitial radiation therapy (J)

Stage IV (G) → Palliative radiation with (K)
chemotherapy as
radiation sensitizer

Bulky (L)
cervical
disease → Extrafascial
total abdominal
hysterectomy

Central
recurrence ---→ Pelvic
exenteration

Endometrial Carcinoma

Howard M. Goodman, M.D., and Ross S. Berkowitz, M.D.

(A) Endometrial carcinoma is the most common gynecologic malignancy (40,000 new cases yearly). There is currently no satisfactory screening technique for endometrial carcinoma.

(B) Risk factors include hyperestrogenic states (obesity, estrogen secreting tumors, exogenous estrogen use); reproductive history (low parity, late menopause, anovulatory states); intercurrent illness (diabetes mellitus, hypertension); heredity (family risk); and atypical endometrial hyperplasia (may progress to frank cancer in 25 to 30 percent of cases). A major symptom is abnormal vaginal bleeding (first symptom in 90 percent of women with endometrial carcinoma, usually postmenopausal).

(C) The pelvic examination is usually negative in early disease. Cervical involvement, adnexal enlargement, and parametrial spread are indicative of advanced disease. Ascites may be seen infrequently.

(D) Aspiration curettage is the initial diagnostic procedure. Accuracy approaches that of a formal dilation and curettage (D & C).

(E) Formal fractional D & C remains the standard against which other diagnostic tests are measured. This procedure is usually performed in the operating room with either general or regional anesthesia. Although slightly more accurate than aspiration curettage, the need for hospitalization, anesthesia, and a higher complication rate and cost relegate its use to situations when an office procedure cannot be performed or when an inadequate specimen is obtained, or when symptoms persist after an office aspiration reveals negative pathology.

(F) Preoperative evaluation should include general medical history and physical examination, pelvic examination to assess resectability and evidence of extracorporal spread, chest radiograph, liver and renal blood testing, and routine hematologic testing.

(G) The International Federation of Gynecology and Obstetrics (FIGO) adopted a surgical staging system in 1990. Surgical staging entails exploratory laparotomy with complete assessment of the intraabdominal contents, peritoneal washings, total abdominal hysterectomy and bilateral salpingo-oophorectomy with estimation of grade and depth of myometrial invasion, lymphadenectomy based on these two factors, omental biopsy, biopsy of suspicious areas, and resection of areas of disseminated disease if possible. Assignment of FIGO stage is based on histopathologic findings.

(H) Stage I disease is confined to the uterine corpus (IA, IB, and IC based on depth of myometrial invasion and stratified by grades 1 to 3). The probability of regional metastases depends on histologic subtype, grade, and depth of invasion. There is a 10 percent risk of nodal spread with G3 inner, G2 mid, and G1 outer myometrial invasion. Patients with these or deeper levels of invasion are treated 4 to 6 weeks after hysterectomy with pelvic radiation therapy. Patients with disease confined to the endometrium are at little risk of recurrence and require no adjuvant treatment. Patients with evidence of myometrial invasion less than that noted above are at low risk for pelvic nodal spread but have 10 to 12 times the risk for vaginal apex recurrence. They should receive vaginal radiation postoperatively, which reduces their risk level to 2 percent or less. Reported 5-year survival for over

10,000 patients with stage I endometrial carcinoma was 75 percent. Studies suggest a 5-year survival in excess of 90 percent with the likelihood of cure approaching 100 percent in low-risk patients and 60 to 70 percent in higher risk patients as defined by grade and depth of myometrial invasion.

(I) Stage II is defined as disease confined to corpus and cervix stratified by grades 1 to 3, and involvement of cervical glands (IIA) or cervical stroma (IIB). These patients are at high risk for pelvic nodal involvement (35 to 40 percent). After surgical staging and hysterectomy, these patients are treated with 4500 to 5000 cGy whole pelvic radiation therapy with a boost to the vaginal apex. Five-year survivals ranging from 45 to 80 percent have been reported.

(J) Stage III is stratified into IIIA (serosa, adnexa, positive washings), IIIB (vagina), and IIIC (retroperitoneal nodes) and further stratified by grades 1 to 3. Conventional treatment has been pelvic radiation therapy, uterovaginal radium, followed by total abdominal hysterectomy/bilateral salpingo-oophorectomy, with 5-year survival rates lower than 20 percent. These patients are at high risk for upper abdominal and nodal spread or recurrence and may be considered for more extensive treatment. Cytoreduction and whole abdomen radiation therapy may also be considered in these patients. They have shown improved survivals approaching 50 percent. Patients with metastases to the retroperitoneal nodes are usually treated with radiation therapy. Survivals of 40 to 50 percent

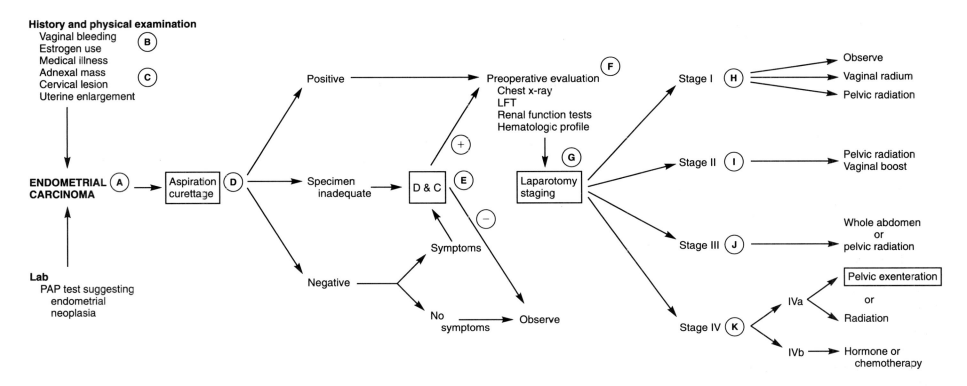

History and physical examination
Vaginal bleeding   (B)
Estrogen use
Medical illness
Adnexal mass   (C)
Cervical lesion
Uterine enlargement

ENDOMETRIAL (A) → **Aspiration curettage** (D)
CARCINOMA

Lab
PAP test suggesting
endometrial
neoplasia

Positive → Preoperative evaluation (F)
Chest x-ray
LFT
Renal function tests
Hematologic profile

Specimen inadequate → D & C (E)

Negative → Symptoms / No symptoms → Observe

(+) / (−)

Laparotomy staging (G)

Stage I (H) → Observe / Vaginal radium / Pelvic radiation

Stage II (I) → Pelvic radiation / Vaginal boost

Stage III (J) → Whole abdomen or pelvic radiation

Stage IV (K) → IVa → Pelvic exenteration or Radiation
IVb → Hormone or chemotherapy

have been achieved with extended field paraaortic irradiation.

(K) Stage IV is divided into IVA (bladder and rectum) and IVB (distal disease) and stratified by grades 1 to 3. Treatment is individualized. Patients with IVA disease may be considered for radiation therapy or supraradical surgery. Women with Stage IVB are usually treated with systemic agents, either hormonal or cytotoxic chemotherapy. Recurrent disease confined to the pelvis can be treated with radiation therapy if overlapping fields are avoided. Patients not eligible for radiation therapy are usually managed with hormones or cytotoxic chemotherapy. The probability of response to progestational agents is related to grade and receptor status. The response rates in patients with well-differentiated tumors range from 30 to 50 percent. The response rate with high-grade tumors is less than 10 percent. Cytotoxic chemotherapy has a role in the management of women with advanced recurrent disease. Adriamycin, Cytoxan, and cisplatin have considerable activity and are frequently used in combination.

REFERENCES

Aalders J, Abeler V, Kolsta P, et al. Postoperative external irradiation and prognostic parameters in Stage I endometrial carcinoma. Obstet Gynecol 1980; 56:419–426.

Creasman WT, Morrow CP, Bundy, BN, et al. Surgical pathologic spread patterns of endometrial cancer. Cancer 1987; 60:2035–2041.

Grimes DA. Diagnostic dilation and curettage: a reappraisal. Am J Obstet Gynecol 1982; 142:1–6.

Jones HW. Treatment of adenocarcinoma of the endometrium. Obstet Gynecol Surv 1975; 30:147–169.

Sant Cassia LJ, Weppelmann B, Shingleton H, et al. Management of early endometrial carcinoma. Gynecol Oncol 1989; 35:362–366.

Adnexal Mass

Tommy N. Evans, M.D.

(A) Any adnexal mass should be considered abnormal and a neoplasm until proven otherwise. One in 70 women will develop ovarian cancer.

(B) Important factors in defining the nature of the mass include its size, consistency, unilaterality, tenderness, fixation, and evidence of spread.

(C) Characteristic symptoms and signs include pain, tenderness, growth, vaginal discharge or bleeding, and fever.

(D) Ultrasound can define the size, location, and bilaterality of the mass. It also determines its outline and consistency (solid or cystic).

(E) Physiologic cysts occur only during reproductive years and are characteristically asymptomatic, unilateral, smooth in contour, and cystic on examination and ultrasound. Cysts less than 6 cm in diameter usually regress spontaneously within 6 weeks. Those greater than 6 cm should be examined laparoscopically. They may require excision.

(F) Ovarian neoplasms are characteristically bilateral, cystic or solid, and larger than 6 cm when discovered. Their nature should be confirmed at laparoscopy if there is any doubt about diagnosis.

(G) A benign ovarian tumor (cystic teratoma or dermoid) should be treated in a way that preserves fertility.

(H) Characteristics of a malignant ovarian tumor include hemorrhage, necrosis, adherence to adjacent structures, ascites, local excrescences, peritoneal studding, and intracystic papillomata.

(I) If malignancy is suspected, the search for extension or metastases should include chest x-ray, computed tomography, or magnetic resonance imaging.

(J) Twisted and infarcted ovarian masses should be excised in toto before untwisting to avoid massive pulmonary embolism.

(K) Staging at the time of laparotomy should include cytology of peritoneal washings (before tumor manipulation), periaortic lymphadenectomy biopsy, omental biopsy, and subdiaphragmatic biopsy. Positive findings indicate a need for postoperative chemotherapy.

(L) Radiation or chemotherapy can prolong survival of patients with unresectable disease.

(M) Tuboovarian abscess no longer always requires total abdominal hysterectomy/bilateral salpingo-oophorectomy.

REFERENCES

DiSaia PJ, Hammond CB et al, eds. Danforth's obstetrics and gynecology, 6th ed. Philadelphia: JB Lippincott, 1990.
Thompson JR, Rock JA, eds. TeLinde's operative gynecology, 7th ed. Philadelphia: JB Lippincott, 1992.
Willson JR, Carrington ER. Obstetrics and gynecology, 8th ed. St. Louis: CV Mosby, 1987.

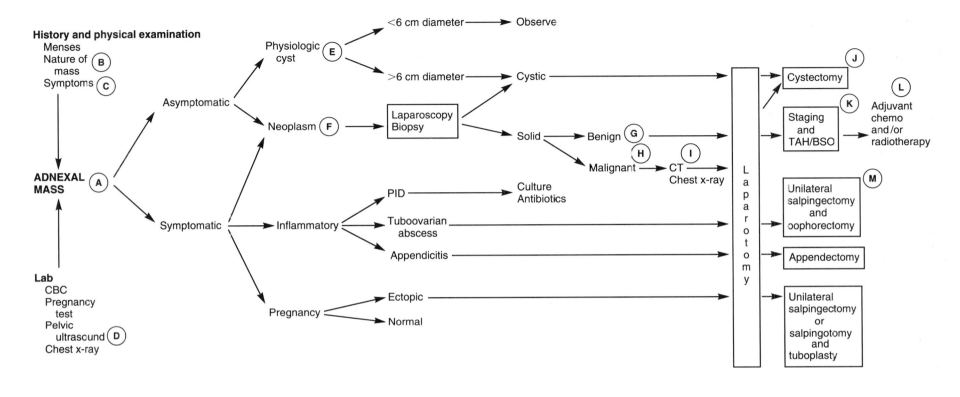

History and physical examination
Menses
Nature of (B)
mass
Symptoms (C)

ADNEXAL MASS (A)

Lab
CBC
Pregnancy
test
Pelvic
ultrascund (D)
Chest x-ray

Asymptomatic

Symptomatic

Physiologic cyst (E)
<6 cm diameter → Observe
>6 cm diameter → Cystic

Neoplasm (F) → Laparoscopy Biopsy
Cystic
Solid → Benign (G)
Malignant (H) → CT (I) Chest x-ray

Inflammatory
PID → Culture Antibiotics
Tuboovarian abscess
Appendicitis

Pregnancy
Ectopic
Normal

Laparotomy

Cystectomy (J)

Staging and TAH/BSO (K)

(L) Adjuvant chemo and/or radiotherapy

Unilateral salpingectomy and oophorectomy (M)

Appendectomy

Unilateral salpingectomy or salpingotomy and tuboplasty

Ovarian Mass

Francis J. Major, M.D.

(A) Any ovarian mass less than 5 cm in diameter is probably functional, whereas any mass greater than 5 cm is likely to be neoplastic.

(B) Pelvic examination can exclude inflammatory disease, pregnancy, or myomata.

(C) Ultrasound delineates cystic vs. solid and unilocular vs. multilocular masses and the relationship of a mass to the uterus.

(D) The Ca-125 serum test is positive in 70 percent of serous malignancies. It can also be positive in endometrial cancer, endometriosis, pregnancy, or inflammations.

(E) If laboratory and radiologic evidence suggests neoplasm, laparotomy should be performed for diagnosis, resection, and staging.

(F) Laparoscopy is valuable if, after other workup, there is still a question as to the nature of the mass.

(G) Masses greater than 5 cm in diameter are more significant in the postmenopausal patient.

(H) Tuboovarian abscess is usually bilateral and requires hysterectomy and bilateral salpingo-oophorectomy. In patients with an intrauterine device, unilateral disease may be found, and in such cases unilateral resection is sufficient.

(I) Functional tumors usually are unilocular. Neoplasms usually are multilocular.

(J) Germ cell and stromal tumors are solid and frequently unilateral. Malignant epithelial neoplasms are a mixture of solid and cystic elements and are often bilateral. The most common solid tumor of the ovary is metastatic cancer from the breast, colon, stomach, or pancreas.

(K) Appropriate staging biopsies permit conservative treatment for early malignancies.

(L) Survival of a patient with ovarian cancer depends primarily on maximal tumor bulk resection at the time of diagnosis.

(M) Linear salpingostomy may preserve fertility.

REFERENCES

Barber HK, Graber EA. The PMPO syndrome (post menopausal palpable ovary syndrome). Obstet Gynecol 1971; 38:921–923.

Buchsbaum HJ, Brady MF, Delgado G, et al. Surgical staging of ovarian carcinoma: a gynecologic oncology group study. Surg Gynecol Obstet 1989; 169:226–232.

Parsons L, Sommers S. Gynecology. Philadelphia; WB Saunders, 1962; 590–601.

Scully RE. Recent progress in ovarian cancer. Hum Pathol 1970; 1:73.

Taylor ES, McMillan JH, Greer BE, et al. Tubo-ovarian abscess with intra-uterine device. Am J Obstet Gynecol 1975; 123:338–348.

Young RC, Walton LA, Ellenberg SS, et al. Adjuvant therapy in Stage I and Stage II epithelial ovarian cancer: results of two prospective randomized trials. N Engl J Med 1990; 322:1021–1027.

History and physical examination

Menses
Bleeding
Mass (A)
Pelvic examination (B)
Rectal examination
Fever
Intrauterine device

OVARIAN MASS

Lab
CBC
ESR
Cervical culture
X-rays of pelvis
and abdomen
Ultrasound (C)
Pregnancy test
CA-125 (D)

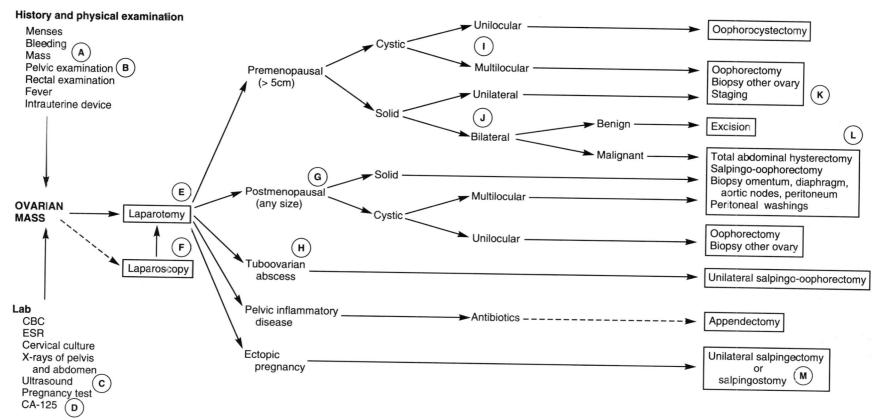

Orthopedic

Cervical Spine Fracture

Robert E. Breeze, M.D.

(A) The optimal management of acute cervical spine fractures first requires recognition of the lesion. Such lesions must be suspected whenever a patient sustains trauma to the head or neck or whenever the mechanism of trauma is in doubt. Motor vehicle accidents, falls, and diving injuries are particularly common causes of neck fracture. Any complaint of neck pain or observed tenderness or spasm in the cervical musculature must also alert the physician. It must be remembered that low cervical fractures often produce pain in the midscapular region.

(B) Early in the decision process, one must decide if neurologic deficits attributable to the cervical spinal cord exist. This information is critical in deciding the subsequent course of the workup. Complete or partial motor or sensory deficits in the arms and legs are the most obvious signs. Other signs must be sought, however, such as absent rectal tone, an absent bulbocavernosus reflex, and priapism. Bradycardia in the face of hypotension also suggests a cord lesion (neurogenic shock). Paradoxical respirations (expansion of the abdomen with contraction of the rib cage on inspiration) is indicative of a lower cervical cord lesion (preservation of phrenic nerve function with loss of intercostal nerve function). Monoplegia and a Horner sign are more suggestive of a plexus lesion. Progressive neurologic deficit usually demands emergent imaging studies (magnetic resonance imaging [MRI] or computed tomography [CT] myelography) followed by surgical intervention. The use of glucocorticoids with cord injuries remains controversial; nevertheless, high-dose steroids employed acutely have recently gained popularity. The presence of a root injury rarely alters the initial management of a cervical spine fracture. Persistent radicular signs and symptoms sometimes lead to delayed surgical intervention.

(C) Awake patients without neck pain or neurologic deficit usually can be evaluated completely with plain films. When an abnormality is noted, one must try to assess the age and stability of the lesion. Older individuals with preexisting cervical spondylosis can often be difficult to assess. Flexion–extension views frequently provide evidence of relative stability. When a question still exists, a plain CT scan through the region of the abnormality usually settles the issue.

(D) When neck pain is present, a thorough and organized search for a fracture must be made. CT scanning is generally reserved for evaluating abnormalities noted on plain films. CT scanning should not be used as a screening examination except in unusual cases where technical problems preclude adequate visualization on plain films. Although it is true that subtle fractures can be missed on plain films, if the algorithm is followed these patients will be treated in a Philadelphia collar despite the initial failure to document the lesion. Such treatment is usually sufficient with such small fractures; persistent pain identifies those patients needing further treatment.

(E) In patients who have neurologic deficits but no plain film abnormalities, nonosseous compressive lesions must be sought. These most frequently take the form of epidural hematomas or acute disc herniations. Although they can sometimes be seen on plain CT scans, MRI and CT myelography are far superior. MRI should be reserved for stable, awake patients, since the patient cannot be monitored as closely in the MRI suite as in the CT scanner.

(F) Patients with marked subluxation generally need to have their fractures reduced. In the absence of neurologic deficit, most clinicians will study the region of abnormality with CT before proceeding. When neurologic deficits are present, it can be argued that closed reduction should be attempted directly, without further delay for CT scanning. In either event, the initial attempt at reduction should be with skeletal traction applied through either Gardner-Wells tongs or a halo ring. Up to 40 to 60 lb can be employed acutely with certain fracture–dislocations. Such a high degree of traction should not be continued after reduction has been achieved, since it may lead to excessive axial distraction and further cord injury. In general, high cervical fractures should not be subjected to high traction forces.

(G) Surgical reduction is generally accomplished using a posterior approach. In the usual lower cervical fracture–dislocation, one or both facets are disrupted and "locked." To reduce such a lesion, the superior facets of the lower vertebra are drilled off, allowing reduction. The involved segments are then wired together and an on-lay fusion graft is placed. Occasionally anterior reduction is preferred. An MRI scan is usually obtained before posterior reductions to rule out a traumatic disk herniation that might be exacerbated by reduction. The patients are generally placed in some type of external orthosis for 8 to 12 weeks after surgery.

(H) When compressive lesions are present, surgical decompression is often indicated. Both anterior and posterior approaches are used, the choice depending on the site of compression. Anterior decompressions usually take the form of a discectomy or vertebrectomy. Posteriorly a laminectomy is performed. Most decompressions are followed by a bony fusion and placement of the patient into some type of external orthosis.

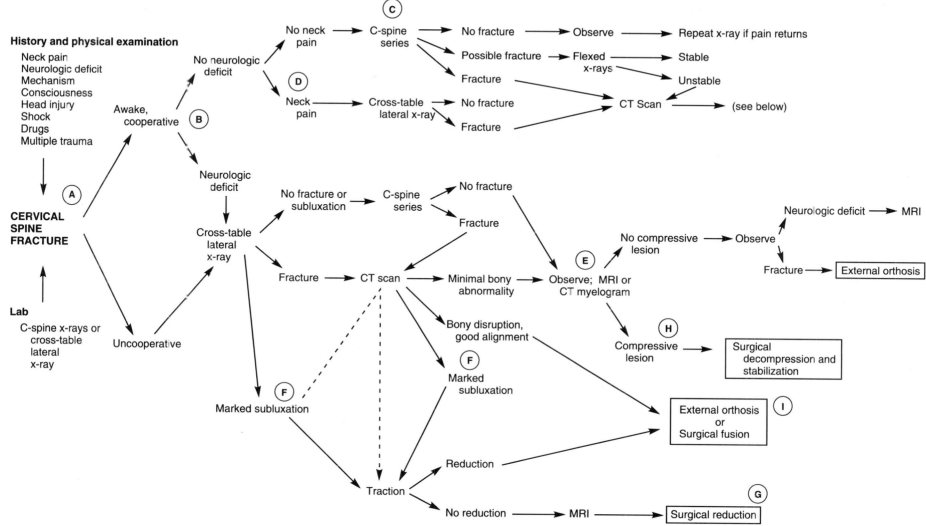

History and physical examination
- Neck pain
- Neurologic deficit
- Mechanism
- Consciousness
- Head injury
- Shock
- Drugs
- Multiple trauma

(A) CERVICAL SPINE FRACTURE

Lab
C-spine x-rays or cross-table lateral x-ray

Awake, cooperative (B)

Uncooperative

No neurologic deficit
- No neck pain → (C) C-spine series → No fracture → Observe → Repeat x-ray if pain returns
  - Possible fracture → Flexed x-rays → Stable
  - Fracture → Unstable
- (D) Neck pain → Cross-table lateral x-ray → No fracture → CT Scan → (see below)
  - Fracture

Neurologic deficit → Cross-table lateral x-ray
- No fracture or subluxation → C-spine series → No fracture
  - Fracture
- Fracture → CT scan → Minimal bony abnormality → (E) Observe; MRI or CT myelogram
  - No compressive lesion → Observe → Neurologic deficit → MRI
    - Fracture → External orthosis
  - Compressive lesion → (H) Surgical decompression and stabilization
- Bony disruption, good alignment
- (F) Marked subluxation
- Marked subluxation (F) → Traction
  - Reduction
  - No reduction → MRI → (G) Surgical reduction

(I) External orthosis or Surgical fusion

REFERENCES

Bohlman HH, Broada E. Fractures and dislocations of the lower cervical spine. In: Bailey RW, ed. The cervical spine. Philadelphia: JB Lippincott, 1983; 247–251.

Harris JH, Edeiken-Monroe B. The radiology of acute cervical spine trauma. Baltimore: Williams & Wilkins, 1987.

Wagner FC. Injuries to the cervical spine and spinal cord. In: Youmans JR, ed. Neurological surgery. Philadelphia: WB Saunders, 1990; 2378–239.

White AA, Panjabi MM. The basic kinematics of the human spine: a review of past and current knowledge. Spine 1978; 3:12–20.

(I) The decision to treat an injury with external fixation or surgical fusion is generally based on the relative degree of bony vs. ligamentous disruption. The greater the bony involvement, the greater the likelihood of adequate fusion with external fixation alone. In situations where the injury is predominately ligamentous or where fracture apposition is inadequate, surgical fusion is frequently necessary. Surgical fusion is performed either anteriorly or posteriorly, depending on where the greatest degree of disruption exists. For example, if the posterior elements alone are disrupted, one would not disrupt that motion segment further by removing the disc to perform an anterior fusion.

(J) **Imaging Studies and Their Relative Costs**

Study	Cost
Cross-table lateral	$ 56
C-spine series	$444
Flexion–extension views	$ 58
Plain CT of cervical spine	$340
Lateral tomograms	$371
MRI	$926

Thoracolumbar Spine Fracture

Robert B. Dzioba, M.D.

(A) Fractures or fracture–dislocations at the thoracolumbar junction are commonly caused by axial compression forces creating burst fractures or by flexion rotation injuries causing fracture–dislocations.

(B) Since the spinal cord ends at the L1–2 level such trauma often results in severe partial neural deficit or paraplegia. The degree of neurologic deficit varies considerably depending on the bony level and severity of injury. Neurologic deficit resulting from fractures between T-10 and L-1 is due to a combination of damage to both the cord and nerve roots. In fractures above T-10 the deficit usually reflects damage to the cord; below L-1 it is an indication of root damage alone.

(C) Initial roentgenograms should include an anteroposterior (AP) and lateral of the complete spine to the sacrum. Computed tomography scanning is standard in determining the extent of the fracture, canal encroachment, and bony instability. With the exception of simple wedge compression fractures in the elderly, all thoracolumbar fractures should be studied by computed tomography scanning.

(D) The treatment of thoracolumbar fractures depends on the stability of the bony elements and the degree of neurologic deficit. Bony stability is viewed as a spectrum, ranging from simple stable wedge compression fractures in osteoporotic vertebrae (Grandma's fracture) to grossly unstable fractures or dislocations in younger patients. Neurologic status is usually directly related to the degree of neural element compression caused by retropulsed bony fragments.

(E) Simple stable thoracolumbar fractures in the elderly or wedge compression fractures in the young with no neurologic deficit are treated by a short period of bed rest and early mobilization.

Spinal orthosis or a Kydex brace may be used to improve stability and provide ambulation.

(F) Unstable thoracolumbar fractures such as three-column burst fractures, shear and chance fractures, or flexion–rotation and flexion–distraction fractures usually cause neurologic deficit and are best treated by surgical methods. These include spinal instrumentation and closed canal decompression.

(G) An unstable fracture in a patient without neurologic complications is treated either by bed rest for 3 to 6 weeks followed by thoracolumbar sacral orthosis or by open reduction and internal fixation followed by early mobilization with or without orthosis.

(H) Incomplete neurologic lesions must be differentiated from complete spinal cord lesions causing paraplegia. Incomplete lesions require immediate reduction of fracture fragments, decompression of neural elements, and maintenance of skeletal alignment by instrumentation and fusion. The only indication for immediate surgical decompression is deterioration of neurologic status or radiologic evidence of gross spinal instability.

(I) Patients who remain paraplegic after early (24 hours) return of reflexes, such as the bulbocavernosus reflex, will be paraplegic for life. Treatment is aimed at skeletal realignment, stabilization of the spine by instrumentation and fusion, usually within 1 week of injury, and rapid rehabilitation with the aid of orthoses and a wheelchair.

(J) Bilateral Harrington rod distraction instrumentation with segmental (Wisconsin) wiring is the single best technique for open reduction and internal fixation of unstable thoracolumbar fractures. Wide decompression laminectomies are no longer performed since they increase fracture instability without benefiting already damaged neural elements. Spinal realignment through fracture reduction and neural decompression by removal of specific offending fracture fragments using anterior or posterolateral approaches will produce the desired results most effectively. Intraoperative fracture fragment reduction may be studied by ultrasound. More recently pedicular screw segmental fixation has allowed for shorter fusion segments.

(K) Braces, casts, or spinal orthoses are useful in protecting relatively stable injuries or when used as immobilizers of the thoracolumbar spine during the postoperative period. The device best suited for this is a molded front and back body jacket (Boston, Rancho, Kydex). By themselves, however, orthoses do not effectively immobilize grossly unstable fractures of the thoracolumbar junction.

REFERENCES

Bryant CE, Sullivan JA. Management of thoracic and lumbar spine fractures with Harrington distraction rods and supplemented with segmental wiring. Spine 1983; 8:532–537.

Davis F. The three column spine and its significance in the classification of acute thoracolumbar spinal injuries. Spine 1983; 8:817–831.

Flesch JR, Leider LL, Erickson DL, et al. Harrington instrumentation and spine fusion for unstable fractures and fracture-dislocations of the thoracic and lumbar spine. J Bone Joint Surg 1977; 59A:143–153.

Jacobs RR, Asher MA, Snikder RK. Thoracolumbar spinal injuries: comparative study of recumbent and operative treatment in 100 patients. Spine 1980; 5:463–477.

Jacobs RR, Casey MP. Surgical management of thoracolumbar spinal injuries: general principles and controversial considerations. Clin Orthop 1984; 189:22–35.

McAfee PC, Hansen AY, Lasda NA. The unstable burst fracture. Spine 1982; 7:365–373.

Post MJD, Green BA, Quencer RM, et al. The value of computed tomography in spinal trauma. Spine 1982; 7:417–431.

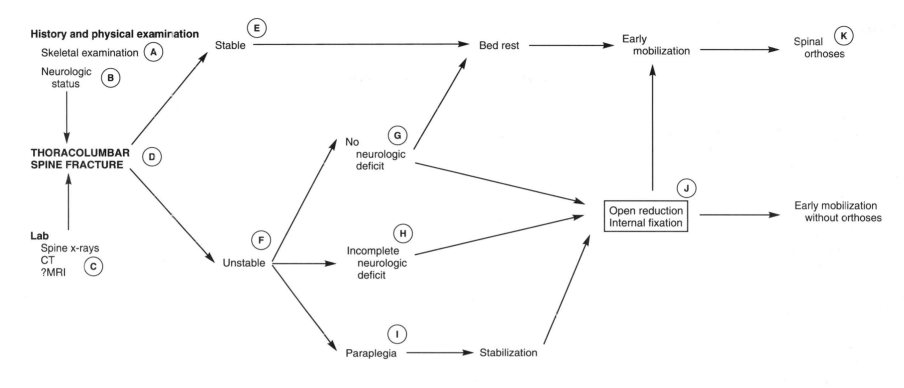

History and physical examination
Skeletal examination (A)
Neurologic status (B)

THORACOLUMBAR SPINE FRACTURE (D)

Lab
Spine x-rays
CT
?MRI (C)

Stable (E) → Bed rest → Early mobilization → Spinal orthoses (K)

Unstable (F)
→ No neurologic deficit (G)
→ Incomplete neurologic deficit (H)
→ Paraplegia (I) → Stabilization

Open reduction Internal fixation (J) → Early mobilization without orthoses

Pelvic Fracture

Alan D. Aaron, M.D.

(A) Concomitant sciatic nerve and lower cord injuries are common in pelvic fracture. Diastasis of the pelvic ring can be associated with bladder or urethral injury.

(B) Inordinate blood loss (more than 1.5 L) can accompany even innocuous-appearing closed pelvic fractures.

(C) Routine radiographs include anteroposterior, inlet, and outlet views of the pelvis. Pelvic instability is suspected with ischial spine avulsions, L-5 transverse process fractures, sacral fractures, posterior gap, or pelvic displacement. Acetabular fractures require internal and external oblique radiographs.

(D) Pulmonary insufficiency due to fat embolism is a serious complication.

(E) Massive electrolyte solution infusion and blood transfusion may be required. Stabilization of the pelvis with an external fixator in the emergency room will minimize blood loss.

(F) Displacement greater than 2.0 mm at the joint surface is significant. If after attempting closed reduction with traction a significant displacement persists, open reduction and internal fixation is necessary.

(G) Open pelvic fractures are often associated with pelvic visceral injuries that require repair. Fracture reduction and external fixation is performed at the time of laparotomy.

(H) Anatomic instability equates with significant pelvic ring displacement.

(I) Positive diagnostic peritoneal lavage is sufficient indication for laparotomy, at which time pubic diastasis can be stabilized.

(J) Angiographic embolization is suitable for bleeding from small vessels. Laceration of major vessels requires early direct operative repair.

(K) Closed reduction is achieved by internal rotation of the femurs or by manipulation of the iliac crests using an external fixator. An external fixator can be used for the reduction and stabilization of lateral compression fractures.

REFERENCES

Dalal SA, Burgess AR, Siegel JH, et al. Pelvic fracture in multiple trauma: classification by mechanism is key to pattern of organ injury, resuscitative requirements, and outcome. J Trauma 1987; 29:981–1001.

Kellam JF, McMurray RY, Paley D, et al. The unstable pelvic fracture: operative treatment. Orthop Clin North Am 1987; 18:25–42.

Mayo KA. Fractures of the acetabulum. Orthop Clin North Am 1987; 18:43–57.

Tile M. Fractures of the pelvis and acetabulum. Baltimore: Williams & Wilkins, 1984.

Tile M. Pelvic ring fractures: should they be fixed? J Bone Joint Surg 1988; 70B:1–12.

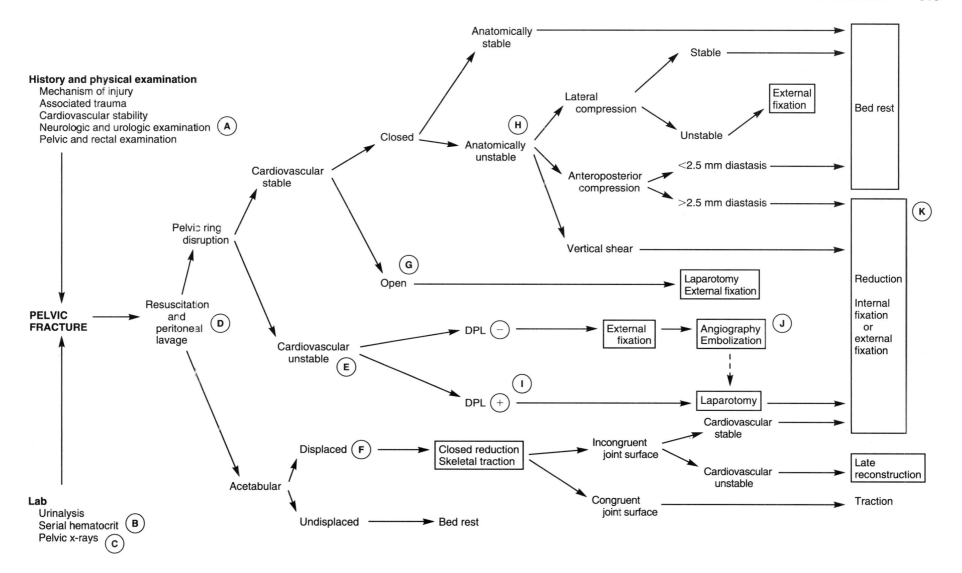

History and physical examination
Mechanism of injury
Associated trauma
Cardiovascular stability
Neurologic and urologic examination (A)
Pelvic and rectal examination

PELVIC FRACTURE

Lab
Urinalysis
Serial hematocrit (B)
Pelvic x-rays (C)

Hip Fracture

Susan L. Jolly, M.D., and Mack L. Clayton, M.D.

(A) The 275,000 hip fractures that occur annually in the United States cost approximately $7 billion. Their care ranks 10th in total hospital days. Because of the aging of the population, the incidence of hip fracture will double or triple by the year 2040.

(B) The usual injury causing fracture in the elderly is a fall at home. Only 19 percent of falls in the elderly lead to a hip fracture, however.

(C) Incidence doubles each decade after age 50 years. Hip fracture is two to four times as frequent in women as in men.

(D) Risk factors include age, white race, history of contralateral fracture, osteoporosis, use of steroids, decreased physical activity, imbalance, confusion, dementia, and alcoholism.

(E) Mortality is often due to cardiorespiratory disease. Morbidity and mortality attributable to deep venous thrombosis have decreased with the routine use of anticoagulation.

(F) Anteroposterior and true lateral radiographs of the hip are indicated. A bone scan is useful in cases of occult fracture.

(G) The volume of blood lost into the fracture site varies with the type of fracture. Extracapsular fracture results in the greatest amount of blood loss and often requires transfusion of 3 to 5 units.

(H) A 1- to 4-day delay in surgical intervention to optimize the patient's medical status can decrease morbidity.

(I) During this time antibiotics, skin traction immobilization, and anticoagulation decrease the probability of pulmonary and fat embolism.

(J) Because of good blood supply to the extracapsular femur through the surrounding soft tissues, prognosis for extracapsular fractures, whether measured by mortality, morbidity, or satisfactory healing, is far better than for intracapsular fractures.

(K) Subcapital fractures occur immediately distal to the femoral head. The head is at risk because of interrupted blood supply. Nondisplaced fractures have a good prognosis. Displaced fractures have a nonunion rate of 10 to 30 percent and an avascular necrosis rate of 15 to 30 percent.

(L) Subtrochanteric fractures, because of biomechanical stress, are difficult to manage. Options for fixation include intramedullary devices, sliding compression screws, and blade plates. The nonunion rate is 5 percent.

(M) Nonoperative management is reserved for patients confined to a wheelchair before fracture or those with a true impacted subcapital fracture. Medically unstable or demented patients may require nonoperative treatment but this is not recommended. Pain control and nursing care are improved and the nonunion rate is decreased with operative intervention.

(N) Reduction of an intertrochanteric fracture requires reduction on a fracture table and fixation with a sliding compression screw. A 4 to 12 percent incidence of loss of fixation is reported.

(O) If unstable, medial displacement of the distal fragment before placement of the compression screw may be required. An alternative is the use of flexible nails passed from the condylar area of the femur. These devices have been associated with a high rate of complication (16 to 71 percent) and a reoperation rate of up to 19 percent.

(P) Multiple screws or pins are used for young, active patients and for nondisplaced fractures.

(Q) Hemiarthroplasty, using a bipolar or fixed head prosthesis, may be used for the elderly. This provides for early weight bearing and minimizes morbidity due to avascular necrosis and nonunion.

(R) Total hip replacement is reserved ordinarily for those who have preexisting, symptomatic degenerative joint disease.

(S) Overall mortality primarily depends on comorbidity factors. It ranges from 15 to 20 percent in the first year with a decrease thereafter. This compares with a mortality rate of 9 percent in matched controls without fracture. Immediate postoperative mortality is reported to be 1.3 to 16 percent.

(T) At the end of a year, approximately 50 to 60 percent of patients regain prefracture levels of ambulation, and 50 to 85 percent are independent ambulators with assistive devices.

(U) Complications average 0.8 to 0.85 per patient. Pulmonary embolism is the most common cause of death perioperatively. Its incidence has decreased through the use of routine anticoagulation. Pneumonia and decubitus ulcer rates are reduced with early operative intervention.

REFERENCES

Einhorn EA. Hip fractures in the elderly. Res Staff Phys 1988; 34:97.

Kenzora JE, McCarthy RE, Lowell JD, et al. Hip fracture mortality. Clin Orthop Rel Res 1984; 186:45–56.

Kumar VN, Redford JB. Rehabilitation of hip fractures in the elderly. Ann Fam Pract 1984; 29:173.

Zuckerman JD. Hip: trauma. In: Orthopaedic knowledge update 3. Park Ridge, IL: American Academy of Orthopaedic Surgeons, 1990:495.

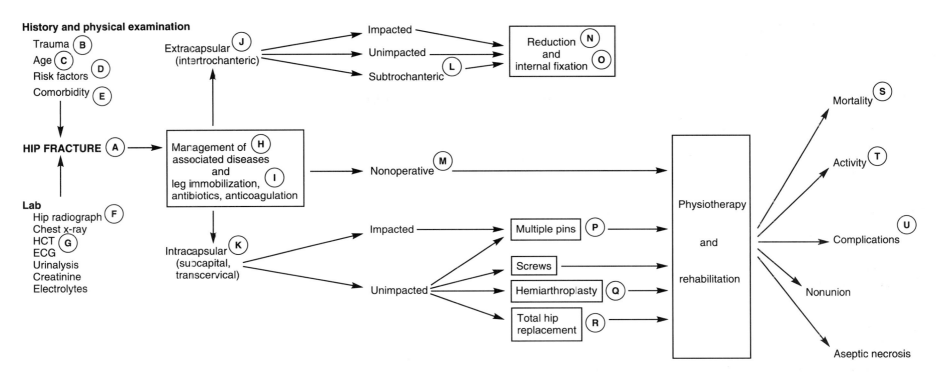

History and physical examination

Trauma (B)
Age (C) (D)
Risk factors
Comorbidity (E)

HIP FRACTURE (A)

Lab
Hip radiograph (F)
Chest x-ray
HCT (G)
ECG
Urinalysis
Creatinine
Electrolytes

Management of (H)
associated diseases
and
leg immobilization, (I)
antibiotics, anticoagulation

Extracapsular (J)
(intertrochanteric)

Impacted
Unimpacted
Subtrochanteric (L)

Reduction (N)
and
internal fixation (O)

Nonoperative (M)

Intracapsular (K)
(subcapital,
transcervical)

Impacted
Unimpacted

Multiple pins (P)
Screws
Hemiarthroplasty (Q)
Total hip
replacement (R)

Physiotherapy
and
rehabilitation

Mortality (S)
Activity (T)
Complications (U)
Nonunion
Aseptic necrosis

Femoral Shaft Fracture

Jerome D. Wiedel, M.D., and Hugh Dougall, M.D.

(A) History is important in considering the mechanism of injury of femoral shaft fracture and the energy involved. Examination of the ipsilateral hip, knee, and tibia is important.

(B) Femoral shaft fractures are common injuries in the multiply traumatized patient. Careful initial assessment and resuscitation are necessary. Alignment of the fracture and portable traction should be applied before radiographs are taken.

(C) Simple fractures are isolated femoral fractures with intact soft tissue envelope.

(D) Ipsilateral fractures of the femoral shaft and tibia (floating knee) occur with approximately 10 percent of all femoral fractures. Mortality and respiratory complications are increased with this combination of fractures, especially if internal fixation is delayed. Open fractures are common with 20 percent of femoral and 50 percent of tibial fractures.

(E) Ipsilateral hip and femoral shaft fractures occur in approximately 5 percent of all femoral fractures. Most common are femoral neck fractures. A high percentage (30 percent) are missed on initial examination. Priority is given to the hip fracture.

(F) A high index of suspicion is required to diagnose ipsilateral knee ligament injury. The incidence is approximately 5 percent. It can be undiagnosed throughout the treatment of the femoral fracture. The ideal time to examine for this injury is immediately after femoral shaft stabilization. Beware of the dislocated knee with its high percentage of arterial and neurologic injury.

(G) Skeletal traction is accomplished through distal femoral or proximal tibial traction pins and balanced traction (90:90, Thomas splint, roller traction). Normally a period of balanced skeletal traction (4 to 6 weeks) is followed by cast bracing.

(H) Most patients are treated with a closed, reamed, locked intramedullary nail. It allows better control of length and rotation than an unlocked nail.

(I) Early stabilization (<24 hours) of a femoral fracture in the multiply traumatized patient decreases respiratory complications, intensive care, hospital stay, and cost of care.

(J) External fixators should be reserved for Gustilo IIIB and grossly contaminated wounds.

REFERENCES

Bone LB, Johnson KD. Early versus delayed stabilization of femoral fractures. J Bone Joint Surg 1989; 71:336–340.

Brumback RJ, Reilly JP. Intramedullary nailing of femoral shaft fractures; part I and II. J Bone Joint Surg 1988; 70A:1441–1451.

Leighton RK, Waddell JP. Open versus closed intramedullary nailing of femoral shaft fractures. J Trauma 1986; 26:923–926.

Swintowski MD. Ipsilateral femoral shaft and hip fractures. Orthop Clin North Am 1987; 18:73–84.

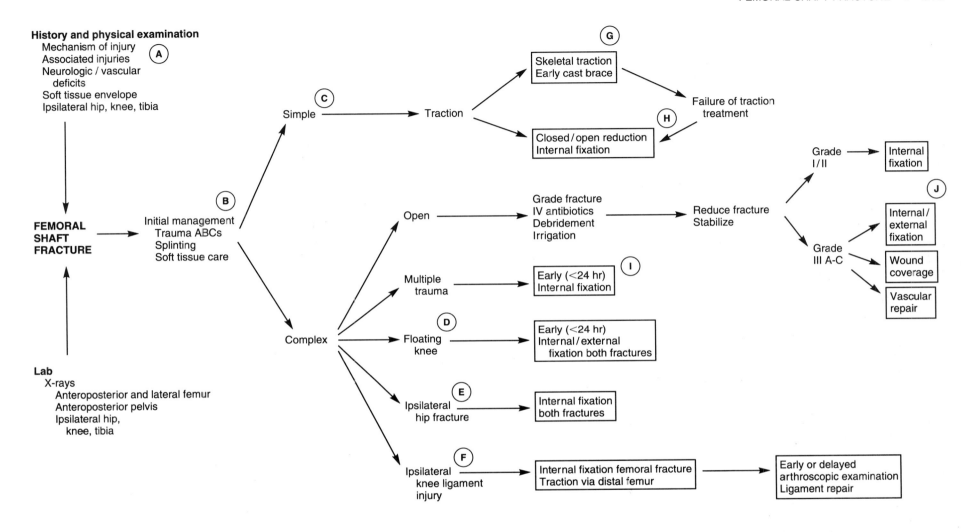

History and physical examination (A)
- Mechanism of injury
- Associated injuries
- Neurologic / vascular deficits
- Soft tissue envelope
- Ipsilateral hip, knee, tibia

FEMORAL SHAFT FRACTURE

Initial management (B)
- Trauma ABCs
- Splinting
- Soft tissue care

Lab
- X-rays
  - Anteroposterior and lateral femur
  - Anteroposterior pelvis
  - Ipsilateral hip, knee, tibia

Simple (C) → Traction

(G) Skeletal traction / Early cast brace → Failure of traction treatment

(H) Closed / open reduction / Internal fixation

Complex

Open → Grade fracture / IV antibiotics / Debridement / Irrigation → Reduce fracture / Stabilize

Grade I / II → Internal fixation

Grade III A-C (J) → Internal / external fixation / Wound coverage / Vascular repair

Multiple trauma → (I) Early (<24 hr) Internal fixation

Floating knee (D) → Early (<24 hr) Internal / external fixation both fractures

Ipsilateral hip fracture (E) → Internal fixation both fractures

Ipsilateral knee ligament injury (F) → Internal fixation femoral fracture / Traction via distal femur → Early or delayed arthroscopic examination / Ligament repair

Tibial Shaft Fracture

Jerome D. Wiedel, M.D., and Hugh Dougall, M.D.

(A) History is important in defining the mechanism and energy of tibial shaft fracture. This helps to determine the extent of injury to the tibia and the surrounding soft tissue envelope and the likelihood of associated injuries.

(B) Assessment and resuscitation are directed initially toward the patient as a whole. The fractured tibia is aligned by longitudinal traction and splinting. This prevents further soft tissue injury and allows examination for open wounds and neurologic and vascular deficit. Radiographs are then obtained in two planes to include the ankle and knee.

(C) Open wounds are cultured and covered by a sterile dressing. Exposed bone is not reduced into the soft tissue envelope. Intravenous antibiotics are started and tetanus immune status is reviewed.

(D) Most tibial fractures are closed (80 to 90 percent) and can be treated nonoperatively.

(E) Grading the open fracture is important in prognosis and treatment. The Gustilo classification of open fractures is used. In grade I the wound is less than 1 cm long, there is minimal soft tissue damage, the fracture is of a simple pattern, and there is little comminution. In grade II the wound is greater than 1 cm long, there is moderate soft tissue damage with crushing injury, and the fracture shows moderate comminution and moderate contamination. In grade III there is extensive damage to soft tissues including muscles, skin, and neurovascular structures; a high degree of contamination; and the fracture is highly comminuted. Three subtypes of each grade are A, adequate soft tissue coverage; B, extensive injury with soft tissue loss, requiring local or free flap; and C, any open fracture associated with an arterial injury.

(F) Grade IIIC open fractures are devastating injuries with high rates of nonunion, infection, and nerve damage, along with vascular injury. A number of these fractures require immediate or delayed amputation.

(G) Surgical management should begin within 6 hours of injury. Debridement eliminates all dead or contaminated tissue. It is followed by irrigation using at least 9 L of normal saline.

(H) There is considerable interest in predicting the viability of limbs at the time of injury (mangled extremity severity score). The decision for immediate amputation vs. salvage procedures has great social and economic impact on the patient.

(I) An acceptable reduction is <5 to 10 degrees flexion–extension deformity, <0 to 5 degrees internal rotation, and <10 degrees external rotation deformity.

(J) The choice of fixation of the fracture is individualized to the patient, the fracture, the surgeon, and the equipment available.

(K) One quarter of all closed tibial fractures undergo primary or secondary open reduction and internal fixation. Intramedullary fixation is considered the safest form of internal fixation.

(L) After most open fractures, a second-look debridement is carried out after 24 to 72 hours depending on the extent of the soft tissue injury and contamination. Most open wounds can be closed by delayed primary closure at 5 to 7 days.

(M) Grade IIIB open fractures require a formal coverage procedure by local muscle flap or free vascularized flap, depending on extent and location of defect.

(N) With closed treatment, healing time averages 20 weeks. There is a 2 to 5 percent nonunion rate and a 5 to 10 percent rate of malunion.

REFERENCES

Bondurant FJ, Cotler HB, Buckle R. The medical and economic impact of severely injured lower extremities. J Trauma 1988; 28:1270–1273.

Gustilo RB, Merkow RL, Templeman D. The management of open fractures. J Bone Joint Surg 1990; 72A:299–304.

Henley MD. Intramedullary devices for tibial fracture stabilization. Clin Orthop 1989; 240:87–96.

Johansen K, Daines M, Howey T. Objective criteria accurately predict amputation following lower extremity trauma. J Trauma 1990; 30:568–573.

Oni OOA, Hui A, Gregg RJ. The healing of closed tibial shaft fractures. J Bone Joint Surg 1988; 70B:787–790.

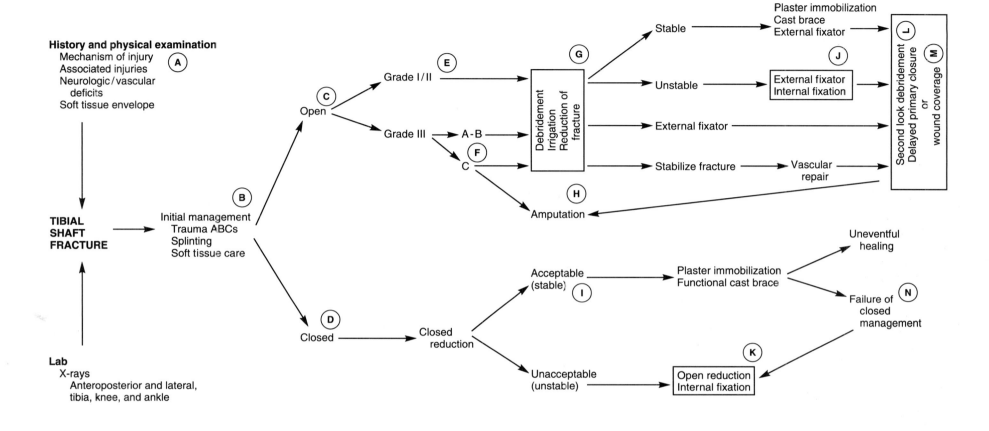

History and physical examination
Mechanism of injury (A)
Associated injuries
Neurologic/vascular
deficits
Soft tissue envelope

**TIBIAL
SHAFT
FRACTURE**

Lab
X-rays
Anteroposterior and lateral,
tibia, knee, and ankle

(B) Initial management
Trauma ABCs
Splinting
Soft tissue care

(C) Open

(D) Closed

Grade I/II (E)

Grade III → A-B

(F) C

Debridement
Irrigation
Reduction of
fracture

(G)

Stable → Plaster immobilization
Cast brace
External fixator

Unstable → (J) External fixator
Internal fixation

External fixator

Stabilize fracture → Vascular repair

(H) Amputation

(L) (M) Second look debridement
Delayed primary closure
or
wound coverage

Closed reduction

Acceptable (stable) (I) → Plaster immobilization
Functional cast brace

Uneventful healing

Failure of closed management (N)

Unacceptable (unstable) → (K) Open reduction
Internal fixation

Knee Fracture

William G. Winter, M.D.

(A) The mechanism of knee injury can suggest which bones are fractured. Adjacent blood vessels and nerves must be evaluated for damage. Joint effusion (lipohemarthrosis) often results from intraarticular fractures and can be relieved by aspiration. The risk of popliteal artery damage in fracture–dislocations or displaced fracture–separations (physeal injuries) around the knee mandates frequent observation or arteriography.

(B) Knee x-rays include anteroposterior, lateral, tunnel, and Merchant (patellar) views.

(C) Undisplaced patellar fractures must be protected from strong quadriceps contraction for 6 weeks. A cylinder cast is desirable in noncompliant patients. In compliant patients, a Velcro-fastened knee immobilizer can be removed for nonweight-bearing active exercises after the first pain and swelling subside, preventing joint stiffness and muscle atrophy. Truly undisplaced tibial plateau fractures are treated nonaggressively by protected weight bearing for 6 weeks.

(D) Plateau or tibial spine fractures depressed or displaced more than 0 to 5 mm are best reduced and fixed by open means. X-rays can be difficult to read. Sagittal tomograms in two planes can clarify fracture deformity. Borderline cases, or those wherein ligament injury is suspected, demand individual, specialized treatment. Small marginal plateau fragments often signal major capsular or ligamentous injury. Displaced fractures of the patella are treated operatively. Severely comminuted fractures of the patellar body require patellectomy. Two large patellar fragments can be reduced and fixed. Small fragments are excised. Displaced fractures of the femoral condyles are treated best by open reduction and internal fixation.

(E) Displaced fractures of the femoral condyles are treated best by open reduction and internal fixation.

(F) If osteochondral fragments are in the joint, arthroscopy is indicated to remove smaller fragments and to replace large fragments. Patellar dislocation can cause osteochondral fragments.

(G) After any knee fracture, rehabilitation, increasing activities, stretching, and exercise (RISE) are mandatory.

REFERENCES

Bray TJ, Marder RA. Patellar fractures. In: Chapman MW, ed. Operative orthopedics. Philadelphia: JB Lippincott, 1988; 413–420.

Ceron HS, Tremmlet J, Casey P, et al. Fractures of the distal third of the femur treated by internal fixation. Clin Orthop 1974; 100:160–170.

Hohl M. Tibial condylar fractures. J Bone Joint Surg 1967; 49A:1455–1467.

Hoover NW. Injuries of the popliteal artery associated with fractures and dislocations. Surg Clin North Am 1961; 41:1099–1112.

McLenna JG. The role of arthroscopic surgery in the treatment of fractures of the intercondylar eminence of the tibia. J Bone Joint Surg 1982; 64B:477–480.

Milgram JE. Osteochondral fractures of the articular surfaces of the knee. In: Helfet AF, ed. The management of internal derangements of the knee. Philadelphia: JB Lippincott, 1988; 421–434.

Schatzker J. Fractures of the tibial plateau. In: Chapman MW, ed. Operative orthopedics. Philadelphia: JB Lippincott, 1988; 421–434.

Smillie IS. Injuries of the knee joint. New York: Churchill Livingstone, 1978.

Waddell JP, Johnston DW, Nadre A. Fractures of the tibial plateau. J Trauma 1981; 21:376–381.

Weber MJ, Janecki CJ, McLeaod P, et al. Efficacy of various forms of fixation of transverse fractures of the patella. J Bone Joint Surg 1980; 62A:215–220.

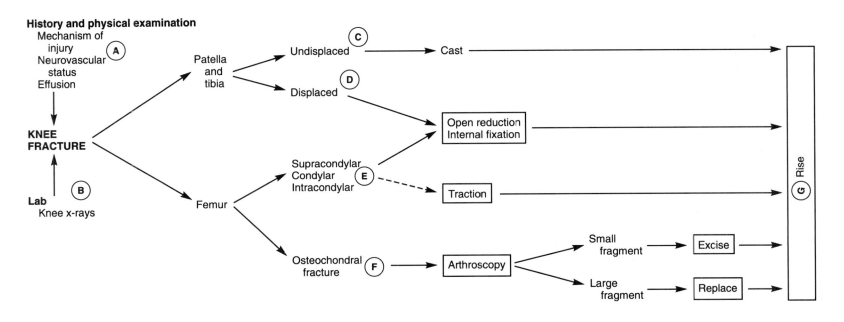

History and physical examination
Mechanism of
  injury   (A)
Neurovascular
  status
Effusion

KNEE FRACTURE

Lab   (B)
Knee x-rays

Patella and tibia
  Undisplaced (C) → Cast
  Displaced (D) → Open reduction Internal fixation

Femur
  Supracondylar Condylar Intracondylar (E) → Open reduction Internal fixation
  → Traction
  Osteochondral fracture (F) → Arthroscopy
    Small fragment → Excise
    Large fragment → Replace

(G) Rise

Ankle Injury

William G. Winter, M.D.

(A) The mechanism of ankle injury can suggest the type of damage sustained. Pain, swelling, tenderness, and hesitancy to bear weight are symptoms and signs of significant ankle injury.

(B) The goals of treatment of all ankle injuries are a stable, congruent fit of the talus within the ankle mortise and prompt rehabilitation.

(C) All ankle injuries should be evaluated by anteroposterior, lateral, and mortise x-rays. If the mortise appears widened but no fracture of the fibula is seen, physical examination and x-ray of the entire proximal fibula should be undertaken.

(D) Acute subluxation of the peroneal tendons is detected by resistance to active eversion of the injured ankle. Tendons subluxate laterally when the superior peroneal ligament is torn.

(E) Rupture of the Achilles tendon is confirmed by the Thompson test. Squeezing the calf causes the suspended foot to assume the equinus position if the Achilles tendon is intact.

(F) Transosteochondral fractures are evaluated by x-ray, tomography, computed tomography, magnetic resonance, or arthroscopy. Undisplaced osteochondral fractures with partially intact cartilage can be treated by cast or brace, preferably with no weight bearing for 3 to 4 weeks. Displaced osteochondral fractures are treated by open replacement or excision of the fragment.

(G) A mild (first-degree) sprain causes pain and slight swelling. The patient can walk. Treatment, if needed, is symptomatic—*rest, ice, compression, elevation* (RICE). Weight bearing and function are allowed as needed.

(H) A second-degree sprain causes more pain, swelling, and limping. Treatment includes RICE together with splinting by tape, brace, or cast. Crutches may be needed. Severe swelling or ecchymosis suggests a third-degree sprain.

(I) A third-degree sprain is a complete ligament tear with temporary subluxation and partial or complete joint instability. Ecchymosis and severe swelling suggest the diagnosis. Positive anterior drawer or inversion stress tests or x-rays confirm it. Treatment is a brace or cast to hold ligament ends together for 3 or more weeks. Surgical repair is rarely chosen. For athletically active patients, proprioceptive and muscle-strengthening exercises, with or without other physical therapy modalities, may be appropriate.

(J) Undisplaced fractures of the medial or lateral malleolus are usually treated by a below-the-knee walking cast for 6 weeks.

(K) When perfect anatomic reduction cannot be obtained by manipulation or maintained in plaster, open reduction with internal fixation is indicated. Isolated posterior malleolar fractures are immobilized if less than 25 percent of the tibial articular surface is involved. Fracture–dislocations generally require operation.

(L) Rehabilitation by increasing activities, stretching, and exercises (RISE) is vitally important after ankle injury.

(M) Stable ankle injuries involve only one of the five mortise elements (two collateral ligaments, two malleoli, and the interosseous tibiofibular ligaments). Unstable injuries involve two or more components. Even if undeformed on initial x-rays, unstable injuries must be x-rayed after cast application and at least once again when swelling has subsided in 5 to 10 days.

(N) Persistent pain and instability suggest the possibility of ankle laxity, subtalar laxity, chondral damage, peroneal tendinitis, or interosseous sprain.

REFERENCES

Berndt AL, Hardy M. Transchondral fractures (osteochondritis dissecans) of the talus. J Bone Joint Surg 1955; 41A:988–1020.

Dabezies W, Dabezies E, D'Ambrosia RD, et al. Classification and treatment of ankle fractures. Orthopedics 1978; 1:365–373.

Eckert WR, Davis EA. Acute rupture of the peroneal retinaculum. J Bone Joint Surg 1976; 58A:670–672.

Niedermann B, Andersen A, Andersen SB, et al. Rupture of the lateral ligaments of the ankle: operation or plaster cast? Acta Orthop Scand 1981; 52:579–587.

Percy EC, Hill RO, Callaghan JE. The sprained ankle. J Trauma 1969; 9:972–986.

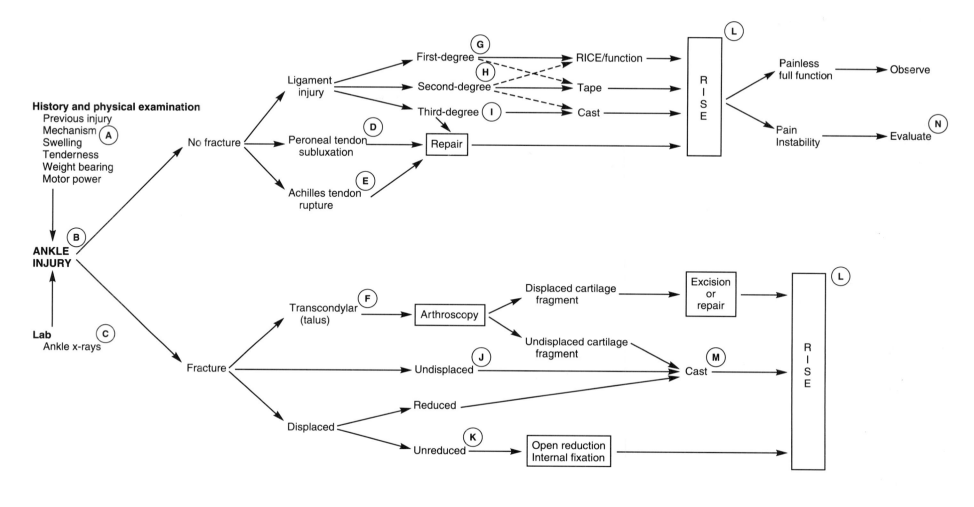

Hand Fractures

Francis G. Wolfort, M.D.

(A) The incidence of fracture of the phalanx is greater distally than proximally or in the middle. Central digit fractures are more common than border fractures. Metacarpal fractures are more frequent on the borders (index most common). Small metacarpals are fractured more frequently than the thumb metacarpal. Twenty-three percent of adult metacarpal fractures, 75 percent of phalangeal fractures, and 66 percent of children's hand fractures are stable. Nonunion is usually due to unstable internal fixation. The treatment is stabilization. Malunion is due to unrecognized condylar fractures and malrotations.

(B) Metacarpal fractures are often caused by a direct blow. Phalangeal fractures result from rotary twisting. Age, occupation, and hand dominance are important etiologic factors. It is critical for diagnosis and treatment to determine function, time, and location of injury and degree of contamination.

(C) Treatment emphasizes the one-scar concept and early motion. There is a high incidence of nonunion in crush fractures, especially phalangeal fracture secondary to soft tissue mangle.

(D) Pathologic fractures occur in the hand because of benign or malignant bone tumors, bone dysplasia, or AV malformation. Metabolic bone disease (osteomalacia, osteoporosis) is the most frequent cause of pathologic fractures. Methods of treatment include curettage, bone grafting and stabilization, and excision and stabilization. Recurrence can occur. Nonunion is uncommon.

(E) In spiral and oblique fractures, rotational deformity of the metacarpals and phalanges is common. To evaluate this, partially flex the fingers. If a rotational deformity exists at the fracture site, scissoring (overlapping), splaying, or unparallel nail plates are present. Be certain to compare findings with the normal hand to exclude congenital rotational deformities. Proximal phalanx fractures are notorious for malrotation and shortening. If unstable, they should be wired. Middle phalangeal fractures are usually oblique and in the midshaft. Stabilization with a Kirschner wire may be necessary. Distal phalanx oblique fractures not uncommonly result in nonunion. Prolonged splinting or percutaneous Kirschner wire fixation is then necessary. A little angular deformity is acceptable, especially in the proximal phalanx, but no rotational deformity is allowable. Splinting should include the joints proximal and distal to the fracture. The adjacent digit can be used to effect a buddy splint. The wrist should be held in 30- to 40-degree extension, the metacarpal phalangeal joint in 70- to 90-degree flexion, and the proximal interphalangeal joint in 20-degree flexion. Metacarpal spiral and oblique fractures require closed reduction and Kirschner wire fixation or open reduction and internal fixation. These fractures tend to shorten and rotate rather than angulate. Shortening of 3 mm is acceptable. Minimal dorsal displacement alone is not an indication for open reduction. Nonunions may require fixation or bone grafting.

(F) The volar plate is the volar part of the joint capsule. A proximal interphalangeal joint injury with hyperextension instability should be treated by reattaching the volar plate. A proximal interphalangeal joint dislocation–fracture that is irreducible suggests entrapment by the volar plate, lateral band, or collateral ligament and requires open reduction and internal fixation. In metacarpal phalangeal joint dislocation (dorsal), the volar plate ruptures in a two-sided tear that prevents the metacarpal head from returning to normal position. Treatment is open reduction. A metacarpal phalangeal joint volar dislocation is rare. The dorsal capsule is avulsed and the distal volar plate is sometimes avulsed. Treatment is open reduction. A distal interphalangeal joint dislocation with volar plate, tendon, or ligament interposed is complex and rare. Open reduction is necessary. Simple distal phalangeal joint dislocations are more common and readily reducible.

(G) Bennett's fracture is a displaced intraarticular fracture through the base of the thumb metacarpal. It is a very unstable fracture because the abductor pollicis longus tends to pull the metacarpal shaft proximally and radially, causing the thumb to assume a position of adduction. Accurate reduction of the intraarticular fracture using traction, pressure, and minimal pronation with percutaneous Kirschner wire fixation of the first metacarpal to the second metacarpal or the trapezium is commonly accepted treatment. If necessary, open reduction and internal fixation are performed with screw or pins. Bone grafting may be needed for a comminuted fracture. Even with articular incongruity the prognosis is good if one accepts minimal stiffness. Nonunion is rare.

(H) The scaphoid is fractured by forcing the wrist into extension and radial deviation. It is the most common wrist fracture. Pain in the anatomic snuff box suggests a navicular fracture even if an initial x-ray is normal. Pain justifies splinting. Early diagnosis and treatment of acute scaphoid fractures result in virtually 100 percent union. Delay in diagnosis and treatment leads to nonunion and aseptic necrosis (70 percent of fractures through the wrist, 20 percent through proximal pole, 10 percent through distal pole). Scaphoid fracture should be treated initially with a long-arm cast with the wrist in neutral. The thumb should be palmar abducted using a thumb spica that includes the interphalangeal joint. Distal one third fractures are immobilized for at least 4 to 8 weeks, middle one

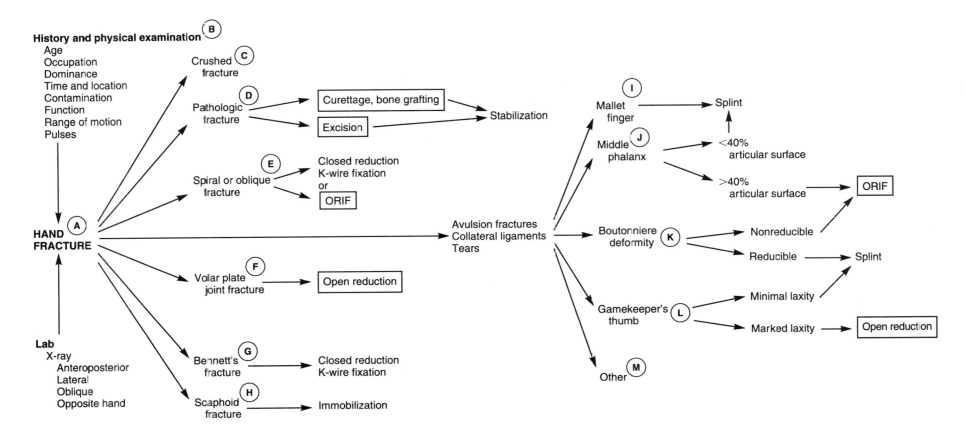

History and physical examination (B)
- Age
- Occupation
- Dominance
- Time and location
- Contamination
- Function
- Range of motion
- Pulses

HAND FRACTURE (A)

Lab
- X-ray
  - Anteroposterior
  - Lateral
  - Oblique
  - Opposite hand

third for 6 to 12 weeks, and proximal one third for 12 to 20 weeks. Unusual distal-to-proximal blood supply in the scaphoid accounts for 20 percent of instances of nonunion and aseptic necrosis. These complications are treated by prolonged casting (4 to 9 months), bone grafting, Herbert screw, vascularized radial graft, proximal row carpectomy, limited arthrodesis, or excision.

(I) Simple mallet finger (extensor disruption from the dorsal tip) can be treated with a dorsal distal interphalangeal splint for 6 weeks. Treatment is the same for a large dorsal articular fragment with no volar subluxation of the distal phalanx. It is anatomically reduced and immobilized by a dorsal splint with or without Kirschner wire fixation.

(J) Avulsion fracture of the middle phalanx usually occurs at the volar base (proximal interphalangeal joint). When the fracture is stable (less than 40 percent articular surface), it is reduced in flexion and immobilized in a dorsal extension block splint for 6 weeks. When the fracture is unstable (more than 40 percent articular surface), open reduction and internal fixation are required.

(K) If a closed acute boutonniere deformity (central slip tear or avulsion fracture from middle phalanx base dorsally) is reducible, it can be treated by splint or extension for 6 weeks. If it is not reducible, the avulsion fracture may need open reduction and internal fixation.

(L) Gamekeeper's thumb (ulnar collateral ligament tear—avulsion fracture of the thumb) is a common injury. Do not perform a stress examination before x-rays. After x-rays, stress test the metacarpal phalangeal joint in 10- to 20-degree flexion to demonstrate disruption. The opposite (normal) side should be tested to determine normal tone. Local anesthesia may be necessary for pain relief. If laxity is more than 45 degrees, or 15 degrees more than normal, open reduction is necessary. If laxity is minimal, a thumb spica is used for 4 to 6 weeks.

(M) Displaced intraarticular fractures, condylar fractures of proximal and middle phalanges, corner avulsion fractures of the base of the proxi-

Hand Fractures (Continued)

mal phalanx (if more than 10 to 15 percent of articular surface), and avulsed collateral ligament fractures from the neck of the metacarpal (if non-displaced) require immobilization for 3 weeks and close x-ray follow-up. Patients should be advised that joints become very stiff after these injuries. Self-therapy and directed hand therapy are crucial for recovery of normal range of function after healing.

REFERENCES

Amadio P. Fractures of phalanges and metacarpals. Third Annual Review Course in Hand Surgery. American Society for Surgery of the Hand. 1991:1–14.

American Society for Surgery of the Hand. The Hand, Primary Care of Common Problems, 1st ed. Aurora, CO: American Society for Surgery of the Hand, 1985.

Barton NJ. Fractures of the shafts of the phalanges of the hand. Hand 1979; 11:119–133.

Barton NJ. Fractures of the phalanges of the hand in children. Hand 1979; 11:134–143.

Green DP, Rowland SA. Fractures and dislocations in the hand. In: Rockwood CA, Green DP, eds. Fractures in adults, 2nd ed. Philadelphia: JB Lippincott, 1984.

O'Brien ET. Fractures of the metacarpals and phalanges. In: Green DP, ed. Operative hand surgery. New York: Churchill Livingstone, 1982.

Stricklan JW, Steichen JB, Kleinman WB, et al. Phalangeal fractures: factors influencing digital performance. Orthop Rev 1982; 11:39–50.

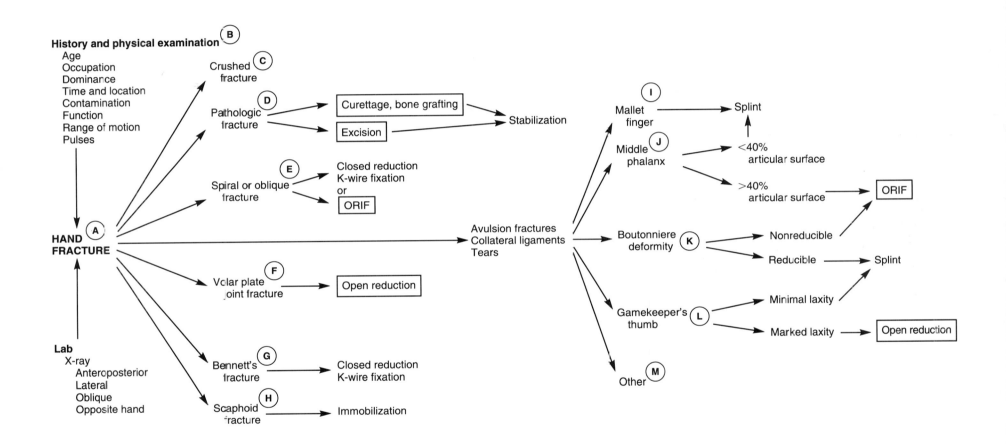

History and physical examination (B)
Age
Occupation
Dominance
Time and location
Contamination
Function
Range of motion
Pulses

HAND FRACTURE (A)

Lab
X-ray
Anteroposterior
Lateral
Oblique
Opposite hand

Crushed (C)
fracture

Pathologic (D)
fracture → Curettage, bone grafting → Stabilization
→ Excision → Stabilization

Spiral or oblique (E)
fracture → Closed reduction
K-wire fixation
or
ORIF

Volar plate (F)
joint fracture → Open reduction

Bennett's (G)
fracture → Closed reduction
K-wire fixation

Scaphoid (H)
fracture → Immobilization

Avulsion fractures
Collateral ligaments
Tears

Mallet (I)
finger → Splint

Middle (J)
phalanx → <40% articular surface
→ >40% articular surface → ORIF

Boutonniere (K)
deformity → Nonreducible → ORIF
→ Reducible → Splint

Gamekeeper's (L)
thumb → Minimal laxity → Splint
→ Marked laxity → Open reduction

Other (M)

Flexor Tendon Injuries of the Hand

Lawrence L. Ketch, M.D.

A Severed flexor tendons in the hand must be treated as major injuries despite their often benign appearance. The potential for disability can be out of proportion to the immediate appearance of the injury. Important management factors include repair in the operating room using proper anesthesia, tourniquet control, meticulous wound care, atraumatic technique, use of fine instruments and small-caliber synthetic monofilament suture on a tapered needle, sutures placed under no tension, and postoperative dynamic splinting.

B Treatment and prognosis depend on location of the injury, which is classified by zones (see the illustration). Primary repairs in Zone II fail as a result of adhesions beneath the area of the A_2 pulley. This is a result of limited space and critical tolerances resulting from the profundus passing between the chiasm of the superficialis slips. The profundus is also less well perfused at the proximal portion of the sheath. Repair requires expert judgment and ideal conditions and techniques.

C Only contaminated wounds require culture before cleansing and debridement. Tetanus prophylaxis and broad-spectrum antibiotics are routine.

D Delayed primary repair of contaminated injuries is performed 72 hours or more after trauma when a decrease in the bacterial count has been documented by quantitative cultures. Zone II tendon injuries require staged tendon reconstruction.

E Inflammatory or fibroblastic response within the fibroosseous canal (Zone II) results in scarring of both the superficial and deep flexors with subsequent compromised function. It is often necessary to create a pseudosheath by silastic rod implantation reconstruction to preserve gliding function.

F Any suture placed within a tendon weakens it. Therefore, a partial laceration less than 50

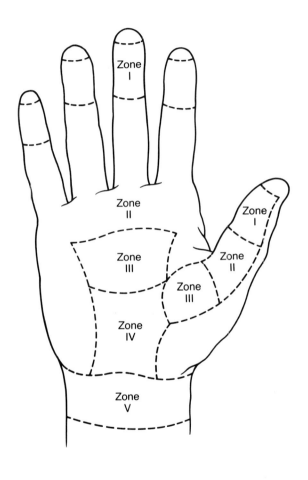

Flexor Tendon Injuries of the Hand (Continued)

percent may go unrepaired if there is no triggering. If there is, repair improves gliding function.

(G) Nerve injuries seriously compromise prognosis and with soft tissue loss must be managed before tendon repair. Pulley destruction requires silastic rod implantation and staged repair.

(H) Tenorrhaphy is used when there is less than a 1.5- to 2-cm gap in tendon substance. A free tendon graft is contraindicated when there is gross contamination, skin loss, extensive pulley destruction, comminuted raw bone, or a severe crush injury. Return of sensation and motor function to an injured digit is the criterion for determining success regardless of the quality of the tenor-

rhaphy. Arthrodesis is for salvage in a severe injury or failed reconstruction.

(I) Definitive treatment of superficial and deep flexor injuries in so-called no man's land is difficult and should immediately be referred to an experienced hand surgeon for repair.

(J) If a tendon is severed less than 1 cm proximal to its insertion, it may be advanced and reinserted into bone. If it is severed more than 1 cm from its insertion, intratendinous repair is suitable.

(K) Repair after 4 weeks results in muscle shortening. This necessitates tendon grafting with

its resultant decreased excursion and incomplete flexion.

(L) Immobilization significantly decreases tendon tensile strength. Guarded, passive range-of-motion exercise increases healing, minimizes contracture and joint stiffness, and decreases adhesions. This results in a greater return of function with fewer ruptures.

REFERENCES

AASH. The hand—primary care of common problems, 1st ed. New York: Churchill Livingstone, 1985.

Green DP. Operative hand surgery, 2nd ed. New York: Churchill Livingstone, 1988.

Hunter JM, Schneider LH, Mackin EJ, Callahan AD. Tendon surgery in the hand. St. Louis: CV Mosby, 1987.

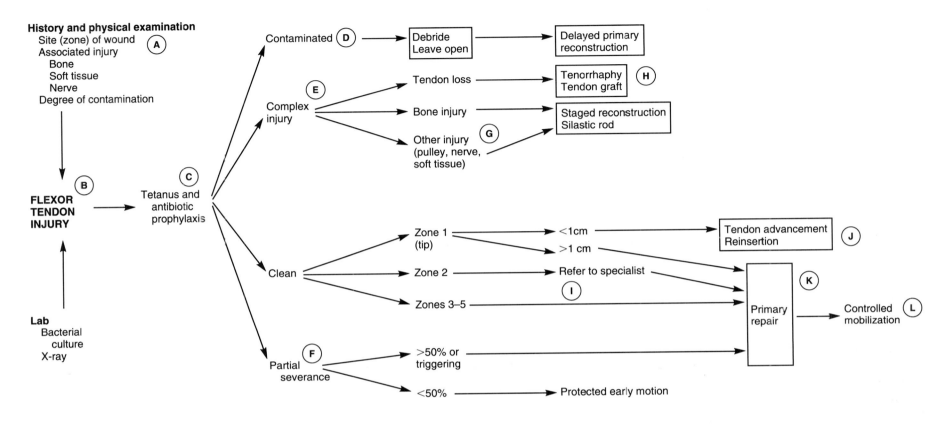

History and physical examination
  Site (zone) of wound ⒶＡ
  Associated injury
    Bone
    Soft tissue
    Nerve
  Degree of contamination

FLEXOR TENDON INJURY Ⓑ

Lab
  Bacterial
    culture
  X-ray

Ⓒ Tetanus and antibiotic prophylaxis

Contaminated Ⓓ → Debride / Leave open → Delayed primary reconstruction

Complex injury Ⓔ
  → Tendon loss → Tenorrhaphy / Tendon graft Ⓗ
  → Bone injury → Staged reconstruction / Silastic rod
  → Other injury (pulley, nerve, soft tissue) Ⓖ → Staged reconstruction / Silastic rod

Clean
  → Zone 1 (tip)
      → <1cm → Tendon advancement / Reinsertion Ⓙ
      → >1 cm → Primary repair Ⓚ
  → Zone 2 → Refer to specialist → Primary repair
  → Zones 3–5 → Primary repair Ⓘ

Primary repair Ⓚ → Controlled mobilization Ⓛ

Partial severance Ⓕ
  → >50% or triggering → Primary repair
  → <50% → Protected early motion

Back Pain

Byron Young, M.D.

(A) Back pain affects 70 to 80 percent of all people at some point in their lives.

(B) Leg pain does not necessarily indicate nerve root compression. Facet joint disease without nerve root compression can cause referred leg pain. Referred pain usually stops at the midposterior thigh. Sciatica caused by root compression causes pain to the midcalf or heel.

(C) Posteroanterior and lateral lumbar spine x-rays should give evidence of degenerative osteoarthritis (lumbar spondylosis), the most frequent mechanical spine disorder. This causes structural weakness, disc herniation, bony hypertrophy, ligamentous facet joint instability, and susceptibility to injury.

(D) Systemic diseases associated with low back pain include ankylosing spondylitis, osteoporosis, and spinal osteomyelitis.

(E) Local diseases associated with low back pain include urinary tract tumors and infection, abdominal aortic aneurysm, and retroperitoneal infections or neoplasms.

(F) Complete bed rest for more than 2 days does not increase rapidity of return to work. Transcutaneous electrical nerve stimulation, exercise, heat, cold, traction, and ultrasound are of no proven benefit.

(G) High field strength magnetic resonance imaging has largely replaced both myelography and computed tomography scanning for confirming disc herniation and diagnosing other causes of root compression.

(H) Rehabilitation consists of exercises to improve the strength of abdominal muscles and to stretch back muscles.

(I) Indications for operative treatment of a herniated disc are no improvement in 4 to 6 weeks, unilateral sciatica, positive straight leg raising test, neurologic findings indicating nerve root compression (weakness, sensory loss, and reflex diminution), and magnetic resonance imaging or computed tomography findings consistent with the clinical examination.

(J) Myelography combined with computed tomography, magnetic resonance imaging, and EMG can disclose lesions that compress nerve roots missed by magnetic resonance imaging alone. Pelvic magnetic resonance imaging can show neoplasm invading the lumbosacral plexus.

(K) Operative discectomy and laminectomy are performed with the aid of the microscope. Results depend on patient selection. About 70 to 90 percent of patients are improved by the operation.

(L) Automated percutaneous discectomy is performed under local anesthesia and results in about 60 percent improvement.

(M) Chemonucleolysis involves needle introduction of chymopapain into the disc space. It provides about 75 percent improvement.

REFERENCES

Deyo RA, Walsh NE, Martin DC, et al: A controlled trial of transcutaneous electrical nerve stimulation (TENS): an exercise for chronic low back pain. N Engl J Med 1990; 322:1627–1634.

Frymoyer JW. Back pain and sciatica. N Engl J Med 1988; 318:291–300.

Macnab I. Backache. Baltimore: Williams & Wilkins, 1977.

Wiesel RW, Feffer HL, Borenstein DG, et al. Low back pain, 2nd ed. Charlottesville: The Michie Co, 1989.

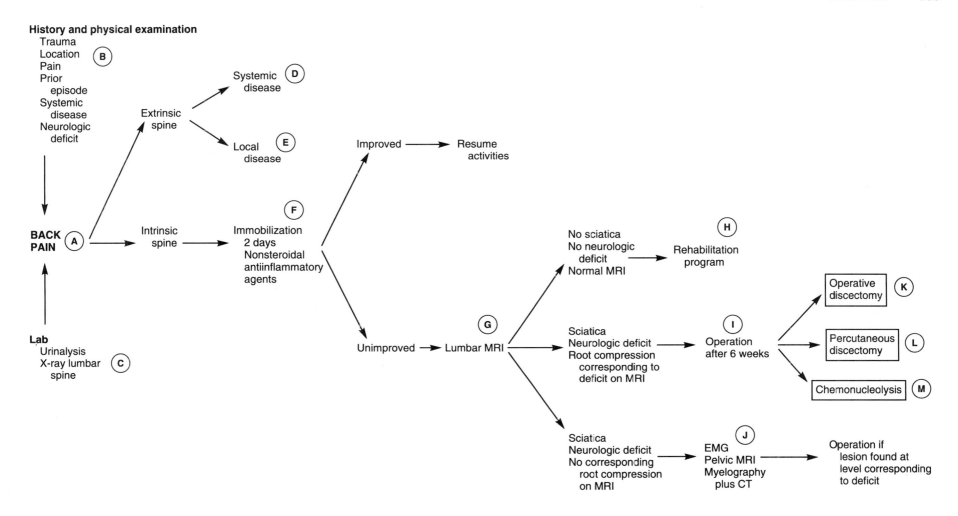

History and physical examination
Trauma
Location (B)
Pain
Prior
episode
Systemic
disease
Neurologic
deficit

Systemic (D)
disease

Extrinsic
spine

Local (E)
disease

Improved → Resume
activities

BACK (A)
PAIN

Intrinsic
spine

Immobilization (F)
2 days
Nonsteroidal
antiinflammatory
agents

Lab
Urinalysis
X-ray lumbar (C)
spine

Unimproved → Lumbar MRI (G)

No sciatica
No neurologic
deficit
Normal MRI

Rehabilitation (H)
program

Sciatica
Neurologic deficit → Operation (I)
Root compression   after 6 weeks
corresponding to
deficit on MRI

Operative (K)
discectomy

Percutaneous (L)
discectomy

Chemonucleolysis (M)

Sciatica
Neurologic deficit
No corresponding
root compression
on MRI

EMG (J)
Pelvic MRI → Operation if
Myelography   lesion found at
plus CT   level corresponding
                 to deficit

Index

Note: Page numbers in *italics* refer to algorithms.

Abdomen, aortic aneurysm of, 226, *227*
  gunshot wound to, 92, 98
  right lower quadrant of, pain in, 154, *155*
  trauma to, blunt, 90–91, *91*
    penetrating, 92–93, *93*
Abscess, anorectal, 168, *169*
  lung, 64, *65*
Achalasia, 102, *103*
Achilles tendon, rupture of, 324
Acidosis, metabolic, in cardiopulmonary resuscitation, 12
Acquired immune deficiency syndrome (AIDS), surgery and, 26, *27*
Adie's tonic pupil, 34–35
Adnexal mass, 304, *305*
Adolescent, varicocele in, 284
Adrenal hemorrhage, in neonates, 252
Adrenocortical cancer, 194
Airway maintenance, in head injury, 32
Alagille syndrome, 250
Aneurysm, abdominal aortic, 226, *227*
Angiography, in gastrointestinal bleeding, 8
  in preoperative cardiac evaluation, 4
  in pulmonary embolism, 60
  in renal mass, 272
Anisocoria, 34–35, *35*
  cocaine test in, 34
  lesion localization in, 35
  pilocarpine test in, 34
  simple, 34
  sympathetic innervation and, 34
Ankle injury, 324, *325*
Ann Arbor classification system, for Hodgkin's disease, 191
Anorectal abscess, 168, *169*
Anorectal fistula, 168, *169*
Antibiotics, prophylactic, in colon injury, 98
Anus, cancer of, 166, *167*
  imperforate, 248–249, *249*
Aorta, abdominal, aneurysm of, 226, *227*
  coarctation of, 70, *71*, 76
  rupture of, 58
Aortic valve stenosis, 76, 84–85, *85*
Aortopulmonary window, 78, *79*
Arrhythmia, acute myocardial infarct and, 80
  perioperative, 6–7, *7*

Arrhythmia (Continued)
  causes of, 6
  risk factors in, 6
Arterial blood gas levels, in preoperative laboratory evaluation, 2
Arterial embolism, peripheral, 224, *225*
Arterial insufficiency, 220
  ulcers due to, 234
Arterial thrombosis, 224
Associated trauma index (ATI), in abdominal injury, 98
Asystole, in cardiopulmonary resuscitation, 10, 12
  ventricular, 6
ATI (associated trauma index), in abdominal injury, 98
Atrial fibrillation, 6
Atrial flutter, 6
Atrial tachycardia, paroxysmal, 6
Atrioventricular block, first-degree, 6
  second-degree, 6
  third-degree, 6
Atrioventricular junctional tachycardia, 6–7
Atropine, 10

Back pain, 334, *335*
Barium sulfate, 238
Bennett's fracture, 326
Bezoars, gastric, postoperative, 114
Bile duct(s), atresia of, extrahepatic, 250
  cancer of, 122
  common, obstruction of, 134
    stones in, 126, *127*, 128, *129*, 132
Bilirubin level, elevated, 250
Biopsy, in anal and rectal cancer, 166
  needle, of prostate, 278
  of lung abscess, 64
  rectal mucosal, 246
Bladder. See *Urinary bladder*.
Blalock-Taussig operation, for cyanotic congenital heart disease, 74
Bleeding, adrenal, in neonates, 252
  disorders of, 16, *17*
  from esophageal varices, 118, *119*
  from nose, 40, *41*

Bleeding (Continued)
  gastrointestinal, lower, 160, *161*
    upper, 116, *117*
  vaginal, in nonreproductive years, 294, *295*
    in reproductive years, 290, *291*, 292, *293*
Blind loop syndrome, 114, *115*
Blood components, 18
Blood counts, complete, in preoperative laboratory evaluation, 2
Blood gas(es), arterial, in preoperative laboratory evaluation, 2
Blood transfusion, 18–20, *19*, *21*
  alternatives to, 19
  complications of, 19–20
  oxygen consumption in, 18
  platelet hemostasis in, 18
  prothrombin/activated partial thromboplastin time in, 18–19
Bowel obstruction, neonatal, 242, *243*, 244, *245*
  duodenal atresia or stenosis in, 242, 244
  jejunal and ileal atresia in, 244
  meconium in, 242
  necrotizing enterocolitis in, 244
  small, 142, *143*
Breast cancer, advanced, 182, *183*, 184, *185*
  early, 180–181, *181*
  recurrent, 186, *187*, 188, *189*
Breast mass, solitary, 178, *179*
Bretylium tosylate, 12
Bronchopleural fistula, 62
Bronchus, rupture of, 58
Burns, 198–199, *199*
  biologic dressings for, 198, 199
  body surface area and mortality rate in, 198
  debridement in, 198–199
  Ringer's lactate volume calculation in, 198

Calcium levels, in cardiopulmonary resuscitation, 12
  in hypercalcemia, 208
Calf claudication, 222
Cancer, of adrenal cortex, 194
  of anus, 166, *167*
  of bile duct, 122
  of breast, advanced, 182, *183*, 184, *185*

Cancer *(Continued)*
  early, 180–181, *181*
  recurrent, 186, *187*, 188, *189*
  of colon, 164, *165*
  of endometrium, 294, 302–303, *303*
  of esophagus, 104–105, *105*
  of larynx, 54–55, *55*
  of lip, 46, *47*
  of liver, 130
  of lung, 66, *67*
  of oral cavity, 48–49, *49*
  of prostate, 282, *283*
  of rectum, 166, *167*
  of testis, 286, *287*
  of thyroid, 206, *207*
  of urinary bladder, 274–276, *275*, *277*
  of uterine cervix, 300, *301*
  renal cell, 272
Carcinoma. See *Cancer.*
Cardiac. See also under *Heart.*
Cardiac anomalies, congenital obstructive, 76, 77
Cardiac contusion, 58
Cardiac evaluation, preoperative, 4, *5*
Cardiac output, in shock, 14
Cardiac tamponade, 58
Cardiopulmonary resuscitation, 10, *11*, *12*, *13*
  asystole in, 10, 12
  calcium levels in, 12
  chest compressions in, 10
  defibrillation in, 10
  electromechanical dissociation in, 10
  metabolic acidosis in, 12
  obstruction relief in, 10
  tracheal intubation in, 10
Cefotetan, 296
Cefoxitin, 296
Ceftriaxone sodium, 296
Cerebrovascular insufficiency, 228, *229*
Cervical spine fracture, 310–311, *311*
Cervix, uterine, cancer of, 300, *301*
Chagas' disease, 102
Chemotherapy, for Hodgkin's disease, 191–192
  in advanced breast cancer, 182
  in urinary bladder cancer, 274, 276
Chest, flail, 58
Chest compressions, in cardiopulmonary resuscitation, 10
Chest injury, 58–59, *59*
  aortic rupture in, 58
  cardiac contusion in, 58
  cardiac tamponade in, 58
  intubation for, 58
  pulmonary contusion in, 59
  ruptured diaphragm in, 58
  tracheal rupture in, 58
Chest tubes, 58
Chest x-ray, of ruptured diaphragm, 58
  preoperative, 2

Children. See also *Infants; Neonates.*
  acute otitis media in, 36
  congenital obstructive cardiac anomalies in, 76
  congenital septal defects in, 78–79
  cyanotic congenital heart disease in, 74–75
  hepatoblastoma in, 130
  Hirschsprung disease in, 246–247, *247*
  insulinoma in, 210
  kidney transplantation in, 256
  liver transplantation in, 260
  neck mass in, 52
  patent ductus arteriosus in, 68
  pilonidal disease in, 172
  small bowel obstruction in, 142
  static scrotal hydrocele in, 284
  testis cancer in, 286
  varicocele in, 284
Cholecystitis, acute, 124
  chronic, 124
Cholelithiasis, 124–125, *125*
Cholesteatoma, 36
Clark's classification system, for melanoma, 196
Claudication, intermittent, 222
  leg, 222–223, *223*
Clindamycin, 296
Coagulopathy, consumptin, 16
Coarctation, of aorta, 70, *71*, 76
Cocaine test, in anisocoria, 34
Colitis, ulcerative, 162, *163*
Colon, cancer of, 164, *165*
  hepatic metastases in, 164
  intestinal obstruction and, 164
  lung metastases in, 164
  lymph node metastases in, 165
  urinary tract and, 164
  penetrating injury of, 98–100, *99*, *101*
    associated trauma index for, 98
    bowel wall disruption in, 99
    colostomy in, 98–99
    prophylactic antibiotics for, 98
    severity index for, 98
  perforation of, 162
Colostomy, 98–99
Common bile duct(s), obstruction of, 134
  stones in, 126, *127*, 128, *129*, 132
    primary, 126
    residual, 126
Condylomata acuminata, vulvovaginal, 294
Congenital heart disease, cyanotic, 74–75, *75*
Congestive heart failure, 72
Constipation, hemorrhoids and, 170
Consumption coagulopathy, 16
Coronary artery bypass grafting, 82
Coronary artery disease, 82, *83*
  aortic valve stenosis and, 84
Craniotomy, in closed head injury, 32
Creatinine clearance, in preoperative laboratory evaluation, 2

Crohn's disease, 152, *153*
  acute ileitis vs., 152
  anorectal abscess and, 168
Cryoprecipitate, 19
Culdocentesis, 290, 292
Cushing reflex, 32
Cushing syndrome, 216, *217*
Cyanosis, neonatal, 72, *73*
Cyclosporine, in kidney transplantation, 256
Cyst(s), adnexal mass and, 304
  breast, 178
  choledochal, and surgical jaundice in infancy, 250, 251
  in nipple discharge, 176
  pilonidal, 172
  renal, 252, 272
  retroperitoneal, in infancy, 252

Defibrillation, in cardiopulmonary resuscitation, 10
Dexamethasone suppression test, for Cushing syndrome, 216
Diabetes mellitus, necrotizing external otitis and, 37–38
  pancreas transplantation in, 258
Diaphragm, rupture of, 58
Diaphragmatic hernia, in neonate, 72
Diarrhea, in short bowel syndrome, 146–147
Dipyridamole-thallium scan, in preoperative cardiac evaluation, 4
Disc herniation, 334
Diverticulitis, 158, *159*
Dobutamine, 14
Doxycycline, 296
Ductus arteriosus, patent, 68, *69*, 78
Dumping syndrome, 114, *115*
Duodenum, hematoma of, 94
  injury of, 94, *95*
  ulcer of, 112, *113*

Ear(s), external, bacterial infection of, 36
  eczematous inflammation of, 36
  fungal infection of, 36
  necrotizing infection of, 37–38
  middle, malignancies of, 38
  purulent discharge from, 36, *37*, 38, *39*. See also *Otorrhea.*
  swimmer's, 36
Effusion, pleural, 62–63, *63*
Electrocardiography, in preoperative laboratory evaluation, 2
Electrolytes, serum, in preoperative laboratory evaluation, 2
Electromechanical dissociation, 10
  in cardiopulmonary resuscitation, 10
Embolism, arterial, peripheral, 224, *225*
  pulmonary, 60–61, *61*
    angiography in, 60
    deep venous thrombosis and, 60
    surgery and, 60

Emboilism (Continued)
thrombolytic agents for, 61
vena cava filter insertion for, 61
Emphysema, lobar, congenital, 72
Empyema, 62–63, 63
Endometrial cancer, 294, 302–303, 303
Endometriosis, 298, 299
Enterocutaneous fistula, 148, 149
Epinephrine, 10, 12
Epistaxis, 40, 41
Erythromycin, 296
Esophageal myotomy, 102
Esophageal tear, 58
Esophageal varices, bleeding, 118, 119
Esophagomyotomy, 102
Esophagus, cancer of, 104–105, 105
Extrahepatic biliary atresia, 250
Eye(s), injury to, 34
unequal pupils of, 34–35, 35

Famotidine, 116
Femoral shaft fracture, 318, 319
Fever, postoperative, 22, 23
causes of, 22
diagnosis of, 22
Fibrillation, atrial, 6
ventricular, 7
Fibrinolysis, primary, 16
Fistula, anorectal, 168, 169
arteriovenous, congenital, 233
bronchopleural, 62
enterocutaneous, 148, 149
pancreatic pleural, 134
tracheoesophageal, 238, 239
urinary, in imperforate anus, 248
Flail chest, 58
Flexor tendon injury, 330, 331, 332, 333
Flutter, atrial, 6
Fontan operation, for cyanotic congenital heart disease, 74
Fracture, Bennett's, 326
grandma's, 312
Le Fort, 42
of cervical spine, 310–311, 311
of femoral shaft, 318, 319
of hand, 326, 327, 328, 329
of hip, 316, 317
of knee, 322, 323
of mandible, 44–45, 45
of maxilla, 42, 43
of pelvis, 314, 315
of scaphoid, 326–327
of thoracolumbar spine, 312, 313
of tibial shaft, 320, 321
of wrist, 326–327

Fracture (Continued)
open, Gustuilo classification of, 320
transosteochondral, 324
Furosemide, 14, 32

Gallstone(s), 124–125, 125
Gallstone ileus, 142
Gamekeeper's thumb, 327
Gardnerella vaginitis, 294
Gastric bezoars, postoperative, 114
Gastric ulcer, 108–110, 109, 111
arising at gastroesophageal junction, 108–109
bleeding, 108, 109
corporeal, 108
in prepyloric location, 109–110
malignant, 109
medical therapy for, 108
perforation of, 108
with duodenal ulcer, 109–110
Gastrinoma, 112, 212–213, 213
Gastroesophageal reflux, 106, 107
Gastrointestinal bleeding, lower, 160, 161
upper, 116, 117
Gastrointestinal lymphoma, 150, 151
Gentamicin, 296
Glasgow Coma Scale, 32
Goiter, colloid, 204
Goodsall's rule, in anorectal fistula, 168
Grandma's fracture, 312
Gunshot wound, abdominal, 92, 98
Gustuilo classification system, of open fractures, 320

Hand, flexor tendon injuries of, 330, 331, 332, 333
fracture of, 326–328, 327, 329
Head injury, closed, 32, 33
Heart. See also under Cardiac.
congenital disease of, cyanotic, 74–75, 75
congestive failure of, 72
transplantation of, 262–263, 263
Hematoma, duodenal, 94
Hematuria, traumatic, 266, 267
Hemorrhage. See also Bleeding.
adrenal, in neonates, 252
Hemorrhoids, 170, 171
Hemostasis, 18
Heparin, 224
subcutaneous, 234
Hepatoblastoma, in children, 130
Hernia, diaphragmatic, in neonate, 72
incarcerated indirect inguinal, 284
Herniated disc, 334
Hip fracture, 316, 317
Hirschsprung disease, 246–247, 247

HIV (human immunodeficiency virus), surgery and, 26, 27
Hodgkin's disease, 190–192, 191, 193
Ann Arbor classifications for, 191
chemotherapy regimens for, 191–192
staging laparotomy for, 190–191
Horner's syndrome, 34
Human immunodeficiency virus (HIV), surgery and, 26, 27
Hypercalcemia, 208–209, 209
Hyperinsulinism, 210
Hyperparathyroidism, 208–209, 209
Hyperplasia, benign, vaginal bleeding and, 290, 294
in hyperparathyroidism, 208
Hypertension, renovascular, 230, 231
Hyperthyroidism, 202–203, 203
Hyperventilation, in intracranial pressure elevation, 32
Hypoglycemia, in insulinoma, 210
Hypothermia, 28, 29

Ileitis, acute, Crohn's disease vs., 152
Ileus, gallstone, 142
meconium, 242
Immunosuppression, in heart transplantation, 262
in kidney transplantation, 256
in liver transplantation, 260
Imperforate anus, 248–249, 249
Indomethacin, 68
Infants. See also Children; Neonates.
aortopulmonary window in, 78, 79
coarctation of aorta in, 70, 76
congenital lobar emphysema in, 72
congenital obstructive cardiac anomalies in, 76
congenital septal defects in, 78–79, 79
cyanotic congenital heart disease in, 74–75, 75
diaphragmatic hernia in, 72
neonatal cyanosis in, 72
patent ductus arteriosus in, 68, 78
pyloric stenosis in, 240, 241
retroperitoneal mass in, 252–253, 253
surgical jaundice in, 250–251, 251
Infarction, myocardial, acute, 80, 81
coronary artery disease and, 82
Instep claudication, 222
Insulinoma, 210, 211
Intermittent claudication, 222
Intracranial pressure elevation, 32
Intubation, tracheal, in cardiopulmonary resuscitation, 10
Iridoplegia, traumatic, 34
Isoproterenol, 14

Jaundice, diagnostic workup for, 120, 121
obstructive, 122, 123
surgical, in infancy, 250–251, 251
Job-Basedow syndrome, 202

Keratoma, 36
Kidney. See *Renal* entries.
Knee fracture, 322, *323*

Laboratory evaluation, preoperative, 2, *3*
    diagnosis in, 2
    postoperative mortality risk factors in, 2
Laryngeal cancer, 54–55, *55*
Lavage, peritoneal, acute pancreatitis and, 132
    diagnostic, 90, 92
Le Fort fracture, 42
Leg claudication, 222–223, *223*
Leg pain, referred, 334
Levothyroxine, 204
Lidocaine, 10, 12
Lip cancer, 46, *47*
Liver, metastases of, in colon cancer, 164
    in Zollinger-Ellison syndrome, 212
    transplantation of, 260, *261*
    tumors of, 130, *131*
Lung. See also under *Pulmonary.*
    abscess of, 64, *65*
    cancer of, 66, *67*
    metastases of, in colon cancer, 164
Lymph node, metastases of, in colon cancer, 165
Lymphoma, gastrointestinal, 150, *151*

Magnesium aluminum hydroxide, 116
Magnesium sulfate, 12
Malnutrition, 24
    in preoperative laboratory evaluation, 2
Malocclusion, 42, 44
Mammography, 176, 178, 180
Mandibular fracture, 44–45, *45*
Mannitol, 32
Maxillary fracture, 42, *43*
Meconium, in neonatal bowel obstruction, 242
Median bar hypertrophy, 278
Megacolon, congenital, 246–247, *247*
Melanoma, 196–197, *197*
    Clark's classification system for, 196
    common sites of metastases in, 196–197
Mesoblastic nephroma, 252
Metabolic acidosis, in cardiopulmonary resuscitation, 12
Mitral facies, 86
Mitral stenosis, 76, 86, *87*
Mobitz type I AV block, 6
Mobitz type II AV block, 6
Moniliasis, vulvar, 294
MUGA (gated blood scan), in preoperative cardiac
    evaluation, 4
Multiple endocrine neoplasia syndrome, 206, 208
Myocardial infarction, acute, 80, *81*
    coronary artery disease and, 82

Neck, in closed head injury, 32
Neck mass, 52, *53*
Neonates. See also *Children; Infants.*
    adrenal hemorrhage in, 252
    bowel obstruction in, 242, *243*, 244, *245*
    cyanosis of, 72, *73*
    Hirschsprung disease in, 246–247, *247*
    imperforate anus in, 248–249, *249*
    infantile pyloric stenosis in, 240, *241*
    static scrotal hydrocele in, 284
    tracheoesophageal fistula in, 238
Nipple discharge, 176, *177*
Nitroglycerin, 14
Norepinephrine, 14
Nose, bleeding from, 40, *41*
Nutrition, 24–25, *25*
    in burn patients, 198
    parenteral, formulas for, 24–25
        in esophageal cancer, 104
        intubation for, 24
        peripheral, 24–25
    postoperative evaluation of, 8
    total parenteral, 24, 25, *25*
        in short bowel syndrome, 146–147

Ogilvie's syndrome, 156
Omeprazole, 212
Oral cavity cancer, 48–49, *49*
Orbital apex, injury to, 34
Orbital floor, injury to, 34
Otitis externa, bacterial, 36
    eczematous, 36
    fungal, 36
    necrotizing, 37–38
Otitis media, acute, 36
    chronic, 36
Otomycosis, 36
Otorrhea, 36–38, *37*, *39*
    abnormal tissue and, 37
    bacterial otitis externa and, 36
    canal malignancies and, 38
    cerebrospinal fluid in, 37
    cholesteatoma and, 36
    eczematous external otitis and, 36
    fungal otitis externa and, 36
    necrotizing external otitis and, 37–38
    otitis media and, 36
Ovarian mass, 306, *307*
Ovarian tumor, 304, 306

Pain, acute right lower quadrant, 154, *155*
    back, 334, *335*
    in chronic pancreatitis, 134, 135
    renal calculi and, 270

Pancreas, cancer of, 140, *141*
    chronic pancreatitis vs., 134
    injury of, 96, *97*
    transplantation of, 258–259, *259*
Pancreatic necrosis, 138
Pancreatic pleural fistula, 134
Pancreatic pseudocyst, 138, *139*
    hemorrhage and, 138
    in infancy, 252
    internal drainage of, 139
    percutaneous drainage of, 138–139
    secondary infection of, 138
    time factor in, 138
Pancreaticojejunostomy, longitudinal, 135
Pancreatitis, acute, 132, *133*
    peritoneal lavage and, 132
    severity signs of, 132
    chronic, 134–136, *135*, *137*
        common bile duct obstruction in, 134
        complications of, 134
        pain in, 134, 135
        pancreatic cancer vs., 134
        pseudoaneurysms in, 134
Paraplegia, thoracolumbar spine fracture and, 312
Parenteral nutrition, 24, 25, *25*
    formulas for, 24–25
    in esophageal cancer, 104
    intubation for, 24
    peripheral, 24–25
        solutions for, 24–25
    total, 24–25, *25*
        in short bowel syndrome, 146–147
Parotid gland, enlargement of, 50
Parotid tumor, 50–51, *51*
Patent ductus arteriosus, 68, *69*, 78
Patient, unstable, postoperative monitoring of, 8, *9*
    pulmonary embolism and, 61
Pelvic inflammatory disease, 296–297, *297*
Pelvis, fracture of, 314, *315*
    renal, obstruction of, 268
Peripancreatic necrosis, 132–133
Peritoneal lavage, acute pancreatitis and, 132
    diagnostic, 90, 92
Peroneal tendons, acute subluxation of, 324
Phenylephrine, 14
Pheochromocytoma, 214, *215*
Phytobezoars, 114
Pilocarpine test, in anisocoria, 34
Pilonidal cyst, 172
Pilonidal disease, 172, *173*
Platelet disorders, 16
Pleural effusion, 62–63, *63*
Pneumatic dilation, forceful, 102
Postgastrectomy syndrome, 114–115, *115*
Postoperative fever, 22, *23*
    causes of, 22
    diagnosis of, 22
Pregnancy, bacteriuria during, 268

Pregnancy *(Continued)*
  ectopic, 290, 292
  endometriosis and, 298
  molar, 290
  pelvic inflammatory disease and, 296
  thyroid nodules in, 204
  vaginal bleeding during, 290
Probenecid, 296
ProcalAmine, 25
Prostaglandin E_1, 74
Prostate, cancer of, 282, *283*
Prostate nodule, 278, 282
Prostatic hypertrophy, benign, 278
Prostatism, 278, *279*, 280, *281*
  needle biopsy in, 278
  stainless steel stents in, 278, 280
Prostatitis, 278
Prothrombin time test, 16
Pseudoaneurysms, in chronic pancreatitis, 134
Pseudocyst, pancreatic, 138, *139*
  hemorrhage and, 138
  in infancy, 252
  internal drainage of, 139
  percutaneous drainage of, 138–139
Pulmonary. See also *Lung.*
Pulmonary contusion, 59
Pulmonary embolism, 60–61, *61*
  angiography in, 60
  deep venous thrombosis and, 60
  surgery and, 60
  thrombolytic agents for, 61
  vena cava filter insertion for, 61
Pulmonary stenosis, valvular, 76
Pupils, Adie's tonic, 34–35
  size of, sympathetic innervation and, 34
  unequal, 34–35, *35*
Pyelonephritis, 268
Pyloric stenosis, infantile, 240, *241*

Radiation therapy, for prostate cancer, 282
  for recurrent breast cancer, 186
Rectum, cancer of, 166, *167*
Renal calculus, 270, *271*
Renal cell cancer, 272
Renal colic, 270
Renal cyst, 252, 272
Renal mass, 272, *273*
Renal pelvis, obstruction of, 268
Renal transplantation, 256–257, *257*
Renin levels, in renovascular hypertension, 230
Renovascular hypertension, 230, *231*
Resuscitation, cardiopulmonary. See *Cardiopulmonary resuscitation.*
Retroperitoneal mass, 194–195, *195*
  in infancy, 252–253, *253*

Scaphoid fracture, 326–327
Scrotal mass, 284
Seizure(s), after head injury, 32
Seminoma, 286
Sepsis, in imperforate anus, 248
Septal defects, congenital, 78–79, *79*
Shock, 14, *15*
Short bowel syndrome, 146, *147*
  diarrhea in, 146–147
  total parenteral nutrition in, 146–147
Small bowel, Crohn's disease of, 152, *153*
  necrosis of, in acute mesenteric vascular occlusion, 145
  obstruction of, 142, *143*
Sodium bicarbonate, 12
Sodium nitroprusside, 14
Spermatic cord torsion, 284
Spine, cervical, fracture of, 310–311, *311*
  thoracolumbar, fracture of, 312, *313*
Stenosis, aortic valve, 76, 84–85, *85*
  carotid, in cerebrovascular insufficiency, 228
  mitral, 76, 86, *87*
  pulmonary valvular, 76
  pyloric, infantile, 240, *241*
  vertebral artery, 228
Stomach. See also under *Gastric.*
  access to, 24
Stress tests, in preoperative laboratory evaluation, 2
Supraventricular tachycardia, 6
Swimmer's ear, 36
Sympathetic innervation, pupil size and, 34

Tachycardia, atrial, paroxysmal, 6
  atrioventricular junctional, 6–7
  supraventricular, 6
  ventricular, 7
Tamoxifen, for breast cancer, 180, 182
Testis tumor, 286, *287*
Tetracycline, 296
Tetralogy of Fallot, 74, 75
Thigh claudication, 222
Thoracic outlet syndrome, 220–221, *221*
Thoracolumbar spine fracture, 312, *313*
Thromboplastin time test, activated partial, 16
Thrombosis, arterial, 224
  deep venous, pulmonary embolism and, 60
  subclavian vein, 220
  venous, in acute mesenteric vascular occlusion, 144
Thyroid, cancer of, 206, *207*
  nodules of, 204, *205*
Thyroidectomy, complications from, 202–203
Tibial shaft fracture, 320, *321*
Total parenteral nutrition, 24, 25, *25*
  in short bowel syndrome, 146–147
Trachea, rupture of, 58
Tracheoesophageal fistula, 238, *239*

Transosteochondral fracture, 324
Transplantation, of heart, 262–263, *263*
  of kidney, 256–257, *257*
  of liver, 260, *261*
  of pancreas, 258–259, *259*
Trauma, abdominal, blunt, 90–91, *91*
  penetrating, 92–93, *93*
  ankle injury in, 324, *325*
  chest injury in, 58–59, *59*
  colon injury in, 98–100, *99*, *101*
  duodenum injury in, 94, *95*
  eye injury in, 34
  flexor tendon injury in, 330, *331*, 332, *333*
  head injury in, 32, *33*
  hematuria and, 266, *267*
  pancreas injury in, 96, *97*
  urinary bladder injury in, 266
Trauma index, associated (ATI), 98
Trichomoniasis, 294
Tumor(s), in Cushing syndrome, 216
  in pheochromocytoma, 214
  in thyroid, 206
  in Zollinger-Ellison syndrome, 212–213
  malignant. See *Cancer.*
  of breast, 180, 182
  of liver, 130, *131*
  of ovary, 304
  of pancreas, 140, 210
  of parotid gland, 50–51, *51*
  of retroperitoneum, 194–195, *195*
    in infancy, 252
  of small bowel, 142
  of testis, 286, *287*
  of urinary bladder, 274–276, *275*, *277*
  Wilms, 252–253

Ulcer(s), due to arterial insufficiency, 234
  duodenal, 112, *113*
  gastric, 108–110, *109*, *111*
  venous stasis, 234, *235*
Ulcerative colitis, 162, *163*
Unna paste boot, 234
Ureter, obstruction of, 268
Ureteral calculus, 270, *271*
Urinalysis, in preoperative laboratory evaluation, 2
Urinary bladder, in prostatism, 278, 280
  injury to, 266
  tumor of, 274–276, *275*, *277*
    chemotherapy for, 274, 276
    staging of, 274
Urinary fistula, in imperforate anus, 248
Urinary tract, colon cancer and, 164
  infection of, 268, *269*
Uterine cervical cancer, 300, *301*

Vaginal bleeding, in nonreproductive years, 294, *295*
  in reproductive years, 290, *291*, 292, *293*
Vaginitis, 294
Varicocele, in adolescent, 284
Varicose veins, 232–233, *233*
  esophageal, bleeding from, 118, *119*
Vascular disease, mesenteric, 142
Vascular occlusion, acute mesenteric, 144–145, *145*
    clotting profiles in, 144
    small bowel necrosis in, 145
    venous thrombosis in, 144
Vascular resistance, systemic, in shock, 14
Vasopressin, in lower gastrointestinal bleeding, 160
  intravenous infusion of, 116, 118
Venous insufficiency, 220
Venous stasis ulcers, 234, *235*

Venous thrombosis, deep, pulmonary embolism and, 60
  in acute mesenteric vascular occlusion, 144
Ventricular asystole, 6
Ventricular complexes, premature, 7
Ventricular fibrillation, 7
Ventricular tachycardia, 7
Vitamin B_{12}, in short bowel syndrome, 146
Vitamin K deficiency, in bleeding disorders, 16
Vocal cords, cancer of, 54–55, *55*
Volvulus, 156, *157*
Vulvar moniliasis, 294
Vulvovaginal condylomata acuminata, necrotic, 294

Waldeyer's ring, in gastrointestinal lymphoma, 150
Warfarin, 224

Wenckebach AV block, 6
Whipple's diagnostic triad, in insulinoma, 210
Wilms tumor, 252–253
Wound(s), gunshot, to abdomen, 92, 98
Wrist fracture, 326–327

X-ray, chest, of ruptured diaphragm, 58
  preoperative, 2

Zollinger-Ellison syndrome, 212–213, *213*

Little Red Riding Hood

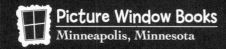
Picture Window Books
Minneapolis, Minnesota

First published in the United States in 2010
by Picture Window Books
151 Good Counsel Drive
P.O. Box 669
Mankato, Minnesota 56002
www.picturewindowbooks.com

©2005, Edizioni El S.r.l., Treiste Italy in CAPPUCETTO ROSSO

Printed in the United States of America.

All books published by Picture Window Books
are manufactured with paper containing
at least 10 percent post-consumer waste.

Library of Congress Cataloging-in-Publication Data
Piumini, Roberto.
[Cappuccetto Rosso. English]
Little Red Riding Hood / by Roberto Piumini; illustrated by Alessandro Sanna.
p. cm. — (Storybook classics)
ISBN 978-1-4048-5647-9 (library binding)
[1. Fairy tales. 2. Folklore—Germany.] I. Sanna, Alessandro, 1975– ill. II. Little Red
Riding Hood. English. III. Title.
PZ8.P717Li 2010
398.20943'02—dc22

[E]   2009010429

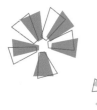

Little Red Riding Hood

Retold by
Roberto Piumini

Illustrated by
Alessandro Sanna

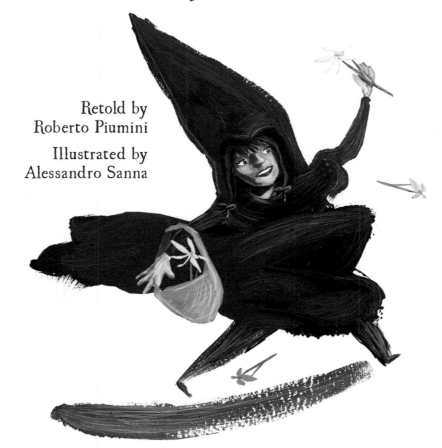

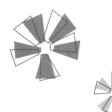

Once upon a time, there was a little girl who lived in a small village with her mother. The little girl often visited her grandmother, who lived deep in the woods.

The grandmother loved the little girl very much and gave her a red velvet riding hood as a gift. The little girl loved her riding hood, and she wore it day and night. So everyone called her Little Red Riding Hood.

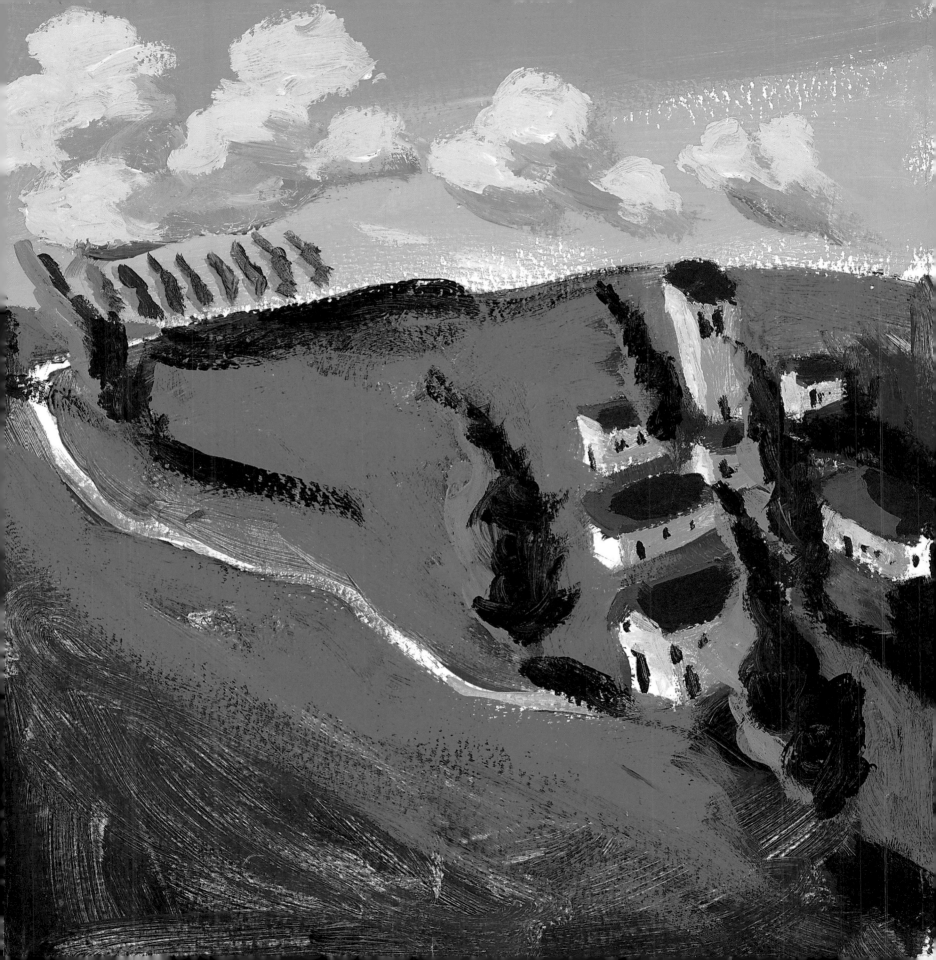

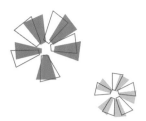

One day, Little Red's mother said to her, "Take this basket of treats to your grandmother. Go right away, walk quickly, and never leave the path."

"Yes, Mother," said the little girl. She picked up the basket and hurried off to her grandmother's house in the woods.

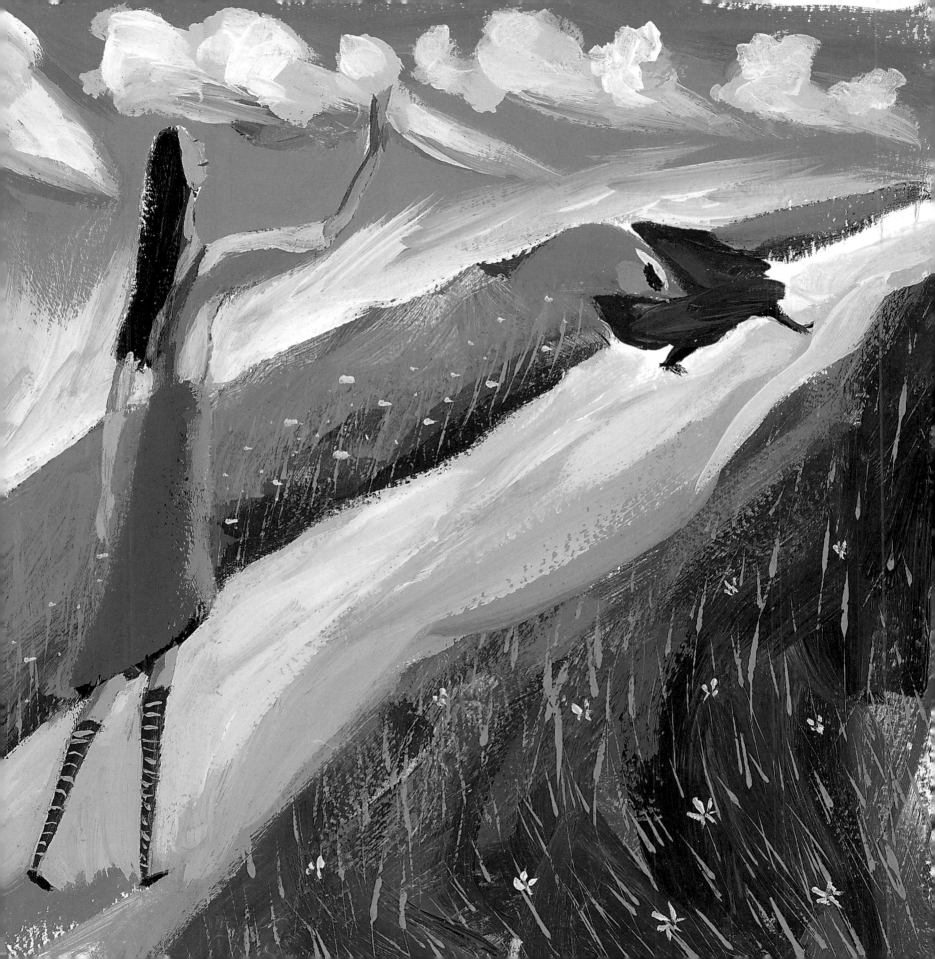

When Little Red was deep in the forest,
a wolf saw her and greeted her.

"What's your name, little girl?" asked the wolf.
"And where are you going all by yourself?"

"I'm Little Red Riding Hood," she said. "I'm
taking some treats to my grandmother."

"Where does your grandmother live?" asked
the wolf.

"Under the big oak tree in the forest," said
the girl.

Ah, what a delicious snack she would make! the
wolf thought to himself, his mouth watering. *If I
am clever and careful, I can eat the grandmother
first and have Little Red for dessert!*

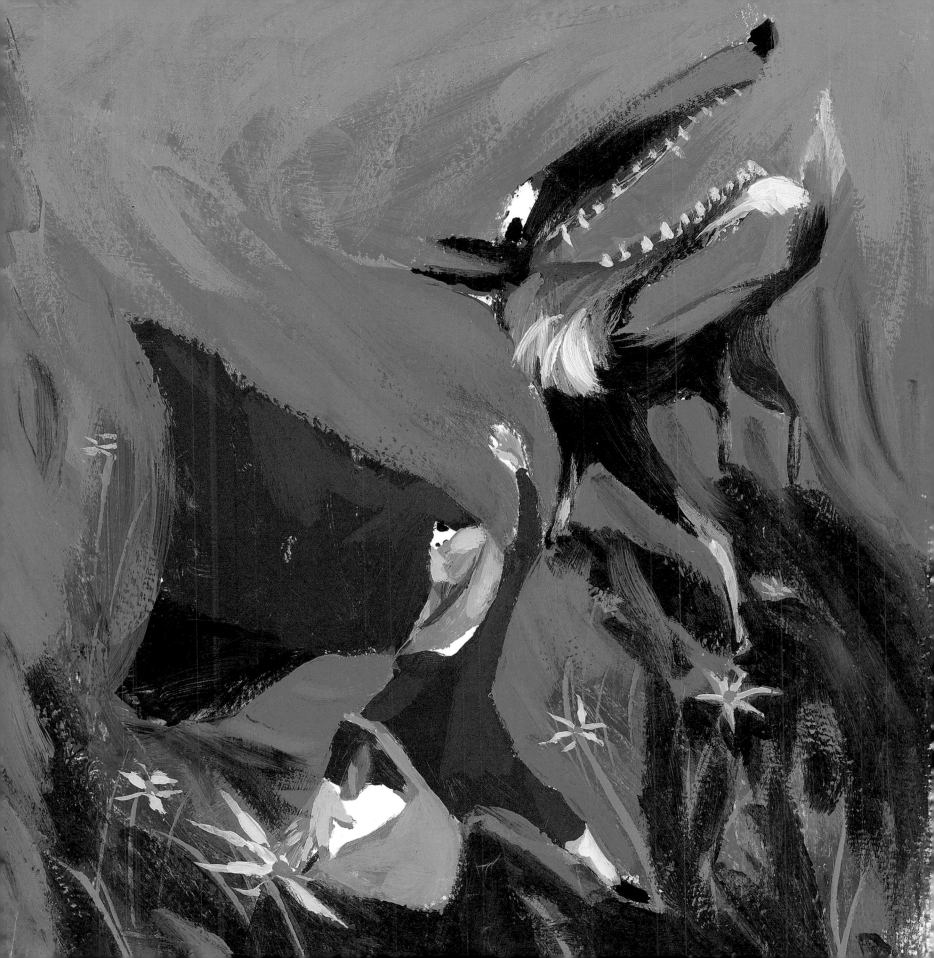

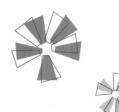

Little Red and the wolf walked together for a while. Then the wolf said, "Look at those lovely flowers! I'm sure your grandmother would love to have some."

Little Red stopped. She loved flowers, and so did her grandmother. The girl picked a few from the side of the path, then a few more a little farther away. With each flower she picked, there seemed to be a more beautiful one just a step away.

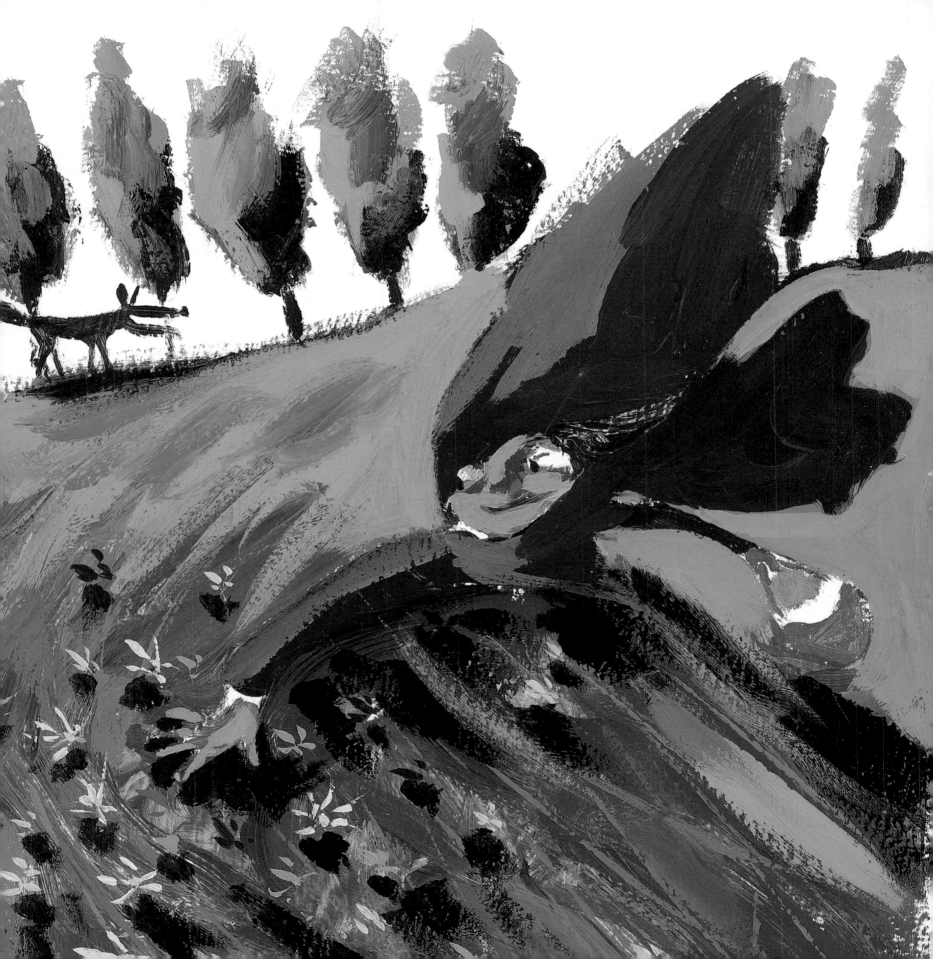

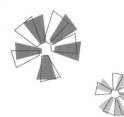

Meanwhile, the wolf ran to the grandmother's house and knocked on the door.

"Who is it?" asked the old woman.

"It's Little Red Riding Hood, Grandmother! I've brought you some treats," the wolf said.

"Open the door and come inside, my dear!" said grandmother.

The wolf opened the door, ran inside, and gobbled up the grandmother whole.

Then he put on her stocking cap, climbed into her bed, and pulled the bedsheets right up to his hairy chin.

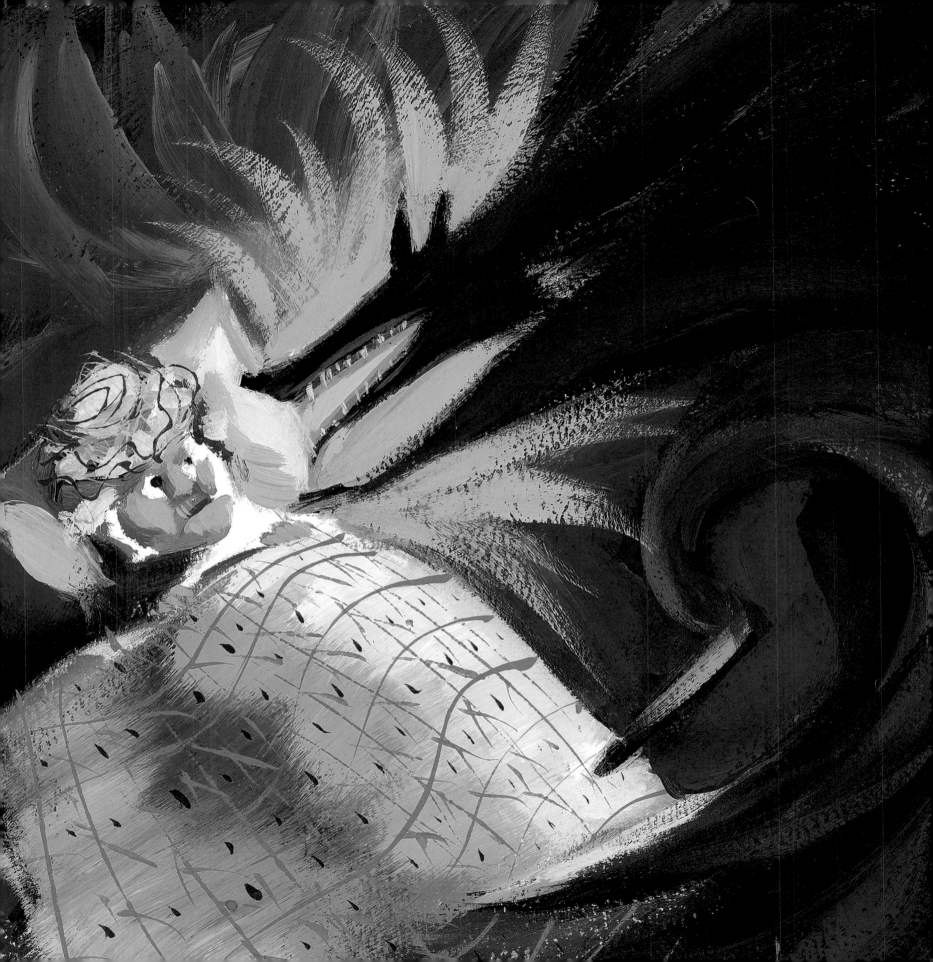

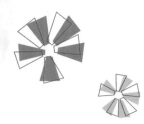

When Little Red Riding Hood's hands were filled with flowers, she went back to the path to hurry toward her grandmother's house.

When she arrived at the house, the door was open so she walked inside. In the dim light, she saw her grandmother in bed with her stocking cap on, looking very different than normal.

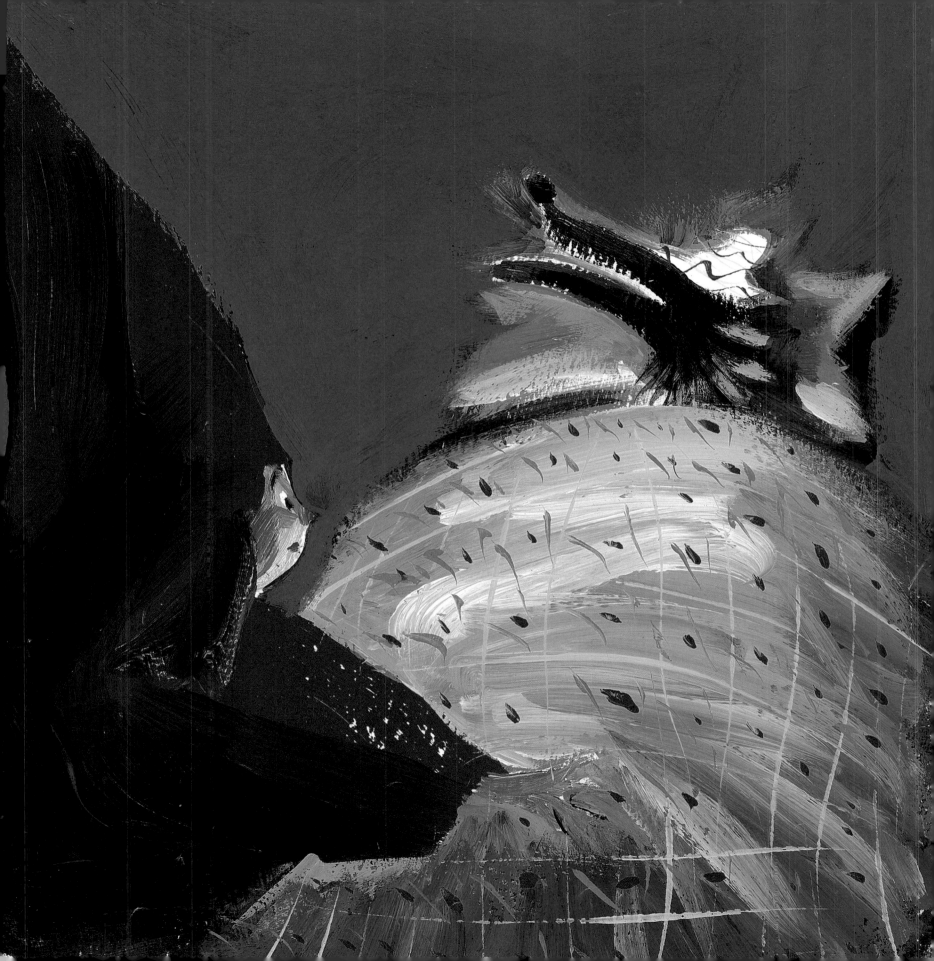

Little Red Riding Hood stepped closer to the bed. "Grandmother, what big ears you have!" she said.

"All the better to hear you with, my dear," said the wolf.

"Grandmother, what big eyes you have!" Little Red said.

"All the better to see you with, my dear," said the wolf.

"And grandmother . . . what big teeth you have!" said Little Red, frowning.

"All the better to eat you with!" howled the wolf.

Then he jumped out of the bed and swallowed Little Red Riding Hood in a single gulp.

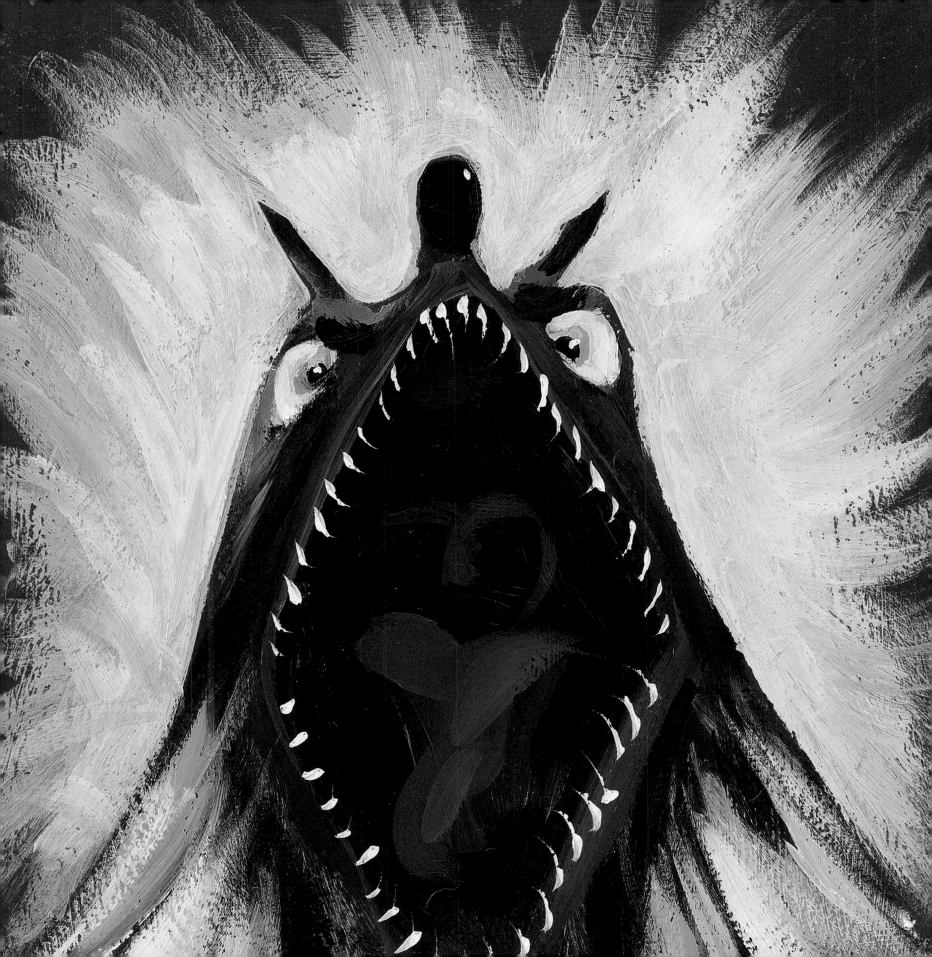

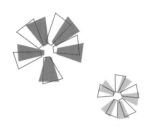

Feeling full, the wolf lay down on the bed again and fell asleep.

A little later, a hunter passed by, and he heard the loud snores. He thought to himself, *The old lady is snoring very loudly! Maybe she's sick. I'd better take a look.*

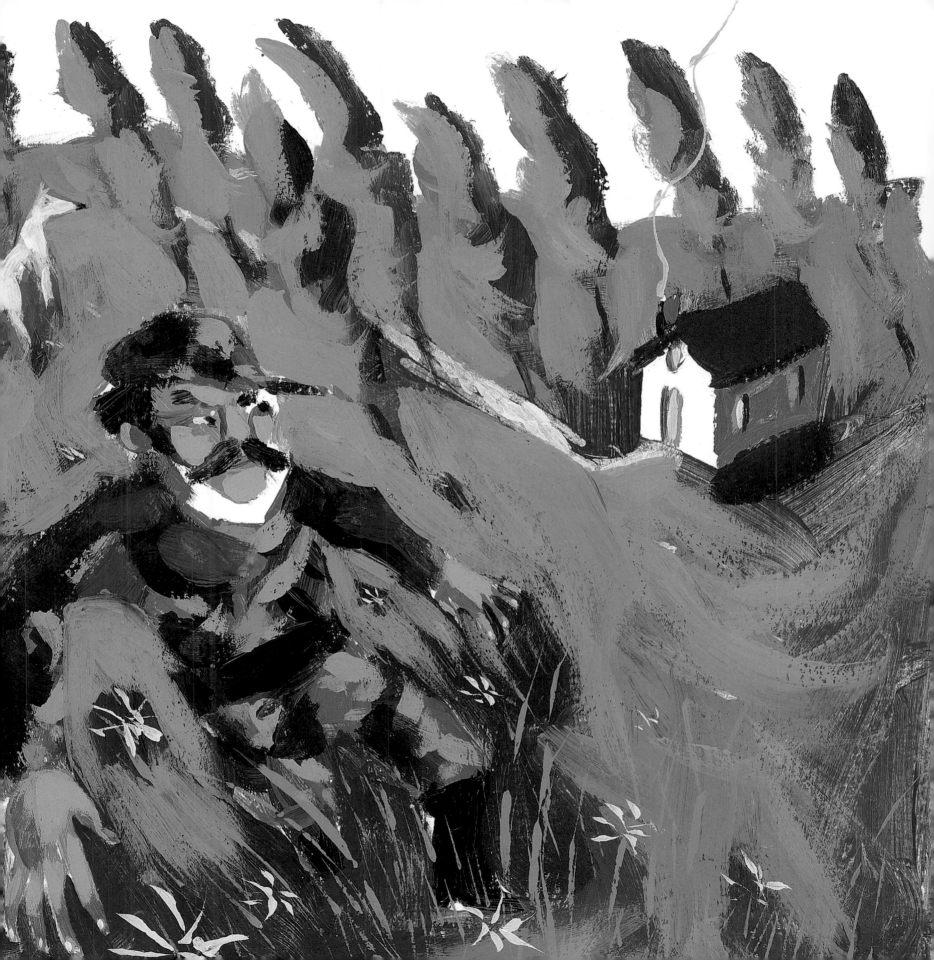

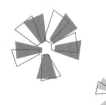

The hunter walked in and saw the wolf lying in bed. He realized that the wolf must have eaten whoever lived in the house. So he cut open the sleeping wolf with his knife. Out hopped Little Red Riding Hood and her grandmother!

"That evil wolf swallowed us up," said Little Red. "Thank you so much for saving our lives!"

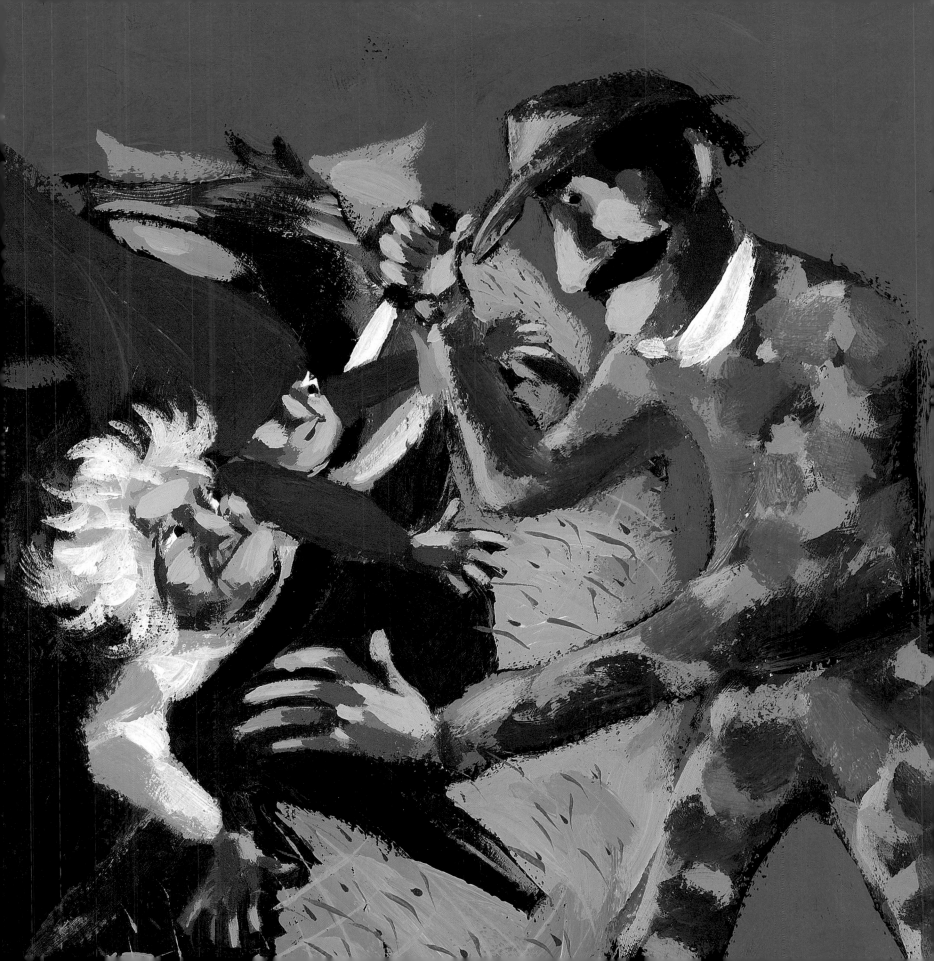

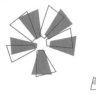

The hunter looked down at the wolf. "We can't let this wolf eat anyone else," he told Little Red. "Go and get some large stones and bring them to me."

So Little Red went outside and walked to a nearby lake. She gathered twelve large stones and brought them, one by one, to the hunter.

The hunter stuffed the stones into the sleeping wolf's belly. Then he stitched up the wolf with a needle and thread.

"That will teach him to eat grandmothers and little girls," the hunter said.

Then the three of them hid and waited.

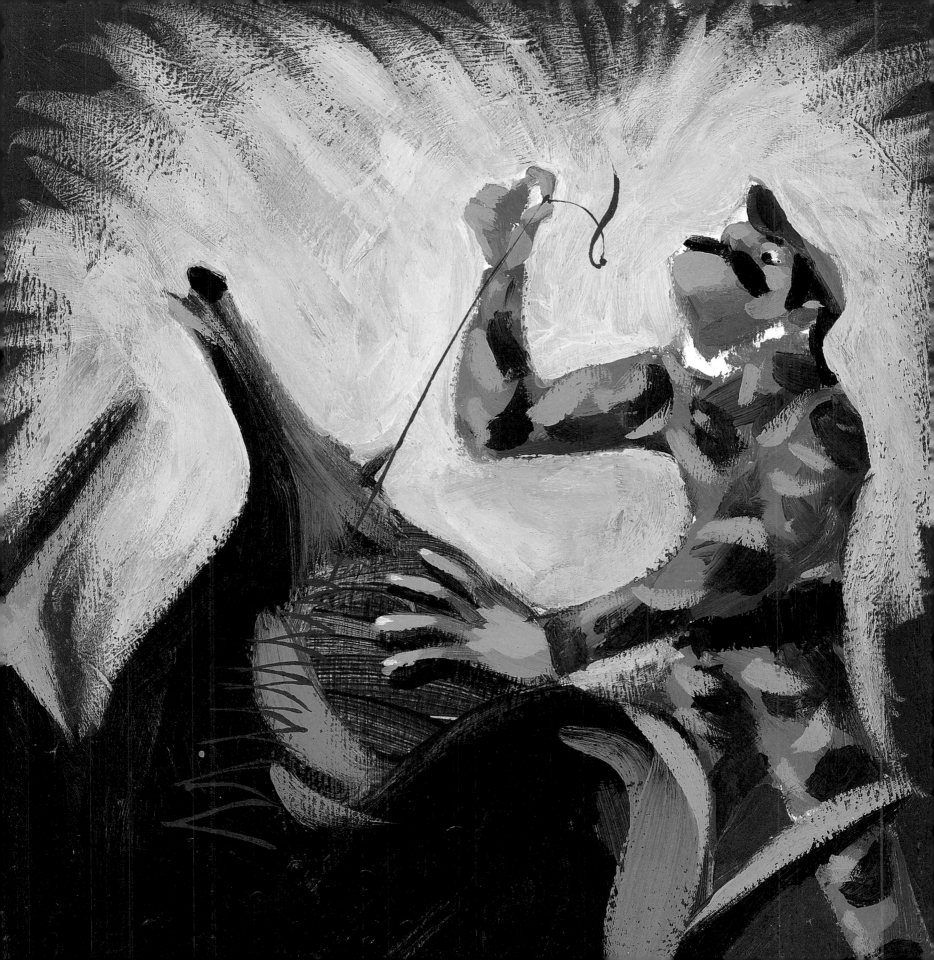

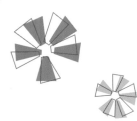

When the wolf woke up, he felt much heavier than before. He dragged himself outside and inched his way down to the lake for a drink. But the stones in his stomach made him so heavy that he fell into the water and sank to the bottom of the lake.

Back at the cottage, Little Red Riding Hood, her grandmother, and the hunter celebrated.

And the wolf was never seen again.

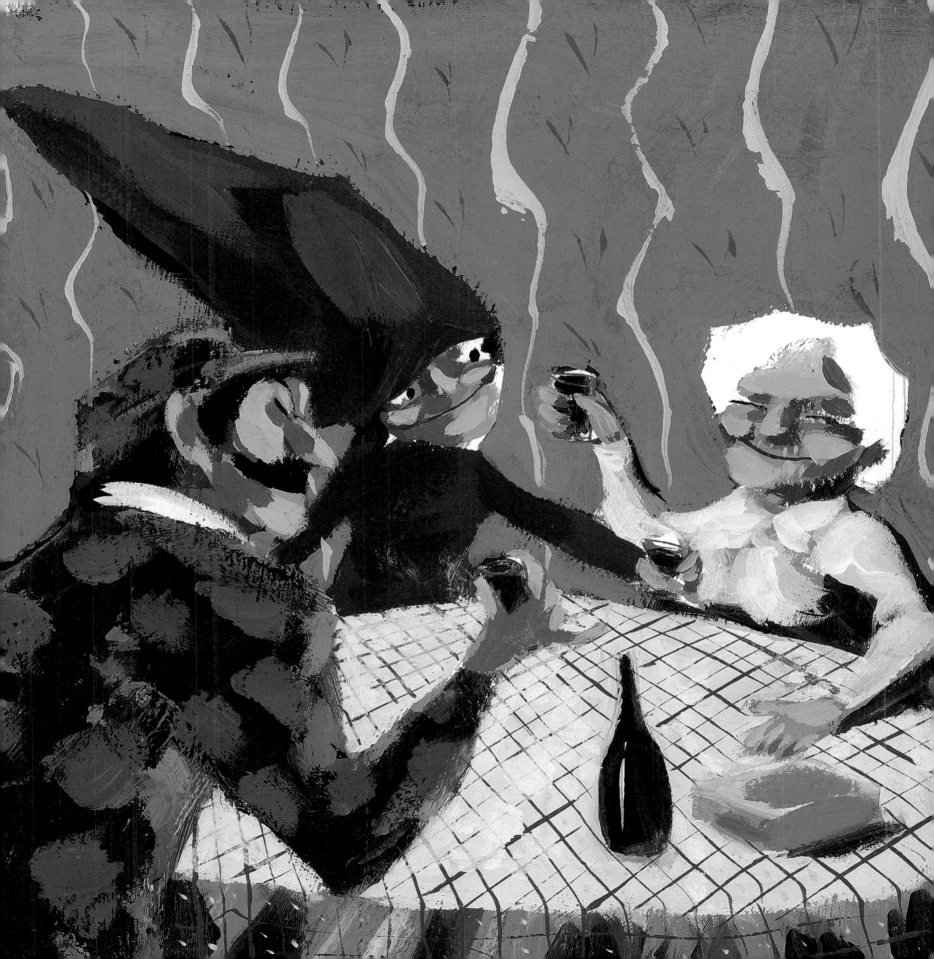

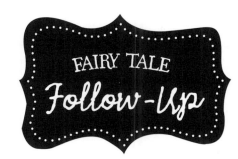

FAIRY TALE
Follow-Up

1. Little Red's mother told her to stay on the path on the way to her grandmother's house, but the girl did not listen. Do you think she would have been safer if she had followed her mother's rule?

2. Was Little Red scared of the wolf? Would you have been scared?

3. Who is the hero of this story? What did he or she do that makes them the hero?

4. Have you ever read another version of Little Red Riding Hood? Was the ending different? Were there other differences?

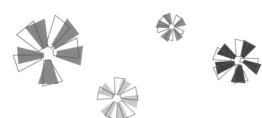

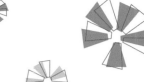

Glossary

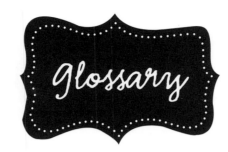

celebrated (SEL-uh-brayt-ed)—did something special, such as had a party

cottage (KOT-ij)—a small house, often in a country setting

delicious (di-LISH-uhss)—very pleasing to taste

gobbled (GOB-uhld)—ate very quickly and greedily

howled (HOULD)—cried out like a wolf or dog

WRITE YOUR OWN
Fairy Tale

Fairy tales have been told for hundreds of years. Most fairy tales share certain elements, or pieces. Once you learn about these elements, you can try writing your own fairy tales.

Element 1: The Characters

Characters are the people, animals, or other creatures in the story. They can be good or evil, silly or serious. Can you name the characters in *Little Red Riding Hood*? There is the wolf, the hunter, the grandmother, and the main character — Little Red Riding Hood.

Element 2: The Setting

The setting tells us *when* and *where* a story takes place. The *when* of the story could be a hundred years ago or a hundred years in the future. There may be more than one *where* in a story. You could go from a house to a school to a park. In *Little Red Riding Hood*, the story says it happened "once upon a time." Usually this means that it takes place many years ago. And *where* does it take place? In the forest and at Grandmother's house.

Element 3: The Plot

Think about what happens in the story. You are thinking about the plot, or the action of the story. In fairy tales, the action begins nearly right away. In *Little Red Riding Hood*, the plot begins when the mother tells Little Red to take some treats to her grandmother. She says, "Go right away, walk quickly, and never leave the path." And the story takes off from there!

Element 4: Magic

Did you know that all fairy tales have an element of magic? The magic is what makes a fairy tale different from other stories. Often, the magic comes in the form of a character that doesn't exist in real life, such as a giant, a scary witch, or in the case of *Little Red Riding Hood*, a talking animal.

Element 5: A Happy Ending

Years ago, fairy tales ended on a sad note, but today, most fairy tales have a happy ending. Readers like knowing that the hero of the story has beaten the villain. Did *Little Red Riding Hood* have a happy ending? Of course! The hunter tricked the wolf, who sank to the bottom of the lake with a belly full of rocks. Then Little Red celebrated with her grandmother and the hunter.

Now that you know the basic elements of a fairy tale, try writing your own! Create characters, both good and bad. Decide when and where their story will take place to give them a setting. Now put them into action during the plot of the story. Don't forget that you need some magic! And finally, give the hero of your story a happy ending.

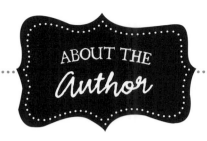

ABOUT THE Author

Roberto Piumini lives and works in Italy. He has worked with children as both a teacher and a theater actor/entertainer. He credits these experiences for inspiring the youthful language of his many books. With his crisp and imaginative way of dealing with every kind of subject, he keeps charming his young readers. His award-winning books, for both children and adults, have been translated into many languages.

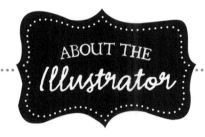

ABOUT THE Illustrator

Alessandro Sanna is a writer and illustrator of children's books. Many of his picture books retell famous stories and plays. He likes experimenting with different techniques, but he loves traditional painting. Often, Sanna's choice of color and style are inspired by famous painters. When he's not working on his own projects, Sanna teaches creative drawing to both children and adults.

More Tales to Treasure

Open a Storybook Classic and experience the world of traditional fairy tales told through simple prose and splendid artwork. These safe and inventive picture books feature beautiful and whimsical illustrations that will charm young and old alike.

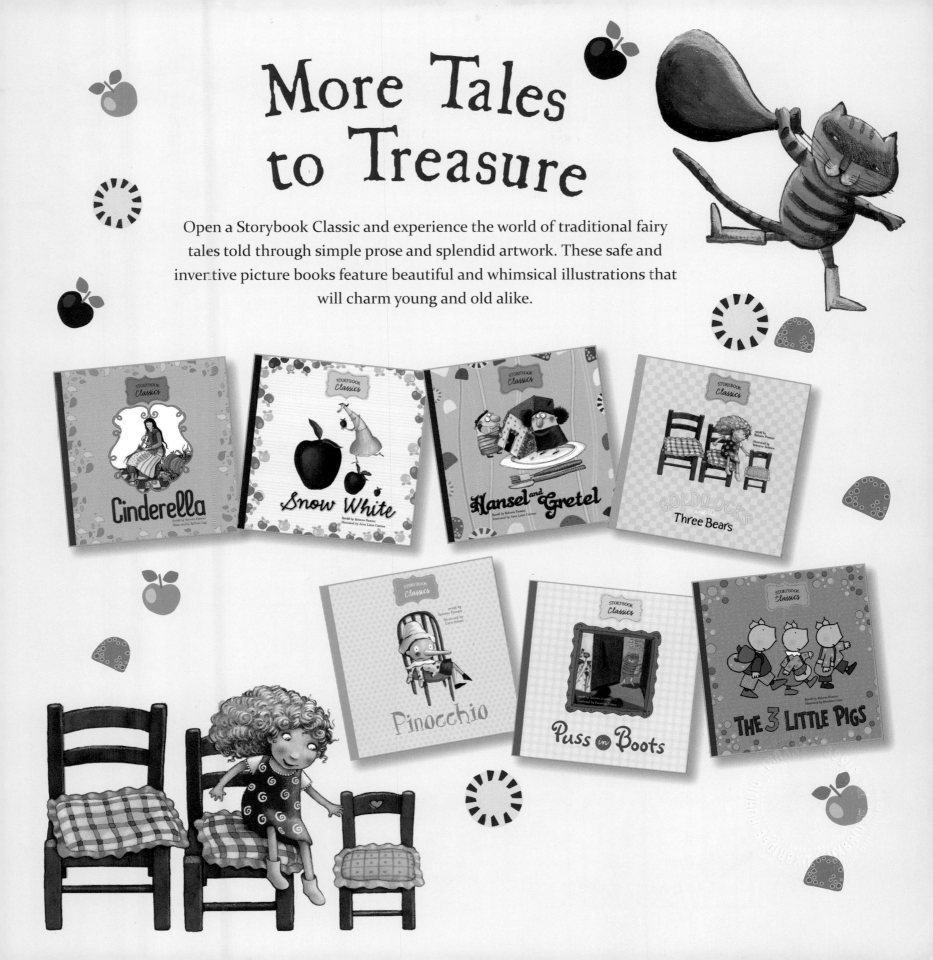

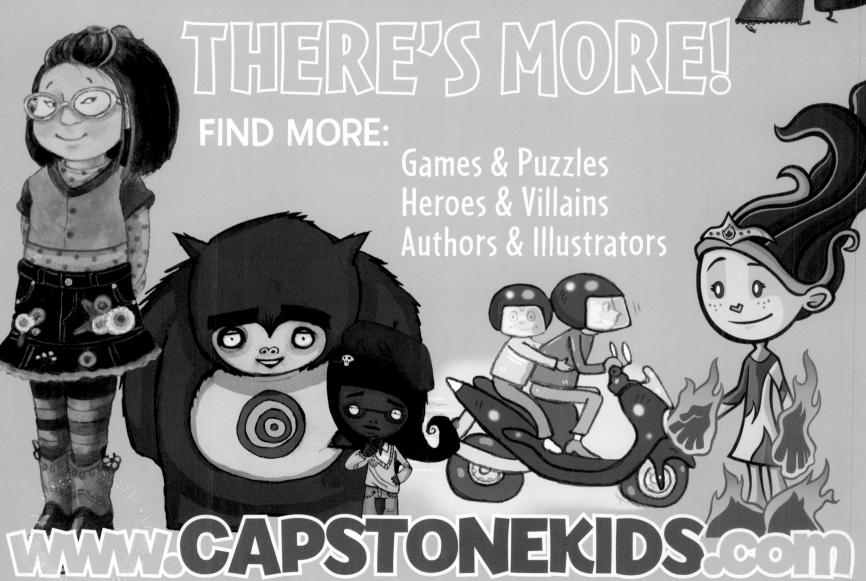